Advances in Parenteral Nutrition

Advances in Parenteral Nutrition

Proceedings of an International Symposium held in Bermuda, 16–19th May, 1977

Edited by
Ivan D. A. Johnston
Department of Surgery, University of Newcastle-Upon-Tyne

Springer-Science+ Business Media, B.V.

Originally published by MTP Press Ltd in 1978
Softcover reprint of the hardcover 1st edition 1978

Library of Congress Cataloging in Publication Data
Main entry under title:

Advances in parenteral nutrition.

Includes bibliographical references and index.
1. Parenteral feeding—Congresses. I. Johnstone, Ivan David Alexander.
RM224.A38 615′.5 77–20198

ISBN 978-94-011-7190-8 ISBN 978-94-011-7188-5 (eBook)
DOI 10.1007/978-94-011-7188-5

Contents

Preface

Parenteral nutrition has been one of the most significant therapeutic advances of the past twenty years. Many patients have survived very serious illness only because of intravenous nutrition for either short or very long periods of time.

The indications for parenteral nutrition are simple and can be summarised as the inability to ingest necessary nutrients for a significant time during increased metabolic demands.

Many problems in the preparation of energy sources and amino acid solutions have been solved so that the time is opportune to review what has been achieved and discuss recent advances and current thinking in the light of future requirements.

The next phase in parenteral nutrition will undoubtedly be the provision of regimens designed for specific situations. The needs of the neonate for example are known to differ from adult requirements.

The choice of carbohydrate for intravenous use has been a matter of much discussion. The supremacy of glucose both in biochemical and clinical terms now seems well established. The value of intravenous fat is well documented, but the interchange of fat and carbohydrate as calorie sources and the effects of prolonged infusions of fat merit further investigation.

The evidence that isotonic amino acids are utilized effectively when given alone due to the availability of endogenous energy sources has led to a greater understanding of the metabolic changes and demands associated with injury and sepsis.

The value of parenteral nutrition in clinical terms will always be assessed in relation to associated complications. Many of the biochemical problems such as hypophosphataemia and hyperosmolar situations can now be anticipated and avoided. The amount and extent of trace element supplementation required during prolonged parenteral nutrition is an interesting and challenging field of study. The most serious drawback to intravenous nutrition has always been the problems associated with access to the circulation. Meticulous attention to details of aseptic technique in all aspects of the preparation and delivery of intravenous nutrients will reduce the hazards of infection to a minimum.

Many chapters in this book and the associated discussions point the way forward to further advances in the understanding of metabolism during illness and the provision of nutritional support.

IVAN D. A. JOHNSTON

List of Contributors

K. G. M. M. ALBERTI
Department of Chemical Pathology and Human Metabolism, University of Southampton

D. BRUCE ALLARDYCE
Department of Surgery, University of British Columbia, 700 West 10th Avenue, Vancouver, British Columbia, Canada

JAMES R. ALLEN
Hospital Infections Branch, Bacterial Diseases Division, Bureau of Epidemiology, Center for Disease Control, US Public Health Service, Dept. of Health, Education and Welfare, Atlanta, Georgia, USA

N. ALLEN
Department of Surgery, Southampton General Hospital, Tremona Road, Southampton

ROBERT K. AUSMAN
Clinical Research, Baxter Travenol Laboratories, Deerfield, Illinois; Clinical Professor of Surgery, Medical College of Wisconsin, Milwaukee, WI, USA

J. BERGSTROM
St Erik¯s Sjukhus, S-112 82 Stockholm, Sweden

GEORGE L. BLACKBURN
Director Nutrition Support Services, New England Deaconess Hospital, Harvard Medical School, 194 Pilgrim Road, Boston, MA 02215, USA

DENIS BOURBEAU
University of Montreal, Hotel Dieu de Montreal, 3840 St Urbain Street, Montreal, Quebec, Canada

ROBERT R. BURNS
Department of Biochemistry, Royal Infirmary, Glasgow, Scotland

E. CANADAS
Ciudad Sanitaria, SS, Principes de Espagna, Barcelona, Spain

YVON A. CARPENTIER
Department of Surgery, Hopital Saint Pierre, University of Brussels, 322 rue Haute, 1000 Brussels, Belgium; Department of Surgery, c/o Professor John M. Kinney, 630 West 168th Street, New York, 10032, USA

H. CONNOR
Department of Pharmacology and Therapeutics, Academic Division of Medicine, The University of Sheffield

EDWARD M. COPELAND III
University of Texas Medical School at Houston, 6400 West Cullen Street, 123 Freeman Building, Houston, Texas 77030; University of Texas System Cancer Center, MD Anderson Hospital and Tumor Institute, Houston, TX 77030, USA

THOMAS D. DARBY
Department of Pharmacology, Travenol Laboratories, Inc., 6301 Lincoln Avenue, Morton Grove, IL 60053, USA

STANLEY J. DUDRICK
Department of Surgery, University of Texas Medical School at Houston, 6400 West Cullen Street, Houston, Texas 77030; University of Texas System Cancer Center, MD Anderson Hospital and Tumor Institute, Houston, TX 77030, USA

A. DURANCEAU
University of Montreal, Hotel Dieu de Montreal, 3840 St Urbain Street, Montreal, Quebec, Canada

A. L. DURST
Hadassah University Hospital, Jerusalem, Israel

M. ELIAKIM
Hadassah University Hospital, Jerusalem, Israel

SUSANNAH EYKYN
Department of Microbiology, St Thomas's Hospital Medical School, London

GORDON S. FELL
Department of Biochemistry, Royal Infirmary, Glasgow, Scotland

KENNETH FOSTER
University of Southampton, Surgical Division, Royal South Hants Hospital, Fanshawe Street, Southampton

URI FREUND
Department of Surgery B, Hadassah Medical Centre, Ein Karem, Jerusalem, Israel

PETER FÜRST
Metabolic Research Laboratory, St Erik¯s Sjukhus, S-112 82 Stockholm, Sweden

ANTHONY GOODE
Department of Surgery, The Royal Postgraduate Medical School, London

A. GOUGOUX
University of Montreal, Hotel Dieu de Montreal, 3840 St Urbain Street, Montreal, Quebec, Canada

GILBERT HARDY
Travenol Laboratories Ltd., Thetford, Norfolk

JOHN T. HARRIES
Institute of Child Health and The Hospital for Sick Children, Great Ormond Street, London

T. HAWKINS
Medical Physics Department, Newcastle General Hospital, Newcastle upon Tyne

RONALD L. HOLLIDAY
Department of Surgery, Victoria Hospital, South Street, London, Ontario, Canada

B. HOLMSTRÖM
St Erik¯s Sjukhus, S-112 82 Stockholm, Sweden

W. P. T. JAMES
Dunn Nutrition Unit, Milton Road, Cambridge; Addenbrookes' Hospital, Trumpington Street, Cambridge

PH. JANNE
Hôpital Universitaire Saint-Pierre, Department of Surgery and Laboratory of Experimental Surgery L. Deloyers, University of Brussels, 322 rue Haute, 1000 Brussels, Belgium

J. JENKINS
Department of Surgery, Southampton General Hospital, Tremona Road, Southampton

BARBARA JENNINGS
Department of Surgery, University of Western Ontario, Victoria Hospital, London, Ontario, Canada

IVAN D. A. JOHNSTON
University of Newcastle upon Tyne, Department of Surgery, Royal Victoria Infirmary, Newcastle upon Tyne

ADRIAN B. JONES
University of Alberta, 4-117 Clinical Science Building, Edmonton, Alberta, Canada

R. M. KAMMERLING
Department of Surgery, Southampton General Hospital, Tremona Road, Southampton

STEPHEN J. KARRAN
Professorial Surgical Unit, Royal South Hants Hospital, Fanshawe Street, Southampton

NICHOLAS J. KARTINOS
Pharmaceutical R & D, Travenol Laboratories, Inc., 6301 Lincoln Avenue Morton Grove, IL 60053, USA

JOHN M. KINNEY
Columbia Presbyterian Medical Center, 168th Street and Ft. Washington Avenue, New York, NY 10032, USA

Y. KRAUSZ
Hadassah University Hospital, Jerusalem, Israel

SIR HANS A. KREBS
Metabolic Research Laboratory, Nuffield Department of Clinical Medicine, Radcliffe Infirmary, Oxford

RUTH B. KUNDSIN
Harvard University School of Medicine, Peter Bent Brigham Hospital, Surgical Bacteriology Laboratory, 721 Huntingdon Avenue, Boston, MA 02115, USA

G. LEMIEUX
University of Montreal, Hotel Dieu de Montreal, 3840 St Urbain Street, Montreal, Quebec, Canada

I. S. LEVIJ
Hadassah University Hospital, Jerusalem, Israel

HAMISH N. MUNRO
Department of Food and Nutrition, Massachusetts Institute of Technology, Cambridge, MA 02138, USA

RONALD L. NEDICH
Pharmacy Department, Travenol Laboratories, Inc., 6301 Lincoln Avenue, Morton Grove, IL 60053, USA

D. NEWTON
Department of Pharmacology and Therapeutics, Academic Division of Medicine, University of Sheffield

IAN PHILLIPS
Department of Microbiology, St Thomas' Hospital Medical School, London

HUGH YOUNG RIENHOFF Jr.
Nutrition/Metabolic Laboratory, Nutrition Support Service, New England Deaconess Hospital, Harvard Medical School, Boston, MA, USA

WILLIAM SCHUMER
Department of Surgery, University of Health Sciences, Chicago Medical School, and Veterans Administration Hospital, North Chicago, IL 60064, USA

B. SHILDT
St Erik¯s Sjukhus, S-112 82 Stockholm, Sweden

HARRY M. SHIZGAL
McGill University; Royal Victoria Hospital, 687 Pine Avenue West, Montreal, Quebec, Canada

A. SITGES-CREUS
Ciudad Sanitaria, SS, Principes de Espagna, Barcelona, Spain

C. SMART
Department of Surgery, Southampton General Hospital, Tremona Road, Southampton

MICHELINE T. STE MARIE
Department of Paediatrics, Le Centre Hospitalier de l'Université Laval, 2705 Boulevard Laurier, Ste. Foy, Quebec, Canada

HUGH N. TUCKER
Travenol Laboratories, Inc., One Baxter Parkway, Deerfield, IL 60015, USA

DAVID E. F. TWEEDLE
University of Manchester; University Hospital of South Manchester, Nell Lane, West Didsbury, Manchester

TONY VIIDIK
Department of Surgery, University of Western Ontario, Victoria Hospital, London, Ontario, Canada

L. VILAR
Ciudad Sanitaria, SS, Principes de Espagna, Barcelona, Spain

PATRICK VINAY
University of Montreal, Hotel Dieu de Montreal, 3840 St Urbain Street, Montreal, Quebec, Canada

E. VINNARS
St Erik¯s Sjukhus, S-112 82 Stockholm, Sweden

R. F. WALLIN
Pharmaceutical and Microbiological Department, Travenol Laboratories, Inc., 6301 Lincoln Avenue, Morton Grove, IL 60053, USA

CARL W. WALTER
Harvard Medical School, 25 Shattuck Street, Boston, MA 02115, USA

DOUGLAS W. WILMORE
Clinical Research, US Army Institute of Surgical Research, Brooke Army Medical Center, Ft. Sam Houston, TX 78234, USA

H. F. WOODS
Clinical Pharmacology and Therapeutics, University of Sheffield, Academic Division of Medicine, Department of Pharmacology, University of Sheffield

NEPOMUK ZÖLLNER
Medezinische Poliklinik der Universitat Muenchen, Pettenkoferstrasse 8a, 8000 Muenchen 2, Germany

Section I
Foundations of Parenteral Nutrition

1
Metabolic foundations of intravenous nutrition

I. D. A. JOHNSTON

INTRODUCTION

Intravenous feeding is required to meet the energy needs of the body when the alimentary canal is unavailable for significant periods of time. The concept of parenteral nutrition is not a new one. Milk was given intravenously to combat the wasting associated with cholera by Hodder[1] in Toronto in 1873. Henriques and Anderson in 1913[2] carried out the first successful experimental studies using goat muscle digested with pancreatic extract and combined with glucose, sodium and potassium. They were able to maintain a positive nitrogen balance in dogs for 6 days using this mixture. The first step in clinical intravenous nutrition was the use of sterile solutions of 5% dextrose during the First World War. By the late 1930s protein hydrolysates were under extensive study by Elman[3] and it was not long until the first fat emulsions were being prepared for intravenous use.

One of the most significant steps forward in intravenous nutrition was the demonstration in 1967 by Dudrick *et al.*[4] that the simultaneous administration to puppies of glucose and amino acids with added vitamins and minerals as the sole source of nourishment allowed normal muscular and skeletal growth to occur. It is now well established that an undernourished patient who cannot eat normally and who is not septic will increase his muscle mass and lay down fat during intravenous feeding. The induction of tissue synthesis in well-selected patients during total parenteral nutrition is one of the most significant therapeutic developments in recent years.

There are however a number of outstanding problems with intravenous feedings. What patients are most likely to benefit from parenteral nutrition? When should it be introduced or when is it meddlesome and unnecessary? What are the exact calorie and nutrient requirements in different clinical situations both in adults and infants? How can the biochemical problems associated with the bypass of the small bowel by nutrients be detected, managed and even prevented? What is the safest technique to maintain uncomplicated access to the circulation for long or short periods of parenteral nutrition? There have been some advances made in the search for answers to the questions which have been posed, and these advances, along with discussion of unanswered problems, form the substance of this symposium.

INDICATIONS

The number of patients who require total parenteral nutrition for any length of time is less than 5% of all admissions to acute hospitals. Alimentary failure leading to intravenous feeding may be acute, temporary or chronic and long term. The most obvious example of acute alimentary failure is the enterocutaneous fistula, and it is a simple matter now to maintain positive nitrogen balance in such patients (Figure 1.1); a significant reduction in mortality from intestinal fistula has been reported by many. In a recent report

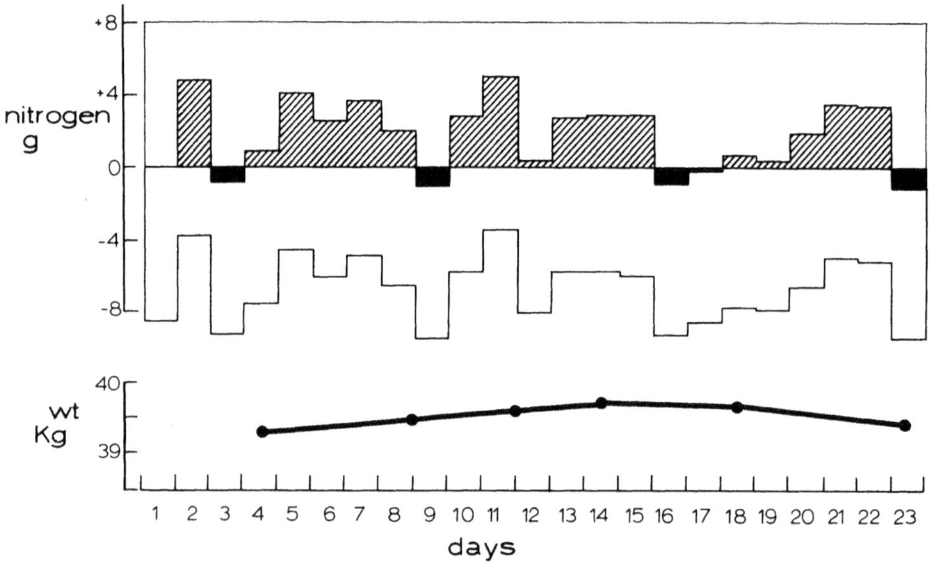

Figure 1.1 Nitrogen balance and body weight during total parenteral nutrition in a patient with an enterocutaneous fistula

of 78 patients with fistulae the spontaneous closure rate was 70% in a mean time of 35 days during total parenteral nutrition with a mortality of 8%[5].

Chronic or permanent alimentary failure occurs when there is permanent loss of the major portion of small intestine. Balance studies from such a patient are shown in Figure 1.2. The colon, and all but 6 inches of jejunum, have been lost following a series of operations for Crohn's disease. The daily fluid and nitrogen losses from the jejunostomy during a period of oral feeding demonstrated clearly the need for permanent parenteral nutrition in this patient. Jeejeebhoy and his colleagues in Toronto[6] have reported the successful delivery of total parenteral nutrition at home to twelve patients for periods ranging from 4 months to 5 years. The route used was a silicone rubber catheter inserted into the superior vena cava. All the patients maintained their ideal weights and all but two were considered to have

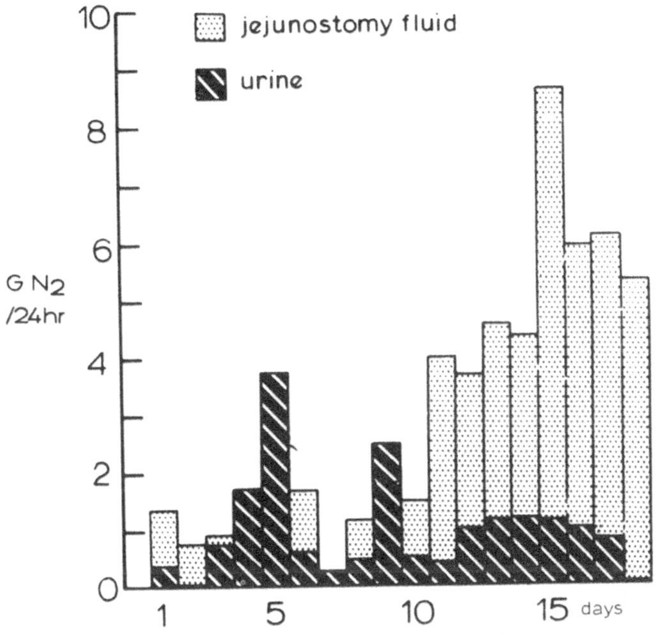

Figure 1.2 Daily urinary and enteral nitrogen losses in a patient with loss of the colon, ileum and most of the jejunum due to Crohn's disease

been socially rehabilitated. Liver function remained normal throughout the treatment periods. Satisfactory nutrient programmes have been worked out for almost indefinite application and the problems of access have been greater than metabolic problems in this long-term use of what is virtually an artificial gut. The exact requirements of vitamins and trace elements remain to be worked out in detail for very prolonged periods of almost complete parenteral nutrition.

The combination of starvation, injury and major sepsis continues to present a challenge, due to extensive catabolism of the lean body mass. The provision of adequate nutrients for such a situation, particularly in undernourished patients, remains difficult. Some of the difficulties are shown in

Figure 1.3 in relation to a patient following multiple thoracic and abdominal trauma. The patient had lost 50% of his ideal weight at the time of his referral to a nutritional care team. The detailed study was therefore carried out in a situation which has a very high mortality rate. During 50 days of parenteral nutrition nitrogen balance remained slightly positive but the calculated lean body mass using a whole body counter fell slightly. The patient was certainly not synthesizing much new tissue at this time, even though he was in zero nitrogen balance. Further surgery was required to deal with loculated intra-abdominal abscesses which were the cause of septicaemia. This operation led to large areas of granulation tissue being exposed within the peritoneum and the problem in many ways was similar to a major burn with associated large protein losses. Nitrogen balance became more and more negative during subsequent total parenteral nutrition and the patient died with a 56% weight loss. The lesson to be learnt from this study is the difficulty of inducing tissue synthesis in a nutritionally depleted and septic patient. The objective in such situations should always be to prevent weight loss from occurring in the immediate post-injury period by appropriate parenteral nutrition. The decision to feed intravenously is all too often delayed until serious malnutrition has developed.

Undernourishment is a serious problem in many patients admitted to hospital, and it tends to be neglected in many plans of management including surgery. Protein calorie malnutrition is associated with impaired humoral and cell-mediated immunity. Copeland and his colleagues in Houston[7] have shown in over 400 patients with cancer that nutritional support has

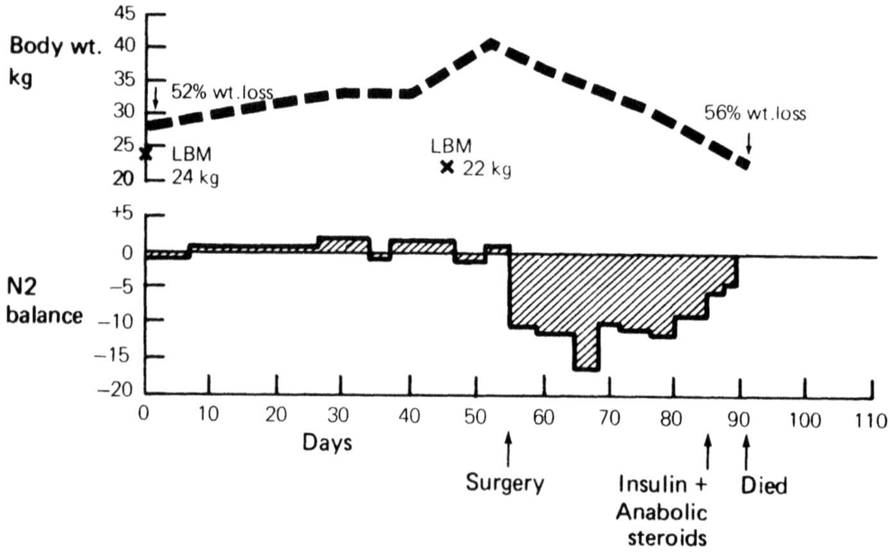

Figure 1.3 Nitrogen balance during parenteral nutrition in a patient with severe sepsis after abdominal injuries with multiple intraperitoneal abscesses and intestinal fistulae

proved effective in allowing adequate treatment to be carried out, often in patients who might have been unsuitable for any form of therapy. Tumour growth appears not to have been enhanced significantly by intravenous nutrition, and sepsis rates are reduced. There appears to be a correlation between adequate nutrition and the potential for a worthwhile response to chemotherapy.

Controlled clinical trials are required in different groups of undernourished cancer patients, to study in detail the effects of replenishing them nutritionally with intravenous hyperalimentation before, during and after various forms of treatment designed either to eradicate or control their malignant disease.

Criteria for undernutrition are difficult to establish but a loss of 15% or more of ideal weight, low serum albumin and serum transferrin and a low lymphocyte count seem to be the most reliable. A recent survey showed that 30% of patients who were undernourished according to these criteria died after admission to hospital. The questions that require to be answered are: Can the nutritional state of these underweight patients be improved rapidly enough to enable them to undergo the most effective treatment (either surgery or chemotherapy) safely, or will the restoration of their nutrition enhance their own basic defence mechanisms?[8]

Supplemental intravenous feeding should be given before operation to patients who fulfil the criteria of undernutrition, particularly patients with upper gastrointestinal cancer.

Enhanced wound healing, reduced post-operative complications and more rapid convalescence are the objectives of such support. The appropriate controlled studies to confirm that these objectives are attainable have not been performed and will be difficult to carry out.

After operation intravenous feeding should be commenced if adequate oral feeding is not possible between 72 and 96 h after surgery. The nett daily loss of lean body mass during complicated post-operative recovery may be as much as 500 g/day without intravenous support.

There is good evidence that intravenous feeding has an important role in the treatment of acute episodes of granulomatous disease of the bowel, and perhaps also of acute ulcerative colitis.

It is difficult to continue to provide an exhaustive list of indications for parenteral nutrition. The introduction of parenteral nutrition when the oral intake is inadequate for days at a time should rather be part of normal management.

REGIMENS

Intravenous nutrition can be provided at two levels by two routes, and this has been the cause of some confusion.

Simple nutritional support can be provided by the use of isotonic solutions of amino acids and dextrose plus fat emulsions using peripheral veins. A daily intake of about 1600 kcal (6.69 MJ) can be given through peripheral veins, and this support is of value as short-term supplementary feeding in post-operative patients.

Total parenteral nutrition through a central venous catheter, on the other hand, is indicated when treatment is likely to be required for more than a week and the oral intake is negligible. The central venous catheter allows the introduction of hypertonic solutions and makes it easier to deal with serious metabolic problems which require the addition of electrolyte and trace elements to the nutrient solutions.

How much is required intravenously and which calorie sources should be used? Patients who are septic and who require prolonged total parenteral nutrition need around 35–40 cal/kg body weight/day to maintain positive nitrogen balance. Long-term support in non-stressed, non-infected patients should include intravenous fat emulsions on a regular basis; the proportion of calories to be provided as fat can range between 5 and 15%.

The metabolic demands of major injury are however much greater. There have to be a number of attempts to produce positive nitrogen balance after elective surgery of moderate severity, and the calories and calorie/nitrogen ratios required are shown in Table 1.1. The needs after major injury are

Table 1.1 Calorie and calorie nitrogen ratios required to achieve positive nitrogen balance after elective surgery

	g N_2/kg	*cal/kg*	*cal/g N_2*	*N_2 balance*
Abbot *et al.*, 1959	0.20	35	175	—
Johnston *et al.*, 1966	0.16	35	219	—
Van Larsen and Brockner, 1969	0.24	32	133	—
Tweedle *et al.*, 1971	0.23	45	196	+

very difficult to meet. The mean daily nitrogen and calorie intakes and associated balance in the first few days after major road traffic accidents are shown in Figure 1.4 and compared with the data obtained from patients undergoing moderate surgical stress. The intakes required to produce positive balance in the major injury patients are clearly very much greater. It must be emphasized that nutritional support after major injury such as severe burns is justified in diminishing the inevitable weight loss which follows serious trauma. There is of course no evidence that the maintenance of positive nitrogen balance after elective surgery of moderate severity confers any clinical benefit in terms of wound healing or accelerated convalescence.

The peripheral infusion of isotonic amino acids alone has been advocated as an effective method of protein sparing in patients[9]. The relative efficacy of amino acids, glucose or fat emulsions as the sole energy substrates to spare

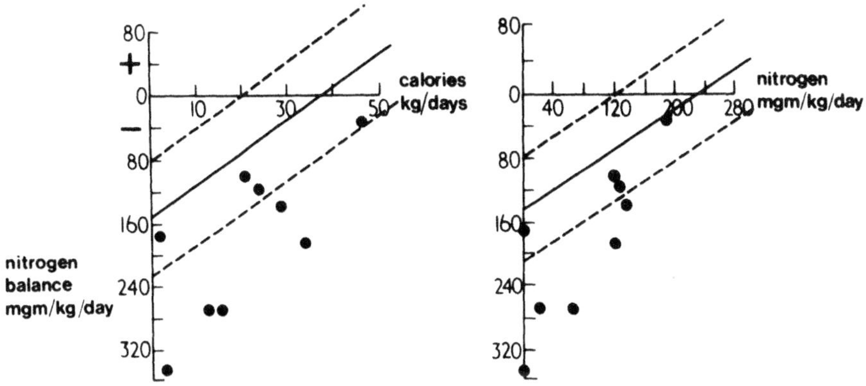

Figure 1.4 Calorie and nitrogen intakes, and associated nitrogen balance, after major injury in nine patients compared to the mean results of twenty-nine patients undergoing vagotomy for peptic ulcer

lean body mass remains controversial, whether during starvation, injury or after severe trauma complicated by sepsis[10]. The effects of equicaloric amounts (2.51 MJ) of glucose, amino acids or soya bean oil emulsion were compared with those of fasting in four groups of male patients during uncomplicated recovery from vagotomy and pyloroplasty[11].

Patients given glucose excreted less nitrogen than the fasting patients, but nitrogen sparing was greatest in the group given amino acids alone (Figure 1.5). There was no evidence of any nitrogen-sparing when fat was the source

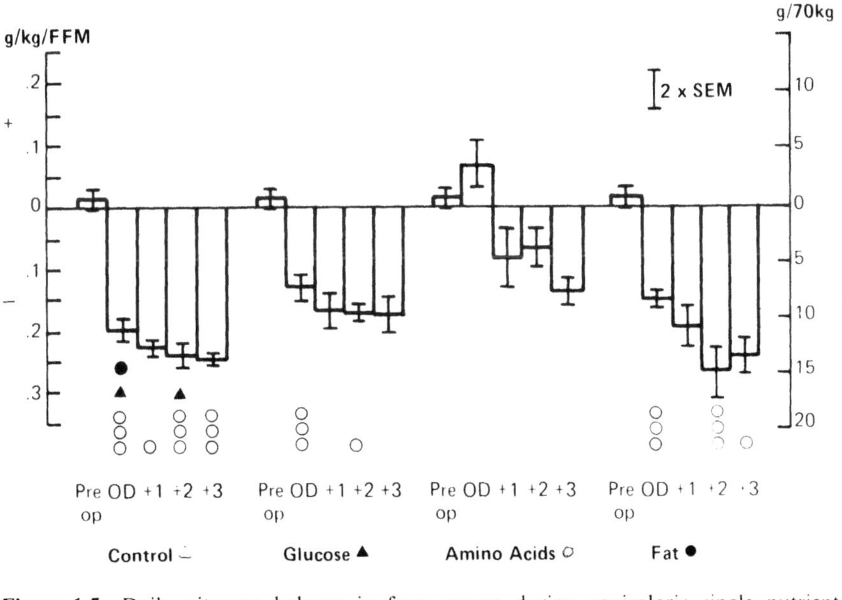

Figure 1.5 Daily nitrogen balance in four groups during equicaloric single nutrient intakes, compared with controls

of calories. There was no difference in blood glucose, free fatty acids and insulin concentrations among the groups. Ketone bodies rose in the fasting and fat-fed groups but remained low in the groups who received glucose and amino acids (Figure 1.6). The protein-sparing effect of amino acids alone in these particular patients appears to be a function of the amino acids alone, and is not related to the degree of fat mobilization.

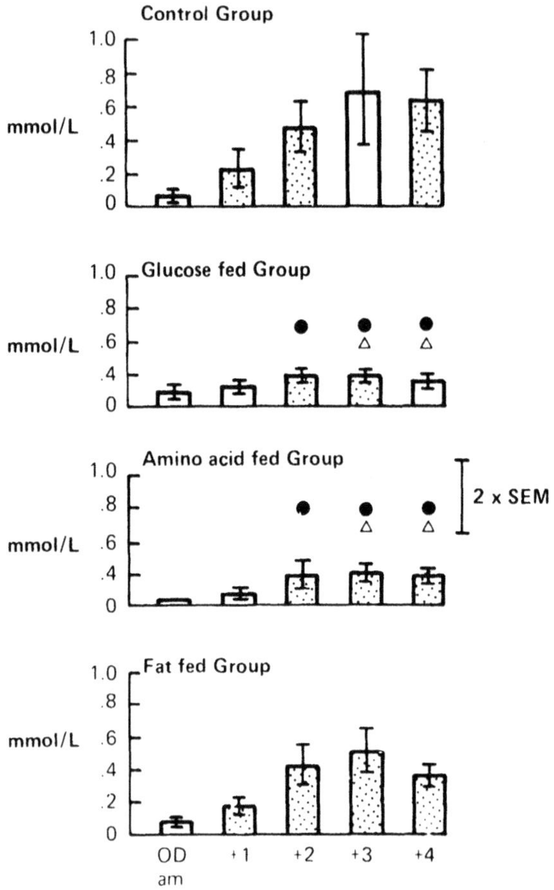

Figure 1.6 Daily ketone body levels in the four groups during equicaloric single nutrient intakes, compared with controls

There is evidence that most of the amino acids infused were converted to glucose.

It is of interest that the administration of intravenous fat had no effect on nitrogen balance compared to the control group. This suggests that perhaps a period of adaptation is required in normally nourished subjects before intravenous fat can be utilized as a calorie source.

These studies should not be confused with the observations in starved, nutritionally depleted subjects where there is good evidence of important nitrogen-sparing when isotonic amino acids alone are infused. Intravenous fat is also a readily available source of calories in such patients.

The formulation of amino acid solutions still depends on the early recommendation of Rose in relation to healthy subjects.

It is however possible to use some clinical situations to make recommendations on the amino acid ratios to be provided in solutions designed for clinical use. Tweedle and his colleagues[12] have compared the utilization of various amino acid mixtures in the immediate post-operative period; one such study is shown in Figure 1.7. The total intake of nitrogen and the calorie nitrogen

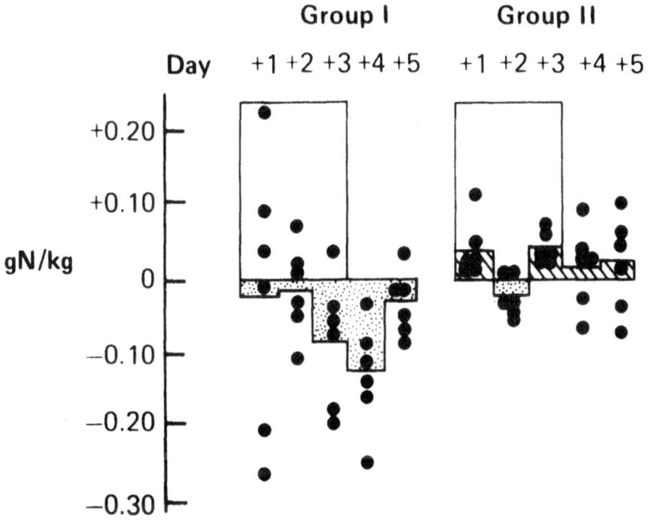

Figure 1.7 Daily nitrogen balances after operation during the infusion of amino acid solutions of different composition

ratios were similar in the infusions for each group, but the effect on nitrogen balance and the amino acid excretion in the urine was quite different. The solution which was associated with larger nitrogen losses had a higher content of glycine and alanine (Table 1.2). Further studies are required in different clinical situations to enable the formulation of amino acid mixtures to be adjusted for specific needs. There is reason to believe, for example, that the amino acid requirements of a neonate are quite different from a malnourished adult without sepsis.

Muscle is the main cellular tissue which is broken down during increased catabolism in injury, and there is evidence of significant changes in cytoplasmic amino acids in muscle cells after injury. Furst and his group[13] have provided information on free intracellular amino acids in different clinical situations. The relationship between plasma amino acid levels and intracellular measurements has yet to be established.

Table 1.2 Percentage of non-essential amino acids in test solutions compared to egg protein

	Egg protein (%)	*Group I* (%)	*Group II* (%)
Alanine	6.6	26.0	11.9
Glycine	3.3	25.0	19.8

There is no simple biochemical measurement of amino acid turnover to give guidance as to the development of protein deficiency. It is hoped that studies of amino acid levels in plasma might provide pointers to appropriate composition of solutions or infusion rates during intravenous feeding. The effect of differing degrees of surgical stress, anaesthesia and post-operative nutrition on plasma amino acid levels were studied before, during and after surgery of varying severity[14]. There is a fall in the plasma concentration of most amino acid solutions immediately after operation (Figure 1.8); the non-essential amino acids (glutamate, proline, glycine, alanine, histidine and arginine) continue to fall during the second post-operative day, whereas the essential amino acids (isoleucine, leucine, phenylalanine and lysine with tyrosine) are at a higher concentration after 48 h than immediately after surgery. Comparison of patients undergoing surgery of moderate severity, such as vagotomy and pyloroplasty, with the more severe procedure of

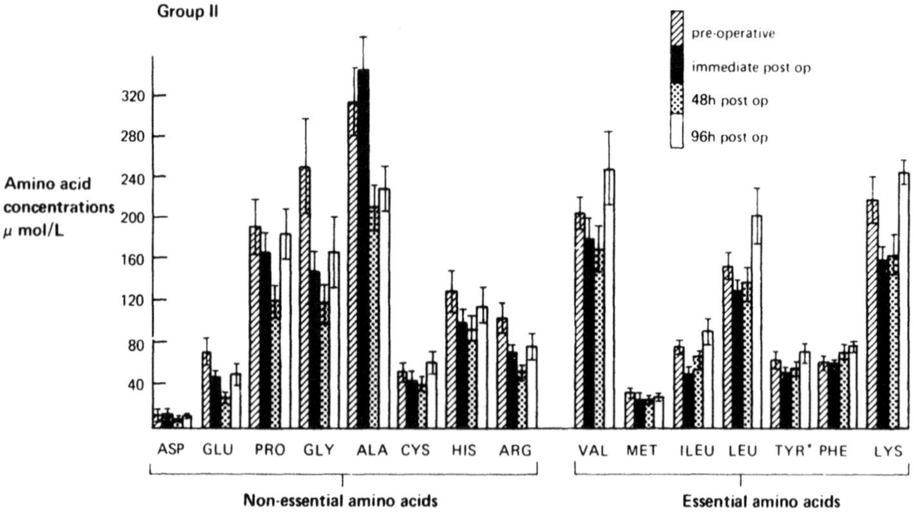

Figure 1.8 Changes in essential and non-essential amino acids in plasma during the first 3 days after elective surgery

resection of aortic aneurysm indicate that these changes in amino acid concentrations are not related to the severity of the trauma, although cystine levels were somewhat lower and phenylalanine levels were higher in the major surgery group. The changes were not found to be related to the effect of anaesthesia alone.

When the calorie intake after surgery was increased by giving intravenous glucose the plasma alanine levels rose and methionine levels fell. Studies of plasma amino acid profiles after injury suggest that in the post-injury state cystine and tyrosine may become essential amino acids, and rises in phenylalanine and methionine may indicate some liver dysfunction. There is evidence of a beneficial effect in terms of amino acid concentrations of a high calorie intake after surgical operation. Much more work is required before we really understand the needs for protein anabolism at a cellular level.

ENDOCRINE BACKGROUND

Intravenous feeding is often required at a time when endocrine function is altered and manipulations of hormone levels and activity have been attempted to enhance the effectiveness of nutritional support.

Insulin levels in the circulation are variable after trauma. Low levels have been recorded in the acute phase of burns and during shock, while inappropriately high levels have been found during the administration of glucose during the first few days after surgery[15]. Wright and Johnston[23] have found the lowest insulin response to a glucose stimulus to occur during major surgery, while significantly raised levels of insulin follow the same stimulus by the second post-operative day (Figure 1.9). A number of insulin antagonists are present in the circulation in increased amounts during stress. ACTH, growth hormone and glucagon are all elevated but catecholamines probably play the major role in the alteration of glucose insulin homeostasis.

Insulin can be infused in quite large amounts during intravenous feeding with improvement in nitrogen balance[16]. Insulin must be given when a hypertonic glucose solution has been established. Plasma and urinary urea levels will fall and the serum potassium will be reduced during insulin administration. Careful monitoring is required to avoid rebound hypoglycaemia and cellular overhydration.

Other anabolic hormones have been used to enhance protein synthesis during intravenous feeding. Wilmore and associates[17] demonstrated the preservation of protoplasmic mass and improved nitrogen balance when human growth hormone was given to burn patients.

Tweedle and Johnston[18] studied the effect of a long-acting anabolic steroid, both on the catabolic and anabolic phases following abdominal surgery when intravenous nutrition was being provided. The post-operative nitrogen balance was improved significantly from the 5th to the 8th post-operative

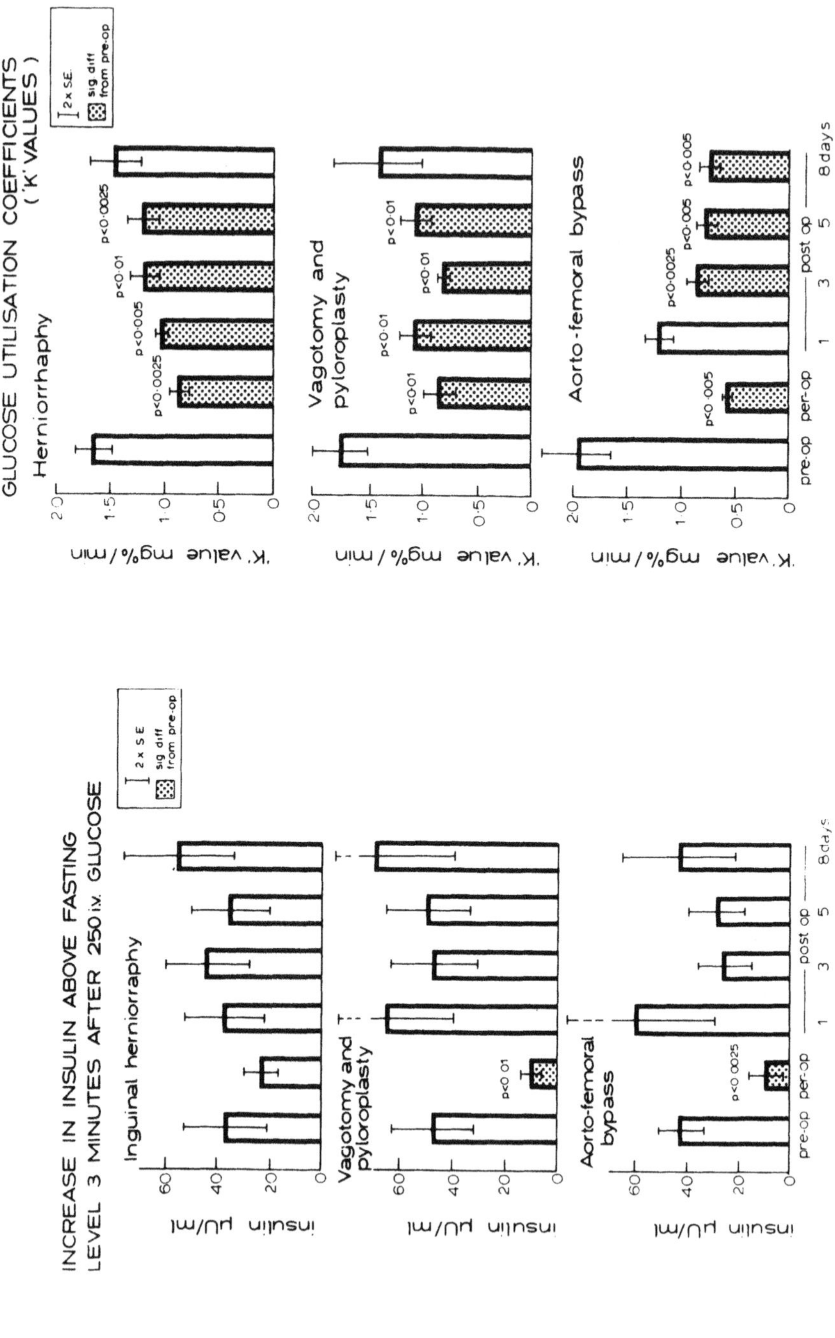

Figure 1.9 Serum insulin and glucose levels at a fixed time interval in response to a glucose load before, during and after surgery

day when an anabolic steroid was given (Figure 1.10). The nett gain in body protein produced by the anabolic steroid was approximately 0.6 kg during 8 days.

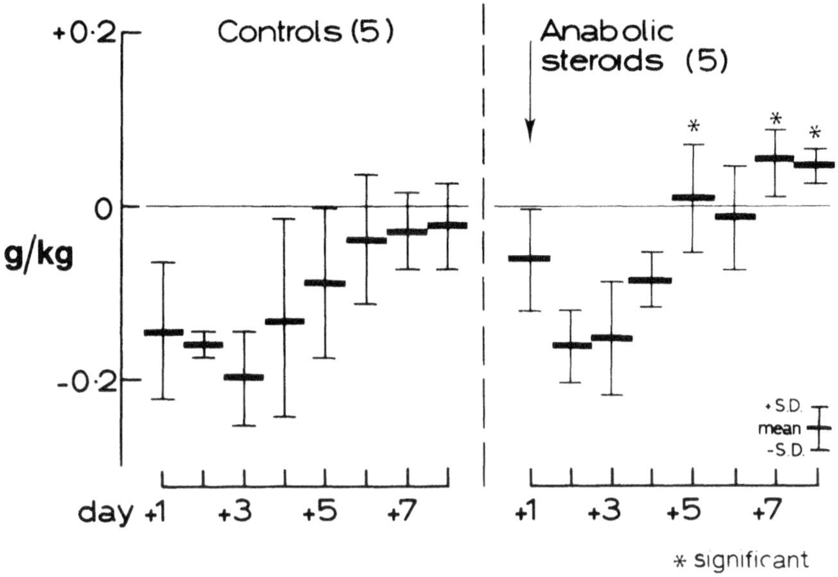

Figure 1.10 The effect of an anabolic steroid on post-operative nitrogen balance after abdominal surgery

The results of these studies indicate that the anabolic drive which begins normally 3–4 days after injury can be increased, as the potential for new protein synthesis under normal conditions may not be utilized fully. Whether or not similar effects can be produced by an increased intake of nutrients by any route during the anabolic phase is uncertain.

METABOLIC PROBLEMS

The introduction of total parenteral nutrition carries with it the need for increased metabolic surveillance to prevent such complications as hyperosmolar states and rebound hypoglycaemia.

One of the most serious biochemical complications of intravenous feeding with essential amino acids and glucose alone is hypophosphataemia. The clinical manifestations of biochemical problems are difficult to recognize in seriously ill patients. Patients who are already nutritionally depleted can develop hypophosphataemia within 24 h of the start of an infusion of hypertonic glucose and amino acids (Figure 1.11). The fall in plasma phosphate may be particularly rapid and profound when insulin is also infused.

The clinical features of hypophosphataemia include neuromuscular inco-ordination, dysarthria, paraesthesia, weakness, disorientation and even coma. There are many enzyme defects which follow hypophosphataemia[18]. The fall in red cell 2:3 diphosphoglycerate shifts the oxygen dissociation curve to the left and diminishes the availability of oxygen to the peripheral tissues. This problem was largely unnoticed when protein hydrolysates and fat emulsions were used for parenteral nutrition because phosphate is present and may be available to the body from these nutrient solutions. Phosphate requirements can be difficult to calculate, but they seem to be related to a combination of the carbohydrate energy intake and renal function. The provision of 25 mEq potassium dihydrogen phosphate daily is usually sufficient to maintain a normal plasma level.

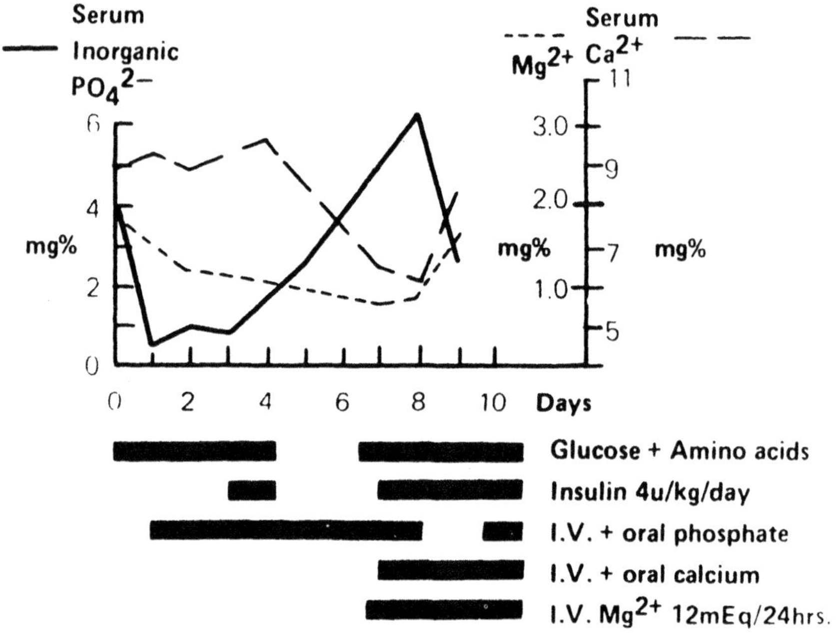

Figure 1.11 Fall in serum inorganic phosphate in nutritionally depleted patient aged 68 given synthetic amino acids and glucose. Patient's weight = 39 kg. Total plasma protein = 6.0 g%

Fructose has been used widely as a substitute for glucose, but its exact role in intravenous feeding remains controversial. There is much evidence that fructose is metabolized more rapidly than glucose; consequently it may be utilized more effectively during stress and after trauma when the utilization of glucose is reduced. There is little information on the effect of injury on fructose metabolism. A comparison of fructose and glucose clearance after surgical operation[19] showed that fructose was cleared much faster during operation (Figure 1.12) but the rate of clearance of fructose had returned to normal by the first post-operative day. However, it must not be forgotten that in quantitative terms 30% of a fructose infusion is converted to glucose. The build-up of lactate and associated metabolic acidosis in ill patients and neonates must be balanced against the evidence of increased clearance during acute stress. The full metabolic significance of these differences in glucose and fructose handling in various clinical situations has yet to be worked out, and there are probably no advantages of fructose compared to glucose in intravenous feeding programmes.

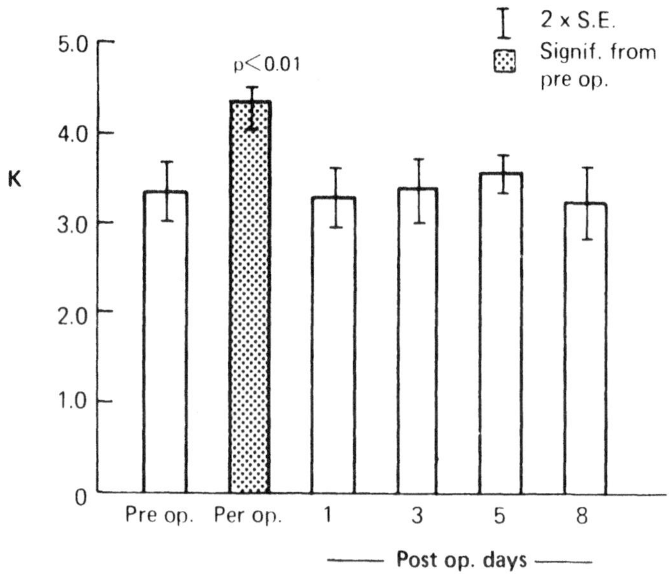

Figure 1.12 Fructose clearance during and after surgical operation of moderate severity

Sorbitol is a sugar alcohol which has been used widely but it is converted to fructose and glucose, and apart from a slightly higher calorie yield it provides no metabolic advantage over glucose.

Alcohol has been provided in some intravenous feeding regimens as a rapid and efficient source of energy. Patients with sepsis, and liver or renal dysfunction, should never be given alcohol. The number of contraindications are now so many that there is no need to include alcohol in parenteral nutrition and its use should be discouraged.

TECHNIQUE OF ADMINISTRATION

Access to the circulation

The success of intravenous feeding depends on easy and safe access to the circulation for as long as is required. Thrombophlebitis and septicaemia are serious problems which have often detracted from the benefits of parenteral nutrition. Poor technique is clearly the cause of infection and thrombophlebitis, and only careful attention to detail of catheter insertion and maintenance of the infusion can overcome the problem.

Parenteral nutrition fluids are effective culture media for organisms, and the addition of electrolytes or the mixing of nutrients must be carried out in the pharmacy by a faultless technique. Organisms can collect in the drip chambers during infusions and Collin *et al.*, 1976[20] have found about 20% of samples from drip chambers which had been in use for more than 48 h were contaminated. Infusion sets should therefore be changed at regular intervals. Millipore filter units have been advocated as a means of reducing the entry of organisms into the circulation, but a prospective controlled study[21] showed no fall in the incidence of thrombophlebitis or positive cannula culture when millipore filters were used. The filters were shown to be inconvenient as well as ineffective.

The junction between the catheter and the skin should be kept bacteriologically clean either by repeated cleansing or with occlusive antiseptic dressings.

A significant advance has been the successful use during total parenteral nutrition at home[6] of the soft silicone rubber catheter introduced into the superior vena cava via a peripheral vein. The catheter is introduced as a surgical procedure and placed in a long subcutaneous tunnel. The catheter has a dacron cuff which becomes fixed in the subcutaneous tissues by fibrous tissue and forms a barrier to the entry of organisms around the catheter. The mean survival of uncomplicated catheters was over 15 months in twelve patients reported by the Toronto group[6]. We have found the early introduction of this catheter to be most valuable when prolonged parenteral nutrition is planned.

It must be emphasized that the parenteral nutrition catheter should never be used for blood sampling, blood transfusion or intermittent intravenous therapy.

A strict aseptic technique is essential when inserting a central venous line. The position of the tip of the catheter must be checked radiologically to ensure that it has not entered the jugular vein or curled up in a peripheral vein.

Local measures may be of value in preventing infection, such as the application of an antibiotic (polybactrin) or Povidine iodine cream around the junction of the catheter and the skin. The advisability of changing the infusion set at frequent intervals has been well established.

Bacterial contamination of the solutions of nutrients is a serious problem and can occur when adding electrolytes or trace elements to bottles of amino acids. Such additions in an open ward or an ill-prepared pharmacy are liable to cause contamination, and this must be avoided.

Patients may develop septicaemia without any local signs of thrombophlebitis. A swinging temperature and positive blood cultures are suggestive of an infected thrombus around the tip of the catheter and septic emboli. A search should be made first for obvious causes of infection and if none are found then the catheter should be removed, the clot cultured and appropriate antibiotics given.

Many organisms have been found in patients with catheter sepsis but infection with *Candida albicans* has been the most serious. Some amino acid solutions are known at body temperature to support the growth of this organism. While blood-borne organisms from infected foci in the patient will undoubtedly settle on a catheter lying in a large vein, careless aseptic techniques by medical and nursing staff add to the hazards.

Organization

It is clear that the provision of parenteral nutrition has been simplified by the reduction of the types of solutions to be used, but it has also in many respects become more complicated. The standards required in prescribing and delivery of intravenous nutrition are probably higher than in any other form of therapy. The patient's requirements of calories, amino acids, trace elements and vitamins can vary from day to day. Daily measurement of urea electrolytes, haemoglobin and urine glucose are essential. Twice-weekly measurements of calcium, phosphorus and liver function tests are also a minimal requirement for good care while zinc, magnesium, folate and B_{12} must be measured at intervals.

Computer technology can be used to provide guidelines in the form of a daily requirement prediction based on body compositional data and plasma concentrations. Once the daily requirements have been calculated the daily prescription can be worked out, based on the types of solutions available in the pharmacy.

The ultimate success of intravenous feeding thus depends on a team of medical staff, nurses and pharmacists. It has been established that a well-defined nutritional care team will ensure the safety and efficiency of the delivery of vital nutritional support to the critically ill[22]. It is hoped that the advances reported in this Symposium will help many clinicians to improve their nutritional care, and alert them as to where further investigative endeavour is required.

References

1. Hodder, E. (1873). Transfusion of milk in cholera. *Practitioner*, **10,** 14
2. Henriques, V. and Anderson, A. C. (1913). Uber parenterale eruchrung durch. Intravenous injecktion. *Hoppe-Seylers Zeitschrift für physiologische chemi*, **42,** 357
3. Elman, R. (1939). Time factor in retention of nitrogen after intravenous injection of mixtures of amino acids. *Proc. Soc. Exp. Biol. Med.* **40,** 484
4. Dudrick, S. J., Wilmore, D. W. and Vars, H. M. (1967). Long term parenteral nutrition with growth in puppies and positive nitrogen balance. *Surg. For.*, **18,** 356

5. MacFadyen, B. V. and Dudrick, S. J. (1976). Treatment of enterocutaneous fistulae. *Proceedings of International Conference on Parenteral Nutrition*, Montpellier
6. Jeejeebhoy, R. N., Longer, B., Tsallas, G., Chu, R. C., Kaksis, A. and Anderson, G. H. (1976). Total parenteral nutrition at home. *Gastroenterology*, **71,** 943
7. Copeland, E. M. and Dudrick, S. J. (1976). Nutritional aspects of cancer. Current problems in cancer. *Year Book*. (Chicago: Medical Publishers)
8. Copeland, E. M., MacFadyen, B. V. and Dudrick, S. J. (1976). Effect of intravenous hyperalimentation on hypersensitivity in the cancer patient. *Ann. Surg.*, **184,** 60
9. Blackburn, G. L., Flatt, J. P. and Clowes, G. H. A. (1973). Peripheral intravenous feeding with isotonic amino acid solutions. *Am. J. Surg.*, **125,** 447
10. Greenberg, G. R., Marliss, E. B., Anderson, G. H., Longer, B., Spence, W., Toree, E. B. and Jeejeebhoy, K. N. (1976). Protein-sparing therapy in postoperative patients. *New Engl. J. Med.*, **294,** 1411
11. Craig, R. P., Tweedle, D. E. F., Davidson, H. A. and Johnston, I. D. A. (1977). Intravenous glucose, amino acids and fat in the post operative period. *Lancet*, **ii,** 8
12. Tweedle, D. E. F., Spivey, J. and Johnston, I. D. A. (1972). Choice of intravenous amino acid solution for use after surgical operation. *Metabolism*, **22,** 173
13. Vinars, E., Bergstrom, J. and Furst, P. (1975). Influence of the post operative state on the intracellular free amino acids in human muscle tissue. *Ann. Surg.*, **182,** 665
14. Dale, G., Young, G., Latner, A. L., Goode, A. W., Tweedle, D. E. F. and Johnston, I. D. A. (1977). The effect of surgical operation on venous plasma free amino acids. *Surgery*, **81,** 295
15. Ross, H., Johnston, I. D. A., Welborn, T. A. and Wright, A. D. (1966). The effect of surgical operation on glucose tolerance and serum levels of insulin and growth hormone. *Lancet*, **ii,** 563
16. Allison, S. P. (1974). In H. A. Lee (ed.). *Carbohydrate and Fat Metabolism in Acute Metabolic Illness*, pp. 167–175. (New York: Academic Press)
17. Wilmore, D. W., Moyton, J. A., Bristow, B. F., Mason, A. D. and Prouitt, B. A. (1974). Anabolic effects of human growth hormone following thermal injury. *Surg. Gynecol. Obstet.*, **138,** 855
18. Sheldon, G. F., Plzak, L. F. and Watkins, G. M. (1971). Inorganic phosphate and the the oxygen dissociation curve. *Surg. For.*, **22,** 81
19. McCarthy, D. O'B., Wright, P. D. and Johnston, I. D. A. (1975). Plasma clearance of fructose during and after surgical operation. *Br. J. Surg.*, **62,** 658
20. Collin, J., Constable, F. L., Johnston, I. D. A. and Hall, R. I. (1976). Comparison of PVC and glass containers in the prevention of contamination and thrombophlebitis in intravenous therapy. *Br. J. Clin. Practice*, **30,** 17
21. Collin, J., Tweedle, D. E. F., Venables, C. W., Constable, F. L. and Johnston, I. D. A. (1973). Effect of a millipore filter on complications of intravenous infusions. *Br. Med. J.*, **2,** 456
22. Ellis, B. W., Stanridge, R. de L., Fielding, L. P. and Dudley, H. A. F. (1976). A rational approach to parenteral nutrition. *Br. Med. J.*, **1,** 1388
23. Wright, P. D. and Johnston, I. D. A. (in press)

Section II
Carbohydrates in Parenteral Nutrition

2
Some general considerations concerning the use of carbohydrates in parenteral nutrition

H. A. KREBS

Within the last decade several symposia have dealt with parenteral nutrition[1–6]. My own experiences relating to the subject stem, apart from studies of intermediary metabolism, from the 'feeding' of isolated organs in laboratory experiments. In studying metabolism and its regulation we have made much use of isolated perfused organs, especially the liver, kidney, heart and the hind-limb of rats (the latter presenting mainly the musculature). More recently we have also used isolated hepatocytes whose metabolic competence is almost identical with that of the intact perfused organ[7]. In such experiments it is essential to 'feed' the organs in order to keep them in a normal functional state. This means in the first instance supplying a source of energy in the form either of carbohydrate, or carbohydrate derivatives, or fatty acids or ketone bodies. It may also be essential to provide special blood plasma constituents such as amino acids or hormones[8,9]. These experiences, then, are my credentials for participating in this Symposium. They imply that I must limit myself to comments on principles derived from basic biochemistry.

A principle which may serve as a key-note is the following: when we are forced to do something artificial we must aim at remaining as close as possible to the natural situation. In laboratory experiments we often *must* use artificial conditions because many quantitative aspects of organ function can be studied only in the isolated organ, fed by an artificial circulation with a chemically well-defined fluid—better defined than blood plasma. In patients we must resort to something artificial, when the function of the digestive tract is so disturbed that oral feeding is inadequate.

In the efforts to remain close to the natural situation, we must bear in mind that parenteral nutrition means not only the circumvention of the gastrointestinal tract, but also circumvention of the liver. It is the function of the gastrointestinal tract to degrade, by hydrolysis, macromolecules such as proteins, nucleic acids, lipids, starch and glycogen into the readily soluble, low-molecular building blocks, and also hydrolyse smaller molecules such as peptides, oligosaccharides, triglycerides and nucleotides to the smallest molecules which can be obtained by simple hydrolysis. Hydrolysis solubilizes the ingested material and disposes of toxic properties without a major loss of energy. It is one of the important functions of the liver, through the portal circulation, to clear the portal blood of materials which might be harmful to the peripheral tissues and from which other tissues must be protected.

A striking illustration of this protective action is the effect of the liver on ethanol, a substance acutely toxic to the brain. The liver is the only major organ which can detoxicate ethanol relatively rapidly by oxidizing it to acetate. Moderate amounts of ethanol in the food are filtered off, as it were, by the liver. In all vertebrate species the liver is the only tissue with a high activity of alcohol dehydrogenase, the main enzyme responsible for the disposal of alcohol. It is remarkable that the activity of alcohol dehydrogenase is very high even in animals, such as the horse, which do not partake of alcoholic drinks. However, not consuming alcoholic beverages does not mean that some animals are not faced with the problem of detoxicating alcohol. Alcohol can be produced in significant quantities in the gastrointestinal tract by fermentations, mainly by micro-organisms occurring in the rumen, colon or caecum. This applies, for example, to African elephants and to African wart-hogs when feeding on the decaying fruit of the Marula tree and to the ring-tailed lemur when feeding on the fermenting pods of the tamarind tree. Drunken elephants and lemurs, just like humans, lose balance and control over their muscles. They stumble and are liable to fall into rivers and drown. Alcohol has also been found as a major product in the caecal fermentation of birds; e.g. willow ptarmigans and bullfinches. Drunken birds kill themselves by flying against walls and windows, misjudging distances[10].

Glucose coming from the intestine is another example of the importance of the liver as a clearing organ. Much of the glucose arising in the gut is taken up by the liver and deposited either as glycogen or converted to fatty acids, so that the concentration of blood sugar is kept below the renal threshold.

Apart from removing glucose from the portal blood and regulating the concentration of blood glucose, the liver takes up other carbohydrates and related substances such as fructose, galactose, sorbitol, xylitol, lactate and glycerol and converts them into glucose. Although the liver does not entirely eliminate these substances from the blood during a single passage, it substantially decreases their plasma concentrations.

Most of the carbohydrate derived from food reaches the peripheral organs in the form of glucose. There are also some peripheral organs which can

Table 2.1 Glucose formation from various precursors in rat kidney cortex

Precursor	*Glucose formed*
None	0.25
L-Lactate	1.71
D-Fructose	7.05
D-Galactose	0.93
D-Mannose	0.83
Sorbitol	1.33
Xylitol	1.77
Glycerol	1.32

Glucose formation is expressed as μmol min/g dry wt. The tests were carried out on kidney cortex slices[11].

convert fructose, galactose or polyols into glucose but the liver is the most important site of the conversion. The rates of conversion in the kidney cortex are given in Table 2.1. These rates are of the same order of magnitude as for the liver, but as the amount of liver tissue is four to five times that of the kidney cortex, the contribution of the kidneys to the disposal of these substances is relatively small.

It is also true that some specialized tissues use fructose even in preference to glucose. This applies to spermatozoa which are supplied with fructose by the secretion of the seminal glands[12]. It also holds for embryonic tissues of ungulates (e.g. cattle, sheep, goats). The fetal fluids of these animals contain fructose as the main carbohydrate. The reasons for this are not understood. Fetal membranes of other species can readily convert fructose to lactic acid under anaerobic conditions, the rates being almost as fast as with glucose[13]. Among adult tissues, the anaerobic degradation of fructose is relatively rapid in kidney and testis, the rates being between 20% and 30% of that of glucose degradation. The majority of adult tissues do not readily utilize the fructose directly, but only after conversion to glucose by liver or kidney[13].

Such special situations do not imply that fructose is a generally useful energy source to man. The fact that excess fructose can deplete the liver of adenine nucleotides[14] is a powerful argument against the use of major amounts of fructose in parenteral nutrition. If, then, in parenteral nutrition we attempt to keep as closely as possible to the natural situation, we must consider glucose as the carbohydrate nutrient of choice. Other carbohydrate derivatives should not be major constituents of infusion fluids, a conclusion also reached by others, in particular by Froesch[15-18]. This holds in the first instance for patients whose metabolic status is reasonably normal. In special situations, such as in the diabetic, there may be a case for variations from this principle.

It has been argued that the infusion of precursors of glucose, such as xylitol or sorbitol, provides a gradual rise in blood glucose and this somehow simulates the natural rate of glucose supply. This is not a convincing argument; moreover polyols, because of their rapid utilization, may disturb the redox state of the pyridine nucleotides in the direction of reduction, and this may be harmful. As it is unnecessary to use unphysiological substances they should be avoided.

A carbohydrate derivative included in some solutions for parenteral feeding is lactate. L-lactate has the advantage of contributing to the acid–base balance as a precursor of bicarbonate. This function is discharged by acetate in some infusion fluids. Acetate has the advantage of being cheaply available in the purity required for intravenous infusion. It may be a disadvantage that it is not a major normal metabolite and that it is therefore rather slowly utilized. To judge from the experience with the rat, only two tissues—cardiac muscle and kidney cortex— burn acetate at a high rate. The liver can burn some acetate (arising in this tissue when alcohol is oxidized) but the rates are relatively low. Acetate moreover is not a good source of energy. It yields up to 10 molecules of ATP per molecule with an O_2 consumption of 2 molecules. Lactate gives up to 18 ATP for three molecules of O_2. Lactate has the disadvantage of not being cheaply available at present in the required degree of purity but I believe that this problem can be solved. We have recently worked out a procedure whereby the cheap lactic acid marketed by Boehringer-Ingelheim consisting almost entirely of the physiologically natural L-isomere can be converted readily into crystalline L-lactic acid. All the other commercial samples of lactic acid tested by us contained major amounts of D-lactate which is utilized much more slowly than L-lactate. So I think that the use of L-lactate in place of acetate deserves serious consideration.

Straying away from carbohydrate to amino acids, I would like to comment that the intestinal wall is now known to convert glutamate, glutamine and aspartate arising from protein digestion largely to alanine. This involves oxidation of the amino acids to pyruvate and transamination of the latter with glutamate. Pyruvate can also be derived from carbohydrate[19–22]. The physiological significance of this conversion may lie in the fact that glutamate and aspartate, unlike most other amino acids, do not readily enter the liver cell because of their negative charge. Amino nitrogen as well as the greater part of the carbon skeleton in the form of alanine can be dealt with by the liver. It is also known that glutamate can be toxic to the central nervous system[23,24]. The flooding of the peripheral circulation with glutamate should therefore be avoided. Thus the simulation of the physiological situation in parenteral infusion fluids suggests exclusion of the dicarboxylic amino acids and their replacement by alanine, a principle not adhered to in the formulation of Vamin or Aminosol. Travasol* is better in this respect, relying essentially on alanine and on glycine as precursors of the non-essential amino acids. In fact, all the non-essential amino acids are readily formed from alanine and I am therefore not at all sure whether the relatively large

* Sythamin

amounts of glycine are useful, considering that glycine is neither an efficient source of energy nor an effective precursor of non-essential amino acids. Its main asset is its cheapness.

The importance of keeping close to the physiological situation was brought home to me recently in a related field. The Institute of Scientific Information in Philadelphia, which publishes the *Citation Index* and *Current Contents* informed me a few weeks ago that a paper I published in 1932 describing the ornithine cycle of urea synthesis[25] was one of the most frequently quoted papers in the period between 1960 and 1970, 30 years after the publication, and they asked me to comment on this. When I looked into the reason for the frequent quotation it turned out that this paper was not quoted because it reported a discovery of general interest, but because it described a new saline solution replacing the old Ringer solution. I had designed this saline for the study *in vitro* of a synthetic process—the synthesis of urea—using liver slices, something which had not been attempted before. In order to have the most favourable conditions I used as a guide for the composition of the suspension medium the normal concentrations of the ionic constituents of blood plasma. Subsequently, this saline solution has proved optimal in biochemical, physiological and pharmacological studies. The wide use of the solution is the only reason for the frequent quotation of the paper. The previous saline solutions employed as a blood substitute, such as the Ringer solution, were obtained by trial and error while observing the beat of a frog heart fed with saline solutions of different composition. The solution of 1932 was based, not on the trial and error principle, but on chemical analyses of the inorganic plasma constituents and contained bicarbonate and CO_2 in physiological quantities, as well as phosphate, chloride, magnesium, sodium, potassium and calcium. When basing my design of the solution on the given physiological situation, I was guided by the conviction that it was no accident that the plasma concentrations of ions are not only the same in all mammalian species, but are also carefully regulated and maintained within narrow ranges against varying intakes.

I think this is a powerful demonstration of the importance of keeping closely to the natural situation when we experiment, either in the laboratory or in the course of treatment of patients. Although the body possesses regulatory mechanisms adapting metabolic processes according to circumstances, it would be unwise in situations of stress, as in the sick patient, to rely on such regulatory mechanisms. Efforts should be made to stretch them minimally.

In summing up, I would like to express the view that basic biochemistry may still suggest improvements in the practice of parenteral nutrition.

References

1. Wilkinson, A. W. (ed.). (1972). *Parenteral Nutrition.* (Edinburgh and London: Churchill Livingstone)

2. Ghadimi, H. (ed.). (1975). *Total Parenteral Nutrition: Premises and Promises.* (New York: Wiley Biomed-Health Publications)
3. Allen, P. C. and Lee, H. A. (1969). *A Clinical Guide to Intravenous Nutrition*, (Oxford: Blackwell)
4. Cowan, G. S. M. and Scheetz, W. L. (eds.). (1972). *Intravenous Hyperalimentation.* (Philadelphia: Lea & Febiger)
5. Alberti, K. G. M. M. (ed.). (1974). *Parenteral Nutrition. A Clinical Conversation*
6. Fischer, J. E. (ed.). (1976). *Total Parenteral Nutrition.* (London: Little, Brown)
7. Krebs, H. A., Cornell, N. W., Lund, P. and Hems, R. (1974). Isolated liver cells as experimental material. In F. Lundquist and N. Tygstrup (eds.) *Regulation of Hepatic Metabolism*, Alfred Benzon Symposium VI, pp. 726–750 (Copenhagen: Munksgaard; North and South America: Academic Press, New York)
8. Cornell, N. W., Lund, P. and Krebs, H. A. (1974). The effect of lysine on gluconeogenesis from lactate in rat hepatocytes. *Biochem. J.*, **142,** 327
9. Krebs, H. A., Hems, R. and Tyler, B. (1976). The regulation of folate and methionine metabolism. *Biochem. J.*, **138,** 341
10. Krebs, H. A. and Perkins, J. R. (1970). The physiological role of liver alcohol dehydrogenase. *Biochem. J.*, **118,** 635
11. Krebs, H. A. and Lund, P. (1966). Formation of glucose from hexoses, pentoses, polyols and related substances in kidney cortex. *Biochem. J.*, **98,** 210
12. Mann, T. (1964). *Biochemistry of Semen and of the Male Reproductive Tract.* (London: Methuen & Co. Ltd.; New York: John Wiley & Sons Inc.)
13. Walker, D. G. (1968). Developmental aspects of carbohydrate metabolism. In F. Dickens, W. J. Whelan and P. J. Randle (eds.). *Carbohydrate Metabolism and its Disorders*, p. 465. (London and New York: Academic Press)
14. Woods, H. F., Eggleston, L. V. and Krebs, H. A. (1970). The cause of hepatic accumulation of fructose-1-phosphate on fructose loading. *Biochem. J.*, **119,** 501
15. Froesch, E. R. (1976). Comparison between the metabolism of xylitol, sorbitol, fructose and glucose. In R. Ritzel and G. Brubacher (eds.). *Monosaccharides and Polyalcohols in Nutrition, Therapy and Dietetics*, p. 239. (Bern, Stuttgart, Wien: Verlag Hans Huber)
16. Froesch, E. R., Zapf, J., Keller, U. and Oelz, O. (1971). *Eur. J. Clin. Invest.*, **2,** 8
17. Froesch, E. R. (1974). In H. A. Lee (ed.). *Parenteral Nutrition in Acute Metabolic Illness*, p. 73. (London: Academic Press)
18. Froesch, E. R. and Jakob, A. (1974). In H. L. Sipple and K. W. McNutt (eds.). *Sugars in Nutrition*, p. 241 (New York: Academic Press)
19. Windmueller, H. G. and Spaeth, A. E. (1976). Metabolism of absorbed aspartate, asparagine and arginine by rat small intestine *in vivo. Arch. Biochem. Biophys.*, **175,** 670
20. Windmueller, H. G. and Spaeth, A. E. (1975). Intestinal metabolism of glutamine and glutamate from the lumen as compared to glutamine from blood. *Arch. Biochem. Biophys.*, **171,** 662
21. Sleisenger, M. H., Pelling, D., Burston, D. and Matthews, D. W. (1977). Amino acid concentrations in portal venous plasma during absorption from the small intestine of the guinea pig of an amino acid mixture simulating casein and a partial enzymic hydrolysate of casein. *Clin. Sci. Mol. Med.*, **52,** 259
22. Watford, M., Lund, P. and Krebs, H. A., unpublished work.
23. Pizzi, W. J., Barnhart, J. E. and Fanslow, D. J. (1977). Monosodium glutamate administration to the newborn reduces reproductive ability in female and male mice. *Science*, **196,** 452
24. Lemkey-Johnston, N. and Reynolds, W. A. (1974). Nature and extent of brain lesions in mice related to ingestion of monosodium glutamate. A light and electron microscope study. *J. Neuropathol. Exp. Neurol.*, **33,** 74
25. Krebs, H. A. and Henseleit, K. (1932). Untersuchungen über die Harnstoffbildung im Tierkörper. *Z. Physiol. Chem.*, **210,** 33

3
Metabolic pathways for carbohydrates in parenteral nutrition

D. NEWTON, H. CONNOR AND H. F. WOODS

INTRODUCTION

Parenteral nutrition involves the infusion of complex mixtures of nutrients in sufficient quantities and in such proportions as to facilitate the preservation of tissue integrity. Treatment regimens usually include a nutrient which acts as a source of energy providing fuel to meet the basal energy requirements of tissues, together with that needed to support the synthesis of cell constituents. The introduction of alternatives to glucose as energy sources was stimulated by those who found certain objections to the use of glucose. The objections were of two main types: (a) practical: glucose was thought to be more 'damaging' to veins than other substrates; and (b) metabolic. The metabolic objections have been based on two main lines of evidence. First, that alternative substrates are metabolized more rapidly than glucose and thus are 'better'; and second, that the presence of insulin is required for glucose utilization and that trauma together with some disease states are associated with glucose intolerance.

An examination of the literature reveals that much of the reasoning behind the introduction of the alternatives to glucose is faulty. It is our intention in this paper to consider the metabolic pathways for carbohydrates in a quantitative manner, giving special emphasis to rate-limiting reactions and their relevance to the pathogenesis of the metabolic complications sometimes encountered during parenteral nutrition.

It is important in this introduction to deal briefly with the 'practical' objection to glucose. The incidence of damage to veins is more related to the carę with which the initial cannulation is performed and that with which it is maintained on a day-to-day basis rather than to the nature of the solution being infused.

PATHWAYS AND SITES OF CARBOHYDRATE UTILIZATION

Four substrates will be considered: fructose, sorbitol, xylitol and glucose. In all cases the pathways of utilization in man and other mammals are well established and will be outlined.

Fructose

The pathways of fructose metabolism in liver are shown in Figure 3.1. The

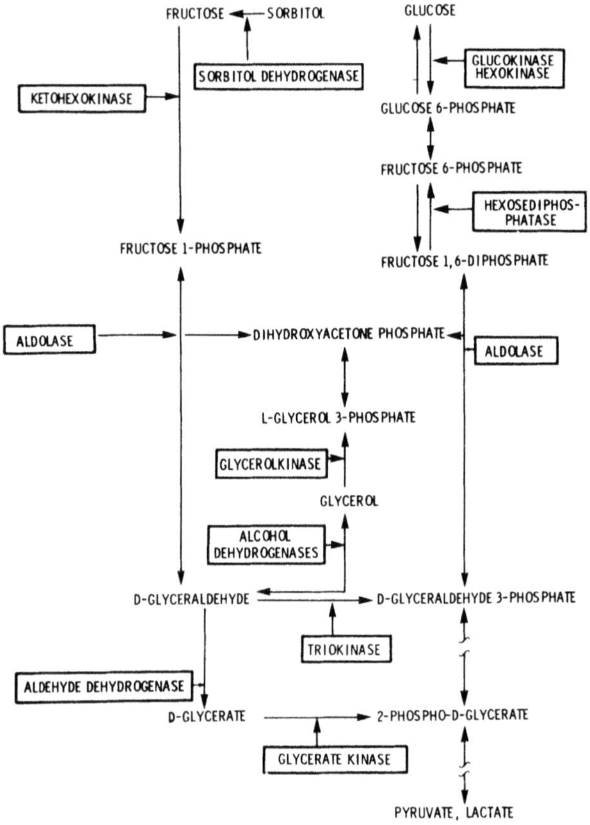

Figure 3.1 The pathway of hepatic fructose metabolism

initial step in fructose breakdown is catalysed by fructokinase (ketohexokinase) and results in the formation of fructose-1-phosphate.

$$\text{Fructose} + \text{ATP} \rightleftharpoons \text{Fructose-1-phosphate} + \text{ADP} \qquad (1)$$

The fructose-1-phosphate is further metabolized via the ketose-1-phosphate aldolase reaction to form dihydroxyacetone phosphate and D-glyceraldehyde.

$$\text{Fructose-1-phosphate} \rightleftharpoons \text{Dihydroxyacetone phosphate} + \text{D-glyceraldehyde} \quad (2)$$

The main proportion (approx. 90%) of the D-glyceraldehyde thus formed is phosphorylated via the triokinase reaction to give glyceraldehyde-3-phosphate[1]. The overall reaction for the first stages of fructose utlization is

$$\text{Fructose} + 2\text{ATP} \rightleftharpoons \text{Dihydroxyacetone phosphate} + \text{glyceraldehyde-3-phosphate} + 2\text{ADP} \quad (3)$$

The liver is the main site of fructose metabolism[2,3]. Quantitatively less important sites are muscle[4], adipose tissue[4], kidney[5] and gut[6]. In adipose tissue and muscle the activity of fructokinase (reaction (1) above) is low[4], and fructose is metabolized to fructose-6-phosphate by hexokinase[7]. This is a possible route of utilization in the liver, but the properties of hepatic hexokinase are such that it is of little quantitative importance in that organ[8].

Sorbitol

Sorbitol is oxidized to fructose by sorbitol dehydrogenase (polyol dehydrogenase) and thereafter its metabolism is the same as that of fructose.

$$\text{Sorbitol} \underset{\text{NADH}}{\overset{\text{NAD+}}{\rightleftharpoons}} \text{D-Fructose}$$

The main sites of sorbitol oxidation are the liver and to a lesser extent the kidney.

Xylitol

Xylitol is a five-carbon alcohol which, as in the case of sorbitol, has oxidation by polyol dehydrogenase as the initial step in its metabolism. The product of this reaction is D-xylulose which, under the action of D-xylulose kinase, is converted to xylulose-5-phosphate.

$$\text{Xylitol} \xrightarrow{\text{Polyol dehydrogenase}} \text{D-xylulose} \xrightarrow{\text{D-xylulose kinase}} \text{Xylulose-5-phosphate}$$

The xylulose-5-phosphate then enters the pentose phosphate pathway which is outlined in Figure 3.2. The work of Bassler *et al.*[9] demonstrated that although many tissues, including gut, testis and brain, have polyol dehydrogenase activity, the capacity of the liver to metabolize xylitol (and sorbitol) far outweighs that of all the extrahepatic tissues.

It would be expected that as xylitol and sorbitol share a common enzyme for their initial metabolism the infusion of one would alter the utilization of the other. This has been shown by Bässler and Bickel[10] who infused sorbitol at a rate of 0.75 g/kg/h and when a steady-state blood concentration had been achieved infused xylitol in addition at the same rate and saw the establishment of a new higher steady-state sorbitol concentration.

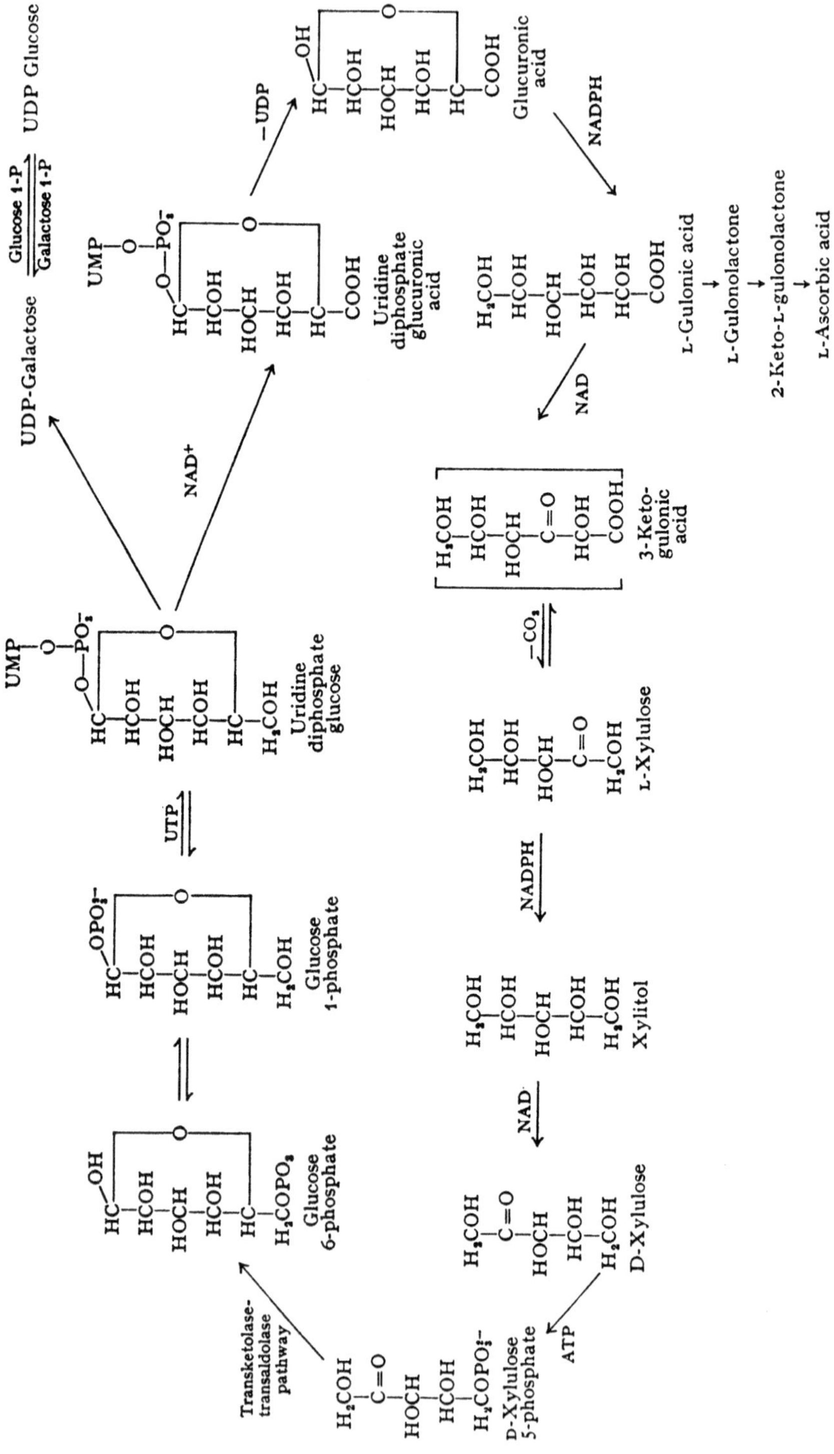

Figure 3.2 The pathway of xylitol metabolism

Glucose

The pathways for glucose utilization are well established and need minimal comment. Glucose enters the glycolytic pathway, and the pyruvate produced can either be oxidized via the tricarboxylic acid cycle or may be used as a substrate for glucose synthesis. Oxidation of pyruvate occurs after its transport into the mitochondria and conversion to acetyl CoA. The synthesis of acetyl CoA from pyruvate is controlled by the enzyme pyruvate dehydrogenase, the activity of which is regulated, in part, by insulin.

Quantitative aspects of substrate utilization

It will be clear from a consideration of the metabolic pathways described above that each substrate is metabolized by a complex series of reactions, each of which can be influenced by controlling factors.

It has often been assumed that the provision of energy during parenteral nutrition can be considered in terms of a 'black box' (see Figure 3.3). This concept considers only the rate of removal of the substrate and the free energy

Figure 3.3 Substrate utilization—the black box. In this figure the utilization of an energy providing substrate has been represented as a 'black box'. S represents the substrate and ΔF the free energy released during its metabolism

liberated within the tissues as a result of substrate utilization which is then available to fuel the reactions involved in the synthesis of tissue components. Thus the use of alternatives to glucose has often been advocated on the grounds that a particular substrate was removed from the blood more rapidly than was glucose. Fructose, for example, is removed twice as rapidly as glucose[11].

It must be realized however that this type of argument, based solely on substrate removal rates, can be misleading. The difficulties arise because the

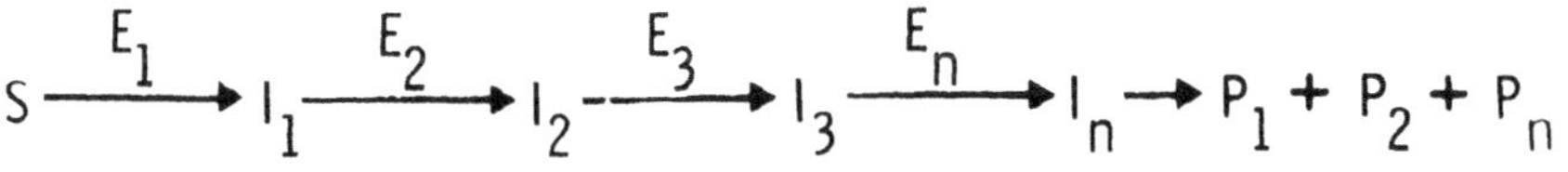

Figure 3.4 Substrate utilization—a theoretical pathway. The figure shows a theoretical pathway via which an energy-providing substrate is metabolized. S represents the substrate, E_{1-n} the enzymes in the pathways, I_{1-n} the intermediates and P_{1-n} the products of metabolism

carbohydrate substrates used in parenteral nutrition undergo a series of reaction steps during their utilization and if a theoretical pathway is considered (Figure 3.4) it will be seen that the simple 'black box' concept can mislead the clinician for the following reasons:

1. The first enzyme in the sequence (E_1) may not be the rate-limiting enzyme within the sequence of reactions.
2. Both intermediates and products may accumulate or be lost in the urine and thus the overall rate of flux of carbon through the pathway depends in part upon the rates of removal of those intermediates and products which accumulate or are lost in the urine.

In the remainder of this chapter we will discuss the numerical data relating to substrate utilization in relation to these problems of interpretation.

SOME KINETIC CONSIDERATIONS

Estimates of substrate utilization rates in man are usually derived from measurement of the rate at which the substrate disappears from blood or plasma after an oral or intravenous load. The rate of removal can be expressed in several ways and it is important to appreciate that these different expressions give different information. The usual expressions of removal rate are the half-life ($T\frac{1}{2}$), the fractional rate removal constant (K) and the clearance.

Half-life and fractional rate removal constant

These two expressions are considered together because they provide similar information and are closely related.

$$K = \frac{0.693}{T\frac{1}{2}} \qquad \text{(i)}$$

The half-life is the time which it takes for the concentration of a substrate in the blood to fall by half. The fractional rate removal constant is the percentage of substrate removed in unit time. The two expressions are therefore similar in that they are both functions of time and the change in blood concentration of the substrate. If the blood concentration following an infusion of a substrate is known, these values can then be used to predict the concentration in blood at a subsequent point in time or to predict how long it will take the substrate concentration to fall to a given level. This may be of value when threshold concentrations are involved. For example, if a substrate is excreted in urine when the concentration is above a certain threshold level the total urinary loss of substrate will depend on the length of time for which the threshold concentration is exceeded, as well as on the absolute concentration of substrate in blood.

Neither $T\frac{1}{2}$ nor K take any account of the volume of distribution of the infused substrate. They should not, therefore, be used for comparisons of removal rates in different subjects unless it is known that the volume of distribution of the infused substrate is the same in all the subjects studied.

Clearance

Clearance is defined as the volume of blood from which the substrate is completely removed in unit time. It can be calculated as:

$$\text{Clearance} = V \times K \qquad \text{(ii)}$$

where V is the apparent volume of distribution of the infused substrate and K is the fractional rate removal constant. If V is expressed in litres per kg body weight and K as a constant per minute then the units of clearance are litres per minute.

Because clearance is a function of distribution volume, as well as of blood concentration and time, it can be used as an expression of total elimination of substrate from the body. In the absence of any loss of unmetabolized substrate in urine, bile, sweat, etc. clearance is therefore a measure of the rate of metabolic removal. It must be understood that it is not an index of the actual quantity of removal because it contains no expression of concentration. The actual quantity of removal or total removal (TR) at a given substrate concentration, (S), is given by:

$$\text{TR} = S \times V \times K \qquad \text{(iii)}$$

If S is expressed in mmol/l and V and K as in (ii) above, then the units of total removal are mmol/kg body weight/min.

There are many potential pitfalls in the interpretation of kinetic data. Two are considered below. After the infusion of a substrate its concentration decay curve in blood may be a single or multi-exponential. This is most easily appreciated if the change in concentration with time is plotted semilogarithmically. In the example given in Figure 3.5 there are three exponentials (α, β, γ) representing three different fractional rate removal constants (K_1, K_2, K_3) for the removal of substrate from blood. If clearance is calculated from a mathematical model of the infusion protocol, it is essential that all three values for K should be taken into account. However, if sampling is not continued for long enough or if the sensitivity of the substrate assay is inadequate to detect low concentrations, the final exponential might not be detected. The calculated value for clearance might then be a serious overestimate of the true value and could lead to metabolic problems if it were used to calculate a safe infusion rate for use in clinical practice.

Particular care is needed in interpreting data obtained from studies in which tracer doses of radioactive substrate have been used. Even when attempts are made to allow for recycling of label and for exchange reactions, the validity of the conclusions may still be suspect. The problems arising from the study of human glucose and lactate metabolism in this way have been reviewed by Cohen and Woods[12].

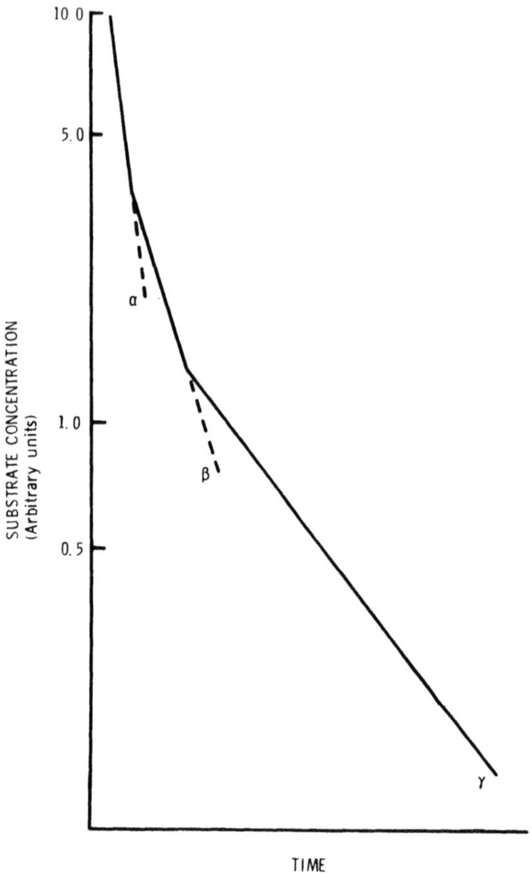

Figure 3.5 The time-course of substrate removal from blood

THE QUANTITATIVE DATA

Some values selected for the clearance and maximum metabolic capacity of human subjects for fructose, sorbitol, xylitol and glucose are quoted in Table 3.1, together with recommendations for a maximum infusion rate.

SOME PROBLEMS OF INTERPRETATION

Although the data for the various substrates listed in Table 3.1 are derived from studies carried out under comparable conditions they represent an overall value for the whole organism. In many cases the substrate, as outlined in the Introduction, can be metabolized by several tissues and thus the clearance is a complex quantity made up of a number of individual tissue clearances.

Table 3.1 The capacity for metabolism of carbohydrate substrates in man

Substrate	*Clearance* (ml/kg/min)	*Maximum metabolic capacity* (g/kg/h)	*Suggested maximum safe infusion rate* (g/kg/h)
Glucose	—	1.5	variable
Fructose	18.4 (1.26)	1.5	0.25
Sorbitol	11.0 (2.10)	0.5	0.25
Xylitol	12.8 (2.11)	0.5	0.25

The data are derived from studies in normal subjects and are mean values. In all cases the metabolic clearances and capacities have been calculated from 'steady state' studies and the figures in parenthesis in the clearance column are the plasma concentrations (mmol/l) at which the clearances were calculated. The data are abstracted from the papers of Bässler[13] and Heukenkamp[14].

Some of the data are difficult to explain in terms of the known controlling factors governing the rates of metabolism of some substrates. Thus from Table 3.1 it is apparent that fructose is removed from the circulation more rapidly than is sorbitol when infused at the same rate. This implies that sorbitol dehydrogenase is a rate-limiting enzyme in sorbitol metabolism. This is incompatible with the finding that fructose is detectable in the blood of patients during sorbitol infusion, the concentration being dependent on the rate of sorbitol infusion[15,16]. There is also a lack of relationship between calculated maximal metabolic capacity and the dosage recommended for practical use. It would appear, as Bässler[13] has pointed out, that safe infusion rates for clinical use are considerably less than the calculated maximal turnover rates. He does not suggest why this is the case. The discrepancy is too great to be accounted for by any errors in the calculation of maximal turnover rates and the most likely explanations are:

1. That the maximal turnover rates for the most part have been determined using normal healthy subjects and thus are not applicable to the sick patients receiving parenteral nutrition.
2. The rate of removal of the infused nutrient is only one of the quantities that are important. There must be additional information relating to (a) the rate of formation and loss of intermediates, (b) the rate of formation of metabolic end products, (c) the effects of underlying disease on the metabolic pathways involved, (d) the rate of removal of major metabolic products, and (e) the modifying effect of other nutrients infused at the same time.

Some of these factors can be illustrated by reference to fructose, sorbitol and lactate metabolism.

Under normal conditions 30% of a fructose load is converted to lactate and pyruvate and 70% to glucose[17]. The rate of hepatic fructose metabolism is increased under anaerobic conditions but the only product is lactate[18]. Thus when there is tissue hypoxia there may be a greatly increased lactate production.

So far as the removal of end products is concerned the metabolism of lactate is a good example. A substantial proportion of infused fructose and sorbitol is metabolized to lactate and accumulates in the blood. The full utilization of fructose or sorbitol thus depends on the metabolism of the lactate produced, and it is clear that this constitutes a rate-limiting step in the utilization of these substrates. It is also a factor involved in the pathogenesis of metabolic complications. The occurrence of lactic acidosis during parenteral nutrition with fructose and sorbitol is well recognized[19]. In this condition the accumulation of lactic acid is sufficient to disturb acid–base homeostasis and in the case of fructose and sorbitol infusion the accumulation is mainly due to lactate generation at a rate much greater than its rate of removal.

The utilization of sorbitol is impaired in patients with liver disease[20]. If the half-life were the only controlling factor in sorbitol metabolism a lowered rate of lactate production and hence a lower incidence of lactic acidosis would be expected in patients with liver disease. In practice lactic acidosis is more likely to occur in patients with liver disease[21]. An explanation for this can be found if the kinetics of lactate in man are examined.

The lactate infusion studies of Connor *et al.*[22], Table 3.2, have shown that the metabolic clearance rate for lactate is significantly impaired in liver

Table 3.2 The metabolic clearance rate for lactate—the effect of liver disease

Subjects studied	*K* (*per minute*)	*V* (*l/kg body weight*)	*MCR* (*mmol/kg body weight/min*)
Normal $n = 8$	0.056 ± 0.002	0.379 ± 0.089	0.021 ± 0.002
Liver disease $n = 26$	0.044 ± 0.003	0.363 ± 0.125	0.015 ± 0.001
p value	<0.01	N.S.	<0.01

The data refer to normal subjects and patients with a wide range of liver disease and were obtained using the lactate infusion described by Connor *et al.* (1977)[22]. The metabolic clearance rate (MCR) $= K \times V$ where K is the fractional rate removal constant and V is the volume of distribution. The MCR refers to a notional blood lactate concentration of 1.0 mmol/l. The p value refers to the significance of the difference between the mean values for the two groups and N.S. signifies no significant difference.

disease. It follows that the complete utilization of sorbitol carbon after conversion to fructose is impaired in liver disease and, in spite of the lowered rate of sorbitol removal, the lactate produced may accumulate.

The underlying metabolic state of the patient is also relevant to lactate accumulation. In seriously ill patients there are widespread metabolic abnormalities. Figure 3.6 shows the distribution of resting venous blood lactate and pyruvate concentrations in a series of twenty-three such patients. It can be seen that many of them (57%) had an increased lactate concentration, the upper limit of normal being 1.2 mmol/l. It follows that a relatively small additional load of lactic acid derived from sorbitol or fructose metabolism may be sufficient to precipitate lactic acidosis.

Two types of metabolic interaction may occur during parenteral nutrition. One is the effect of disease upon the metabolism of infused nutrients, and the other is the way in which the metabolism of one constituent of an infusion mixture may modify that of another. The first has already been mentioned above and the second has recently been considered by Woods and Marston[23]. These authors described the interactions involving fructose (and thus sorbitol). Two groups of interactions occur; those between fructose and ethanol and those between fructose and amino acids. These are summarized below and show the way in which ethanol and amino acids act on the pathways of fructose utilization.

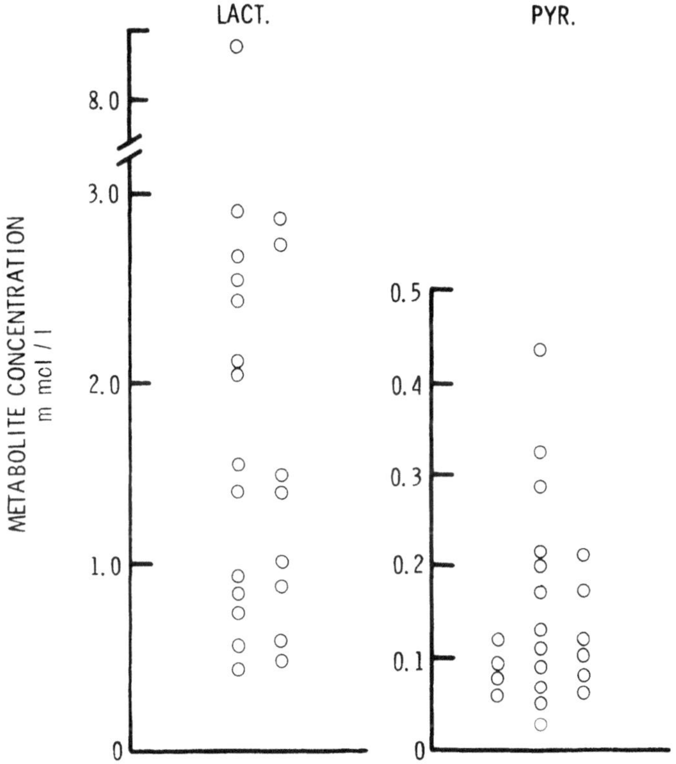

Figure 3.6 Blood lactate and pyruvate concentrations in patients about to be fed intravenously. The determinations were performed using venous blood collected without stasis from a series of patients who were about to be fed by the intravenous route. In the majority of cases the patients had been starved overnight. In our laboratory the upper limit of normal for a normal-fed subject is 1.2 mmol/l for lactate and 0.13 mmol/l for pyruvate

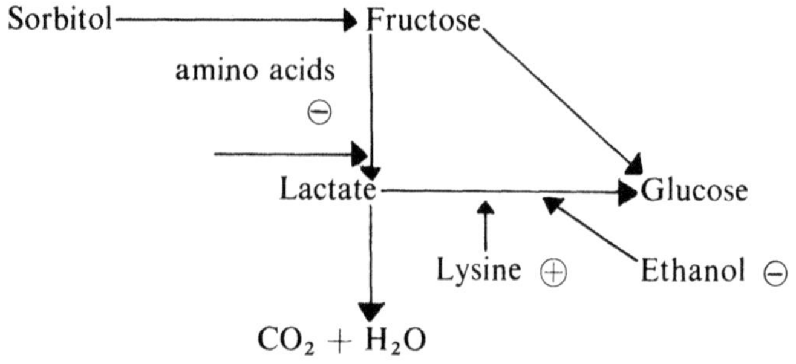

The accumulation of intermediates within organs which are the major site of the metabolism of a particular substrate is probably never sufficient to influence the total clearance of that substrate. However, such accumulation may have important metabolic consequences. The hyperuricaemia and increased urinary uric acid excretion caused by fructose infusion in normal subjects and patients with hereditary fructose intolerance has been shown to be due to increased adenine nucleotide breakdown in liver[17,24] leading to adenine nucleotide depletion. This depletion arises because fructose-phosphate accumulates in the liver following fructose loading and causes a decrease in the inorganic phosphate (Pi) content of the tissue. Both ATP and Pi are essential in stabilizing the hepatic AMP concentration because they inhibit the enzymes that cause the irreversible degradation of AMP. When the ATP and Pi concentrations fall this inhibition becomes less effective and AMP is degraded to form uric acid[25].

The transient hyperuricaemia may not be harmful but there is evidence that ATP depletion can inhibit energy-dependent processes within the liver. Thus there is experimental evidence that protein synthesis, triglyceride synthesis and RNA synthesis are inhibited by acute fructose loading[26].

SAFE MAXIMUM INFUSION RATES–TWO CASE REPORTS

Included in Table 3.1 are recommended maximum infusion rates, and it is clear from the preceding paragraphs that these figures will be altered by a large variety of factors. Two case reports will serve to illustrate this point.

Case I The patient was a woman aged 48 and her clinical progress is summarized below.

Clinical progress

(a) Diagnosis: Intestinal obstruction. Gross weight loss. Gram-negative septicaemia

(b) Treatment: Defunctioning Colostomy. Antimicrobials

(c) Progress: *Day 3*—Metabolic acidosis corrected with intravenous sodium bicarbonate. Subtotal colectomy and ileostomy performed.

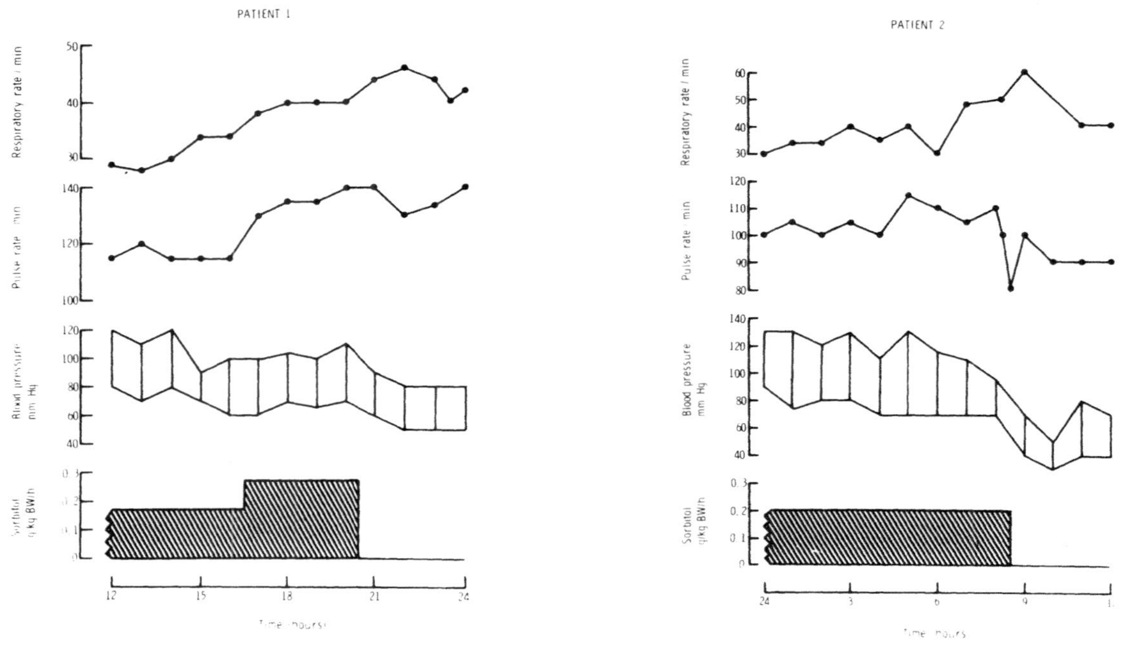

Figure 3.7 Lactic acidosis during sorbitol infusion. The two figures show the time-course of changes in the vital signs recorded for the two patients described in the text

Day 4—Hyperglycaemia treated with soluble insulin (i.m.)
Day 5—Parenteral nutrition started. The carbohydrate infused was sorbitol at a rate of 0.17 g/kg/h.
Day 6—Sorbitol infusion rate increased to 0.27 g/kg/h. Lactic acidosis developed.

The changes in vital signs recorded during the time when the sorbitol infusion rate was increased are shown in Figure 3.7. The respiratory rate and the pulse rate increased and the patient was noticed to have an 'acidotic' breathing pattern. The results of the biochemical investigations at the time of onset of the lactic acidosis are recorded in Table 3.3

Table 3.3 Investigations at onset of lactic acidosis

	Patient		
Investigation	*No. 1*	*No. 2*	*Normal values*
Lactate	8.0	6.7	0.4–1.2 mM/l
L/P ratio	20	21.6	7–14
Base excess	−12	−10	<-5 mM/l
Bilirubin	45	99	3–17 μM/l
SGOT	42	78	10–50 i.u./l
Albumen	25	28	35–50 g/l
Prothrombin	—	46%	>70%
Urea	23	12.2	2.5–6.7 mM/l
Creatinine	198	180	70–150 μM/l

The data are those relating to the two cases described in the text.

(d) Comments: In this case we concluded that the extra lactic acid load produced by a small increase in sorbitol infusion rate was sufficient to precipitate lactic acidosis in a patient with widespread metabolic abnormalities including liver disease.

Case II This patient was a male aged 42, who one year before admission had undergone a vagotomy and pyloroplasty.

Clinical progress

(a) Diagnosis: Pyloric stenosis
(b) Treatment: Partial gastrectomy of the Polya type
(c) Progress: *Day 3*—Pancreatitis leading to a further laparotomy. A metabolic acidosis then developed in the immediate post-operative period which was corrected with intravenous sodium bicarbonate. Parenteral nutrition was started using glucose (with insulin) as the energy source.
Day 7—Intravenous regimen changed to include a solution containing sorbitol and ethanol in the place of glucose. The

sorbitol infusion rate was 0.2 g/kg/h.
Day 8—Lactic acidosis was diagnosed.

Figure 3.7 shows the changes in the vital signs in this patient and as in the first case there was an abrupt rise in the respiratory rate when lactic acidosis developed. It would appear that the change to sorbitol and ethanol as energy sources resulted in lactic acid accumulation. In this case and the previous one the sorbitol infusion rates at which the acidosis occurred were close to that listed in Table 3.1 as maximum 'safe' rate.

The investigations at the onset of lactic acidosis (Table 3.3) showed that in both cases there was biochemical evidence of hepatic and renal disease.

FINAL CONCLUSIONS

The metabolic complications which sometimes arise during infusion of energy sources other than glucose have led to their use being forbidden in some countries. It should however be clear from the contents of this paper that a safe maximum infusion rate for an individual substrate is a metabolic characteristic of each particular patient. The clinician needs reliable methods which he can use to decide which substrate is the most suitable in each case. The ideal energy source (Table 3.4) does not exist.

Table 3.4 The ideal energy source for use in parenteral nutrition

A SPECIFICATION
1. No chemical reaction with other substrates in solution or during heat sterilization
2. Will not support microbial growth
3. Non-irritant to vessel walls
4. No reaction with plastic materials
5. Utilized by all tissues in health and disease
6. Tissue utilization independent of insulin
7. High calorific value
8. No metabolic side-effects
9. Very high renal threshold

Acknowledgement

D.N. is a Travenol Research Fellow.

References

1. Sillero, M. A. G., Sillero, A. and Sols, A. (1969). Enzymes involved in fructose metabolism in liver and the glyceraldehyde metabolic crossroads. *Eur. J. Biochem.*, **10**, 345
2. Weischelbaum, T. E., Margraf, H. W. and Elman, R. (1953). Metabolism of intravenously infused fructose in man. *Metabolism*, **2**, 434

3. Topping, D. L. and Mayes, P. A. (1972). The immediate effects of insulin and fructose on the metabolism of the perfused liver. *Biochem. J.*, **126**, 295
4. Adelman, R. C., Ballard, F. J. and Weinhouse, S. (1967). Purification and properties of rat liver fructokinase. *J. Biol. Chem.*, **242**, 3360
5. Raivio, K. O., Kekomaki, M. P. and Mäenpää, P. H. (1969). Depletion of liver adenine nucleotides induced by D-fructose; dose-dependence and specificity of the fructose effect. *Biochem. Pharmacol.*, **18**, 2615
6. Deuel, H. J. (1936). The intermediary metabolism of fructose and galactose. *Physiol. Rev.*, **16**, 173
7. Hers, H. G. (1955). The conversion of fructose-1-^{14}C and sorbitol-1-^{14}C to liver and muscle glycogen in the rat. *J. Biol. Chem.*, **214**, 373
8. Woods, H. F. (1973). Hepatic accumulation of metabolites after fructose loading. *Acta Med. Scand.*, 542 (Suppl.), 87
9. Bässler, K. H., Stein, G. and Belzer, W. (1966). Xylitstoffwechsel und Xylitresorption. Stoffwechsel-adaptation als Ursache für Resorptionsbeschleunigung. *Biochem. Z.*, **346**, 171
10. Bässler, K. H. and Bickel, H. (1972). The use of carbohydrates alone and in combination in parenteral nutrition. In A. W. Wilkinson (ed.). *Parenteral Nutrition*, pp. 99–104. (London: Churchill Livingstone)
11. Smith, L. H., Ettinger, R. H. and Seligson, D. (1953). A comparison of the metabolism of fructose and glucose in hepatic disease and diabetes mellitus. *J. Clin. Invest.*, **32**, 273
12. Cohen, R. D. and Woods, H. F. (1976). *Clinical and Biochemical Aspects of Lactic Acidosis*, p. 234. (Oxford: Blackwell Scientific Publications)
13. Bässler, K. H. (1976). Quantitative aspects of the metabolism of glucose, fructose, sorbitol and xylitol. In G. Ritzel and G. Brubacher (eds.). *Monosaccharides and Polyalcohols in Nutrition, Therapy and Dietetics*, pp. 22–30. (Bern: Hans Huber)
14. Heuckenkamp, P.-U. (1976). Comparison of glucose, fructose and xylitol for parenteral alimentation in metabolically healthy men. In G. Ritzel and G. Brubacher (eds.). *Monosaccharides and Polyalcohols in Nutrition, Therapy and Dietetics*, pp. 170–176. (Bern: Hans Huber)
15. Schultis, K. and Beisbarth, H. (1972). Posttraumatic energy metabolism. In A. W. Wilkinson (ed.). *Parenteral Nutrition*, pp. 255–265. (London: Churchill Livingstone)
16. Aynsley-Green, A., Baum, J. D., Alberti, K. G. M. M. and Woods, H. F. (1974). Hyperlactataemia during intravenous feeding in childhood. *Arch. Dis. Childh.*, **49**, 647
17. Woods, H. F., Eggleston, L. V. and Krebs, H. A. (1970). The cause of hepatic accumulation of fructose 1-phosphate on fructose loading. *Biochem. J.*, **119**, 501
18. Woods, H. F. and Krebs, H. A. (1971). Lactate production in the perfused rat liver. *Biochem. J.*, **125**, 129
19. Cohen, R. D. and Woods, H. F. (1976). *Clinical and Biochemical Aspects of Lactic Acidosis*, p. 194. (Oxford: Blackwell Scientific Publications)
20. Brachtel, D., Popp, J. and Richter, E. (1974). Sorbitol elimination in patients with acute hepatitis. *Klin. Wochenschr.*, **52**, 101
21. Woods, H. F. (1971). Some aspects of lactic acidosis. *Brit. J. Hosp. Med.*, **6**, 668
22. Connor, H., Woods, H. F., Murray, J. D. and Ledingham, J. G. G. (1977). Lactate metabolism in liver disease. Presented at the *11th Annual Meeting of the European Society for Clinical Investigation*, Rotterdam.
23. Woods, H. F. and Marston, A. (1977). Metabolic interactions during intravenous feeding. In D. G. Grahame-Smith (ed.). *Drug Interactions*, pp. 251–263. (Macmillan Press Ltd.)
24. Bode, C., Schumacher, H., Goebell, H., Zelder, O. and Pelzel, H. (1971). Fructose induced depletion of liver adenine nucleotides in man. *Horm. Metab. Res.*, **3**, 289
25. Woods, H. F. (1975). Some metabolic aspects of parenteral feeding. In S. C. Truelove and J. Trowell (eds.). *Topics in Gastroenterology* 2, pp. 191–207. (Oxford: Blackwell Scientific Publications)
26. Woods, H. F. (1975). Energy provision during intravenous feeding. *Clin. Trials J.*, 12 (Suppl.), 62

4
Short-term parenteral nutrition with and without fructose

P. VINAY, D. BOURBEAU, G. LEMIEUX, A. DURANCEAU AND A. GOUGOUX

INTRODUCTION

Total parenteral nutrition (TPN) is useful in patients unable to feed by the oral route and undergoing the catabolic stress of an acute disease, surgery, or neoplasia. This procedure implicates the simultaneous administration of nitrogen, to provide essential and non-essential amino acids for protein synthesis, and calories to meet energy requirements and minimize or reverse the peripheral protein mobilization. The caloric sources used for TPN are mainly carbohydrates and fatty acids. Both glucose and fructose have been used in the past as a source of carbohydrates. Fructose administration has been recommended in various studies because of its rapid utilization[1,2], lack of dependence on insulin for its metabolism[3,4], and a reduced stimulation of endogenous secretion of insulin[5,6] which is considered to be beneficial[7] as it may reduce the risk of hypoglycaemia after abrupt cessation of TPN[1].

Recent biochemical studies, however, have demonstrated that fructose bypasses a major regulatory site of the glycolytic pathway, the phosphofructokinase step, and that acute administration leads to a rapid accumulation of fructose-1-phosphate in the liver[8-10], kidney[8], and the gastrointestinal tract[11] with simultaneous depletion of cell ATP and intracellular sequestration of inorganic phosphate[9]. A depression of the protein synthesis[12] by the liver follows. These changes, on theoretical grounds, seem undesirable and potentially dangerous for critically ill patients. It is not clear however if the prolonged administration of small amounts of fructose is less beneficial to patients on parenteral nutrition than similar amounts of

* With technical assistance of Mrs. C. L'Homme.

glucose. A study was planned to compare nitrogen balance during 10 consecutive days of intravenous nutrition with two different protocols providing similar amounts of nitrogen, carbohydrates, lipids, vitamins, and electrolytes. Fructose made up 25% of the carbohydrates in the first protocol while none was given in the second.

METHODS

Patients

Patients who were unable to achieve adequate nutrition via the oral route and referred to the Surgery Service of the Hôtel-Dieu Hospital of Montreal were selected for this study (Table 4.1). Patients with chronic or acute renal

Table 4.1 Patients in protocols I and II

	Patients	*Sex*	*Age*	*Weight* (kg)	*Height* (m)	*Primary diagnosis*
I Travasol* ($n = 7$)						
	L.A.	M	60	61.5	1.67	Gastroduodenal stenosis
	P.O.	M	72	72.0	1.76	Acute pancreatitis
	R.C.	F	52	54.0	1.60	Ileitis; ileovaginal fistula
	S.A.	M	49	56.6	1.83	Chronic pancreatitis
	M.G.	F	72	54.0	1.62	Biliary fistula
	P.J.	M	28	75.4	1.70	Ruptured Meckel's diverticulitis
	L.R.	F	65	55.7	1.57	Carcinoma of pancreas
mean ± SEM			56.9 ± 5.9	61.3 ± 3.4		
II Vamin ($n = 8$)						
	V.H.	F	61	70.8	1.61	Ruptured diverticulitis
	D.R.	F	64	37.0	1.57	Radiation ileitis
	P.J.	F	46	38.5	1.60	Crohn's disease
	A.V.	M	41	68.5	1.72	Dermatomyositis (acute)
	D.M.	M	22	56.1	1.87	Crohn's disease
	L.J.	M	63	38.7	1.69	Carcinoma of pancreas
	D.A.	F	21	37.8	1.58	Crohn's disease
	R.P.	M	65	70.2	1.72	Gastric adenocarcinoma
mean ± SEM			47.9 ± 6.5	52.2 ± 5.6		

failure, insulin-dependent diabetes or active infections were excluded. The majority of patients underwent surgery either shortly prior to or after TPN and all patients had total parenteral nutrition. The patients were followed by the same medical team, and a special nurse supervised the TPN administration, care of the catheters, and the collection of the various specimens.

* Synthamin

Solutions

All solutions were prepared in a sterile fashion by a clinical pharmacist. The latter ensured the exact formulation and provision of the infusions. No nutrients were given by mouth for 4 days prior to and during the parenteral nutrition.

Experimental design

Seven patients were placed on a parenteral nutrition protocol without fructose (protocol I) and eight with fructose (protocol II). The patients placed on a fructose-free regimen received a 10% amino acid solution (Travasol, Baxter Laboratories, Malton, Ontario, Canada) as the nitrogen source while the patients given fructose received a 7% amino acid solution containing fructose (Vamin, Pharmacia Canada Ltd, Montreal, Canada). Fructose was added to the parenteral regimen in the latter group to provide 25% of the carbohydrate intake.

Both regimens were designed to give similar fluid volume, nitrogen, carbohydrate, and lipid intake (Table 4.2). Electrolytes and vitamins were added to

Table 4.2 Daily intake during TPN

	Protocol I (Travasol)	*Protocol II (Vamin)*
Calories (cal/kg)	58.0 (49–66)	69.4 (52–98)
Carbohydrates (g/kg)	12.2 (10–14)	14.4 (11–20)
Lipids (g/kg)	1.6 (1.4–1.9)	1.9 (1.4–2.6)
Nitrogen (g/kg)	0.21 (0.18–0.23)	0.24 (0.18–0.33)
Composition of the fixed regimen (per day)		
Volume (ml/day)	4562	4653
Nitrogen (g/day)	12.6	12.6
Amino acids (g/day)	75.4	94.9
Protein equivalent (g/day)	78.7	79.4
Glucose (g/day)	750	565
Fructose (g/day)	0	185
Lipids (g/day)	100	100
Calories (non-prot) (cal/day)	3558	3621
N/K	2.9	2.9

provide similar amounts of sodium, potassium, magnesium, chloride, phosphate, calcium and vitamins (Bourbeau *et al.*, chapter 25). No trace metals were given. All patients received a fixed intake irrespective of body weight. The intake of carbohydrate was 0.51 g (0.43–0.58)/kg/h in protocol I and 0.60 g (0.47–0.81)/kg/h in protocol II (Table 4.2). 12.6 g of nitrogen, i.e. 0.01 g (0.007–0.014)/kg/h was given in both protocols. The amounts of individual amino acids given with both protocols are given in Table 4.3. Because of the different amino acid mixtures, different amounts were given

Table 4.3 Daily intake of amino acids during parenteral nutrition with protocols I and II

	Protocol I *Travasol* (0.75 l.)	*Protocol II* *Vamin* (1.35 l.)
Essential amino acids (g/day)		
L-Leucine	4.65	7.16
L-Phenylalanine	4.65	7.43
L-Methionine	4.35	2.57
L-Lysine	4.35	5.27
L-Isoleucine	3.60	5.27
L-Valine	3.45	5.81
L-Threonine	3.15	4.05
L-Tryptophane	1.35	1.35
Cysteine–cystine	—	1.89
Total Essential AA	29.55 (39%)	40.80 (43%)
Non-essential amino acids		
L-Histidine	3.30	3.24
L-Aspartate	—	5.54
L-Alanine	15.60	4.05
L-Serine	—	10.13
Glycine	15.68	2.84
L-Arginine	7.80	4.50
L-Proline	3.15	10.94
L-Tyrosine	0.30	0.68
L-Glutamate	—	12.15
Total Non-essential AA	45.83 (61%)	54.07 (57%)
Total amino acids	75.4	94.9

in both protocols: 75.4 g/day in protocol I and 94.9 g/day in protocol II. A total of 3600 non-protein calories per day were provided which represents between 2.4 and 2.9 cal/kg/h. 28% of the calories were given as lipids in both groups (Intralipid, Pharmacia Canada Ltd., Montreal, Canada) which represents between 0.07 and 0.08 g/kg/h.

The patients were studied for 4 days (referred to as −4 to −1) before TPN and for 10 days (referred to as +1 to +10) during TPN. Four patients underwent abdominal surgery either on the first or on the 10th day of parenteral nutrition. In these patients a liver biopsy was obtained during surgery as well as in five control patients undergoing surgery for cholecystectomy. Informed consent was obtained from all patients.

Nitrogen balances

In all patients 24 h collection of urine, stools, fistula fluids, and gastrointestinal drainage were made with the appropriate preservatives. Twenty-four hour urinary creatinine excretion was measured daily to check the completeness of the collections. Nitrogen was determined by an Auto-Analyzer micro-kjeldahl technique[13].

Blood sampling

Blood was obtained twice before and at least three times during parenteral nutrition for measurements of plasma total calcium, phosphate, glucose, urea, uric acid, creatinine, cholesterol, total proteins, albumin, and enzymes GOT, GPT, LDH, and alkaline phosphatase, as well as for the determination of insulin, lactate, pyruvate, β-hydroxybutyrate, aceto-acetate, triglycerides, total transferrin, red and white cell counts, and prothrombin time.

Special biochemical methods

Blood for analysis of pyruvate, lactate, β-hydroxybutyrate and aceto-acetate was deproteinized immediately with equal volume of chilled 10% (wt/vol) perchloric acid. These organic acids were measured enzymatically by spectrophotometry[14]. Transferrin was measured according to Mancini *et al.*[15]. Insulin was measured by radioimmunoassay[16]. Hepatic biopsies were frozen immediately in liquid nitrogen and analysed for ATP, ADP, AMP[17], lactate and pyruvate[14].

RESULTS

The total nitrogen output before and during parenteral nutrition is presented in Figure 4.1. A total nitrogen output of around 5–6 g/day was observed during the control period with both protocols. During parenteral nutrition, this nitrogen output rose significantly in both groups, but slightly more with Vamin than with Travasol. This difference was not statistically significant. The faecal contribution to the total nitrogen output remained between 1 and 2.5 g/day (Figure 4.1).

Complete nitrogen balance was obtained for 85/90 days of study in patients on protocol I and for 100/112 days in protocol II (Figure 4.2). A similar negative balance of around −6 g/day was observed during the 4 control days. Following TPN a positive nitrogen balance was established of around 2 g/day in the Travasol group and 1 g/day in the Vamin group. This difference however is not statistically significant. A mean delta nitrogen balance of +8.9 was observed in the Travasol group and +6.9 in the Vamin group. The mean cumulative balance of nitrogen after 10 days of TPN reached +22.2 g and +16 g in each group respectively. This implicates a positive change in fat-free protoplasm of 283 g and 222 g[18]. This should represent a mean gain of lean body mass of 1.1 kg in Travasol patients and 0.9 in the Vamin patients[18]. The observed gain in body weight was in fact of +3 kg in both groups (Tables 4.4 and 4.5). This suggests that some fat was

Table 4.4 Effect of TPN with Travasol (protocol I) on body weight and various blood parameters

	Day				
Blood parameter	−3	−1	+2	+5	+8
Body weight (kg)	60 ± 2.9	60 ± 2.7	60 ± 2.7	61 ± 2.5	63 ± 2.8
Plasma transferrin (mg/100 ml)	210 ± 56	229 ± 39	151 ± 45	214 ± 38	183 ± 22
Total proteins (g/100 ml)	5.6 ± 0.3	5.4 ± 0.3	5.5 ± 0.2	5.5 ± 0.2	5.5 ± 0.2
Albumin (g/100 ml)	2.9 ± 0.2	2.7 ± 0.2	2.9 ± 0.2	2.7 ± 0.2	2.8 ± 0.1
Urea (mg/100 ml)	17 ± 2.8	14 ± 2.4	19 ± 1.9	22 ± 1.8	28 ± 1.8
Creatinine (mg/100 ml)	0.7 ± 0.09	0.8 ± 0.07	0.8 ± 0.06	0.8 ± 0.05	0.9 ± 0.06
Uric acid (mg/100 ml)	3.8 ± 0.3	3.5 ± 0.5	2.9 ± 0.4	2.4 ± 0.3	3.4 ± 0.3
Total calcium (mg/100 ml)	8.3 ± 0.3	8.2 ± 0.3	8.5 ± 0.2	8.8 ± 0.2	8.4 ± 0.2
Bilirubin (mg/100 ml)	1.1 ± 0.2	1.2 ± 0.3	1.4 ± 0.3	1.5 ± 0.3	1.3 ± 0.2
Prothrombin time (s)	13 ± 1.4	12 ± 0.7	11 ± 0.6	11 ± 0.4	12 ± 0.3
LDH (mU/ml)	174 ± 15	177 ± 9	229 ± 25	214 ± 15	249 ± 13
GOT (mU/ml)	44 ± 8.5	38 ± 6.1	47 ± 7.0	73 ± 5.0	85 ± 8.0
Alk. phosphatase (mU/ml)	147 ± 40	158 ± 39	149 ± 25	206 ± 35	201 ± 27
Haemoglobin (g/100 ml)	11.6 ± 0.8	11.7 ± 0.5	10.4 ± 0.6	11.1 ± 0.7	9.8 ± 0.8
White blood cells ($\times 10^3$ cells/mm^3)	9.7 ± 1.4	14 ± 4.7	11 ± 1.7	12 ± 1.2	11 ± 2

Values are ± SEM

produced with both protocols as well as a slight expansion of the extracellular fluid.

Body weight is thus not a reliable index of the effectiveness of parenteral nutrition during short-term studies.

The significant scattering of the nitrogen balance values around the mean is in part due to the administration of a fixed regimen independent of the patient's weight and to the presence of three patients who were critically ill (one in the Travasol and two in the Vamin group) and who never reached a positive balance. These patients were also the heaviest subjects of the study: 68.5, 70.2 and 75.4 kg. If these patients are excluded the mean daily positive nitrogen balance following 10 days of TPN is 3.85 with the Travasol group and 3.84 in the Vamin group. The nitrogen balances are thus comparable in both groups. The mean weight of the patients placed on the fixed Vamin regimen was smaller than those on Travasol, ensuring 15–20% greater

Table 4.5 Effect of TPN with Vamin (protocol II) on body weight and various blood parameters

Blood parameter	*Days* −3	−1	+2	+5	+8
Body weight (kg)	54 ± 20	52 ± 5.6	53 ± 5.5	56 ± 5.6	57 ± 5.6
Plasma transferrin (mg/100 ml)	199 ± 20	190 ± 21	176 ± 18	143 ± 17	162 ± 31
Total proteins (g/100 ml)	5.9 ± 0.5	5.8 ± 0.2	5.7 ± 0.2	5.4 ± 0.2	5.5 ± 0.2
Albumin (g/100 ml)	2.7 ± 0.3	3.0 ± 0.2	2.8 ± 0.2	2.6 ± 0.1	2.7 ± 0.1
Urea (mg/100 ml)	25 ± 3.6	23 ± 2.5	24 ± 3.7	19 ± 3.7	23 ± 2.1
Creatinine (mg/100 ml)	0.9 ± 0.08	0.8 ± 0.08	0.8 ± 0.07	0.9 ± 0.09	0.8 ± 0.06
Uric acid (mg/100 ml)	4.2 ± 0.6	3.8 ± 0.4	3.0 ± 0.3	2.8 ± 0.3	3.7 ± 0.3
Total calcium (mg/100 ml)	8.4 ± 0.4	8.5 ± 0.2	8.3 ± 0.2	8.2 ± 0.2	8.3 ± 0.2
Bilirubin (mg/100 ml)	2.1 ± 0.6	2.3 ± 0.5	1.0 ± 0.2	0.9 ± 0.2	1.3 ± 0.4
Prothrombin time (s)	13 ± 0.7	13 ± 0.7	12 ± 0.5	11 ± 0.4	11 ± 0.6
LDH (mU/ml)	210 ± 22	183 ± 21	180 ± 15	208 ± 28	200 ± 14
GOT (mU/ml)	37 ± 14	28 ± 6.0	32 ± 7.0	33 ± 6.0	48 ± 8.0
Alk. phosphatase (mU/ml)	129 ± 48	104 ± 27	119 ± 14	147 ± 19	187 ± 32
Haemoglobin (g/100 ml)	10.4 ± 0.3	11.4 ± 0.6	9.7 ± 0.6	10.4 ± 0.5	9.9 ± 0.3
White blood cells ($\times 10^3$ cells/mm^3)	11.6 ± 1.7	11.5 ± 1.5	10.3 ± 1.7	12.4 ± 2.5	11.7 ± 2.9

Values are means ± SEM

quantities of calories, carbohydrates, lipids and nitrogen intake in the former group (Table 4.2).

Mean blood glucose rose to 250 mg/100 ml in patients placed on protocol I and 300 mg/100 ml with protocol II after 5 days of parenteral nutrition (Figure 4.3). Simultaneously glycosuria of similar magnitude appeared in both groups during the first 5 days of TPN and virtually disappeared later. Plasma insulin rose with both protocols and was slightly higher in the Travasol than in the Vamin group. The difference however was not statistically significant. Exogenous insulin was given to some patients during the first days of TPN if the blood glucose was greater than 300 mg/100 ml. This probably raised the plasma insulin level on day +2.

Serum cholesterol was stable around 120 mg/100 ml in the control period and rose steadily to between 250 and 300 mg/100 ml at the end of the study (Figure 4.3). Plasma triglycerides also rose slightly.

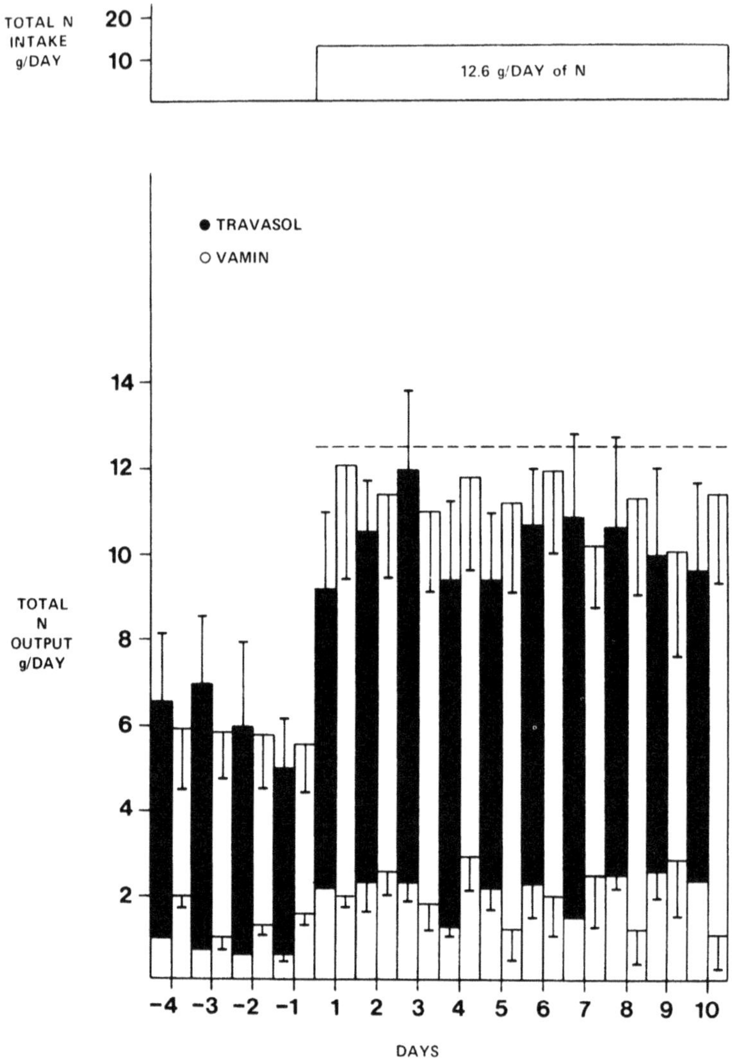

Figure 4.1 Total nitrogen intake and output before and after administration of parenteral nutrition with protocols I and II. The upper part of each bar represents urinary and lower part faecal nitrogen excretion. Values are means ± SEM

Blood ketone bodies were elevated moderately during the control days and nearly disappeared during TPN. Inversely, blood lactate and pyruvate rose significantly during the carbohydrate load and were slightly higher in the Vamin than in the Travasol group (Figure 4.4). The net effect of these changes was a slight accumulation of organic anions in the extracellular fluids in both groups (Bourbeau *et al.* Chapter 25).

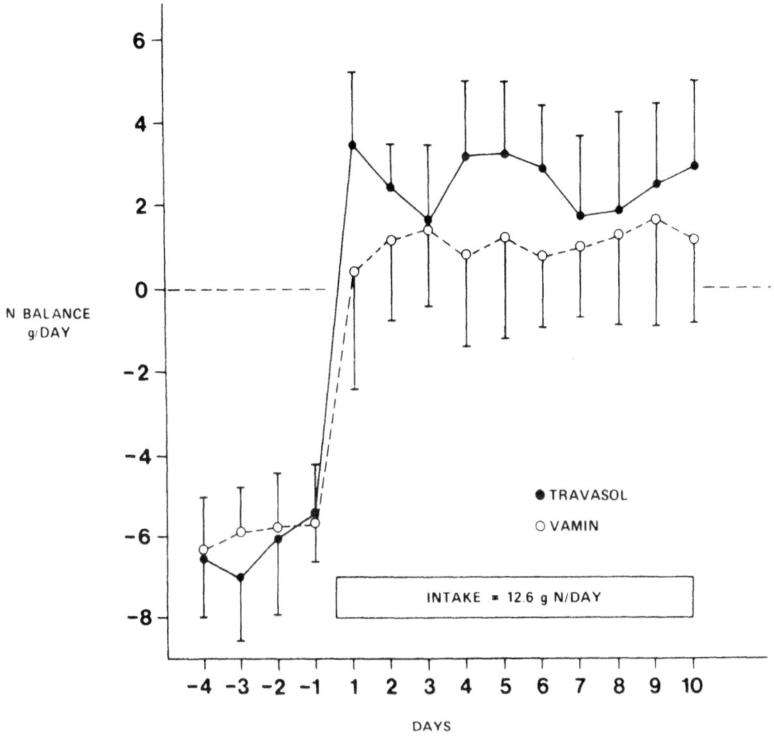

Figure 4.2 Nitrogen balance before and after parenteral nutrition with protocol I and II. Values are means ± SEM

Table 4.6 shows the liver adenine nucleotides content after 1 or 10 days of parenteral nutrition. The lactate : pyruvate ratio was also measured as an index of adequacy of the rapid freezing procedures. The hepatic ATP concentration was lower in the patient biopsied at the end of the first day of the fructose protocol than in the control group. Comparable data were not obtained in the patient on a fructose-free regimen. After 10 days of fructose, the ATP concentration was normal in the only patient biopsied, but the total adenine nucleotides were lower than in the control. This was also observed following 10 days of fructose-free regimen in two patients and thus might not be due to fructose administration.

Transferrin, total proteins and albumin were studied as indicators of liver protein synthesis. No difference in the plasma level of these three proteins

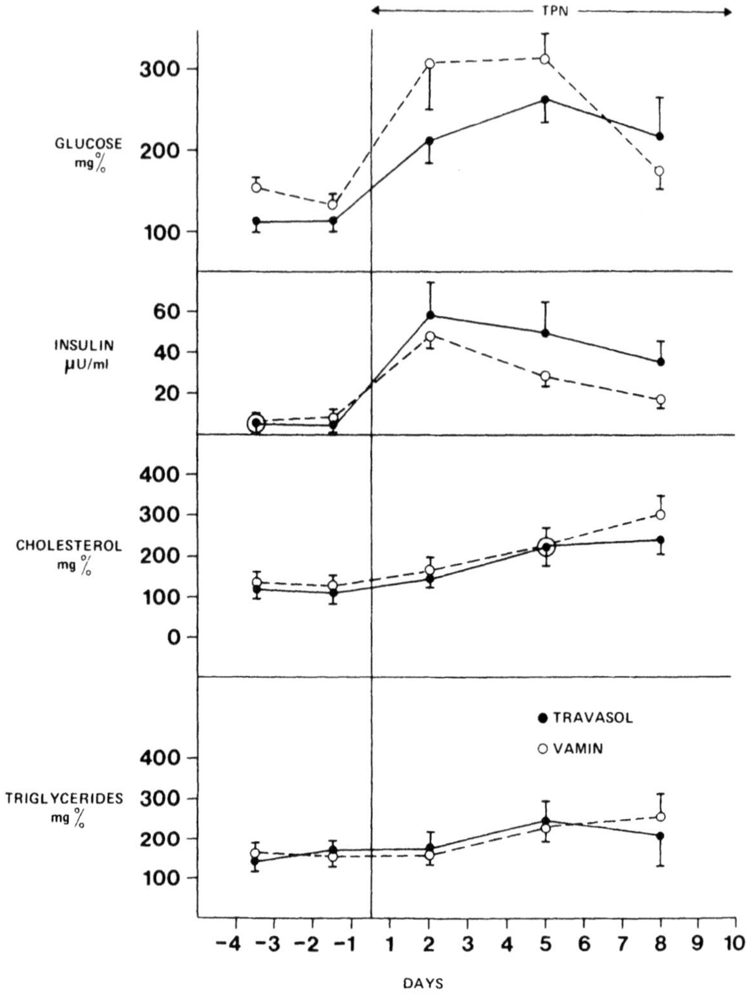

Figure 4.3 Plasma levels of glucose, insulin, cholesterol and triglycerides before and after parenteral nutrition with protocol I and II. Values are means ± SEM

Table 4.6 Lactate, pyruvate and adenine nucleotides in liver biopsies of four patients following TPN with protocols I or II

	Controls ($n = 5$)	*Protocol I*		*Protocol II*	
		Day +1	*Day* +10	*Day* +1	*Day* +10
Lactate (μm/g)	2.11 ± 0.39	—	1.65; 2.70	3.96	1.59
Pyruvate (μm/g)	0.20 ± 0.04	—	0.13; 0.20	0.25	0.17
L/P	10.6 ± 0.77	—	12.8; 13.5	15.8	9.4
ATP (μm/g)	2.86 ± 0.22	—	2.10; 1.7	1.46	2.9
ADP (μm/g)	1.81 ± 0.19	—	1.04; 0.54	2.10	1.42
AMP (μm/g)	1.43 ± 0.31	—	0.61; 0.23	0.93	0.39

Results are expressed as μmol/g of fresh tissue

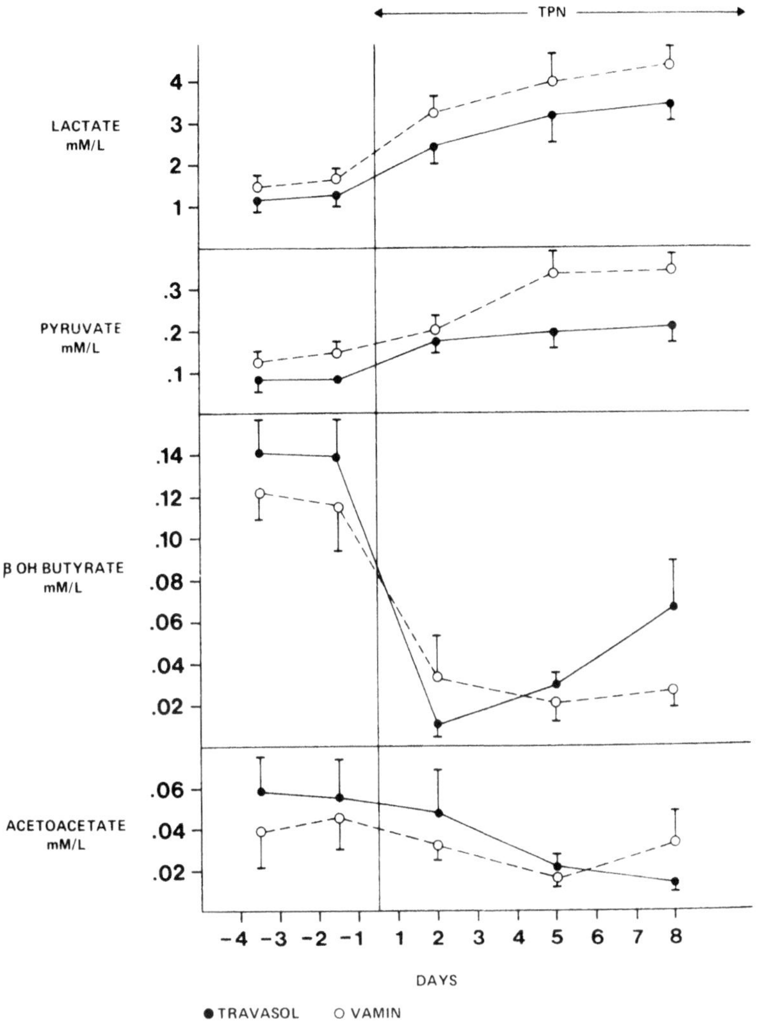

Figure 4.4 Blood organic anions before and after parenteral nutrition with protocols I and II. Values are means ± SEM

was observed following parenteral nutrition with both protocols (Tables 4.4 and 4.5).

Blood urea did not rise significantly either, but a significant amount of the total nitrogen output was due to an increased excretion of urea in the urine.

Figure 4.5 presents the only significant difference between both protocols: plasma phosphate was stable around 3.5 mg/100 ml in the control period, and tended to stay in a similar range during TPN with Travasol while a significant decrease in plasma phosphate was observed in the fructose Vamin group ($p < 0.05$).

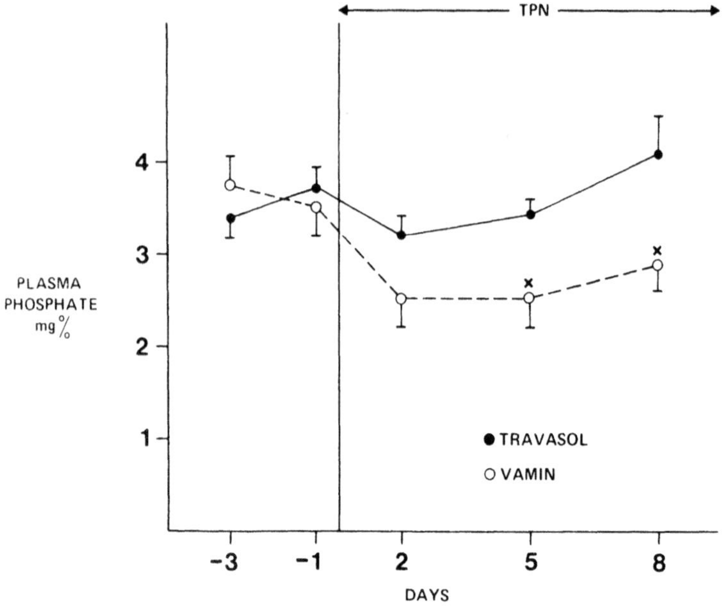

Figure 4.5 Plasma phosphate levels during and after parenteral nutrition with protocols I and II. Values are means ± SEM. An asterisk indicates a significant difference between Travasol and Vamin groups. $P < 0.05$

Tables 4.4 and 4.5 present various parameters measured before and following TPN with both protocols. No significant changes were observed for bilirubin, LDH, GOT, alkaline phosphatase, prothrombin time, haemoglobin, or white blood cell count.

DISCUSSION

The study was designed to investigate if the administration of part of the total carbohydrate intake as fructose would modify the overall effect on nitrogen balance. Two protocols providing similar calories, carbohydrates, lipids and nitrogen intake with and without fructose were compared. A second variable was introduced, as the nitrogen sources were different in both regimens, the fructose protocol providing more essential and non-essential amino acid than the fructose-free protocol to achieve an identical nitrogen intake. This difference is further emphasized by the different distribution of patients in both protocols, patients on protocol II tending to be younger and to be less heavy than patients on protocol I. Consequently, the mean amount of calories, carbohydrates, lipids and nitrogen given to patients receiving fructose was slightly higher than in patients placed on a fructose-free regimen. In both protocols however the essential amino acid intake was 4–7 times the normal dietary requirements.

Nitrogen balances

No significant differences could be shown in the nitrogen balance in both groups. This is specially clear if the three patients who did not achieve a positive nitrogen balance during TPN are excluded. Thus, the presence of 0.1 g/kg/h of fructose did not improve nor impair a positive balance during parenteral nutrition. This positive balance was of the magnitude expected in view of data obtained by other workers[19,20] including a study by Gazzaniga[21] in which similar amounts of fructose were provided as carbohydrates. We thus confirm that administration of 12.6 g of nitrogen/day together with 3500 cal is able to reverse the catabolic state of most patients on TPN. However in three critically ill patients, the fixed protocol did not supply enough calories to reverse the catabolic state and induce a positive balance. Two of these patients died shortly after the study. This emphasizes the need to have day-to-day nitrogen balance as we might have obtained a positive balance if greater amounts of calories could have been given to these patients.

Effect of fructose

Fructose administration has been favoured in the past because fructose metabolism is more rapid than glucose metabolism[12], is not insulin dependent[3,4] and therefore is not impaired during stress[3]. Less hyperglycaemia and less glycosuria have also been observed during short-term administration of 0.5 g/kg/h of fructose[7]. As fructose may not stimulate insulin secretion[4], it was hoped that less hypoglycaemia would be seen after sudden cessation of TPN[1]. It was also thought that the stimulation of insulin secretion caused by glucose infusion was detrimental by suppressing fat mobilization at the expense of body protein stores[22]. However, these views might be incorrect and have been challenged by Felig[23] in the light of recent data showing that insulin enhances the muscle uptake[24,25] of the branched-chain amino acids which stimulate protein synthesis in muscle[24]. Hyperinsulinaemia might therefore enhance nitrogen retention[25,26] as well as reducing protein catabolism[27,28] which is the very aim of parenteral nutrition. The finding by Wolfe *et al.* that arterial levels of these amino acids were lower following glucose infusion than fructose is in accord with this view[26]. Blood glucose was not lower in this study when 25% of the carbohydrate was given as fructose and a similar elevation of plasma insulin was observed with both protocols. This is probably related to the rapid hepatic[26,29] and renal[30] transformation of fructose into glucose. In no case however was this hyperglycaemia a significant clinical problem, its only disadvantage being the induction of glycosuria and renal losses of calories.

There are no findings suggestive of a superiority of fructose over glucose in this study but numerous points can be raised concerning the risks of fructose administration due to the rapid phosphorylation of fructose through the ketohexokinase reaction in the liver, kidney, and digestive tract leading to a rapid utilization of fructose[1]. A significant, and potentially dangerous, lacticacidaemia consequently follows fructose administration[31]. Lactate accumulation was not significantly greater with fructose in our study but this is probably related to the small amounts given. Fructose administration also leads to the accumulation of fructose-1-P in the liver, kidney, and digestive tract due to the rapid phosphorylation, and inhibition of the fructose-1-phosphate aldolase through simultaneous accumulation of AMP and IMP[8-11] in the cells. This results from the effect of ATP depletion and P_i sequestration on the metabolism of cell adenine dinucleotides[9]. These biochemical changes have been observed in man following acute fructose administration[32] as well as in the hepatic biopsy of our patient on the first day of protocol II. They have been shown to be associated with a reduction of protein synthesis in the liver[12] of the rat.

Less is known on the effect of chronic administration of fructose. The only obvious difference between the two protocols in our study was the hypophosphataemia observed during fructose administration. This is in accordance with the findings of others[33] and probably reflects the Pi sequestration in tissues metabolizing fructose. This hypophosphataemia was seen throughout the period of fructose administration. The total adenine nucleotide content of a liver biopsy after 10 days of the fructose protocol was subnormal, but not different from the values obtained after 10 days of glucose. While it is well established that the acute administration of fructose leads to a rapid depletion of hepatic and renal ATP, it is not clear if chronic administration produces the same results. Further studies with the administration of greater quantities of fructose may show a different pattern.

Hereditary fructose intolerance

It is well known that the administration of fructose to patients with hereditary fructose intolerance due to a genetic defect of the F-1-P-aldolase generates several problems. A proximal tubular acidosis[34-36], an aminoaciduria[36-38], hyperuricosuria[34] and phosphaturia[36-38] together with hypercalciuria[34] are observed. This picture resembles an acquired and reversible Fanconi syndrome[36]. Lacticacidaemia[34], and secondary hyperuricaemia[34], as well as hypophosphataemia[36] also appear. Most of these effects are not seen when an acute load of fructose is given to normal subjects[37]. It is not known however if prolonged administration of significant quantities of fructose could cause these various disturbances. It is certainly not the case with a prolonged small intake of fructose, as used in this study, as no systemic acidosis appeared, and the distal H^+ secretion appeared to be intact as indicated by an elevation of the urinary $p\text{CO}_2$ well above the plasma $p\text{CO}_2$ during a bicarbonate load (results not presented). No significant hypercalciuria or phosphaturia was noted. We have not measured the aminoaciduria in these groups, but the similarity of the urinary nitrogen excretion in patients presenting a positive nitrogen balance during both protocols suggests that both groups were similar. It is known that some of the changes induced by fructose administration can be minimized by simultaneous phosphate administration. This is probably not the case in our study as one mole of fructose was given daily while the phosphate load was around 50 mmol.

Toxicity of TPN solutions

No evidence for systemic toxicity was found for the protocol I with Travasol + Intralipid or protocol II Vamin + Intralipid, if one excludes the slight hypophosphoraemia observed in the latter regimen. The only clinical problems encountered during TPN were infection associated with catheters (one), fluid overloading (three) and hyperkalaemia induced by abrupt cessation of TPN (one).

ACKNOWLEDGEMENTS

The authors are grateful to Y. Courchesne, S. Desjardins, D. Donaldson, L. Tessier, and J. Sénécal for their kind assistance, as well as to all the physicians and nurses who were involved in this study. Travasol solution was kindly provided by Baxter Laboratories Canada, Ltd.

References

1. Thoren, L. (1962). Parenteral nutrition with carbohydrate and alcohol. *Acta Chir. Scand.*, **325**, 75
2. Bergström, J. and Hultman, E. (1967). Synthesis of muscle glycogen in man after glucose and fructose infusion. *Acta Med. Scand.*, **182**, 93
3. Miller, M., Craig, J. W., Drucker, W. R. and Woodward, H. (1956). The metabolism of fructose in man. *Yale J. Biol. Med.*, **29**, 335
4. Leuthardt, F. (1960). Der stoffwechsel der Fruktose. *Schw. Med. Wochenschr.*, **90**, 455
5. Hager, D., Pipeleers, D. G., Herchvelz, A. and Malaisse, V. J. (1973). Effects of fructose and other sugars on islet function in vitro. *Acta Med. Scand.*, **542**, (Suppl.), 159
6. Mehnert, H., Forster, H., Gejer, C. A., Haslbeck, M. and Dehmel, K. H. (1970). Clinical use of carbohydrates in parenteral nutrition. In H. C. Meng and D. H. Law (eds.). *Parenteral Nutrition*, p. 122. (Springfield, Ill.: Charles C. Thomas Publishers)
7. Hessov, I. (1975). Utilisation of intravenous glucose and fructose in the postoperative period. *Acta Chir. Scand.*, **141**, 467
8. Burch, H. B., Lowry, O. H., Meinhardt, L., Max, P. and Chyu, K. (1970). Effect of fructose, dihydroxyacetone, glycerol and glucose on metabolites and related compounds in liver and kidney. *J. Biol. Chem.*, **245**, 2092
9. Woods, H. F., Eggleston, L. V. and Krebs, H. A. (1970). The cause of hepatic accumulation of fructose-1-phosphate on fructose loading. *Biochem. J.*, **119**, 501
10. Sestoft, L., Tonnesen, K., Hansen, F. V. and Damgaard, S. E. (1972). Fructose and D-glyceraldelyde metabolism in the isolated perfused pig liver. *Eur. J. Biochem.*, **30**, 542
11. Nisell, J. and Linden, L. (1968). Fructose-1-phosphate aldolase and fructose-1, 6-diphosphate aldolase activity in the mucosa of the intestine in hereditary fructose intolerance. *Scand. J. Gastroenterol.*, **3**, 80
12. Maenpaa, P. H., Raivio, K. O. and Kekomaki, M. P. (1968). Liver adenine nucleotides: fructose-induced depletion and its effect on protein synthesis. *Science*, **161**, 1253
13. Ferrari, A. (1960). Nitrogen determination by a continuous digestion and analysis system. *Ann. N.Y. Acad. Sci.*, **87**, 792
14. Bergmayer, H. U. (1974). *Methods of Enzymatic Analysis*, p. 1446. (New York and London: Academic Press)

15. Mancini, G., Carbonara, A. O. and Hevemans, J. F. (1965). Immunochemical quantitation of antigens by single radial immunodiffusion. *Int. J. Immunochem.*, **2,** 235
16. Hales, C. N. and Randle, P. J. (1963). Immunoassay of insulin with insulin antibody precipitate. *Biochem. J.*, **88,** 137
17. Bergmayer, H. U. (1974). *Methods of Enzymatic Analysis*, p. 2101. (New York and London: Academic Press)
18. Reifenstein, E. C. Jr., Fuller, A. and Wells, S. L. (1945). The accumulation, interpretation, and presentation of data pertaining to metabolic balances, notably those of calcium, phosphorus and nitrogen. *J. Clin. Endocrinol.*, **5,** 367
19. Anderson, G. H., Patel, D. G. and Jeejeebhoy, K. N. (1974). Design and evaluation by nitrogen balance and blood aminograms of an amino acid mixture for total parenteral nutrition of adult with gastrointestinal disease. *J. Clin. Invest.*, **53,** 904
20. Van Way, C. W., Meng, H. G. and Sandstead, H. H. (1975). Nitrogen balance in postoperative patients receiving parenteral nutrition. *Arch. Surg.*, **110,** 272
21. Gazzaniga, A. B., Bartlett, R. H. and Shobe, J. B. (1975). Nitrogen balance in patients receiving either fat or carbohydrate for total intravenous nutrition. *Am. Surg.*, **182,** 163
22. Flatt, J. P. and Blackburn, G. L. (1974). The metabolic fuel regulatory system: implications for protein-sparing therapies during caloric deprivation and disease. *Am. J. Clin. Nutr.*, **27,** 175
23. Felig, P. (1976). Intravenous nutrition: fact and fancy. *N. Engl. J. Med.*, **294,** 1455
24. Fulks, R. M., Li, J. B. and Goldberg, A. L. (1975). Effect of insulin, glucose and aminoacids on protein turnover in rat diaphragm. *J. Biol. Chem.*, **250,** 290
25. Sherwin, R. S., Rosenzweig, J., Soman, V., Hendler, R. and Felig, P. (1976). Effect of insulin and diabetes on protein and branched chain amino acid utilization. *Diabetes*, **25,** (Suppl. 1), 332
26. Wolfe, B. M., Ahuja, S. P. and Marliss, E. B. (1975). Effects of intravenously administered fructose and glucose on splanchnic amino acid and carbohydrate metabolism in hypertriglyceridemic men. *J. Clin. Invest.*, **56,** 970
27. Tata, J. R. (1966). Hormones and the synthesis and utilisation of ribonucleic acids. *Prog. Nucleic Acid Res. Exp. Biol.*, **5,** 191
28. Wool, I. G., Stirewalt, W. S. and Kurihara, K. (1968). Mode of action of insulin in the regulation of protein biosynthesis in muscle. *Recent Prog. Horm. Res.*, **24,** 139
29. Froesch, E. R. (1973). Concluding remarks. *Acta Med. Scand.*, **542,** (Suppl.), 239
30. Salomon L. L., Lanza, F. I. and Smith, D. E. (1961). Renal conversion of fructose to glucose. *Am. J. Physiol.*, **200,** 871
31. Sahebjami, H. and Scalettar, R. (1971). Effect of fructose infusion on lactate and uric acid metabolism. *Lancet*, **i,** 366
32. Bode, J. Ch., Bode, C., Rumpelt, H. J. and Zelder, O. (1974). Loss of hepatic adenosine phosphates and metabolic consequences following fructose or sorbitol administration in man and in the rat. In K. F. Lunquist and N. Tygstrup (eds.). Alfred Benzon Symposium VI—*Regulation of Hepatic Metabolism*, p. 267
33. Rowlands, B. J. and Giddings, A. E. B. (1976). Postoperative hypophosphataemia. *Lancet*, **ii,** 1077
34. Morris, R. C. Jr. (1968). An experimental renal acidification defect in patients with hereditary fructose intolerance: II. Its distinction from classic renal tubular acidosis: its resemblance to renal acidification defect associated with the Fanconi syndrome of children with cystinosis. *J. Clin. Invest.*, **47,** 1648
35. Levin, B. and Snodgrass, G. J. D. (1965). Fructosemia another inborn error of metabolism. *Clin. Red.*, **4,** 605
36. Morris, R. C., Ueki, I. and Wegienka, E. (1968). An experimental renal acidification defect in patients with hereditary fructose intolerance. I—Its resemblance to renal tubular acidosis. *J. Clin. Invest.*, **47,** 1309
37. Froesch, E. R., Wolf, H. P., Baitsch, H., Prader, A. and Labhart, A. (1963). Hereditary fructose intolerance; inborn defect of hepatic fructose-1-phosphate aldolase. *Am. J. Med.*, **31,** 151

5
Evaluation of non-glucose carbohydrates in parenteral nutrition

N. ZÖLLNER

If those who required parenteral nutrition were healthy there would be no need to discuss the choice of carbohydrate because glucose is the main energy substrate for the brain. It prevents excessive losses of sodium and water and stimulates the secretion of insulin, thus enhancing anabolism. However, in patients who are very ill or who have sustained a severe injury or operation, there is an increased secretion of adrenaline and noradrenaline which inhibits insulin release. Glucose metabolism could be controlled in most of these conditions by the careful administration of insulin. This is not always accomplished however even by experts. Hence the search for carbohydrates and carbohydrate-like substances which are metabolized independent of insulin.

In order to evaluate carbohydrates and polyols used in parenteral nutrition, the rate of utilization of these substances must be known as well as their metabolic effects other than that of supplying the cells with energy.

Studies of the utilization of sugars in parenteral nutrition must consider amounts and rates. If 2500–3000 kcal (10–12 MJ) are to be supplied daily, the amount of carbohydrate to be administered (if amino acids are neglected) is 600–800 g or 300–400 g, depending on whether intravenous fat is given or not. From these basic assumptions one can calculate (Table 5.1) that infusion rates between 0.2 and 1.5 g/kg/h must be used if reasonable conclusions are to be drawn. We shall see that only glucose and fructose can be infused with rates in the upper part of this range.

In order to compare the utilization of different carbohydrates, infusion studies have to be carried out under identical conditions. One prerequisite for a prolonged and accurately timed intravenous infusion is the use of a pump, as introduced by Woodyatt *et al.*[1] in 1915. The infusion time must be

Table 5.1 Metabolic requirements

Basal daily energy requirement 2500–3000 kcal (10–12 MJ)	
600–750 g of carbohydrates without fat	
300–400 g of carbohydrates with fat	
Reference person 70 kg body weight	
average 9 or 5 g carbohydrate/kg body weight	
Infusion time 6 or 24 h	
Infusion rates	1.5 or 0.4 g/kg/h without fat
	0.9 or 0.2 g/kg/h with fat

long enough to assure a steady state. Experiments with several administration rates should be carried out. It is also obvious that blood and urine must be checked at regular intervals for the concentration of the infused carbohydrates, and possibly for intermediary products. And finally, the group of subjects to be investigated should be homogeneous in regard to health or disease.

Strack *et al.*[2] in Leipzig were the first to perform reproducible experiments in rabbits; these experiments were based upon the above requirements. We have adopted their model and applied it to man.

Our studies extending from 1965 until now were aimed primarily at the utilization of sugars under physiological conditions. The utilization can be assessed in the steady state, if the inflow (i.e. the infusion rate), and the urinary outflow of the sugar under investigation are known.

At first we were interested in our main dietary carbohydrates, i.e. glucose, fructose and galactose. Later we performed studies using xylitol, sorbitol and ethanol, which are widely used in parenteral nutrition in some countries. Recently we have become interested in intravenous maltose. I shall describe part of our results and some of the literature, excluding glucose and ethanol. For a review of these refer to Heuckenkamp and Zöllner, 1975[3]. The technical details have been described by Zöllner *et al.* 1968[4]. Calculations were made according to Dost (1953).

FRUCTOSE

If fructose is infused intravenously a constant plasma level is reached 60–90 min after the beginning of the infusion. There is no early peak (Figure 5.1) as is seen during the administration of glucose (compare Figure 5.5).

Fructosuria reaches constant values after 2 h. For that reason steady state calculations can be performed best after 120 min. As shown in Table 5.2 fructose is slightly better utilized at high infusion rates, whereas glucose is better utilized at low rates. The total clearance is listed in Table 5.3.

There are linear relationships between plasma fructose and the infusion rates of 0.5–1.5 g/kg/h. Taking fructose as an example, we emphasize the importance of steady-state conditions for quantitative evaluations. If there is a linear relationship between the rate of administration and the plasma level it is possible to predict the amount of fructose which is utilized if the

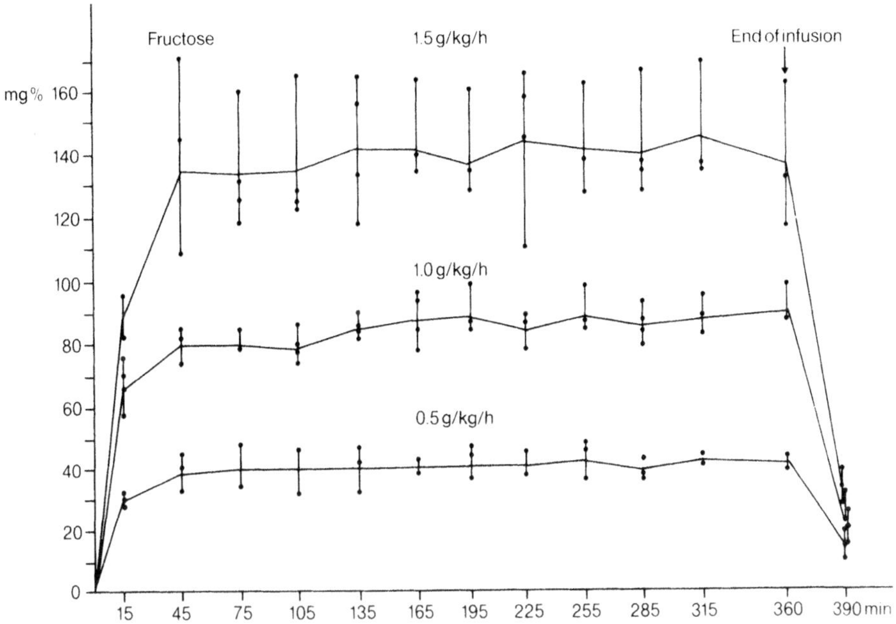

Figure 5.1 Plasma fructose levels in healthy subjects receiving fructose infusions with three different rates. The vertical lines represent the range of all measurements

Table 5.2 Comparison of utilization of glucose and fructose for three different infusion rates during the steady state

Infusion rate (g/kg/h)	*Utilization of glucose* (mg/kg/h)	*Utilization of fructose* (mg/kg/h)
0.5	499	488.8
1.0	985	947.4
1.5	1390	1409.6

Table 5.3 Values for the total clearance of fructose

Infusion rate (g/kg/h)	*Total clearance* (ml/kg/min)
0.5	19.8
1.0	19.2
1.5	18.3

administration rate is increased. An increase of the administration rate by, for example, 0.1 g/kg/h leads to a rise of the plasma level by 9.0 mg/100 ml and an addition urinary fructose loss of 7.6 mg/kg/h (compare Figure 5.2). The utilization is enhanced under these circumstances by 0.092 g/kg/h. These values are in good agreement with those by Strack *et al.*[2] in the rabbit.

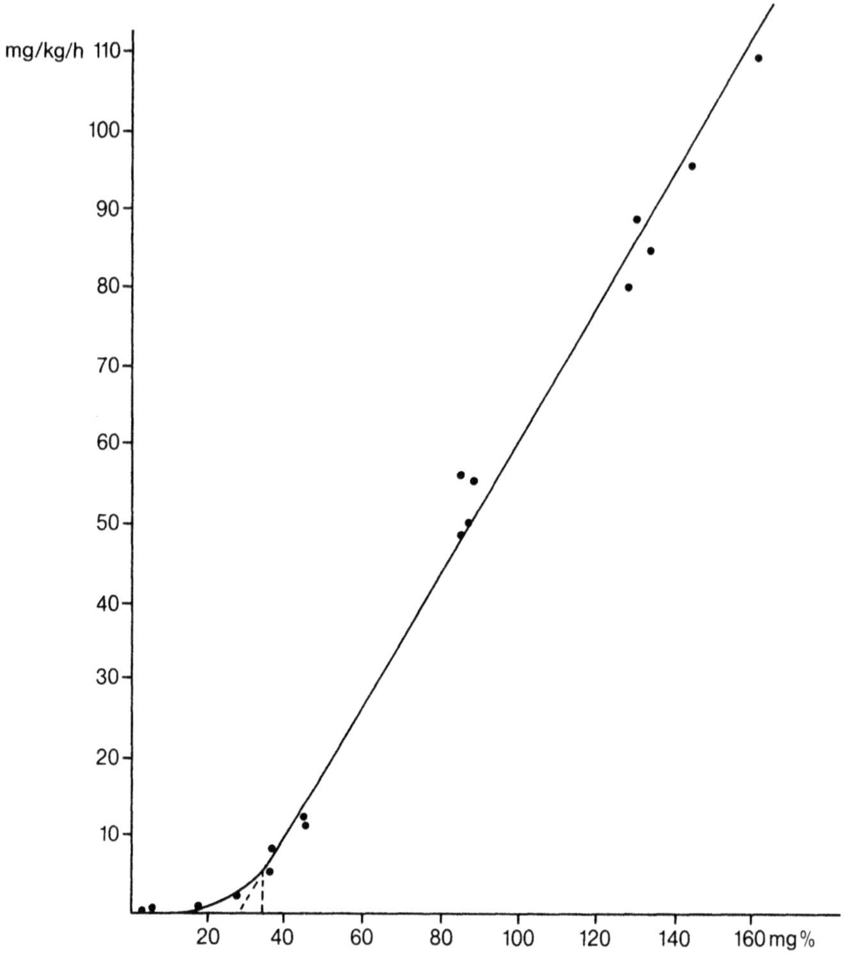

Figure 5.2 Plasma fructose level (abscissa) and urinary fructose excretion (ordinate) (compare Figure 5.1). There is a linear relationship between the rates of 0.5–1.5 g/kg

After the intravenous administration of labelled fructose (0.5 g/kg) to man[5], sizeable amounts of radioactivity were recovered in the subjects' plasma glucose although the level of plasma glucose rose only slightly. This demonstrates that in man as well as in animals fructose is rapidly converted to glucose. In the rat it appears that fructose is converted to glucose quantitatively before oxidation[6,7].

These findings explain why fructose leads to a rise of blood glucose and increased losses of glucose in the urine in patients with severe diabetes. In a case of Felber *et al.* (1959)[8] the total loss of fructose infused at a rate of 0.5 kg/h amounted to 50% after 8 h of infusion and probably would have risen further if the experiment had not been terminated. Obviously, the utilization of non-glucose carbohydrates by patients with a deranged glucose metabolism (i.e. in diabetes, severe illness, stress, etc) cannot be predicted from experiments in volunteers or patients with a normal glucose metabolism.

GALACTOSE

Galactose differs in many respects from glucose and fructose. First of all, administration rates could not be raised beyond 0.75 g/kg/h due to pronounced abdominal discomfort[9]. A steady state is obtained with infusion rates up to 0.4 g/kg/h only (Figure 5.3). Above that rate galactose in blood rises constantly within a 6 h infusion period (Figure 5.4), accompanied by an increasing galactosuria.

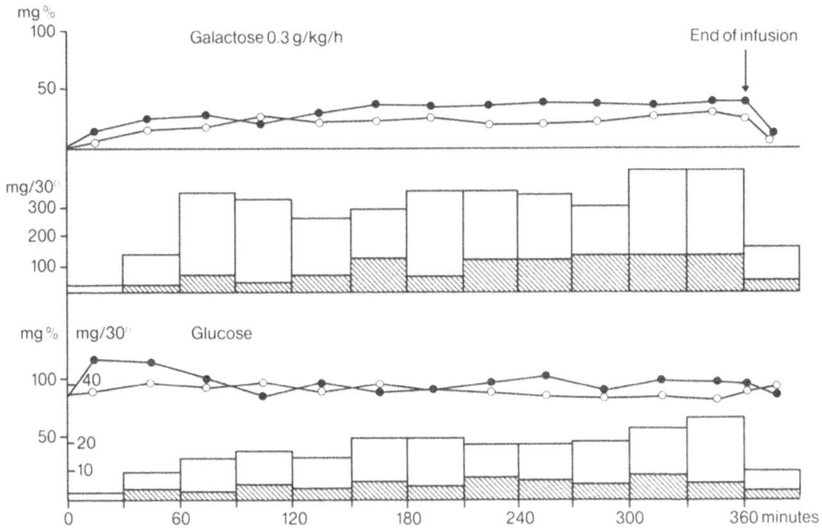

Figure 5.3 Plasma galactose levels and blood glucose levels in two healthy volunteers receiving galactose infusions at a rate of 0.3 g/kg body weight/h. The columns represent galactose and glucose excretion, respectively

The total clearance for the rate of 0.3 g/kg/h gives a value of 17.8 ml/kg/min and lies between the data calculated for glucose and fructose.

Galactose infusions lead to a small but definite glucosuria, a phenomenon not observed during fructose infusions. This is due to the fact that galactose and glucose compete for the same receptor site for reabsorption within the kidney tubules[10].

Galactose and glucose, infused together at a rate of 0.5 g/kg/h for each substance, lead to an increase in blood galactose which is only half of that observed during an infusion of galactose alone at a rate of 0.5 g/kg/h (Figure 5.5), whereas glucose behaves as if it were infused alone. Moreover, the mixture causes glucosuria to increase but galactose excretion to decrease. According to Levine (1961)[11], glucose stimulates insulin secretion and by this galactose is carried into the muscle cells together with glucose. Levine was able, on the other hand, to show that later galactose returns into the extracellular space. From our observations we see no reason for further consideration of galactose in parenteral nutrition.

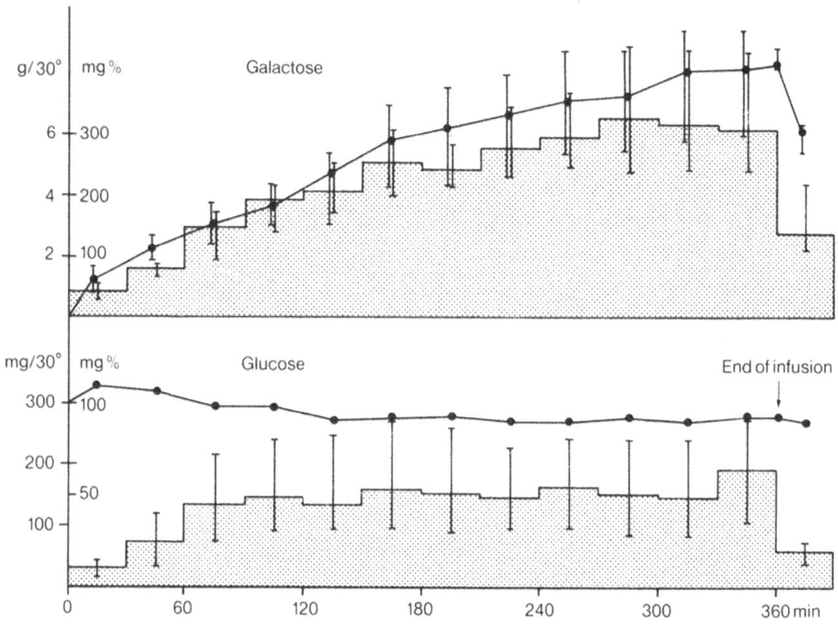

Figure 5.4 Galactose level in plasma and blood glucose in five healthy subjects receiving galactose infusions at a rate of 0.75 g/kg body weight/h. There is a rising galactose level accompanied by a rising galactosuria (hatched area). Note that galactose infusions lead to an increasing glucosuria (lower half of the figure)

XYLITOL

Xylitol is a polyol with five C-atoms which is used in some countries in cases of impaired utilization of glucose such as occurs after surgery[12]. Figure 5.6 shows the results obtained from ten healthy men to whom xylitol was given at a rate of 0.5 g/kg/h. A steady state is reached only at the end of the infusion period of 5 h[13].

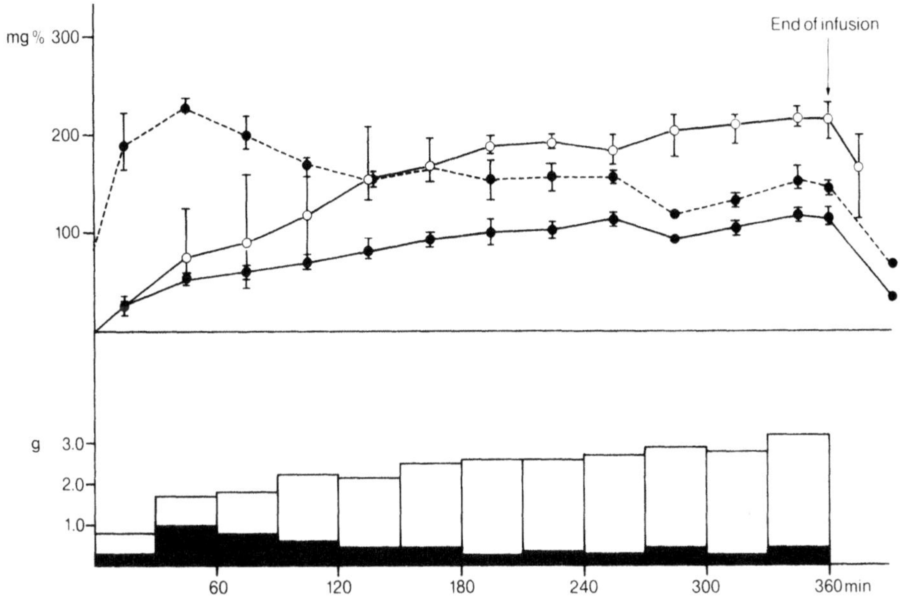

Figure 5.5 Results of an infusion experiment where two subjects received a mixture of glucose and galactose at a rate of 0.5 g/kg body weight/h for each sugar. Blood galactose level (●—●) in compared with galactose level in subjects receiving galactose at a rate of 0.5 g/kg body weight/h alone (○—○). The dotted line represents blood glucose during the glucose–galactose mixed infusion. The black columns indicate glucose, the white columns galactose excretion in the urine

There is a considerable loss of xylitol in the urine, amounting to 22% on the average of the administered dose. The difference between fructose and xylitol excretion during their infusion at a rate of 0.5 g/kg/h is shown in the lower half of Figure 5.6. But even with lower infusion rates the urinary losses make up 15% of the administered dose on the average. The comparatively high losses of xylitol are due to the fact that pentitols are not reabsorbed in the kidney tubules[14]. This is not unique to xylitol, but occurs with other polyols as well.

Bickel *et al.* (1973)[15] claim that in some but not all surgical patients, shortly after an operation, the utilization of xylitol is greater than in healthy controls. However in their cases the losses in the urine ranged between 8 and 20%.

Like fructose, xylitol converted readily to glucose in the liver. Keller and Froesch[6] conclude that this conversion consists of 60–75% of the xylitol administered. If this is the case and if the urinary losses are considered, the immediate catabolism of xylitol without conversion through the pentose phosphate shunt plays a very minor role. The considerations relating to patients with a decreased ability to utilize glucose which were mentioned in the section on fructose apply also to xylitol.

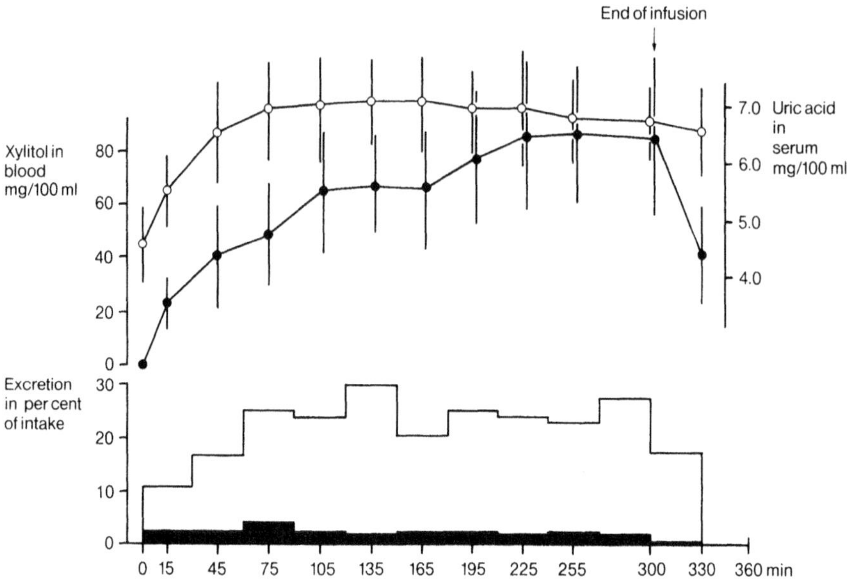

Figure 5.6 Blood xylitol level (●—●) and plasma uric acid level (○—○) in ten healthy volunteers receiving xylitol infusion at a rate of 0.5 g/kg/h. The xylitol excretion in the urine is given as a percentage of the dose administered (white columns) and compared with the fructose excretion (hatched area) which we observed during fructose infusions at a rate of 0.5 g/kg/h

SORBITOL

The utilization of sorbitol has been studied by Bickel *et al.* (1973)[12]. A steady state is reached after 90 min with administration rates of 0.5 g/kg/h, and the urinary losses average 11%. If the administration rate is raised further, sorbitol concentration rises continuously and blood fructose increases. All the observations agree with the basic biochemical assumption that in man sorbitol is metabolized via fructose and that this conversion may become rate-limiting. However, fructose space is considerably larger than that of sorbitol (or xylitol) and, at similar rates of administration, urinary losses of fructose are smaller than those of sorbitol.

MALTOSE

The utilization of intravenous maltose has been studied[16,17]. A kind of steady state is obtained after 4½ h at a rate of 0.5 g/kg/h. At the end of a 6 h experiment (Figure 5.7) the renal carbohydrate loss is between 50 and 60% of the amount administered. Not all of it is maltose; there is a significant glucosuria in the face of normoglucosaemia. From Finke and Reinauer[17] one can estimate that the maximal utilization of maltose is 35 mg/kg/h. Sprandel's results[16] suggest however that these results may be too low.

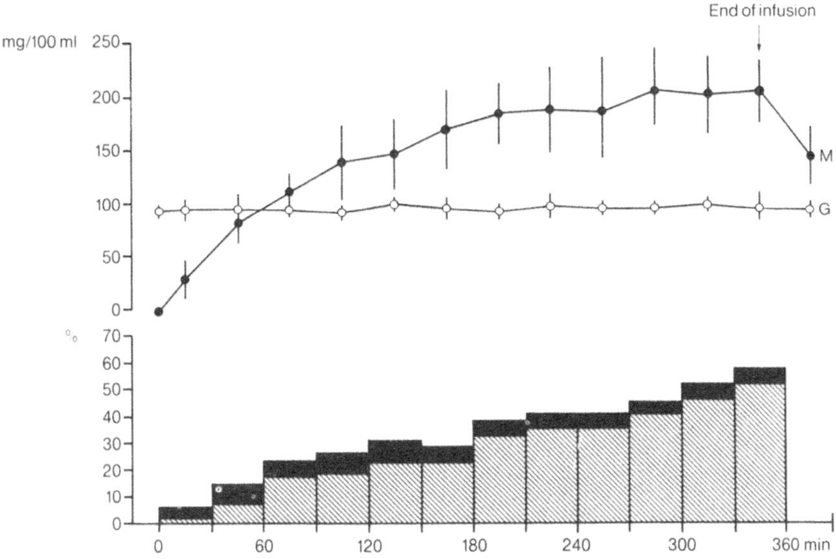

Figure 5.7 Average blood level and urinary excretion of maltose and glucose during maltose infusion with a rate of 0.5 g/kg body weight/h ($n = 10$). The open dots represent glucose, the closed dots maltose blood levels. The vertical lines describe SEM. In the lower half of the figure maltose (hatched columns) and glucose (black columns) excretion is illustrated as a percentage of maltose administered

At the moment, maltose only has an academic interest. However, it is a very interesting substance, which merits further study. Finke and Reinauer[17] consider that maltose is predominantly broken down by the kidney, which explains glucosuria. However, Sprandel *et al.* (1976)[18] have shown that the perfused rat liver as well as isolated hepatocytes break down maltose to glucose. Certainly further studies are necessary.

UTILIZATION OF NON-GLUCOSE CARBOHYDRATES

One of the main purposes of parenteral nutrition is the maintenance of energy balance, occasionally over long periods of time. At the same time essential nutrients must be administered in amounts necessary to avoid the development of deficiencies, and both these aims should be accomplished without adverse reactions.

If one compares glucose, fructose, galactose and maltose as well as sorbitol and xylitol with respect to maximal utilization under steady-state conditions (Table 5.4), these 'carbohydrates' fall into three groups. Glucose and fructose can easily meet the energy requirements of the body, sorbitol and xylitol can barely do it, while galactose and maltose cannot. These conclusions are based on measurements in the steady state and do not use other criteria.

Table 5.4 Comparison of maximal carbohydrate utilization during steady state. From Tables 5.1 the caloric requirement may be calculated. It is 1.6 cal/kg/h

Sugar	*Infusion rate* (g/kg/h)	*Utilization* (g/kg/h)	*Calories* (cal/kg/h)
Glucose	1.5	1.390	5.5
Fructose	1.5	1.409	5.5
Xylitol	0.5	0.483	1.9
Sorbitol	0.5	0.436	1.7
Galactose	0.3	0.290	1.1
Maltose	0.5	0.35	0.15

Berg *et al.* (1974)[19] using a different approach arrived at somewhat different conclusions which are presented in Table 5.5 with which we do not agree. It should also be mentioned that the maximal utilization of ethanol is better than that of sorbitol and xylitol and in our experience amounts to 2.8 cal/kg/h at an administration rate of 0.4 g/kg/h.

Table 5.5 Maximal rate of advisable carbohydrate administration[19] (g/kg/h)

Glucose	0.75
Fructose	0.25
Sorbitol	0.25
Xylitol	0.25

The selection of the carbohydrate(s) of choice for parenteral nutrition depends on two considerations, namely the utilization in specific clinical situations and on the severity or importance of the side effects which may occur.

SPECIFIC EFFECTS IN CERTAIN DISEASES

It is well known that in certain clinical situations the utilization of glucose is severely impaired. During cardiac surgery in hypothermia blood glucose levels of 1000 mg/100 ml have been measured as well as plasma insulin levels which were very low. After severe surgical trauma the administration of usual amounts of intravenous glucose leads to hyperglycaemia, possibly with pathological consequences but certainly with increased requirements for insulin. The reasons for this are not completely understood. Some authors favour the idea that the secretion of insulin is decreased, others consider that increased lipolysis and ketone body formation reduce the sensitivity to insulin.

Precise balance studies are lacking. So far hyperglycaemia has been considered by most to indicate that glucose is not utilized. From this it is concluded by some that non-glucose carbohydrates should be given, while others prefer to use fat emulsions as an alternative.

It is hard to conceive how a body which cannot utilize glucose can live on xylitol, sorbitol or fructose, substances which are predominantly metabolized in the living cell where they are converted to glucose. It appears more probable that these carbohydrates are of limited nutritive value in all metabolic states in which glucose cannot be utilized, their value being restricted to their beneficial effect on the liver cell and the production of substrate for the periphery, e.g. by lactic acid formation. Under these considerations intravenous fat is a very good alternative.

SIDE-EFFECTS OF INTRAVENOUS CARBOHYDRATES

The main side-effects are an increased production of lactate leading to acidosis, an increased formation of uric acid indicating an increased turnover of purine nucleotides in the liver, loss of body water and electrolytes possibly due to osmotic diuresis, and the formation of increased amounts of oxalate.

The production of lactate from fructose and xylitol has been known for some time and the mechanisms have been described, by Froesch (1975)[7] and by Woods and Krebs (1973)[20] as well as by others.

The effects of fructose, sorbitol, xylitol and ethanol on purine metabolism, originally described with respect to uric acid only, are now well known to be predominantly the consequence of an increased breakdown of purine nucleotides in the liver, notably of ATP, leading to a temporary depletion of the organ which by no means can *a priori* be considered harmless[21].

The famous German physician Bombastus Theophrastus von Hohenheim (Paracelsus) was the first to enunciate clearly, in the sixteenth century that the dose determines whether a substance is a benefit or a poison. Thus, publications and evaluations not considering dose as well as rate of administration may be meaningless. To explain that point let me present a comparison of the effects of fructose and xylitol on serum uric acid levels. Fructose infusions at a rate 0.5 g/kg/h, in contrast to an acute intravenous loading, do not change serum uric acid levels. At a rate of 1.0, and in particular at 1.5 g/kg/h, there is, however, a definite increase in serum uric acid[22]. In contrast, xylitol at a rate of 0.5 g/kg/h leads to an increase of serum uric acid from 4.65 mg/100 ml $\pm$ 0.78 to 7.16 mg/100 ml $\pm$ 0.92[13]. This serum uric acid elevation (Figure 5.8) is more pronounced than that observed with fructose infusions using a rate of 1.5 g/kg/h, i.e. the threefold load. Moreover, xylitol with infusion rates of only 0.3 and 0.4 g/kg/h causes serum uric acid to rise. In most subjects Heuckenkamp (1974)[23] was able to demonstrate that serum uric acid levels measured 24 h after the end of the infusion were still above those obtained immediately before the infusion. The reason for the latter phenomenon is not quite clear, but it makes unlikely the assumption that a breakdown of preformed adenine nucleotides may be the sole cause for the xylitol-induced hyperuricaemia.

It must also be realized that metabolic consequences of the administration

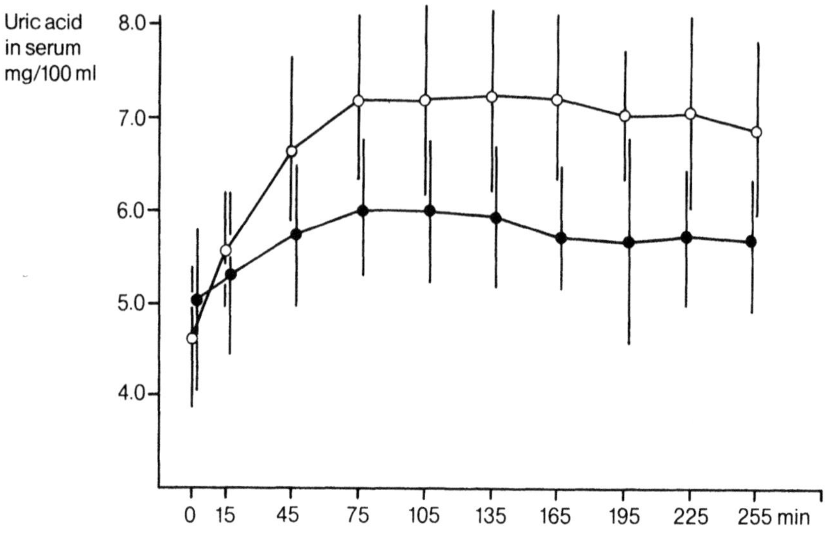

Figure 5.8 Comparison of serum uric acid levels in ten healthy volunteers (○—○) during xylitol infusions at the rate of 0.5 g/kg body weight/h with fourteen healthy volunteers (●—●) receiving fructose infusions at a rate of 1.5 (threefold load!) g/kg body weight/h

of substances which do not belong to man's normal food may uncover differences in biochemical individuality, related to genetics or disease states. Thomas *et al.* (1972)[24,25] have described complications of xylitol infusions which could not always be reproduced. This has caused considerable debate. Clinical research has often shown that differences are more often caused by faulty interpretation than by experimental errors.

CONCLUSIONS

Considering the available evidence, no case can be made for the use of sorbitol and xylitol in parenteral nutrition. In all respects, both substances are inferior to fructose, at all dose levels investigated.

Pending further studies there is no reason to accept claims that the polyols are utilized outside the liver in states where insulin-dependent glucose utilization is impaired, and the failure of the polyols to produce hyperglycaemia in these states may argue against their use.

From available evidence there is no reason to assume that mixtures of hexoses and polyols have any advantages over the administration of hexoses alone. This conclusion refers to energy supply as well as to the avoidance of side-effects.

The criticisms just raised are not final, but they reflect current thought, based on today's knowledge.

Again, considering the quantities involved, there is no serious reason against using limited amounts of polyols, for example in amino acid solutions administered in reasonable amounts at reasonable rates. However the committee on drugs of the German Medical Associations (Bundesärztekammer) has issued a warning against the extended use of xylitol. Possibly this warning is a reason for the use of mixtures.

There are no recognizable indications for galactose and maltose in parenteral nutrition. This leaves us with fructose and glucose. As an internist and nutritionist I consider that glucose remains the carbohydrate of choice in parenteral nutrition. In situations where its use may have to be limited, an increase in the amount of fat emulsions given should be considered as the first alternative source of energy. However, these may be indications for fructose given at reasonable rates, of not more than 0.2 g/kg/h over 24 h, provided biochemical monitoring of the patient is carried out frequently. And of course fructose solutions remain a useful way of giving water in most diabetics in whom carbohydrate metabolism is not severely deranged.

References

1. Woodyatt, R. T., Sansum, W. D. and Wilder, R. M. (1915). Prolonged and accurately timed intravenous injections of sugar. *J. Am. Med. Assoc.*, **65,** 1067
2. Strack, E., Reinhold, H. and Müller, F. (1962). Blutspiegel und Ausscheidung von Fructose bei intravasaler dauer infusion. *Z. ges. exp. Med.*, **135,** 431
3. Heuckenkamp, P.-U. and Zöllner, N. (1975). Quantitative comparison and evaluation of utilization of parenteral administered carbohydrates. *Nutr. Metab.*, **18** (Suppl. 1), 209
4. Zöllner, N., Heuckenkamp, P.-U. und Nechwatal, W. (1968). Über die Verwertung und renale ausscheidung von Fructose während ihrer langdauernden intravenösen Zufuhr. *Klinische Wochenschrift*, **46,** 1300
5. Keller, U. and Froesch, E. R. (1972). Vergleichende Untersuchungen über den Stoffwechsel von Xylit, Sorbit und Fructose beim Menschen. *Schweiz. med. Wschr.*, **102,** 1017
6. Keller, U. and Froesch, E. R. (1971). Metabolism and oxidation of U-^{14}C-glucose, xylitol, fructose and sorbitol in the fasted and in the streptozotocin-diabetes rat. *Diabetologia*, **7,** 349
7. Froesch, E. R. (1975). Umsatz und Verwertung von Glukose und Glukose austauschstoffen bei Mensch und Tier. *Nutr. Metab.*, **18** (Suppl. 1) 30
8. Felber, J.-P., Renold, A. E. and Zahnd, G. R. (1959). The comparative metabolism of glucose, fructose, galactose and sorbitol in normal subjects and disease states. *Mod. Probl. Paediat.*, (Karger) **4,** 467
9. Heuckenkamp, P.-U. und Zollner, N. (1970). Über das Verhalten von Galaktose, Glucose, Insulin und der freien Fettsauren im Plasma sowie der renalen Ausscheidung von Galaktose und Glucose während mehrestündiger Galaktoseinfusionen beim Menschen. *Z. ges. exp. Med.*, **153,** 136
10. Kleinzeller, A., Kolinská, J. and Benes, I. (1967). Transport of glucose and galactose in kidney cortex cells. *Biochem. J.*, **104,** 843
11. Levine, R. (1961). Concerning the mechanisms of insulin action. *Diabetes, N. Y.*, **10,** 421
12. Bickel, H., Bunte, H., Coats, D. A., Misch, P., von Rauffer, L. und Scranowitz, P. (1973). Die Verwertung parenteral verabreichter Kohlenhydrate in der postoperativen Phase. *Dtsch. med. Wschr.*, **89,** 809
13. Heuckenkamp, P.-U. und Zöllner, N. (1972). Xylitbilanz während mehrstündiger Infusionen mit konstanten Zufuhrraten bein gesunden Menschen. *Klinische Wochenschrift*, **50,** 1063

14. Müller, F., Strack, E., Kuhfahl, E. und Dettmer, D. (1967). Der Stoffwechsel von Xylit bei normalen und alloxandiabetischen Kaninchen. *Z. ges. exp. Med.*, **142,** 338
15. Bickel, H., Matzkies, F., Fekl, W. und Berg, G. (1973). Verwertung und Stoffwechselverhalten von Sorbit während parenteraler Langzeitinfusion. *Dtsch. med. Wschr.*, **98,** 2079
16. Sprandel, U., Heuckenkamp, P.-U. and Zöllner, N. (1975). Utilization of intravenous maltose. *Nutr. Metab.*, **19,** 96
17. Finke, C. und Reinauer, H. (1976). Uber den Abbau von infundierter Maltose beim Menschen. *Z. Ernahrungswiss.*, **15,** 231
18. Sprandel, U., Wolfram, G. and Scholz, R. (1976). Metabolism of maltose in perfused rat liver and in isolated hepatocytes. *Res. Exp. Med.*, **168,** 157
19. Berg, F., Matzkies, F. and Bickel, H. (1974). Dosierungsgrenzen bei der Infusion von Glucose, Sorbit, Fructose, Xylit und deren Mischungen. *Dtsch. med. Wschr.*, **99,** 633
20. Woods, H. F. and Krebs, H. A. (1973). Xylitol metabolism in the perfused rat liver. *Biochem. J.*, **134,** 437
21. Bode, J. Ch. (1973/74). Unerwünschte Stoffwechselwirkungen bei Gabe höherer Dosen von Fruktose und Sorbit. *Infusionstherapie*, **1,** 558
22. Heuckenkamp, P.-U. and Zöllner, N. (1971). Fructose-induced hyperuricaemia. *Lancet*, **i,** 808
23. Heuckenkamp, P.-U. (1974). Xylit in der parenteralen Ernährung. *Ernährungs-Umschau*, **21,** 70
24. Thomas, D. W., Edwards, J. B., Gillingan, J. E., Lawrence, J. R. and Edwards, R. G. (1972). Complications following intravenous administration of solutions containing xylitol. *Med. J. Aust.*, **1,** 1238
25. Thomas, D. W., Gilligan, J. E., Edwards, J. B. and Edwards, R. G. (1972). Lactic acidosis and osmotic diuresis produced by xylitol infusion. *Med. J. Aust.*, **1,** 1246

Panel Discussion

P. Vinay: (Canada) I should like to comment on the effect on uric acid metabolism of these analogues of glucose. Dr Zöllner has shown that hyperuricaemia is observed after the administration of xylitol or the administration of fructose. This is due not only to increased uric acid synthesis, but is also due to an acute suppression of uric acid secretion by the kidney. As more than 90% of daily uric acid excretion is through the kidney, if renal secretion is reduced significantly, then levels of urate in the plasma will automatically rise even if the rate of synthesis of uric acid is not increased. Both mechanisms work together to cause hyperuricaemia.

H. A. Krebs: (UK) I suppose that means that the xylitol also has an effect on renal function.

Vinay: Yes, through lactate formation. The lactate inhibits urate secretion.

Krebs: I would like to comment that in the isolated rat liver xylitol is not as effective as fructose in depleting the adenine nucleotides, ATP, ADP and AMP, and the blood level is the balance of the rate of formation and rate of secretion.

N. Zöllner: (Germany) We have also studied the renal retention of uric acid, and it is of a similar magnitude with fructose and with xylitol. I think that this is due to the fact that lactate is the common mediator, but also it is the shift in NAD, NADH relationship in the kidney tubule which inhibits the uric acid secretion.

J. T. Harries: (UK) In addition to histidine, there is some reason to believe that alanine may be an essential or semi-essential amino acid in the human newborn. Has Professor Krebs any information on metabolism of alanine in the tissues of experimental animals?

Krebs: I have no information on newborn animals, but I think that alanine is a very important intermediate metabolite because we know that alanine not only arises from proteolysis of ingested food and proteolysis when tissue proteins are broken down, but as C. A. Hill and his colleagues[1–5] have shown, much of the nitrogen which is set free by proteolysis in tissues leaves the tissue not in the form of the amino acid in which it is primarily released, but in the form of glutamine or alanine. Alanine and glutamine are carriers of nitrogen from the peripheral tissues to the liver. Not only are they carriers of nitrogen—which is converted eventually into urea—but the carbon skeleton of alanine can readily be converted after transamination, into pyruvate, and many other substances, in particular the non-essential amino acids, via pathways that are well established. Let me emphasize again that I am referring to adult animals. I have no information on the newborn.

G. L. Blackburn: (USA) I would join in the enthusiasm for carbohydrate but would make the point that it cannot be the complete fuel to meet the energy requirement.

Workers in Philadelphia[6] have looked at the $^{14}CO_2$ production using ^{14}C glucose continuous infusion technique and [^{14}C] glucose by single injection provided by 5% or 10% glucose. They then worked in the hyperalimentation range (25%) in both traumatized individuals and patients with cancer (Figure 1).

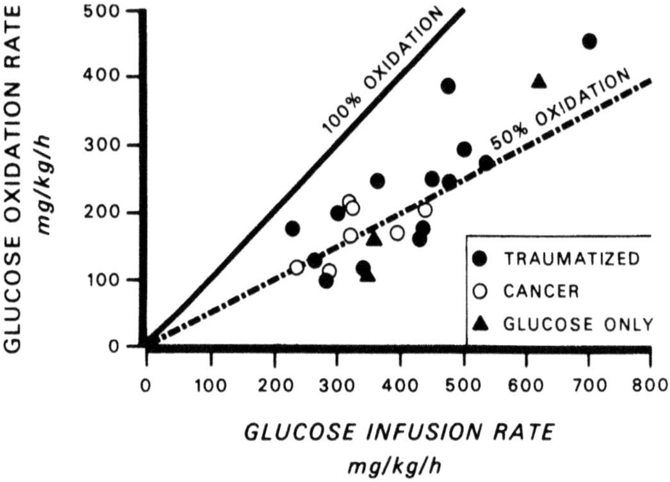

Figure 1 The relationship between glucose oxidation and glucose infusion rates after trauma, and in patients with cancer

At no level of infusion can a theoretical 100% oxidation (a complete recovery of the label in expired CO_2) be accomplished.

Most of the solutions used in standard hyperalimentation regimens provide about 16–20% of the energy requirement from protein. But even with hypertonic (25%), 600–700 g glucose intake, there is an obligatory requirement for energy that must come from lipid. Since none was provided, even at very low free fatty acid levels, approximately 20% of the energy expenditure did come from endogenous lipid stores. This situation may support those who suggest that a combination of lipid, protein and carbohydrate fits best with body requirements, even when the entire exogenous fuel source for energy expenditure is provided as glucose only. More glucose is being provided than is being expended, so this must be stored, first as glycogen, which has a finite limit.

Our work [7,8] shows that we must give more calories as glucose than we can account for by oxidation in order to obtain nitrogen balance (i.e. nitrogen infused retained in the body cell mass). Again a theoretical calculation of the thermogenesis or the specific dynamic action of the conversion of glucose to triglyceride would come up with a value considerably higher than observed in published measurements, and more fitting with the calories required for nitrogen balance. Many people such as Kinney, Shizgal, Wilmore and others have shown that 35–45 cal/kg must be provided, and yet the energy expenditure is more like 30 cal/kg; therefore the other glucose calories must be stored as triglyceride at a cost.

This forced hepatic lipogenesis does take work and is thermogenic. The resulting increased core temperature may have an effect on enzymatic pathways: the so-called thermogenic coefficient.

Glucose is a marvellous fuel but it cannot be the optimal source to meet the energy requirement during hyperalimentation. Particularly if visceral protein metabolism is the goal of therapy (*Anesthesiol.*, **47**, 101–114 (1977).)

Krebs: I should like to emphasize what has been said. We know that the majority (from the quantitative point of view) of tissues in the mammal primarily use fat as a fuel. Only the brain and its derivatives, the retina and peripheral nerves, the blood cells and a few other tissues, such as the renal medulla, depend on glucose as a fuel of respiration and cannot use fat or other substances in major quantities. But the majority of tissues such as the kidney, the liver, and muscle except in very severe exercise, use fat for preference, derived from circulating free fatty acids attached to plasma proteins.

Much of the glucose which eventually serves as a fuel of respiration goes through fat. The store of energy in the form of glycogen is limited and much of the glucose ingested on a high-carbohydrate diet is converted into fat before it is utilized, with the fat serving as a store. We all agree on the importance of fat as a fuel, which has to be borne in mind in parenteral nutrition.

Zöllner: If the energy is given as fat, very little carbohydrate is needed to make a negative balance positive.

H. F. Woods: (UK) It is important at this stage to separate out the different functions of carbohydrate. I presume that Dr Blackburn referred to uniformly-labelled glucose. One would not expect a 100% recovery of all the carbon as radioactive labelled carbon dioxide. We must remember that a very important function of the C_6 carbohydrate skeleton, is the provision of building blocks. Going down the glycolytic chain, for example, a lot of the carbon is siphoned off down side pathways to provide skeletons for amino acids and to base the argument on not recovering 100% of the carbon from carbohydrate does not necessarily hold. Some of that carbohydrate is utilized for the synthesis of other compounds which are themselves tissue constituents.

Blackburn: Not only was uniformly ^{14}C-labelled glucose used, but it was a steady state system, and one priming infusion of [^{14}C] glucose was also used to confirm that indeed the other pathways were filled and a steady state obtained, and yet 100% clearance and oxidation of the glucose to CO_2 was not obtained.

Vinay: I should like to emphasize the point made by Professor Woods. Some of the carbon chain will be retained as building blocks in the body and will therefore not be recovered as ^{14}C. Isotopic exchange occurs, and 100% of the carbon cannot appear as ^{14}C or CO_2 even if 100% of the glucose went to CO_2. Because of the isotopic dilution problem one must be cautious in interpreting such data.

Woods: Professor Krebs and Dr Weideman, in 1968[9], showed quite conclusively the pitfalls of even these steady state infusions using radioactive levels. One cannot necessarily make firm conclusions about total turnover of radioactively labelled compounds because of the metabolic exchanges to which Dr Vinay has been alluding.

To go back to uric acid over-production, it is important to realize that the acute depletion of ATP has effects other than that emphasized by Dr Vinay. More recent work from Germany has shown an inhibition of RNA synthesis in regenerating liver if fructose is infused. Presumably this is in some way related to the ATP depletion. Walton and I have shown that triglyceride synthesis can also be inhibited by fructose. This is rather anomalous as it is said that high-fructose-containing diets promote triglyceride synthesis. If enough fructose is given under certain circumstances, triglyceride synthesis from fatty acid can be inhibited.

I should also like to emphasize that the mechanism is common to all three substrates and it does not matter whether xylitol, sorbitol or fructose is used. It has nothing to do with demand for ATP to phosphorylate the primary product. The extra ATP requirements per gram of liver to phosphorylate each of those substrates at its maximal rate can be calculated. Even at the fastest rates of phosphorylation, that extra demand for ATP is no more than 20% of the total ATP turnover in unit time in the liver.

Each of those compounds gives rise to a build-up within the liver of a phosphorylated intermediate; fructose-1-phosphate in the case of fructose. If glycerol is given then it is α-glycero-phosphate and with xylitol it is α-glycero-phosphate.

I have argued against the massive sudden infusion of these compounds because I do not see the logic in infusing a compound which will lower ATP concentrations, possibly inhibit protein synthesis, RNA synthesis and triglyceride synthesis in a situation where one is trying to benefit the patient by promoting tissue synthesis.

P. Fürst: (Sweden) One of the most important points should be to supply the patient with glyconeogenic substrate in an attempt to produce glycogen in the post-traumatic situation.

Using direct *dissemination* of glycogen in muscle tissue, the glycogen content drops 4 or 5 days after an uncomplicated operation—despite the fact that 200 g glucose is infused daily.

We have tested glycogen synthesis in post-operative patients compared with normal healthy volunteers and the rate of synthesis is significantly lower after operation. Normal individuals synthesize about 3.5 g glycogen whereas the post-traumatic patients synthetize about half this amount. Perhaps one of the most important problems is the block to glycogen synthesis in these patients.

I have a question for Professors Krebs and Woods. What is their opinion about direct utilization of fructose in muscle? Some recent articles suggest this possibility. All recent evidence is based on experiments where the glucose concentration in the *media* was kept as high as the physiological extracellular concentration. At this level the constant from the K-enzyme inhibits the direct utilization of fructose. However, the glucose concentration in muscle cells is very low. I would therefore like to ask whether it is a possible route for fructose following infusion.

Krebs: I cannot remember any specific information about the utilization of fructose by muscle tissue. Many years ago, in the early 1930s, Dickens and Greville[10, 11] published a number of papers on the utilization of fructose by different animal tissues, especially the anaerobic formation of lactate, which was relatively low in most tissues, except the liver, compared with lactate production from glucose.

Woods: The arguments follow exactly what Dr Fürst has said. The muscle can utilize fructose *in vitro*, not by the keto *hexokinase* pathway, but by phosphorylating the fructose to fructose-6-phosphate using hexokinase.

The objectors to the story that muscle must be a major tissue for fructose utilization—an argument that I have used myself in the past—have based their argument on the fact that if glucose is present, the K_m for hexokinase for fructose is very high, in the region of 12–15 mmol/l. Under those circumstances in the presence of reasonable physiological concentrations of glucose, one would not expect major phosphorylation of fructose to fructose-6-phosphate.

However, I am aware that those who have been doing work on freshly obtained muscle biopsy material show that the intracellular concentration of glucose is not, as we have assumed, quite high, but reasonably low. Under those circumstances, it is quite possible that a substantial proportion of fructose would be utilized directly via the hexokinase pathway.

Vinay: I was a bit surprised after analysing two biopsies, one taken from a patient who had received a small amount of fructose, and who demonstrated normal levels of ATP, compared to those in patients that had received equivalent amounts of glucose. What about the long-term administration of fructose? It is possible that this rapid and acute depletion in cell ATP that Professor Woods and others have demonstrated is an acute phenomenon, reversible with time, and after 2–3 weeks the liver restores its nucleotide content to normal?

Woods: That suggestion is possible. Some of Dr Vinay's own results could be very nicely explained on that basis.

It is certainly true that in isolated perfused tissue, the adenine nucleotides do in fact return to normal within 2 h. The trouble is that the rate of utilization of the primary substrate, be it fructose, xylitol, or glycerol, has decreased.

That in itself does not matter. It is whether the concentration of the phosphorylated intermediate has decreased. In our hands it does not. What does happen is that the inorganic phosphate concentration of the liver recovers. I would suspect that one possible mechanism would be the re-inhibition of adenosine diaminase and 5-nucleotidase because phosphate gets back into the cell.

The provision of phosphate with fructose or xylitol, or glycerol, prevents to some extent the ATP depletion, which would support that argument. The eventual recovery has nothing to do with the rate of metabolism of fructose, but rather shows that the phosphate is getting back in again.

Vinay: So in fact we do not know whether chronic administration of fructose is as bad as we always thought that it was.

Woods: I do not like the word 'bad'. What we ought to say is that it is not always an advantage in every situation.

D. E. F. Tweedle: (UK) I should like to revert to the points made by Professor Krebs about alanine and glycine.

He asked why there was so much glycine in various amino acid solutions. I suspect that the answer has two parts. First, as Professor Krebs himself pointed out, the incorrect belief that glycine is a particularly potent gluconeogenic amino acid; and second, that it is the cheapest amino acid available commercially.

As to alanine, he made the point that it is the best gluconeogenic amino acid, and that was a good reason for putting a large quantity of alanine in the solutions. However, I must make a cautionary comment about that. Johnston and I reported some studies in patients infused with various amino acid solutions after operation. Whilst the nitrogen balances differed we found that large quantities of nitrogen were excreted in the urine with certain solutions. Using high-voltage electrophoresis it became apparent that not only were large quantities of glycine excreted, but with some of the solutions, large quantities of alanine were also being lost. With one particular solution, when 25% of the amino acids were in the form of alanine, large quantities came out, when the alanine content was reduced to 15%, alanine could no longer be detected in the urine. There must therefore be a limit to the amount of alanine that can with certainty be infused after operation.

Fit and healthy subjects can probably synthesize the necessary non-essential amino acids. However, some work done in Newcastle shows that after operation in adults, and also in the newborn, the ability to synthesize some of the so-called non-essential amino acids is different from healthy adults; as we are usually treating sick patients with impaired synthetic pathways, I suggest that there is a good reason for including various non-essential amino acids in these solutions, for example tyrosine and cystine.

Krebs: I quite agree that we do not know how metabolically competent the organism is as a whole immediately after an operation. My considerations were concerned with a situation where the individual was reasonably healthy from the metabolic point of view, where disturbances in the gastrointestinal tract alone were responsible for the need for parenteral nutrition.

As for the inclusion of glycine, I rather put that in the form of a question. I said that I was not sure what the case for it would be. I take it that the Travasol* formulation was devised quite a long time ago. If I were to be asked to design such a solution of amino acids, it would be—from the point of view of basic biochemistry—very similar except for the glycine.

N. J. Kartinos: (USA) I believe that we started to develop the Travasol formula in about 1970. In 8.5% Travasol about 20% of the total amino acids is as alanine and 20% as glycine or amino-acetic acid.

One of the reasons for the glycine content was to provide some non-essential amino acids. We were also persuaded that glycine is one of the rate-limiting acids in haemoglobin and some plasma protein synthesis, as demonstrated in Italy by Giordano and his colleagues[12]. We felt that it was beneficial and innocuous, in view of the data that they had produced.

Our original formula did not have tyrosine, but we were persuaded that there are difficulties, particularly in neonates, of converting phenylalanine to tyrosine, so we modified the formula and introduced a low level of tyrosine. I have not heard that it is an inadequate level.

Krebs: It is true that glycine is essential for haemoglobin synthesis but it can be very easily obtained from *serine*, which can itself be obtained from carbohydrate and transamination processes. So there are alternatives.

* Synthamin.

References

1. Felig, P., Owen, O. E., Wahren, J. and Cahill, G. F. (1969). Amino acid metabolism during prolonged starvation. *J. Clin. Invest.*, **48,** 584
2. Pozefsky, T., Felig, P., Tobin, J. D., Soelchner, J. S. and Cahill, G. F. (1969). Amino acid balance across tissues of the forearm in postabsorptive man. Effects of insulin at two dose levels. *J. Clin. Invest.*, **48,** 2273
3. Marliss, E. B., Aoki, T. T., Pozefsky, T., Most, A. S. and Cahill, G. F. Muscle and splanchnic glutamine and glutamate metabolism in postabsorptive and starved man. *J. Clin. Invest.*, **50,** 814
4. London, D. R. and Foley, R. H. (1965). Evidence for the release of individual amino acids from the resting human forearm. *Nature* (*Lond.*) **208,** 588
5. Carlsten, A., Hallgren, B., Jagenburg, R., Svanborg, A. and Werkö, L. (1967). Arterio-hepatic venous differences of free fatty acids and amino acids. Studies in patients with diabetes or essential hypercholesterolemia, and in healthy individuals. *Acta Med. Scand.*, **181,** 199
6. Myers, R. N., Smink, R. D., Skutches, G. L., Paul, P. and Reichard, G. A. Jr. *J. Can. Res.* (in press)
7. Rutten, P., Blackburn, G. L., Flatt, J. P., *et al.* (1975). Determination of optimal hyperalimentation infusion rate. *J. Surg. Res.*, **18,** 477
8. Blackburn, G. L. (1975). Nitrogen conservation using fat as a non-protein calorie source. *Proceedings AMA Symposium on Fat Emulsion in Parenteral Nutrition.* (Chicago)
9. Krebs, H. A., Hems, R., Weideman, M. J. and Speake, R. N. (1966). *Biochem. J.*, **101,** 242

10. Dickens, F. and Greville, G. D. (1932). The conversion of fructose and glucose to lactic acid by embryonic tissues. *Biochem. J.*, **26**, 1251
11. Dickens, F. and Greville, G. D. (1933). Respiration in fructose and in sugar-free media. *Biochem. J.*, **27**, 832
12. Giordano, C. *et al.* (1970). Histidine and glycine indispensable amino acids for globin synthesis in uraemia. Private communication

Section III
Amino Acids in Parenteral Nutrition

6
Intracellular amino acids and energy metabolism in catabolic patients with regard to muscle tissue

P. FÜRST, J. BERGSTRÖM, E. VINNARS, B. SCHILDT AND B. HOLMSTRÖM

INTRODUCTION

Weakness and tiring easily are the most common symptoms of surgical convalescence. This response is more severe and prolonged than the associated bed-rest and decreased nutrition can account for. A prominent feature of acute surgical catabolism is an obligatory negative nitrogen balance, associated with protein breakdown. Despite the repeated confirmation of these findings since the first reports in 1930, the underlying mechanism and physiological significance remains obscure. The observed clinical weakness and fatigue may be the result of the negative nitrogen balance which is largely due to the breakdown of muscle protein.

Clinical observation has confirmed that practically every condition which is associated with weight loss is also associated with muscle wasting. The accelerated muscle protein breakdown in catabolic patients suggests an alteration of the cytoplasmic amino acid profile in muscle, which could affect protein synthesis at the cellular level in the ribosomes.

The weakness and fatigue of surgical convalescence may also be related to abnormalities in glycolysis or the TCA cycle and the associated production of high energy bonds, such as ATP and phosphocreatine (PC). The pathways of ATP resynthesis occur simultaneously in the muscle and are in equilibrium with the rate of ATP breakdown. This equilibrium is dependent on the rate of energy expenditure in the muscle cell in different pathological conditions.

Analysis of skeletal muscle tissue provides the best estimation of the average intracellular solute composition in the whole organism, since skeletal muscle is by far the most abundant cellular tissue in the body and relatively uniform as to cellular composition.

Sampling muscle tissue in man and the methods of biochemical determination are still difficult. This is probably the reason why intracellular solute studies in human muscle have not been performed previously. A technique for percutaneous needle biopsy of skeletal muscle was developed by Bergström, which permits repeated sampling of muscle tissue[1].

The new biopsy technique was used originally for studies of intracellular water and electrolyte metabolism in muscle tissue. It was, however, soon apparent that the method could also be used for the study of other tissue constituents. In the last 10 years various aspects of energy, carbohydrate, lipid, protein, and mineral metabolism under normal and pathological conditions have been studied. The method has also proved to be suitable for the study of muscle morphology by light and electron microscopy.

The technique of obtaining samples and the diagnostic and research opportunities offered by this technique have been discussed extensively in two current reviews[2,3]. In the present communication we present a survey of clinical research in which percutaneous needle biopsy has been used successfully in an attempt to investigate intermediary energy metabolism and intracellular muscle free amino acid metabolism in the catabolic state. Direct measurements of muscle intracellular amino acid patterns and concentrations of energy intermediates in surgical catabolism may provide a better understanding of post-injury intracellular metabolism and assist in the development of guidelines for improved timing and composition of nutritional support.

Methods

The biopsy needle consists of a sharp-tipped hollow outer needle with a small opening 'window' near the tip (Figure 6.1). A cylinder with a sharp edge fits tightly into the needle. The needle is inserted under local anaesthaesia through a small incision into the muscle (usually the vastus lateralis muscle) and one or more pieces of tissue bulging into the 'window' are punched out with the sharp cylinder. This method of sampling is rapid and only slightly traumatic. It can be repeated therefore several times in the same individual.

With a biopsy needle 4.5 mm in diameter, about 20–100 mg of muscle tissue is obtained. When fresh muscle is needed, the sample is weighed immediately on a sensitive electrobalance, and the weight curve extrapolated to zero time to compensate for water evaporation.

The technique for muscle sampling from the quadriceps femoris, the method for weighing the specimens, and the methods for determinations of neutral fat, water, chloride, sodium, potassium, magnesium and free amino acids in

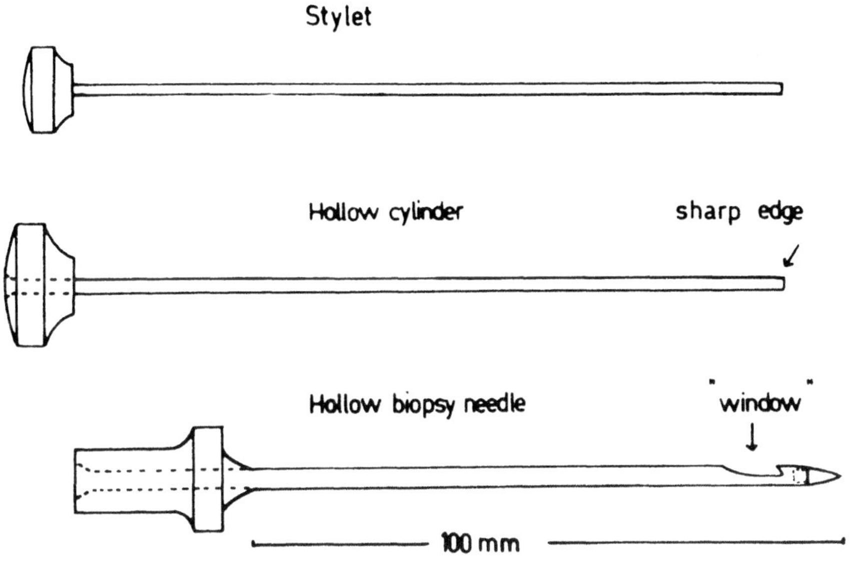

Figure 6.1 Punch biopsy needle, hollow cylinder with sharp edge and the stylet for pushing out biopsy specimens from the cylinder

muscle tissue and plasma have been described earlier in detail[1,4–6], and are illustrated schematically in Figure 6.2.

The calculation of the extra- and intracellular distribution of water and the intracellular concentration of electrolytes and amino acids is based on the chloride method using Nernst's equation where the chloride distribution constant is a function of the membrane potential[1,5–7].

A reliable method must be used for the estimation of the extracellular fluid volume in order to enable the calculation of the intracellular concentration of an individual solute in muscle tissue. The chloride method is generally used for this purpose. The reliability of the chloride method, however, requires that the transmembrane potential is known or else assumed to be normal. This potential has been measured directly and found to be about −88 mV[8] in healthy subjects. However, it has been shown that severely ill patients[9], severely uraemic patients[10,11] and experimental animals[12,13] may have a decreased negative transmembrane potential.

As direct measurements of the membrane potential were not made a computer program was developed to estimate the effect of a decreased potential on the water distribution and the distribution of the different substances studied. In this equation the different variables (water, electrolytes and free amino acids) and the membrane potential are expressed according

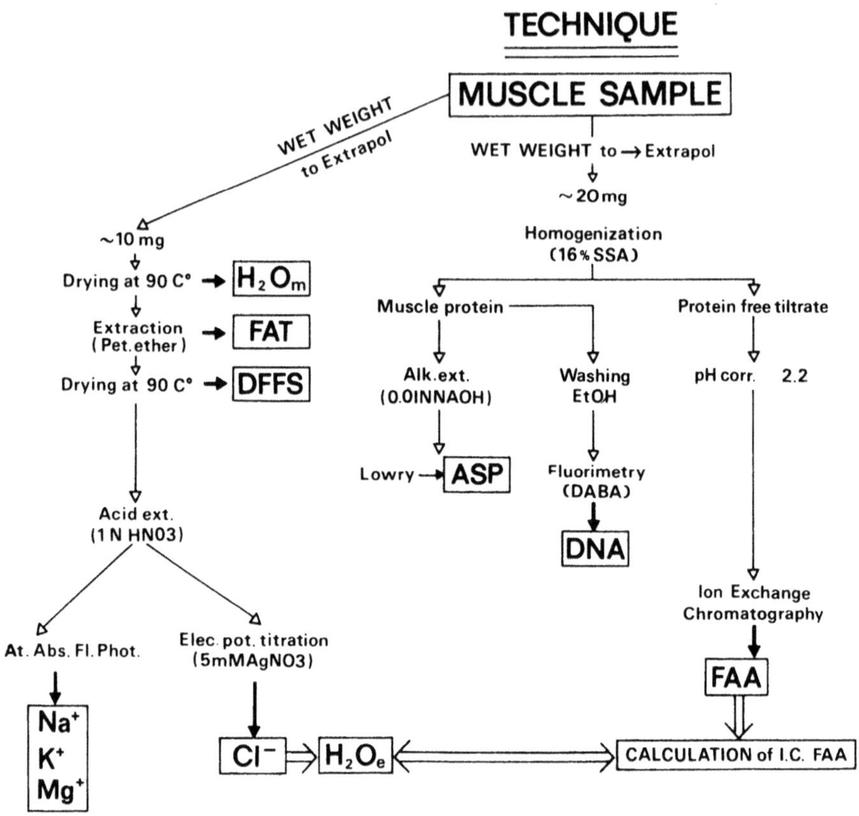

Figure 6.2 Schematic illustrations of the procedure used.

Abbreviations: ↓ Preparations and processes
⬇ Direct determinations
⇓ Calculations

DFFS = Dry, fat free solids
H_2O_m = Muscle water
H_2O_e = Extracellular water
ASP = Alkaline soluble protein
FAA = Free amino acids
DABA = 3,5-diaminobenzoic acid
SSA = Sulphosalicylic acid

to exponential functions where the membrane potential is used as a stepless variable from −50 to −100 mV.

$$[A_i] = \frac{e^{E/26.7}\left[1000\,A_m - \frac{[A_p]\,Cl_m\,0.96\,(984 - 7.18\,P)}{[Cl_p]}\right] - 1000\,A_m + [A_p]\,H_2O_m}{e^{E/26.7}\cdot H_2O_m - \frac{Cl_m\,0.96\,(984 - 7.18\,P)}{[Cl_p]}}$$

A_i = the concentration of the amino acid in intracellular muscle water
A_m = the content of the amino acid in muscle
A_p = the concentration of the amino acid in plasma
Cl_m = the content of chloride in muscle
Cl_p = the concentration of chloride in plasma
P = the concentration of protein in plasma
H_2O_m = the content of water in muscle
E = the membrane potential
e = the base of the natural logarithms

If labile metabolites are to be measured it is essential that the samples are frozen as quickly as possible (1–2 s) by plunging the biopsy needle into liquid freon maintained at its melting point −150 °C. The samples are stored in liquid nitrogen. The frozen samples are then lyophilized by freeze drying, and usually weigh 30–80 mg. The dried samples are powdered and all visible connective tissue removed. The amount of connective tissue varies from sample to sample and its removal is of the greatest importance. The further preparation, the analytical technique, and normal values have been described previously[14]. A schematic presentation of the procedures used is given in Figure 6.3.

Intracellular muscle amino acids

It is known from animal experiments that the concentration of most free amino acids is much higher in cells than in extracellular fluid[15]. For this reason it is not possible to evaluate the total pool of free amino acids by only determining concentrations in plasma. Recently we have adapted ion exchange chromatography for determination of free amino acids in muscle tissue obtained by percutaneous needle biopsy[15–17].

It was possible for the first time using this technique to obtain reliable data on the intracellular concentration and the ratio of intra- to extra-cellular concentration of more than 30 amino acids in normal man (Figure 6.4). It was found that the muscle cells in 32 healthy volunteers contained higher concentrations of amino acids than found in plasma. The concentration gradient was especially high for taurine, glutamic acid and glutamine. The essential amino acids valine, leucine, isoleucine and phenylalanine and the non-essential amino acids citrulline and tyrosine had a gradient below 2. The remainder showed a gradient between 5 and 10. The total pool of intra-cellular free amino acids in muscle tissue was estimated to be about 86.5 g for a 'normal man' (70 kg) assuming a muscle mass of 40% of the body weight.

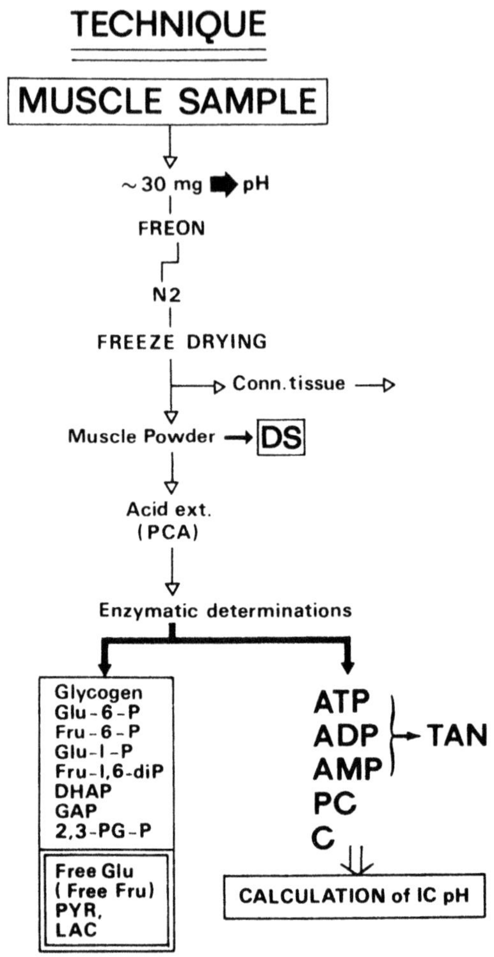

Figure 6.3 Schematic illustration of the procedures used for labile metabolites

Abbreviations: ↓

⬇

⇓

DS = Dry solids

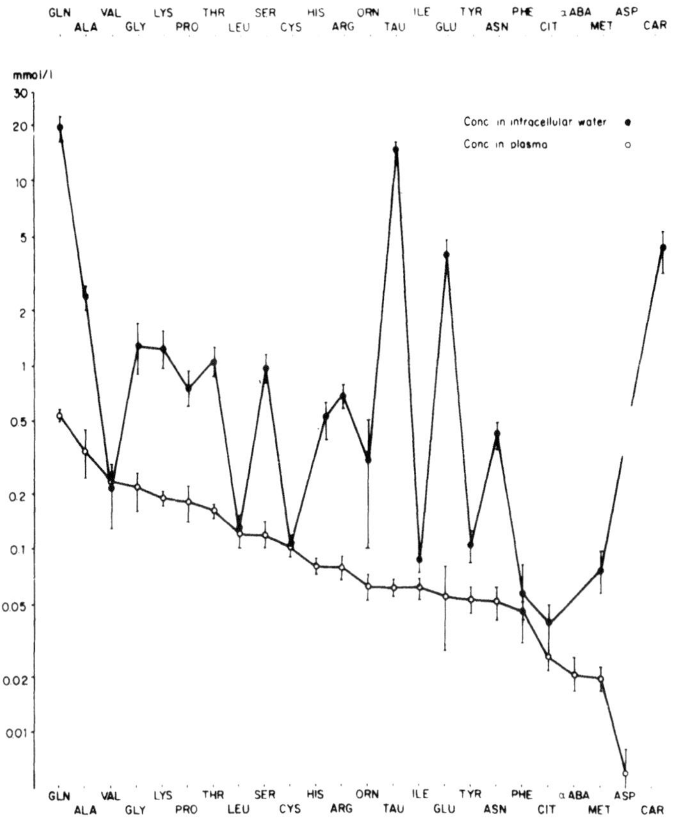

Figure 6.4 Comparison between aminograms in plasma water and intracellular muscle water in 32 healthy subjects. Means ± SD are given

The method has now been used in different catabolic conditions such as the postoperative period[17–19] and severe uraemia[16,20–22]. Abnormal intracellular amino acid patterns have been found in different diseases and the basic knowledge emerging from such experiments may serve as a guideline for improving nutritional therapy in various pathological conditions.

The effect of postoperative trauma

It was reported earlier that the concentration of intracellular free amino acids and the concentrations of amino acids in plasma showed many changes as a result of postoperative trauma[17,18]. Muscle tissue was obtained in these studies before uncomplicated major operations and on the third postoperative day after 8 h overnight fast. The patients were maintained on intravenous feeding (as carbohydrate), electrolytes, and vitamins. No nitrogen or fat was given.

The most significant change in plasma compared with normal controls was an increase in phenylalanine and tyrosine but a decrease in isoleucine and histidine concentrations. The concentrations of serine and proline showed a more moderate decrease while the level of leucine increased slightly.

Many of the changes demonstrated intracellularly were not reflected in the plasma. There was a highly significant decrease in muscle tissue in the concentrations of glutamine, arginine and lysine and a significant fall in proline and glutamic acid concentrations. The increases in the concentrations of taurine, valine and phenylalanine were all highly significant. A significant rise occurred in the concentrations of serine, glycine, alanine and leucine whereas the rise in tyrosine and citrulline concentrations was almost significant.

It has been suggested that an abnormal plasma amino acid profile may be a sign of protein catabolism[23]. It can therefore also be expected that protein catabolism will be reflected in the free muscle amino acid pattern. However, the particular abnormalities in intracellular free amino acid concentrations found in post-traumatic catabolism were not seen in untreated or dietary treated uraemia[20–22], in patients on intermittent peritoneal dialysis[16], or in untreated diabetes[24] (Figure 6.4).

These specific alterations indicate that the abnormalities found after operation cannot simply be explained as a single effect of poor nutrition or general effects of catabolism.

The effect of total parenteral nutrition

To elucidate the effect of total parenteral nutrition including the administration of amino acid solutions, patients were studied[19,25] before and after colon resection.

For 4 days prior to surgery the patients were given a Vivasorb diet only, to provide standardized preoperative nutrition and to obtain a low residue in the intestine at the time of operation. Postoperatively the patients were given total parenteral nutrition for 6 days with fixed energy intake (147 kJ/kg BW/24 h) including both fat and carbohydrates and two different levels of nitrogen intake (145 and 237 mg of amino acid nitrogen, respectively/kg BW/24 h). Two solutions with different amino acid compositions were compared at the lower nitrogen intake (Vamin, and Intramin Forte). At the higher nitrogen intake, only Intramin Forte was used. Three percutaneous muscle biopsies were obtained in each patient, before the synthetic diet, before the operation and on the 4th postoperative day. Nitrogen balance was measured throughout the studies.

These studies show that complete parenteral nutrition results in an improvement of the nitrogen balance in patients with postoperative catabolism, (Figure 6.5). On the other hand, our observations also indicate that intracellular deficiencies are very difficult to correct.

After operation without an amino acid supply highly significant increases were found in valine and leucine concentrations in the intracellular muscle water of all groups studied, whereas the increase in the intracellular isoleucine

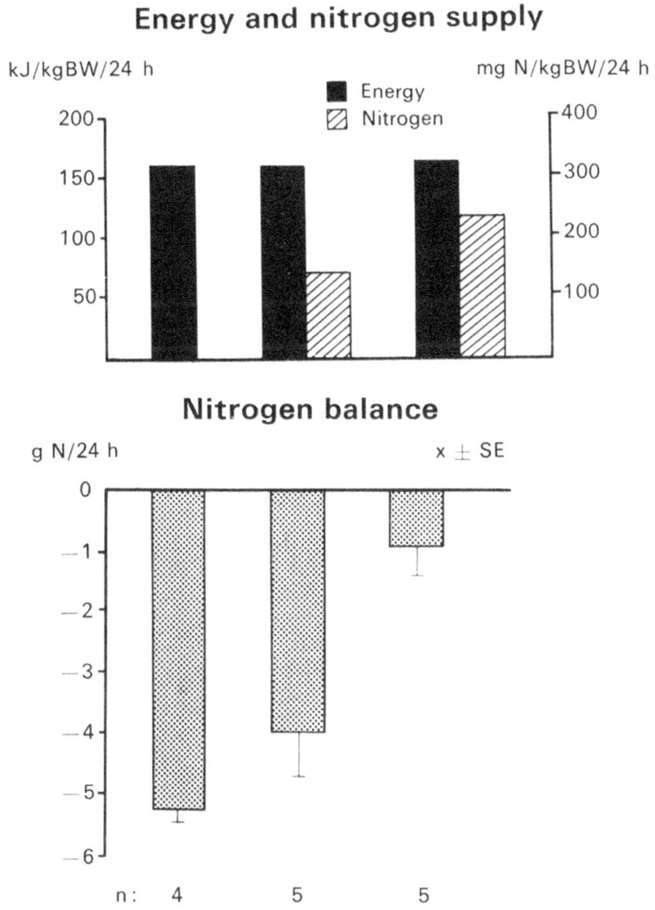

Figure 6.5 Energy and nitrogen supply and the nitrogen balance in patients kept on parenteral nutrition following colon resection. The nitrogen balance is expressed as the mean at the first 6 days after the operation. Post-operatively the patients were given total parenteral nutrition for 6 days with fixed energy intake (147 kJ/kg BW/24 h) including both fat and carbohydrates and two different levels of nitrogen intake. Two solutions with different amino acid compositions (Vamin, and Intramin Forte) were compared at the lower nitrogen intake (145 mg N/kg BN/24 h). At the higher nitrogen intake (237 mg N/kg BN/24 h) only Intramin Forte was used

concentration was not as pronounced. As a consequence the intracellular branched-chain amino acid pool was increased[17,18]. When amino acid solutions were infused the rise in the intracellular compartment involving valine and leucine was still present, whereas isoleucine was unaltered (Figure 6.6). The results suggest that the proportions of amino acids in the solutions used were not optimal for postoperative trauma and suggests that the increases were due to imbalanced composition of the three branched-chain amino acids infused rather than the total amount given.

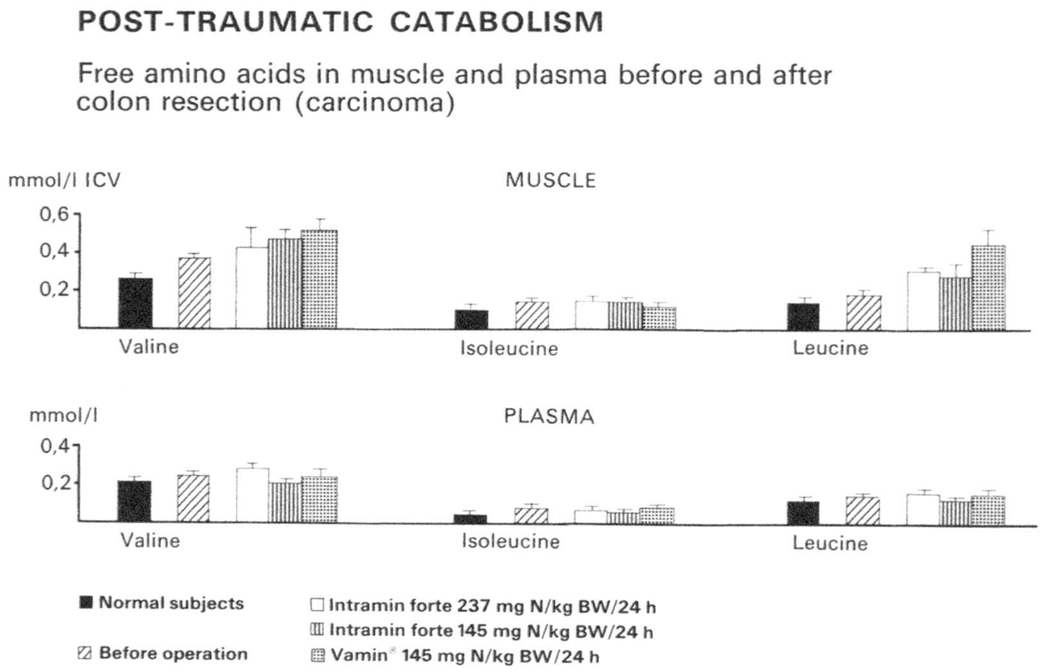

Figure 6.6 The concentration of valine, isoleucine and leucine in plasma and intracellular muscle water in patients before and 4 days after colon resection. (Mean $\pm$ SE)

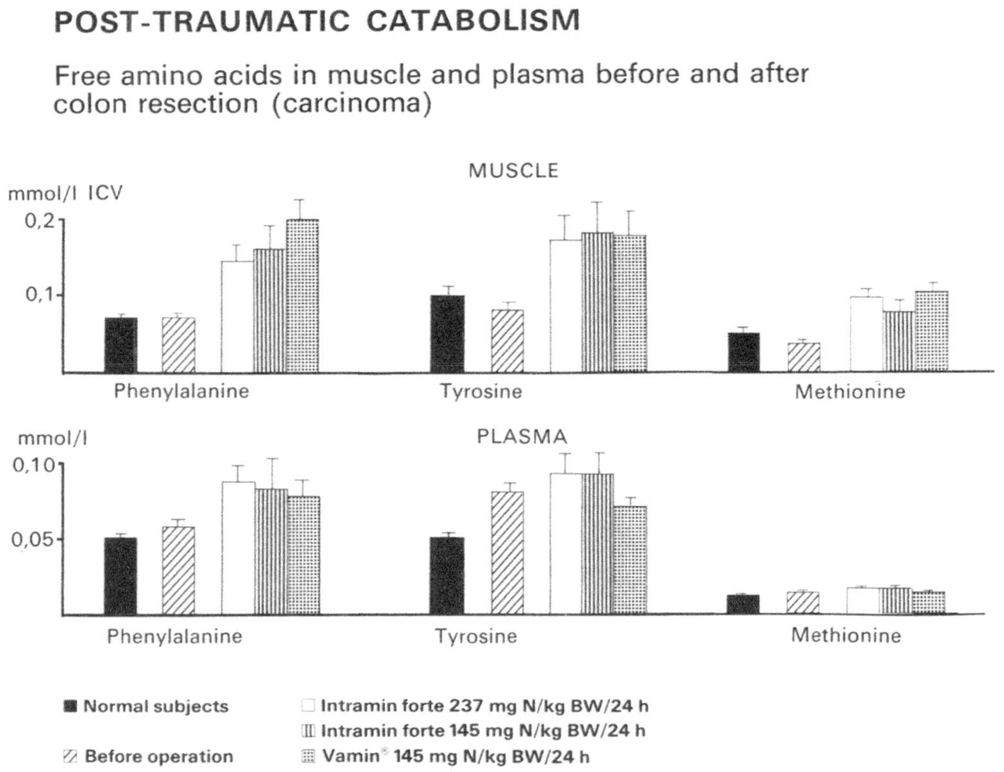

Figure 6.7 The concentration of phenylalanine, tyrosine and methionine in plasma and intracellular muscle water in patients before and 4 days after colon resection. (Mean ± SE)

The essential nature and even antagonism of structurally related amino acids such as leucine, isoleucine and valine have been reported earlier. Excess of any of these amino acids in a rat's diet resulted in depression of growth which could be relieved by adding the other two amino acids. It was also found that excessive intake of leucine depressed the isoleucine and valine levels in plasma and skeletal muscle, which could be corrected by administration of isoleucine and valine[26].

There is evidence that imbalances cause antagonism and increase amino acid requirements. Amino acid antagonism and/or imbalance may stimulate amino acid catabolism and result in a decrease in the pool of amino acids which is already limiting.

It is now recognized that post-traumatic and other forms of catabolism may result in a suppression of protein synthesis rather than an increased protein breakdown[27,28]. Such conditions are associated with high concentrations of branched-chain amino acids in skeletal muscle[28]. It is possible that the high intracellular accumulation of branched-chain amino acids (valine and leucine) in post-traumatic patients and in patients treated with peritoneal dialysis[16] (isoleucine and leucine) may be a consequence of inhibited muscle protein synthesis.

The phenylalanine/tyrosine ratio was also increased postoperatively. The increase was more pronounced in the groups with the lower nitrogen administration. The intracellular concentration of methionine was increased in muscle. This increase was not influenced by the amount of nitrogen supplied or the type of amino acid solution given (Figure 6.7). Cystine has a very low and undetectable intracellular concentration in muscle tissue. It is of interest that following Intramin Forte administration, a normal or slightly elevated plasma cysteine concentration was found, despite the fact that the solution does not contain any cystine.

As reported earlier, a typical feature of post-traumatic catabolism without amino acid nutrition was a decreased glutamine and glutamic acid concentration in muscle tissue. None of the solutions restored the normal intracellular concentration of glutamine. The intracellular concentration was, however, elevated significantly with a higher level of nitrogen intake. The low glutamic acid concentration was raised when the concentrated amino acid solution was given. In contrast, an unchanged low intracellular glutamic acid concentration was found with solutions containing less amino acids (Figure 6.8). The improvement of intracellular glutamine and the normalization of glutamic acid were achieved with a solution lacking glutamic acid. The results indicate that intracellular glutamine depletion following trauma is due to a lack of nonessential nitrogen, an accelerated gluconeogenesis and increased urea synthesis rather than to a specific deprivation of glutamine.

A decreased level of intracellular lysine in muscle tissue was the most consistent finding in postoperative catabolism in patients without amino acid administration. Irrespective of which amino acid solution was given

POST-TRAUMATIC CATABOLISM

Free amino acids in muscle and plasma before and after colon resection (carcinoma)

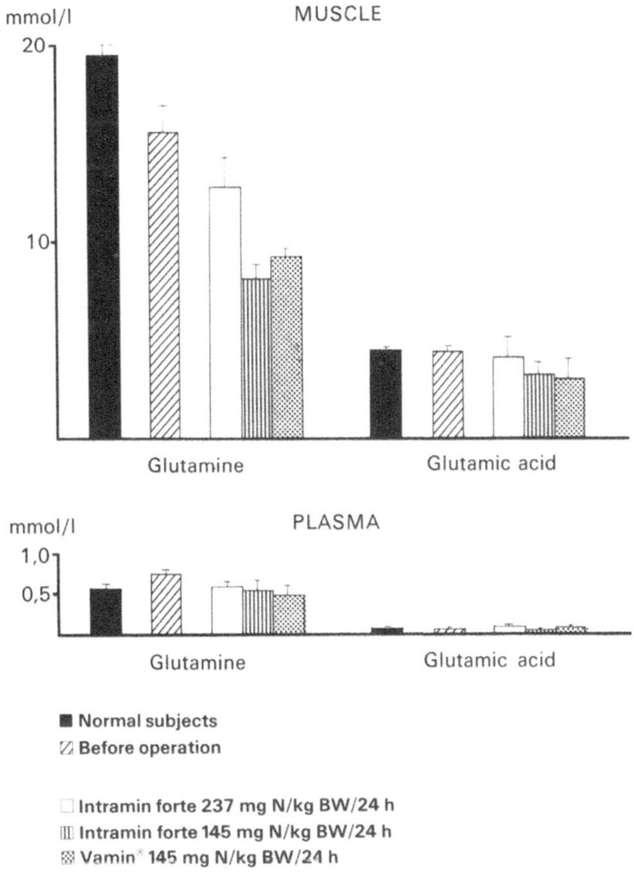

Figure 6.8 The concentration of glutamic acid and glutamine in plasma and intracellular water in patients before and 4 days after colon resection. (Mean ± SE)

at the lower level, only a slight improvement was found in the intracellular lysine concentration. However, the infusion of 237 mg amino acid nitrogen corresponding to 77 mg lysine/kg BW/day resulted in normal intracellular free lysine concentration in muscle (Figure 6.9).

When nitrogen balance data are compared with intracellular muscle free lysine concentrations, a relationship is found between the negativity of the nitrogen balance and the degree of depletion in the intracellular lysine pool.

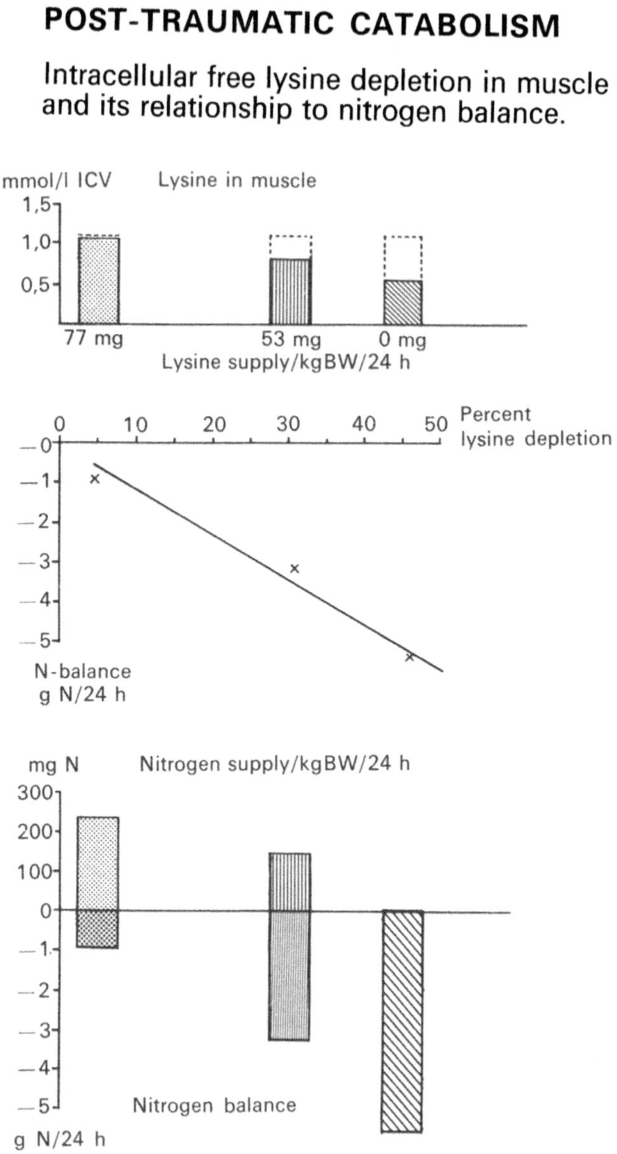

Figure 6.9 The intracellular lysine pool, the lysine and total nitrogen supply, the nitrogen balance and its relationship to the intracellular lysine depletion, expressed as percentage at the normal lysine pool (- - - - - -), in patients 4 days after colon resection

This relationship can be expressed as a linear correlation between the negative nitrogen balance and the rate of intracellular lysine depletion (Figure 7.9). Thus, the improvements in the nitrogen balance, following administration of amino acids, are accompanied by normalization of the intracellular muscle lysine pool.

Clement and Harper[29] postulated that the tissue pool size of the first limiting amino acid had an important effect on the polysome aggregation. Similarly it was reported that protein synthesis in skeletal muscle is regulated by the rate of polysome aggregation[30]. It was also suggested that protein synthesis in skeletal muscle is controlled by the activity of amino acid activating enzymes[31]. Thus, these activities depend on the presence of sufficient amounts of substrate (amino acids) in the cells.

The low concentrations of lysine in intracellular muscle water may suggest that this amino acid is limiting for protein synthesis in trauma.

Intermediary energy metabolism

As in other severely ill patients one might expect that certain fundamental metabolic functions such as energy generation and transmembrane transport may be impaired in postoperative trauma. Our approach towards this problem has been to study the intracellular energy metabolism directly by analysing muscle tissue obtained by percutaneous needle biopsy.

Muscle tissue is considered to be relatively resistant to metabolic insult when compared to the brain or kidney. Therefore, any observed changes in muscle tissue can be correlated with more severe abnormalities in other organs. It thus seemed important to obtain information on the biochemical parameters of muscle during acute diseases and injury and to study the response of nutritional therapy.

Metabolic studies using the needle biopsy technique were performed on patients with circulatory or respiratory failure[32,33]. In these patients an increase in muscle lactate, a decrease in phosphocreatine, and a decrease in ATP and total adenine content was found. Similar results were found in acute cardiogenic shock with pronounced increases of lactate in blood and muscle[34]. Phosphocreatinene values were approaching zero in muscle, while muscle ATP was only mildly decreased. In patients with prolonged catabolic diseases, there was no sign of anaerobic metabolism in the muscle due to hypoxia, but these patients still showed very pronounced changes in the ATP content and in the TA content. For unclear reasons, the normal balance between use and production persisted in these patients.

In discussing the regulation of glycolysis and respiration, the relative concentrations of ADP and ATP in the cell are the most important controlling elements. When ATP is utilized in many biosynthetic reactions, it undergoes pyrophosphatec leavage to yield AMP, whereas in muscular contraction, ADP is the primary production of ATP utilization. At any given moment, a living cell contains not only ATP and ADP but also AMP.

Atkinson[35] proposed the energy change concept for the adenylate pool. The energy charge of the ATP–ADP–AMP system can easily be calculated for any given set of concentrations of ATP, ADP, and AMP by the equation:

$$\text{energy charge} = \frac{1}{2}\,\frac{\text{ADP} + 2\text{ATP}}{\text{AMP} + \text{ADP} + \text{ATP}}$$

Because many regulatory enzymes in both catabolic and anabolic pathways are responsive to AMP, ADP or ATP as modulators, Atkinson has suggested that the regulation of pathways, which produce and utilize high-energy phosphate bonds, is a function of the energy charge of the ATP–ADP–AMP system, which runs optimally in a steady state and which strongly resists any deviation from it.

In severely ill patients and in patients with untreated malnutrition, we found low energy charge potential (ECP) (Table 6.1). This would mean that these patients had a decreased capacity for biosynthetic reactions and for production of energy storage compounds. Such a situation is often referred to as a catabolic state, and it has repeatedly been noted that in the post-operative or post-traumatic situation most patients are 'catabolic'. Possibly the low energy charge seen here is the cellular expression for the 'catabolic state'.

The suggestion has been made that the production of ATP may not parallel the oxidation of substrate during periods of surgical hypermetabolism. This might be due to an abnormal coupling of oxidation and phosphorylation in the mitochondria. However, mitochondrial uncoupling has not been demonstrated in the absence of severe circulatory failure. A second possibility involves 'futile cycles', i.e. an increased turnover of material such as the glycolytic intermediates without a corresponding increase in the net production of ATP. There is consequently increasing evidence that the coupling of oxidation and phosphorylation in the mitochondria may be seriously disturbed in hypermetabolism. The extent to which mitochondria coupling can be reduced and still recover has not yet been determined.

Conclusion

An adequate intracellular amino acid environment requires a certain concentration of intracellular amino acids. Furthermore, efficient protein anabolism requires the simultaneous presence of each amino acid in the correct proportions. The concentration of amino acids in the muscle cell would represent the balance between the rate of production or entry of amino acids into the intracellular pool, and the rate of the utilization of amino acids from this pool. Low intracellular amino acid concentrations may be due either to a decreased uptake from plasma or a reduction in protein catabolism or an increased utilization, or all three, whilst high amino acid concentrations could be due to the opposite effects.

The altered amino acid pattern found in intracellular muscle water should affect protein synthesis occurring in the ribosomes. The mechanism for protein synthesis would then be presented with an amino acid substrate

Table 6.1 Adenine nucleotides (mM/kg dry muscle) and the energy change potential in severely ill patients

	ATP	*ADP*	*AMP*	*TAN*	*ECP*
Healthy subjects (81)	24.0 ± 0.29	3.20 ± 0.06	0.10 ± 0.01	27.40 ± 0.36	0.9392 ± 0.00002
Patients with acute circulatory or respiratory insufficiency (9)	19.4 ± 0.94*	2.92 ± 0.129	0.16 ± 0.038	22.48 ± 1.033*	0.9280 ± 0.0034*
Patients with more prolonged catabolic disease (9)	12.8 ± 1.19*	2.14 ± 0.154	0.18 ± 0.032	15.13 ± 1.142*	0.9134 ± 0.0106*

* $P < 0.001$ compared with the normal mean.

complex, not only low in concentration, but also of unsuitable composition. Therefore, regardless of its initial cause, the imbalance of cellular amino acids in postoperative catabolism may be one of the fundamental inadequacies in cell nutrition adversely affecting normal protein synthesis.

These results indicate that proportions and minimum requirements based on data from healthy subjects and recommended by Rose cannot be applied directly in post-operative catabolism and suggest that patients should be supplied with amino acids in other proportions.

In acutely ill patients with circulatory or respiratory insufficiency, there was an increase in muscle lactate content, a decrease in adenosine triphosphate (ATP) and total adenine (TA) contents. These findings could partly be explained by a relative hypoxia in the muscle, but acute hypoxia alone would not account for the decrease in ATP or TA. These changes in the adenylate pool were even more pronounced in patients with prolonged diseases. In this series the ATP content was only 50% of the normal, despite normal lactate content.

The low adenine nucleotide level in muscle tissue is thought to be due primarily to an increased formation and deamination of adenosine monophosphate during hypoxia in combination with a decreased rate of purine synthesis in the liver and/or a decreased capacity for 'purine salvage' in the muscle. This itself might, in turn, be mediated by a low energy state in muscle or liver, or be due to other metabolic disturbances or tissue damage.

A low energy charge potential was found in patients with prolonged disease, possibly being the cellular expression for the concept of the post-traumatic catabolic state.

Acknowledgements

This investigation was supported by grants from the Swedish Medical Research Council (projects No. B77–03X–4210–04B, B77–19X–1002–12C), Stockholm, Sweden.

References

1. Bergström, J. (1962). Muscle electrolytes in man. *Scand. J. Clin. Lab. Invest.*, **14,** (Suppl.), 68
2. Edwards, R. H. (1971). Percutaneous needle biopsy of skeletal muscle in diagnosis and research. *Lancet*, **ii,** 593
3. Bergström, J. (1975). Percutaneous needle biopsy of skeletal muscle in physiological and clinical research. *Scand. J. Clin. Lab. Invest.*, **35,** 609
4. Bergström, J. and Friden, A. M. (1975). The effect of hydrochlorothiazide and amiloride administered together on muscle electrolytes in normal subjects. *Acta Med. Scand.*, **197,** 415
5. Bergström, J., Fürst, P., Noree, L. O. and Vinnars, E. (1974). The intracellular free amino acid concentration in human muscle tissue. *J. Appl. Physiol.*, **36,** 693
6. Bergström, J., Alvestrand, A., Fürst, P., Hultman, E., Sahlin, K., Vinnars, E. and Widström, A. (1976). Influence of severe potassium depletion and subsequent repletion

with potassium on muscle electrolytes, metabolites and amino acids in man. *Clin. Sci. Mol. Med.*, **51**, 589

7. Cotlove, E. (1963). Determination of the true chloride content of biological fluids and tissues. *Anal. Chem.*, **35**, 101
8. Bolte, H. D., Riecker, G. and Rohl, D. (1963). Messungen des Membranpotentials an einzelnen guergestrieften Musckelzellen der Menshen in situ. *Klin. Wochenschr.*, **41**, 356
9. Cunningham, J. N., Jr., Carter, N. W., Rector, F. C., Jr. and Seldin, D. W. (1971). Resting transmembrane potential in normal subjects and severely ill patients. *J. Clin. Invest.*, **50**, 49
10. Bolte, H. D., Becker, E. and Volker, W. (1972). Changes in ionic permeability of skeletal and heart muscle cellular membranes in renal insufficiency. In R. Kluthe, G. Berlyne and B. Barton (eds.). *Uremia*, pp. 14–18. (Stuttgart: Thieme Verlag)
11. Cotton, J. R., Carter, N. W. and Knochel, J. P. (1976). Muscle membrane potential [Em]; A possible index of adequate dialysis. In *Ninth Annual meeting of the American Society of Nephrology*, p. 29
12. Campion, D. S., Lynch, L. J., Rector, F. C. Jr., Carter, N. and Shires, G. T. (1969). Effect of hemorrhagic shock on transmembrane potential. *Surgery*, **66**, 1051
13. Shires, G. T., Carrico, C. J., Baxter, C. R., Giesecke, A. H. and Jenkins, M. J. (1970). Principles in treatment of severely injured patients. In E. C. Welch (ed). *Advances in Surgery*. Vol. IV, p. 255. (Chicago: Year Book Med.)
14. Harris, R. C., Hultman, E. and Nordesjö, L. O. (1974). Glycogen, glycolytic intermediates and high-energy phosphates determined in biopsy samples of muscles quadriceps femoris of man at rest. Methods and variance of values. *Scand. J. Clin. Lab. Invest.*, **33**, 109
15. Munro, H. (1970). Free amino acid pools and their role in regulation. In H. N. Munro (ed.). *Mammalian Protein Metabolism*, pp. 299–386 (New York: Academic Press)
16. Bergström, J., Fürst, P. and Noree, L. (1972). The effect of peritoneal dialysis on the intracellular free amino acids in muscle tissue from uremic patients. *Proc. Eur. Dial. Transpl. Assoc.*, **9**, 393
17. Vinnars, E., Fürst, P., Bergström, J. and von Francken, I. (1976). Intracellular free amino acids in normal man and in different clinical conditions. In A. W. Wilkinson and D. Cuthbertson (eds.). *Metabolism and the Response to Injury*, pp. 336–350. (London: Pitman Press)
18. Vinnars, E., Bergström, J. and Fürst, P. (1975). Influence of the postoperative state on the intracellular free amino acids in human muscle tissue. *Ann. Surg.*, **182**, 665
19. Fürst, P., Bergström, J., Kinney, J. M. and Vinnars, E. (1977). Nutrition in postoperative catabolism. *Proc. Nutritional Aspects of the Care of the Critically Ill.* (In press)
20. Bergström, J., Fürst, P., Noree, L. O. and Vinnars, E. (1975). Intracellular free amino acids in uremic patients as influenced by amino acid supply. *Kidney Int.*, **7**, S-354
21. Bergström, J., Fürst, P., Ahlberg, M. and Noree, L. O. (1977). Nutrition in renal failure. *Proc. Nutritional Aspects of the Care of the Critically Ill.* (In press)
22. Bergström, J., Alvestrand, A. and Fürst, P. (1977). Amino acids levels and effect of amino acid supplements. *Proc. On Growth Retardation in Children with Kidney Failure* (In press)
23. Munro, H. N. (1964). General aspects of the regulation of protein metabolism by diet and hormones. In H. N. Munro and J. B. Allison (eds.). *Mammalian Protein Metabolism* pp. 412–491. (New York: Academic Press)
24. Roch-Nordlund, A. E., Alinder, I., Ahlberg, M., Fürst, P. and Nerger, G. (1974). Nitrogen metabolism in diabetic patients. *Acta Endocrinol.*, **77**, (Suppl.), 190
25. Vinnar, E., Bergström, J., Fürst, P., Holmström, B. and Schildt, B. (1977). Influence of parenteral nutrition on nitrogen balance and intracellular amino acid pattern in muscle tissue in colon surgery (carcinoma). *Proc. Balanced Nutrition and Therapy*. (In press)
26. Harper, A. E. (1964). Amino acid toxicities and imbalances. In H. N. Munro and J. B. Allison (eds.). *Mammalian Protein Metabolism*, pp. 87–134. (New York: Academic Press)
27. O'Keefe, S. J. D. and Sender, P. M. (1974). 'Catabolic' loss of body nitrogen in response to surgery. *Lancet*, **ii**, 1035

28. Millward, D. J., Garlick, P. J., Dickson, O. N. and Waterlow, J. C. (1976). The relative importance of muscle protein synthesis and breakdown in the regulation of muscle mass. *Biochem. J.*, **156,** 185
29. Clement, C. Y. Ip. and Harper, A. E. (1974). Liver polysome profiles and protein synthesis in rats fed a threonine-imbalanced diet. *J. Nutr.*, **104,** 252
30. Noda, K., Taniguchi, H. and Kitasaka, R. (1975). Effect of amino acid imbalance on protein synthesis of skeletal muscle and liver in rats. *Nutr. Rep. Inter.*, **11,** 129
31. Gaetani, S., Paolucci, A. M., Spadoni, M. A. and Tomassi, G. (1964). Activity of amino acid-activating enzymes in tissues from protein-depleted rats. *J. Nutr.*, **84,** 173
32. Bergström, J., Boström, H., Fürst, P., Hultman, E. and Vinnars, E. (1976). Preliminary studies of energy-rich phosphagens in muscle from severely ill patients. *Critical Care Med.*, **4,** 197
33. Fürst, P., Bergström, J., Hultman, E. and Vinnars, E. (1976). Intermediary energy metabolism for the catabolic state with special regard to muscle tissue. In A. W. Wilkinson and D. Cuthbertson (eds.). *Metabolism and the Response to Injury*, pp. 94–112. (London: Pitman Press)
34. Karlsson, J., Willerson, J. R., Leshin, S. J., Mullins, C. B. and Mitchell, J. H. (1975). Skeletal muscle metabolites in patients with cardiogenic shock or severe congestive heart failure. *Scand. J. Clin. Lab. Invest.*, **35,** 73
35. Atkinson, D. E. (1968). The energy charge of the adenylate pool as a regulator parameter. Interaction with feedback modifiers. *Biochemistry*, **7,** 4030

Discussion

G. L. Blackburn: (USA) The work on which Peter Fürst forms his foundations is primarily Harper's rat data[1]. It would appear that in humans the proportion of protein being given is much smaller than that being created by protein breakdown so that the influence on the pool is dramatically different from that in the rat where a substantial amount of the diet was protein.

Surely most of the problem is not increased catabolism. The 3-methylhistidine data for example do not show, in the type of patient studied, increased rates of breakdown but rather impaired synthesis[2]. Has Dr Fürst any evidence from amino acid fluxes, amino acid synthesis, or nitrogen balance data to support the observation that these intracellular amino acid imbalances are applicable to man?

P. Fürst: (Sweden) I have indirect evidence that imbalances may play a very big role in nutrition in the treatment of the severely ill patient. For several years we have been successfully treating severely uraemic patients with essential amino acid solutions based on the proportions proposed by Rose. However, looking at the intracellular amino acid data during long-term treatment we have found that these patients slowly exhibit a slight negative nitrogen balance after 3–4 months' treatment and simultaneously get imbalances in the intracellular compartment. We have changed the proportions of the essential amino acid preparations according to the findings in the intracellular compartment and some of the imbalances were improved. At the same time the nutrition of these patients also improved. This provides indirect clinical evidence that by changing the proportions of a solution a better utilization of the ingested nitrogen can be achieved.

The imbalances are considerable. If we look at the increase in the intracellular fluid of some of the amino acids or the depletion of lysine and glutamine, we find that these are of considerable quantitative importance. A decrease of 50% in the intracellular glutamine pool means that the body's intracellular free amino acid pool decreases by about 35%. The large increase of up to 200% in other amino acids such as valine and lysine suggests a very severe imbalance of intracellular composition.

P. Vinay: (Canada) Lysine is a cationic amino acid and some of the lysine inside the cell plays a role in matching the anions and cations. There are several ways of diminishing lysine in the cell. One way would be to decrease the negative charge in the cell by decreasing the total amount of intracellular protein, but where that occurs then all the cations in the cell should be diminished, including potassium.

On the other hand, one could decrease the lysine in the cell by increasing other cations in the cells, e.g. sodium. What was the intracellular concentration of sodium and potassium in those biopsies where low lysine levels were found?

Fürst: A normal intracellular potassium was found in these patients and the intracellular sodium was somewhat increased. As is usual in all catabolic situations we had slight edema. However, this increase was not as pronounced as in severe catabolism.

Severe potassium depletion concomitant with alkalosis has a marked effect in the human on intracellular lysine and arginine concentrations, increasing them several times. It is possible that the lysine deprivation may be affected by a decrease in intracellular pH.

W. P. T. James: (UK) Lysine has not been much talked about in the past. Might we hear what is happening to this lysine? As I understood it one tended to have quite a high intracellular concentration of lysine. Cahill and others have recalculated their amino acid exchange on the basis of lysine flux. Are we now saying that a deficit in intracellular lysine is generated as a result of an abnormality of amino acid transport so that the lysine is transported to the liver for catabolism?

Fürst: Unfortunately I have no idea. The patient probably exhibits slight intracellular acidosis which might affect the lysine concentration, but I have no hard evidence.

Tweedle: There is no doubt that the amino acid configuration of the amino acid solutions is of vital importance. Now that Drs Fürst, Vinners and Bergstrom have developed this beautiful technique, I should like to ask about the value of measuring amino acids in plasma.

If a particular amino acid solution is infused, which induces an imbalance in the amino acid configuration in the plasma, is this imbalance not proportional to the concentration at which these amino acids are infused, initially? Can such studies be used to indicate the suitability of the amino acid solutions which were infused?

Fürst: I do not think it can be done. We did a study with Professor Lilledahl in which we investigated patients, with 60–65% burns, or multiple trauma. We looked at both plasma and muscle amino acids. Despite quite a normal plasma amino acid pattern after treatment, we still found severe disturbances in the muscle amino acids. The plasma amino acid pattern gave a false picture and the patients remained in negative nitrogen balance.

References

1. Harper, A. E., Bencuengh, N. J. and Wohlhmeter, R. M. (1970). Effects of ingestion of disproportionate amounts of amino acids. *Physiol. Rev.*, **50,** 128
2. O'Keefe, S. J. D., Sender, P. M. and James, W. P. T. (1974). Catabolic loss of body nitrogen in response to surgery. *Lancet*, **ii,** 1035

7
Biological limiting factors to parenteral amino acid feeding in man

H. N. MUNRO

INTRODUCTION

This chapter will cover two aspects of the factors limiting amino acid utilization in parenteral alimentation. First, the extent to which monitoring of blood amino acid patterns can be helpful in indicating the efficiency of treatment will be covered. Second, it will deal with data recently accumulated on the use of 3-methylhistidine as an index of muscle protein breakdown in a clinical setting. The purpose is to discuss what principles are available for our guidance and what hopeful directions might be exploited in constructing meaningful solutions for the varieties of disease for which parenteral nutrition is appropriate.

HOMEOSTASIS OF BODY FREE AMINO ACIDS

Amino acid pool turnover

Figure 7.1 demonstrates that the body has a large daily turnover of protein and thus can tolerate considerable infusion of amino acids parenterally[1]. Based on ^{15}N studies, total protein synthesis in the body is of the order of 200–300 g/day as against an average protein intake by adults of approx. 90 or 100 g daily. This means that re-utilization of the free pool released by breakdown of body protein and uptake for synthesis is continuously taking place. This free amino acid pool (70 g) is largely made up of non-essential amino acids, particularly four (alanine, glutamic acid, glutamine and glycine), while the essential amino acids constitute about 10 g of which only 0.2 g are present in the plasma. The ratio of plasma free amino acids to daily protein synthesis is such that, if the plasma amino acids were the immediate source for protein synthesis, the turnover time within the plasma would average a few minutes. Thus there is a considerable reserve capacity of the body to accept external amino acid sources, including infusions. Secondly, it can be seen from Figure 7.1 that many of the components of protein synthesis can be identified; later, turnover of one particular component, muscle, will be discussed in detail.

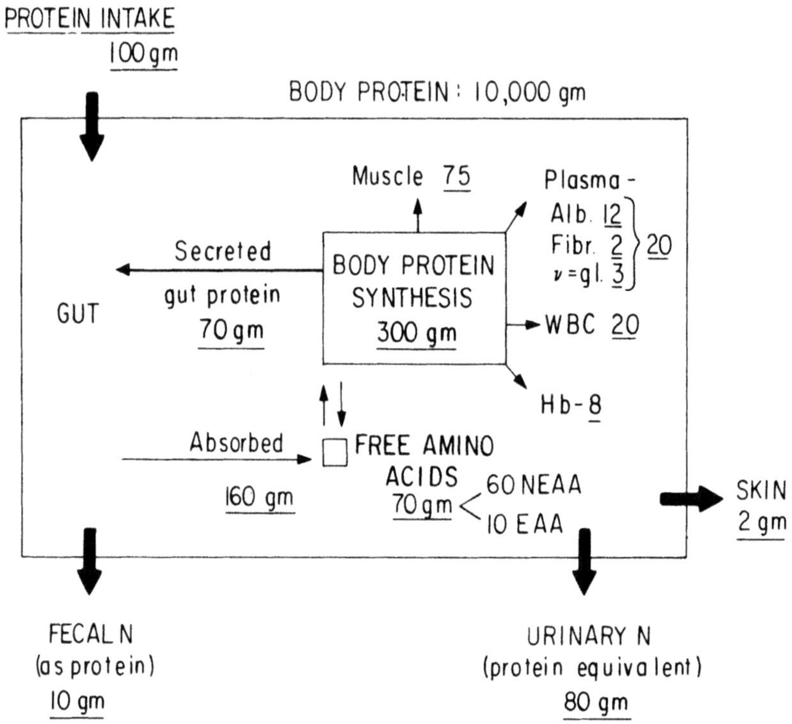

Figure 7.1 Turnover of body protein in a 70 kg man

Role of the gut

The safeguards which are built into the system in order to maintain stable levels in plasma include the gut and the liver, which are bypassed by parenteral nutrition. An important feature of the gut mucosa deserving more attention is its capacity of transamination, particularly for glutamic and aspartic acids. This pathway is capable of utilizing appreciable quantities of glutamic acid and transferring the amino group to alanine. The question, therefore, is whether the parenteral use of fluids containing glutamic and aspartic acid has any particular dangers, due to loss of the protection afforded by the gut mucosa. However, Stegink[2] has demonstrated by perfusion of patients with solutions containing glutamic acid, namely casein hydrolysates, that there is no evident rise in plasma glutamic acid as a result of this parenteral mixture and that there is no evidence of any change in mental function when these hydrolysates are given.

Role of the liver

The next organ which offers protection is the liver. The capacity of the liver to monitor and to remove excess amino acids after a meal has been well attested to[3]. This experiment, which illustrates the capacity to make urea, surprisingly demonstrates, by arteriovenous difference studies across the livers of animals absorbing a large meal of meat, that urea is formed on one transit through the liver to the extent of more than half the total incoming flux of amino acids up the portal vein. Consequently the intervention of the liver is an important component in ensuring homeostasis of amino acid metabolism.

The second important aspect of liver metabolism is the location within this organ of the major or exclusive pathways of degradation for seven of the essential amino acids, the pathways for the branched-chain amino acids being present in kidney and in muscle, while the pathways for non-essential amino acids are widely distributed in the tissues. The presence in the liver of pathways for certain essentials thus makes it a uniquely decisive organ in determining their removal[3].

Harper[4] has shown that when protein intake by the rat is increased, a certain point is reached at which liver enzymes for degradation of a number of essential amino acids undergo induction, whereas in the case of transaminases for non-essential amino acids such as glutamic acid, enzyme activity is proportional to the load of non-essential amino acids in the food consumed. This picture of adaptation to excess is reflected in oxidation studies by Brookes *et al.*[5] in which growing rats were given different levels of lysine. The rate of growth per day was dependent on lysine intake, which varied from insufficient to excess. Following administration of lysine labelled with ^{14}C, labelled CO_2 production was minimal until enough lysine was given to provide optimal growth. Above that level, there was a marked increase in $^{14}CO_2$ production, proportional to the excess of lysine. Thus, above requirements, the liver displays a sensitive monitoring capacity which, however, does not completely prevent increments in peripheral blood levels of the free amino acids such as lysine which are degraded exclusively in the liver[6]. A similar phenomenon has been shown for plasma tryptophan levels in growing and mature rats by Young and Munro[7]. In experiments in which tryptophan was limiting in the diet, addition of more tryptophan to an otherwise adequate diet did not raise blood levels of tryptophan in the young rat until growth became optimal; beyond this point plasma tryptophan levels began to increase steeply. Older animals given graded amounts of tryptophan showed less distinctive absorptive patterns, but there was still a point of inflection when levels of tryptophan were fed which were above requirements. The inflection point was lower than that of the growing animal, thus coinciding with the smaller need for dietary tryptophan for maintenance than for growth (Figure 7.2).

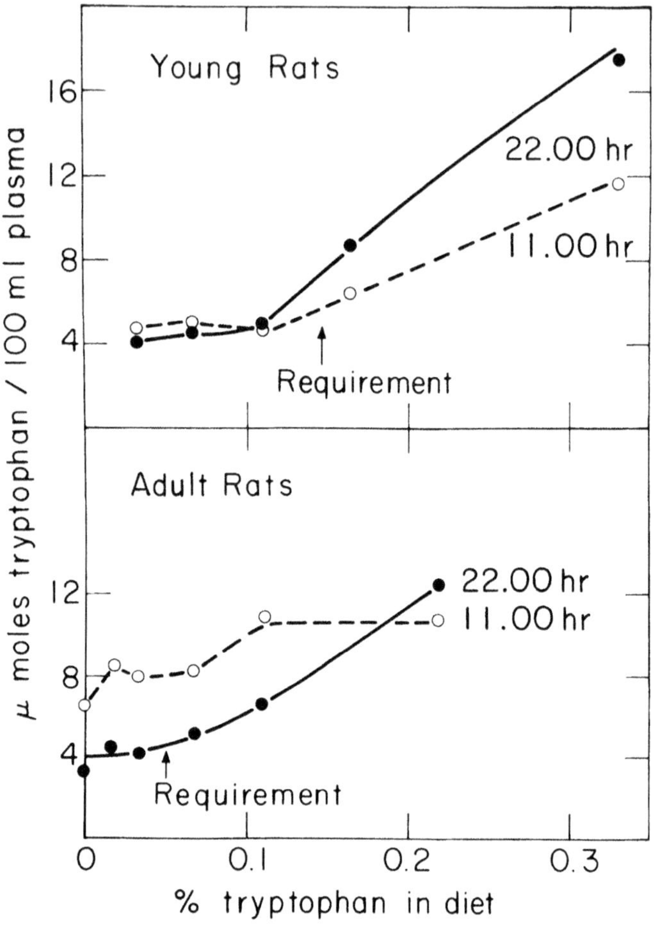

Figure 7.2 Concentrations of tryptophan in the plasma of young and mature rats fed amino acid diets containing various amounts of tryptophan, other nutrients being adequate and constant. The arrows indicate requirements for tryptophan reported in the literature for weanling and adult rats. (Reproduced from ref. 7)

Factors affecting plasma amino acid levels

The above pattern in the rat has encouraged investigators to adopt a similar experimental design in relation to human requirements for amino acids. In some cases such as tryptophan, young adults show a fairly sharp rise in blood tryptophan level beyond the intake providing N equilibrium[8]. However it is not so definitive for all essential amino acids needed by man. Furthermore, in the case of the phenylalanine needs of the rat, catabolism in the liver is regulated not by hydroxylation to tyrosine but by subsequent tyrosine removal. Consequently a rise in the level of tyrosine in plasma indicates when excess of phenylalanine beyond requirements has been given[9].

These observations have two features relevant to parenteral nutrition. First, they allow us to explore changes in needs for individual amino acids caused by disease. Second, they allow us some insight into the evaluation of changes in amino acid metabolism under conditions of parenteral nutrition. In connection with plasma amino acid levels, another factor which has to be taken care of in parenteral feeding is the effect of carbohydrate, which specifically reduces plasma amino acid levels in a distinctive pattern by deposition in a specific tissue, namely muscle, through the intervention of insulin.

In an early study[10], it was shown that, after a dose of 50 g of glucose orally, the plasma levels of tryptophan, histidine and threonine are marginally reduced, whereas the levels of the branched chain amino acids isoleucine, leucine and valine are reduced by about 30%. There is thus an unequal removal of amino acids, a phenomenon that has been repeatedly confirmed. Evidence obtained from diabetic animals, and from administration of radioactive amino acids, indicates that insulin is required and that muscle is the depository into which they are placed[11]. This agrees with much evidence that muscle is selectively sensitive to insulin and that a major response to glucose administration is the transport of amino acids and the stimulation of muscle protein synthesis. This effect must be considered as one consequence of parenteral feeding with glucose, or glucose plus a fat source.

Nutritional effects on brain tryptophan metabolism

Carbohydrate also affects one specific amino acid, namely tryptophan, in a very special way. In plasma, tryptophan circulates partly bound to serum albumin at a specific site on the molecule. This binding is influenced by the competing binding of other substances, of which the commonest competitor is the non-esterified fatty acids. After giving glucose, insulin secretion reduces the flow of non-esterified fatty acids from the fat pads so that their level in plasma falls and there is less competition with tryptophan[12]. Consequently, unbound ('free') tryptophan in plasma falls. However, the significance of this effect for tissue tryptophan content has failed to be established[13]. In particular, an important recipient of nutrients, namely the brain, behaves in a manner which does not reflect the unbound tryptophan level. Rats were either fasted, or briefly fed for 1 h on carbohydrate or carbohydrate and fat (Table 7.1). On feeding glucose, the non-esterified fatty acids declined sharply and, in response to the increased sites on albumin, the albumin-bound tryptophan rose while the non-albumin–bound tryptophan fell from

37 to 18%. However, brain tryptophan level did not fall, but actually rose. This conclusion conflicts with the views of Curzon[14] that the amount of actual free tryptophan determines brain tryptophan levels. Our experiments show that this is not so, an important observation since brain tryptophan is the precursor of serotonin, and rate-limited for its synthesis. Thus, when a meal of carbohydrate is taken, brain serotonin rises. We[15] believe that the uptake of tryptophan to the brain is determined, not by albumin binding, but by competition between neutral amino acids for transport.

Table 7.1 Effects of carbohydrate or carbohydrate–fat diets on serum and brain tryptophan (Modified from Madras *et al.*,[12])

		Diets	
	Fasted controls	*Carbohydrate*	*Carbohydrate + Fat*
Nonesterified fatty acids (mEq/l)	0.831	0.301***	0.615***
Serum total tryptophan (μg/ml)	16.5	19.1***	18.4**
Serum free tryptophan (μg/ml)	6.2	3.4**	5.7*
Free tryptophan (% of total)	37	18	33
Serum bound tryptophan (μg/ml)	10.3	15.7	12.7
Brain tryptophan (μg/g)	2.24	3.45***	3.07***

Groups of twenty-two rats weighing 170–200 g were deprived of food but not water at 2 p.m. and presented with one of the experimental diets at 10.30 a.m. the next day. Two hours later, the animals were decapitated and serum and brains taken for assay. Controls had free access to water and were killed at similar times. The asterisks indicate increasing levels of significance of difference from the control (fasted) group.

This competition is demonstrated when large doses of single amino acids are given to rats[16]. Thus in the case of phenylalanine administration, the plasma levels of most amino acids compared with untreated animals were little changed, except for the phenylalanine which was much elevated, whereas the brain levels of many of the neutral amino acids were depressed. This demonstrates competition when any one of the amino acids is in excess and depresses transport of the remainder. The consequence is that there is a balance between the various neutral amino acids, in which tryptophan and phenylalanine are competing for entry to the brain with branch chains. It will be recalled that, when carbohydrate is given, the levels of the branched chain amino acids fall. When the carbohydrate depresses the branched-chain levels, it allows more tryptophan to enter the brain, so that under these conditions more serotonin is formed.

These features of amino acid supply to the brain for neurotransmitter synthesis are most dramatically seen (Figure 7.3) in the case of the encephalopathy associated with cirrhosis of the liver[17]. Amines from the gut, which are normally metabolized in the liver, pass through in cases of cirrhosis and can give rise to products acting as competitors in the biosynthesis of the catecholamines in the brain. Second, the normal function of the liver to regulate phenylalanine levels is lost, and plasma phenylalanine levels rise

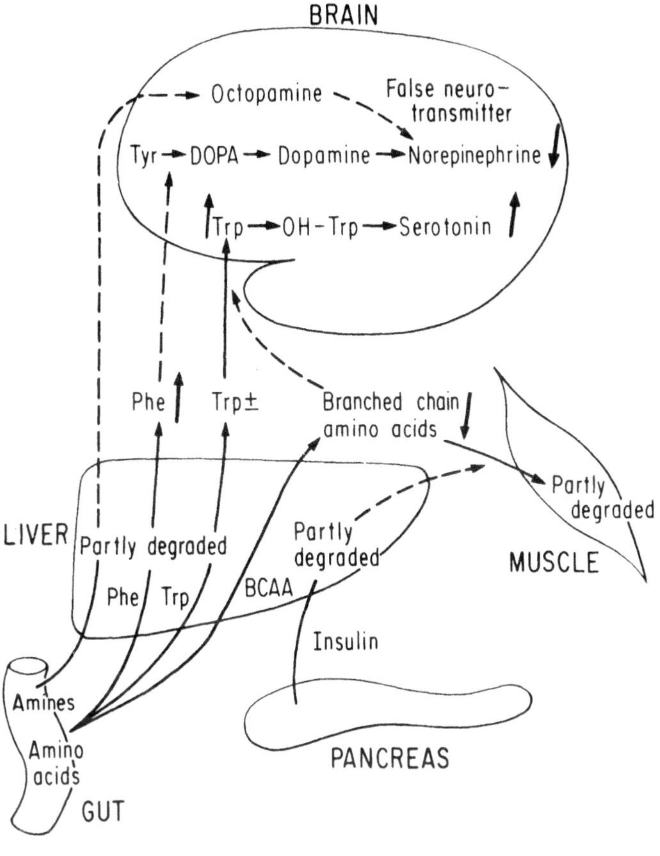

Figure 7.3 Role of branched-chain amino acids in hepatic coma. (Reproduced from ref. 26)

considerably in such cases. In addition, tryptophan levels tend to rise, although not so sharply.

Finally, insulin secreted by the pancreas passes to the liver, where half is removed on each transit. Consequently, removal of liver function in cirrhosis allows insulin levels in the plasma to reach very high concentrations. This accentuates the normal deposition of branched-chain amino acids in muscle and their levels in plasma show considerable reductions. As a result of the reduced competition by branched-chain amino acids, and also the elevated levels of tryptophan and phenylalanine, more of these two amino acids enter the brain. The tryptophan generates serotonin, and this in turn tends to promote drowsiness. The phenylalanine is an inhibitor of the hydroxylation of tyrosine to dihydroxy-phenylalanine and therefore is an inhibitor of the catecholamine pathway. The combination of increased serotonin and reduced catecholamines leads to drowsiness, and in the patient with hepatic failure it promotes and accentuates the tendency to hepatic coma. Evidence of this is provided by the elegant studies of Fischer *et al.*[18], who injected branched-chain amino acids and was able to revive dogs with hepatic coma and also human cases. This implies that great attention must be paid to the plasma patterns of amino acids in terms of the levels obtained with parenteral infusions.

ROLE OF MUSCLE IN AMINO ACID HOMEOSTASIS

Skeletal muscle provides the largest tissue in the body, being some 45% of adult body weight. Accordingly, changes in muscle protein metabolism are likely to have extensive effects on the metabolism of free amino acids. The effect of carbohydrate administration on plasma amino acid levels due to insulin-dependent deposition in muscle has already been described. Accordingly, we need sensitive parameters to demonstrate changes in muscle protein metabolism due to nutritional factors. One such new parameter is excretion of 3-methylhistidine as a specific indicator of myofibrillar breakdown.

Evidence for 3-methylhistidine as a measure of myofibrillar breakdown

Interest in turnover of muscle protein in man has developed in recent years because of the study of arteriovenous differences across the muscles. Applications of this technique to the study of amino acid exchange with muscle have resulted in the exciting finding that alanine is released in quantities far in excess of the amount of alanine in muscle protein, due to synthesis from pyruvate and transamination of other amino acids, and passes to the liver, giving the familiar glucose–alanine cycle[19]. However, it seemed to us desirable to have some simpler measure specific to muscle protein breakdown. In this respect 3-methylhistidine satisfies a number of criteria which are essential, namely that it should be made after synthesis of the peptide chain, that it should be released on breakdown like any other amino acid, that the derived amino acid is not re-utilized, that it is not metabolized to a general metabolite, and that it should be quantitatively excreted in the urine in a form which can be measured easily.

First, synthesis of methylhistidine occurs after completion of the peptides of actin and myosin, with one mole per molecule of actin and a variable amount of myosin in different muscles, no methylation occurring in cardiac myosin. Secondly, 3-methylhistidine released on degradation turns out to be non re-utilizable and to be excreted completely in the urine[20]. On oral or parenteral administration of [^{14}C-methyl]histidine to the rat, there is total recovery of the label in the urine, with only traces in faeces which may represent incomplete separation of urine and faeces, and none in the carbon dioxide exhaled. Most of the excretion occurs in the first 24 h, and on chromatography this shows two radioactive spots, one of which is methylhistidine and the other its N-acetylated derivative. Since the latter can be hydrolysed by heating in acid, it is possible to measure total 3-methylhistidine without difficulty. Similarly, we[21] demonstrated complete recovery of doses of [^{14}C-methyl]histidine administered to human subjects.

The next question is whether the excretion is entirely due to muscle or whether other organs contain and contribute 3-methylhistidine. Analysis of the total content per organ for the skeletal musculature, diaphragm, heart, liver and some other organs shows that the skeletal musculature contains more than 90% of the body content of this histidine derivative[22]. Finally, computation of muscle protein breakdown from urinary excretion requires us to know the average 3-methylhistidine content of muscle. We now have data for muscles sampled from human subjects of various ages. In the mature human, the content is 4.2 μmoles/g protein in muscle. This allows us to compute from the urinary output what the total breakdown of muscle is in man.

Output of 3-methylhistidine at different ages

Regarding the effect of different stages of development on methylhistidine metabolism in man and in the rat, at the time of birth the skeletal musculature is a small component of body weight (23%) compared with the adult, where it represents about 45% of body mass. There is therefore a doubling of the muscle per kg body weight during the process of growth. In the elderly subject, there is a selective erosion of the musculature so that it becomes

Table 7.2 Urinary 3-methylhistidine excretion at various ages in subjects consuming flesh-free diets (unpublished data)

Group	*Number of subjects*	*Age range* (years)	*Body weight* (kg)	*3-methylhistidine (μmoles) per* 24 h	kg body weight	g creatinine
Neonate (premature)	10	1–46 (days)	1.9	8	4.2	253
Young Adult						
Men	4	21–25	77	245	3.2	126
Women	2	23	53	112	2.1	92
Elderly						
Men	7	65–72	74	160	2.2	136
Women	8	67–91	55	70	1.3	96

about 35% of body weight at age 80 years. These changes have to be considered in evaluating changes in 3-methylhistidine output at various ages.

Output of 3-methylhistidine at different ages is shown in Table 7.2. Note that, per kg of body weight, the neonate excretes more than the young adult. When the neonate's small amount of musculature is considered, this increases the difference to threefold greater breakdown. In relation to creatinine output, which provides an approximate measure of muscle mass, output of 3-methylhistidine is double in the neonate compared with the adult. In the elderly subject, output of 3-methylhistidine per kg body weight falls, but per unit of creatinine it does not change. Thus there is a specific loss of muscle during ageing, without a change in output per g muscle.

Effect of dietary protein and energy intake on 3-methylhistidine output

Protein and energy intake affect 3-methylhistidine output by the growing rat[23] and the growing child[24]. Young rats were fed either a diet containing 18% lactalbumin, a diet with 0.5% lactalbumin or a 1% lactalbumin diet at half the energy intake. The first diet was fed for 28 days, whereas the other two diets were given for 14 days followed by 14 days of repletion on the 18%

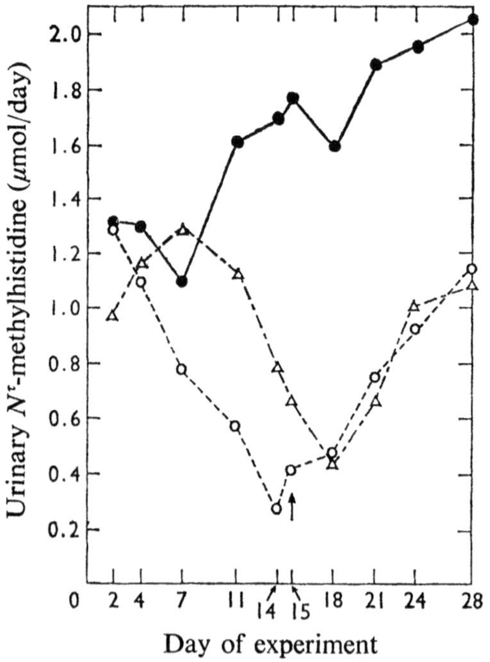

Figure 7.4 Mean urinary N^{τ}-methylhistidine excretion by young rats fed on adequate (●) diet throughout or low-protein (○) or low-protein, low-energy (△) diets for 14 days and then an adequate diet during the subsequent 14 days of repletion. (Reproduced from ref. 23)

lactalbumin diet (Figure 7.4). On the first diet, the rats grew well and showed a progressively increasing output of 3-methylhistidine. The animals on the low protein diet fed *ad libitum* underwent a continuous reduction in 3-methylhistidine output to a low level which was reversed during repletion. The third group, which was subjected to both protein and caloric deficiency, first underwent a slight increase in 3-methylhistidine output followed by a reduction. This fall in output was also reversed on rehabilitation with the 18% protein diet. It will be noted creatinine output did not follow these dramatic changes, but reflected changes in body mass. Thus breakdown of muscle protein is sensitive to malnutrition, such as is imposed by cessation of growth due to inadequate protein intake. Similar observations have been made in malnourished children in India[24] where output of 3-methylhistidine was very low in cases of kwashiorkor and marasmus, and rose on refeeding.

Other factors affecting 3-methylhistidine output

Hormonal factors have recently been examined in unpublished studies. Thyroidectomy of mature rats caused the output of 3-methylhistidine by the rat to fall. Administration of thyroxine to such animals raised output again only when quite substantial doses were given. On the other hand, adrenalectomy did not influence the growth of young rats, nor did it affect their 3-methylhistidine excretion, and was unaffected by small replacement doses of corticosterone. However, large doses of the steroid prevented weight gain and caused a large increase in 3-methylhistidine output.

The effect of injury and infection on 3-methylhistidine output has been confusing. In unpublished studies, we found that fracture of one femur of the rat did not elevate 3-methylhistidine output although N output was increased. On the other hand, Wannemacher *et al.*[25] have observed that 3-methylhistidine output increases during the febrile illness caused by sandfly fever. Again, the magnitude of the change in body protein metabolism may be critical in determining whether muscle protein turnover is affected. Under conditions where muscle protein degradation is increased, it may therefore be possible to use 3-methylhistidine to monitor the benefits of various nutritional treatments.

References

1. Munro, H. N. (1974). Control of plasma amino acid concentrations. In *Aromatic Amino Acids in the Brain*. Ciba Foundation Symposium, p. 6 (New York: Elsevier)
2. Stegink, L. G. and Baker, G. L. (1971). Infusion of protein hydrolysates in newborn infant—plasma amino acid concentrations. *J. Pediat.*, **78,** 595
3. Elwyn, D. (1970). The role of the liver in regulation of amino acid and protein metabolism. In H. N. Munro (ed.). *Mammalian Protein Metabolism*, Vol. 4, pp. 523–571, (New York: Academic Press)
4. Harper, A. E. (1968). Diet and plasma amino acids. *Am. J. Clin. Nutr.*, **21,** 358
5. Brookes, I. M., Owen, F. N. and Garrigus, U. S. (1972). Influence of amino acid level in the diet upon animal acid oxidation by the rat. *J. Nutr.*, **102,** 27

6. Pawlak, M. and Pion, R. (1968). Influence de la supplementation des proteines de ble par des doses croissantes de lysine sur la teneur en acides amines libres du sang et du muscle du rat en croissance. *Ann. Biol. Anim. Biochem. Biophys.*, **8,** 517
7. Young, V. R. and Munro, H. N. (1973). Plasma and tissue tryptophan levels in relation to tryptophan requirements of weanling and adult rats. *J. Nutr.*, **103,** 1756
8. Young, V. R., Hussein, M. A., Murray, E. and Scrimshaw, N. S. (1971). Plasma tryptophan response curve and its relation to tryptophan requirements in young adult men. *J. Nutr.*, **101,** 45
9. Stockland, W. L., Lai, Y. F., Meade, R. J., Sowers, J. E. and Oestemer, G. (1971). L-phenylalanine and L-tyrosine requirements of the growing rat. *J. Nutr.*, **101,** 177
10. Munro, H. N. and Thomson, W. S. T. (1953). Influence of glucose on amino acid metabolism. *Metab. Clin. Exp.*, **2,** 354
11. Munro, H. N., Black, J. G. and Thomson, W. S. T. (1959). The mode of action of dietary carbohydrate on protein metabolism. *Br. J. Nutr.*, **13,** 475
12. Madras, B. K., Cohen, E. L., Fernstrom, J. D., Larin, F., Munro, H. N. and Wurtman, R. J. (1973). Dietary carbohydrate increases brain tryptophan and decreases serum free tryptophan. *Nature (Lond.)*, **244,** 34
13. Madras, B. K., Cohen, E. L., Messing, R., Munro, H. N. and Wurtman, R. J. (1974). Relevance of free tryptophan in serum to tissue tryptophan concentrations. *Metabolism*, **23,** 1107
14. Knott, P. J. and Curzon, G. (1972). Free tryptophan in plasma and brain tryptophan metabolism. *Nature (Lond.)*, **239,** 452
15. Fernstrom, J. D., Madras, B. K., Munro, H. N. and Wurtman, R. J. (1974). Nutritional control of the synthesis of 5-hydroxytryptamine in the brain. In *Aromatic Amino Acids in the Brain.* Ciba Foundation Symposium, p. 153. (New York: Elsevier)
16. Peng, Y., Gubin, J., Harper, A. E., Vavich, M. G. and Kemmerer, A. R. (1973). Food intake regulation: amino acid toxicity and changes in rat brain and plasma amino acids. *J. Nutr.*, **103,** 608
17. Munro, H. N., Fernstrom, D. J. and Wurtman, R. J. (1975). Insulin, plasma amino acid imbalance and hepatic coma. *Lancet*, **i,** 722
18. Fischer, J. E., Funovics, J. M., Aguirre, A., James, J. M., Keane, J. M., Wesdorp, R. I. C., Yoshimura, N. and Westman, T. (1975). The role of plasma amino acids in hepatic encephalopathy. *Surgery*, **78,** 276
19. Pozefsky, T., Felig, P., Tobin, J., Soeldner, J. S. and Cahill, G. F. (1969). Amino acid balance across the tissue of the forearm in post-absorptive man: effects of insulin at two dose levels. *J. Clin. Invest.*, **48,** 2273
20. Young, V. R., Alexis, S. D., Baliga, B. S., Munro, H. N. and Muecke, W. (1972). Metabolism of administered 3-methylhistidine. *J. Biol. Chem.*, **247,** 3592
21. Long, C. L., Haverberg, L. N., Young, V. R., Kinney, J. M., Munro, H. N. and Geiger, J. W. (1975). Metabolism of 3-methylhistidine in man. *Metabolism*, **24,** 929
22. Haverberg, L. N., Omstedt, P. T., Munro, H. N. and Young, V. R. (1975). N^T-methylhistidine content of mixed proteins in various rat tissues. *Biochim. Biophys. Acta*, **405,** 67
23. Haverberg, L. N., Deckelbaum, L., Bilmazes, C., Munro, H. N. and Young, V. R. (1975). Myofibrillar protein turnover and urinary N^T-methylhistidine output. *Biochem. J.*, **152,** 503
24. Narasinga Rao, B. S. and Nagabhushan, V. S. (1973). Urinary excretion of 3-methylhistidine in children suffering from protein-calorie malnutrition. *Life Sci.*, **12** (II), 205
25. Wannemacher, R. W. Jr., Dinterman, R. E., Pekarek, R. S., Bartelloni, P. J. and Beisel, W. R. (1975). Urinary amino acid excretion during experimentally induced sandfly fever in man. *Am. J. Clin. Nutr.*, **28,** 110
26. Crim, M. C. and Munro, H. N. (1976). Protein and amino acid requirements and metabolism in relation to defined-formula diets. In M. E. Shils (ed.). *Defined Formula Diets for Medical Purposes*, p. 5. (Chicago, Ill.: American Medical Association)

8
Isotonic crystalline amino acids for protein sparing

G. L. BLACKBURN AND H. Y. RIENHOFF, Jr.

INTRODUCTION

The formulation of a theory based on models that can be tested and modified accordingly has proved to be a style of reasoning that has provided science with its most spectacular successes. Its power lies in its flexibility to conform to successive revelations that the data may provide. As a postulation–deduction method, hypothesis is never safe, is always tried, and it either matures into formal theory or is soon discarded. The scientific method that has its roots in Descartes and Newton has as its strength and weakness the aspect that only those hypotheses that can be tested by objective reproducible measurements are of value. Those hypotheses that cannot be so tested are not scientific in the strict sense of the word. Hence the hypothesis is the single most creative step in the reductionist process and any logical method, no matter how powerful, is useless without it. From this it is understood that a hypothesis is more sharply defined by its falsifiability. Blackburn and Flatt's hypothesis[1–4] concerning energy substrate regulation is eminently falsifiable because of the specific qualitative and quantitative predictions it makes about substrate concentrations and clinical events[5–7].

ENERGY METABOLISM

The most fundamental biologic characteristic is the constant demand for energy. This is true at every level of organization and it can be stated factually that the greatest proportion of behaviour and activity is a means to procure and conserve energy. Survival in the longer run depends upon reproduction, and to some extent on preservation of the ontologic unit; in the short run, survival is contingent upon energy availability; the organism will begin to consume itself in the absence of exogenous fuel. This preamble is necessary to appreciate the emphasis placed on energy regulation. Energy must be available. The body has energy reserves, in fat; these reserves are used under the proper metabolic circumstances established mostly by diet. A review of the metabolic fuel regulatory system is sufficient to make the point. A precise understanding of the hormonal/substrate enzymatic regulation of energy metabolism provides the foundation for formulation of a nutritional therapy.

ENERGY FUEL STRATEGY

Substrates available for energy come from three general types of nutrients: lipid, protein, and carbohydrate. The extent to which each contributes to energy expenditure depends upon the relative supplies of each and the tissue where they will be consumed. Two remarkable features of metabolism give it the flexibility to deal with deprivation, surfeit, and injury. First, the interconvertibility of carbohydrate and protein allows glucose to be converted to amino acids (non-essentials) and back again. All excess glucose and amino acids that cannot be stored as glycogen or protein or used immediately for fuel are converted to fat, which is an irreversible process. If the supply of glucose is low, amino acids stored as muscle are converted to glucose via gluconeogenesis. Likewise when the supply of protein is low, its conversion to the metabolic fuel glucose is minimized and fat becomes the major source of energy. Because the body cannot synthesize the 'essential' amino acids, effort is made to spare protein.

INSULIN ORCHESTRATION OF SUBSTRATE METABOLISM

The second feature that integrates metabolism is the use of insulin to control the relative levels of carbohydrate, amino acids and fat derivatives in the blood and hence their release or uptake by tissues. Insulin is affected most by glucose. In addition, the level of glucose during fasting provides the set point in the regulation of metabolic fuels. By having the substrates controlled by a single hormone and having several important substrates derived from each other, metabolism can achieve a tremendous flexibility in maintaining homeostasis in the face of a continually changing environment. The preservation of the lean body mass, the 'living' part of an organism, while intake varies, depending upon supply and the degree of stress largely accounts for our success as a species.

Insulin stimulates the conversion of glucose to glycogen and triglycerides in muscle and adipose tissue respectively. In addition the peripheral utilization of glucose is facilitated by insulin. The interaction between glucose and insulin constitutes a negative feedback loop where the fasting blood glucose levels are the physiological norm that this system attempts to maintain. The action of insulin on adipose tissue results in the retention of free fatty acids. The mechanism is thought to be an insulin-induced reduction of activity of a lipase mediated through cyclic AMP in the adipocyte which is also thought to enhance FFA esterification by making glycerol phosphates more available. Because of insulin's known anti-ketogenic and anti-lipolytic effects, high serum insulin concentrations are associated with low free fatty acid and ketone body concentrations. These substrates stimulate the release of insulin and so constitute a negative feedback loop as well. The consumption of free fatty acids and ketone bodies as fuels will spare glucose consumption, as is characteristic of starvation. The feedback loop however is not direct in that if glucose is being spared its concentration will rise, which in turn will stimulate the secretion of insulin[1-3].

The interaction of insulin and amino acids represents a third negative feedback loop in metabolism, though it is mediated through glucose. An increase in serum amino acid levels results in an increased production of

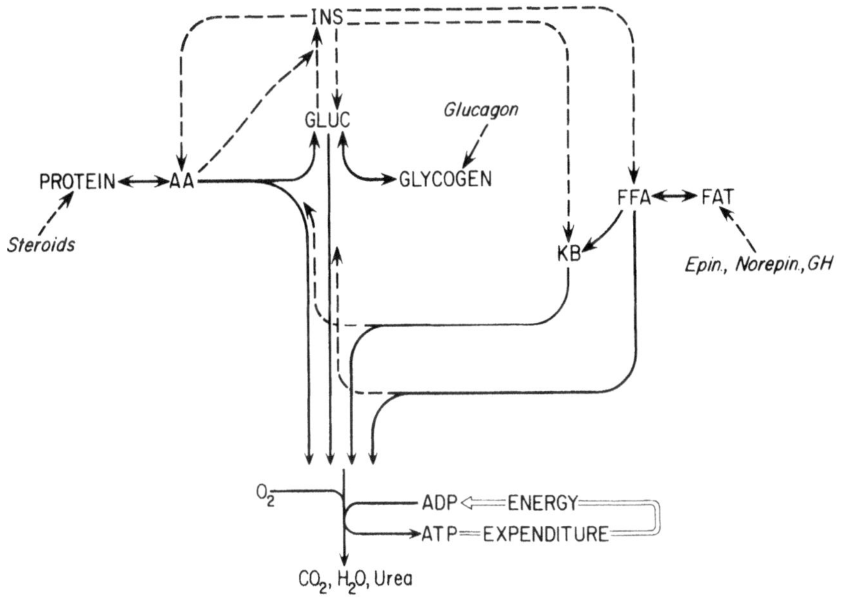

Figure 8.1 Metabolic fuel regulatory system. The arrows indicate the action of substrates or hormones; thus glucose 'pushes up' insulin levels and insulin 'pushes down' serum levels of free fatty acids. Solid lines indicate metabolic pathways; dashed lines indicated hormone/substrate interactions

glucose in the liver by the pathway of gluconeogenesis. This increase in blood sugar elicits an insulin response which promotes among other things the uptake of amino acids. Furthermore some amino acids can directly stimulate insulin secretion. This is most effective when circulating glucose levels are relatively high. These feedback loops are illustrated in Figure 8.1.

CATECHOLAMINES AND OTHER HORMONES

Other hormones that influence energy substrates do not have the global effects that insulin exerts over all sectors of metabolism. Most of these hormones are opposed to the action of insulin. Glucagon is most active in promoting hepatic gluconeogenesis. Specifically, the conversion of alanine to glucose is markedly enhanced. In addition glucagon suppresses the serum level of insulin, the latter inhibiting gluconeogenesis by inhibiting alanine uptake in liver.

Catecholamines are extremely important when discussing trauma and energy metabolism. These hormones enhance glucose and fat mobilization. The adrenal cortical hormones released during stress and injury affect glucose-6-phosphate in the liver and kidneys. This enzyme produces all the blood sugar by both glycogen mobilization and gluconeogenesis. Another major effect of catecholamines is to inhibit the enzyme pyruvate dehydrogenase which is responsible for glucose conversions to CO_2[7,8]. During injury muscle pyruvate dehydrogenase activity is reduced conserving glucose as a fuel for glucose-dependent cells. The energy deficit in muscles promotes the oxidation of branched-chain amino acids. This is the proteolysis commonly associated with severe injury[9,10].

COMPETITION FOR CoA

The relative contribution to the production of ATP by fat, carbohydrate and amino acids is the outcome of a competition for acetyl-CoA by the substrates represented by fat, amino acids and carbohydrate. In muscle the irreversible steps in carbohydrate and branched-chain amino acid (BCAA) degradation are oxidative decarboxylation of an α-keto acid, pyruvate to acetyl-CoA, and the α-keto derivatives of the BCAA to their respective CoA-derivatives. Likewise free fatty acids and ketone bodies are converted to CoA-derivatives before they can be oxidized. The mechanism that determines the relative proportion of CoA-derivatives is poorly understood, but the metabolic events are at least understandable in terms of competition for CoA. This scheme provides a possible explanation for the reduced rates of amino acid degradation that occur after large intakes of carbohydrate. Also competition for CoA by free fatty acids and ketones and amino acids would be nil because of high insulin levels, thereby leaving only carbohydrate to enter the tricarboxylic acid cycle.

KEY TISSUE

Skeletal muscle tissue represents the largest source of stored protein and consumes 30% of resting energy expenditure. The sarcoplasm, owing to its relatively short half-life, makes a greater contribution to the extracellular free amino acid pool than do the more stable structural proteins of muscle, actin and myosin. Several factors contribute to make muscle a readily available source of amino acids. Firstly, because muscle is composed of 20% BCAA, the only free amino acids muscle can consume, the remaining 80% are released into the extracellular pool to be used elsewhere. In addition, muscle protein synthesis involves only constitutional protein, i.e., no secretory proteins are manufactured. Thus muscle represents a sizeable labile pool of amino acids. The oxidation by muscle of isoleucine, valine and leucine, the only amino acids oxidized by muscle in appreciable amounts, is minimized when the more preferred fuels, ketones and fat are mobilized during the convalescent phase of injury[11].

This is in direct contrast to the liver which, while it represents only 1.6% of total body protein, synthesizes up to 50% of all protein made daily. Those proteins include albumin, fibrinogen, α and β globulins, and transferrin. Amino acids, with the exception of the BCAA are also consumed in the gluconeogenic and ureagenic pathways. Furthermore, the structural proteins of the liver have a relatively short half-life of 7–8 days. It is clear that the liver requirement for amino acids is large, and yet following injury the demand is even greater.

An important communication link between liver and muscle is the glucose-alanine cycle. Alanine is formed in muscle tissue by transamination of pyruvate derived from glucose catabolism. From there alanine is transported to the liver where through gluconeogenesis it is converted to glucose. The amine group, in part, derived from the peripheral oxidation of BCAA, and other amino acid transamination is converted to urea. Through insulin the rate of peripheral amino acid oxidation and gluconeogenesis is controlled[12].

FUNCTIONAL REDISTRIBUTION OF BODY CELL MASS

The metabolic response to injury is mediated by hormones directly and by inhibition and induction of enzymes. Most of the work in re-establishing body integrity and homeostasis requires new proteins. Cellular and humoral immune function, erythropoiesis, and new structural protein synthesis all require an adquate supply of precursors, amino acids. Muscle contributes a majority of the amino acids needed. The action of glucocorticoids and catecholamines initiates muscle tissue breakdown, the latter by reducing pyruvate dehydrogenase activity causing imbalances in amino acid mixtures which ultimately slows protein synthesis. Other tissues and organs contribute to the extracellular pool of free amino acids. Collagen tissue in the skin and elsewhere contribute up to 10 g N/day, following injury. The breakdown products of intestinal protein provide up to 15 g N/day. Another source of amino acids following injury is albumin. Figure 8.2 summarizes the sources and uses of endogenous nitrogen[10].

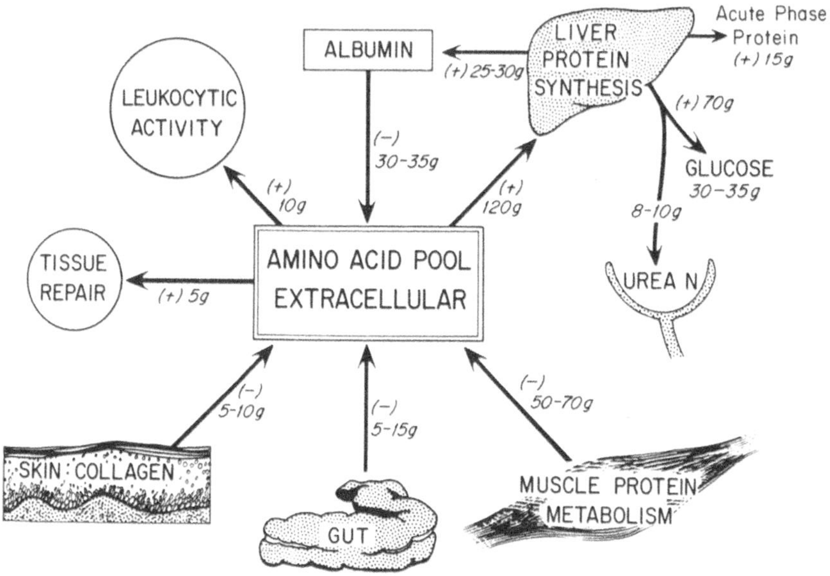

Figure 8.2 Functional redistribution of body cell mass. Following injury there is a response to distribute amino acids from the various tissues that stored protein to the tissues and organs that are involved in the response to injury. [+] indicate net uptake of amino acids, [−] net release.

Note: The body cell mass is defined by Moore as the energy-exchanging, mitotically-active tissue of the body. It is potassium- and phosphate-rich, being contained primarily within muscle and visceral organs (Moore, F. D., Olesen, K. H., McMurrey, J. D., *et al. The Body Cell Mass and Its Supporting Environment: Body Composition in Health and Disease.* Philadelphia: Saunders, 1963)

This mechanism for redistribution has evolved to ensure the most effective use of nitrogen supply, and hence has survival value. In designing post-operative fluid and nutritional support, the clinician should be aware of the substrate and hormonal environment that allows for the efficient use of endogenous protein stores. The appropriate therapy will be one that complements and utilizes the metabolic response to injury rather than one that antagonizes. The administration of 5% dextrose post-operatively is one which antagonizes the normal response to injury. The proteolysis of muscle is inhibited by dextrose infusions, thus depriving the visceral tissue of badly needed protein. Equally important is the inhibition of lipolysis and ketone formation, the effect of which is to deprive the body of an important source of fuel (fat), and forcing the otherwise unnecessary oxidation of amino acids, particularly the essential BCAA in muscle. These considerations require that clinicians be acutely aware of the biochemical and metabolic events following injury.

METHODS

In order to test our hypothesis regarding the primacy of energy a prospective study was designed[13]. Twenty patients were assigned at random to one of two groups, one receiving 5% dextrose solution, the other receiving 3.5% amino acids solution alone. No patients classified as severely depleted nutritionally according to accepted standards were studied, nor were those classified as severely hypermetabolic, determined by urinary urea excretion. Only adults undergoing elective operations for hepatic, biliary, pancreatic disease, or inflammatory bowel conditions requiring intravenous fluid replacement for 6–10 days were eligible. Those patients with diabetes mellitus, heart failure, liver failure, renal failure, shock, or any other disease affecting gross metabolic alterations were excluded.

Each patient received 3 l of solution with vitamin, mineral and electrolyte requirements as tolerated within fluid requirements. All fluid requirements greater than 3 l were met with a balanced electrolyte solution. Serum electrolytes, liver function tests including albumin, and renal function tests were performed on the 1st day and every 2nd day thereafter. In addition glucose, ketone bodies, insulin, and free fatty acids were measured on serum every other day. Urine was collected every 24 h and analysed for urea nitrogen, creatinine, and electrolytes. The presence or absence of ketones and glucose in the urine was determined twice daily. Finally, those parameters of nutritional status—transferrin, delayed hypersensitivity skin tests, and body composition using anthropometric values—were measured at the beginning and end of the study.

RESULTS

Those patients who received amino acid solutions lost a significantly smaller amount of nitrogen compared to those receiving solutions containing only glucose. Amino acid intake on the day of operation was essentially none, and was increased daily in 30 g amounts until those patients were receiving 100 g. The average initial losses then were similar: the amino acid group lost 8.5 ± 0.4 g compared with the dextrose group losses of 10.7 ± 4.3 g of nitrogen. However, net nitrogen losses were significantly less ($P < 0.001$) in the amino acid group, 3.8 ± 1.0 g compared with the dextrose group net losses of 12.3 ± 2.7 g. The results are summarized in Figure 8.3.

The energy fuel substrates and insulin levels were distinctly different. In the amino acid group, ketonuria developed in 1–3 days after operation and persisted while no patient receiving dextrose developed ketonuria. The free

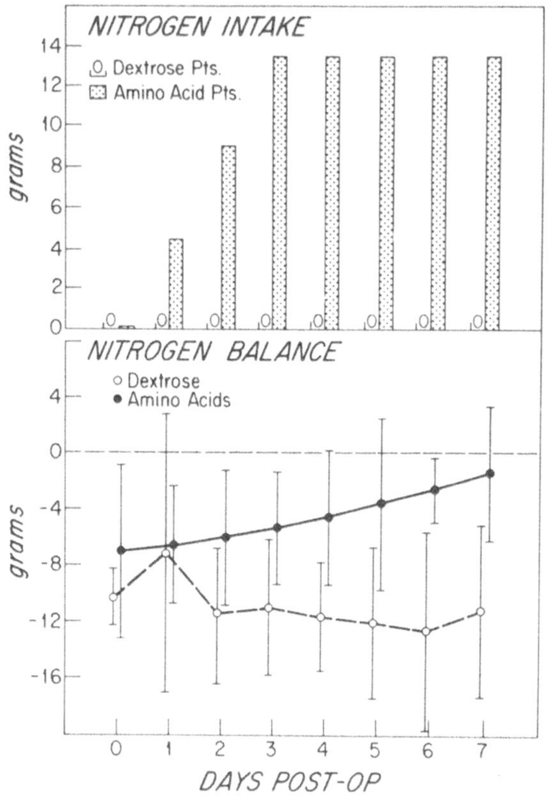

Figure 8.3 Nitrogen intake and balance. Those patients receiving no nitrogen had a consistently negative nitrogen whereas those patients receiving nitrogen in the form of crystalline amino acids had steadily improving nitrogen balances

fatty acid and ketone body levels in the blood reflected the clinical signs. For the dextrose patients, FFA levels did not change over the study period, but remained at 530 mM. For the amino acid group, FFA levels on day 1 were comparable but rose steadily to an average of 1133 mM ($P < 0.001$). For the dextrose group ketone bodies remained at 0.025 mM throughout while the amino acid group showed 0.43 mM on day 1 ($P < 0.005$) and also rose to 1.74 mM ($P < 0.001$) by the conclusion of the study.

In the dextrose group insulin levels decreased from 54 to 28, in the amino acid group from 48 to 15. Only on the day of operation were values in the different groups not significantly different statistically. The blood glucose levels in the dextrose group fell from 146 mg/dl to 128 mg/dl where they remained. In the amino acid group, glucose decreased from 127 to 83 by the 4th day, where they remained. Finally, potassium balances for the two groups over the course of therapy defined curves similar to the nitrogen balances for the two groups (Figure 8.4).

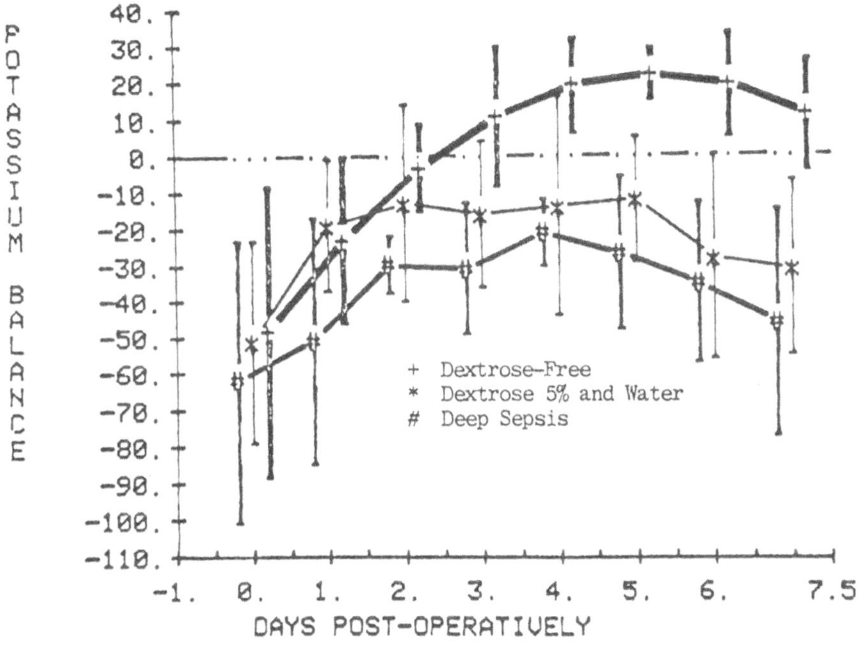

Figure 8.4 Potassium balances. The potassium balance of the group follows closely the behaviour of the nitrogen balance curves

Four patients who developed deep surgical sepsis were given amino acid solutions as well. In these patients, none manifested and maintained ketosis. Figure 8.5 shows that the nitrogen balance of these patients was comparable to that of patients receiving 5% dextrose post-operatively. This would support the hypothesis that unless an alternative source of energy exists, amino acids must and will be oxidized. Catabolism of the lean body mass is indicated by urinary urea nitrogen excretion. Those patients receiving hypocaloric amounts of dextrose or those with a reduced capacity to utilize fat because of sepsis have no alternative other than to use amino acids for fuel[14].

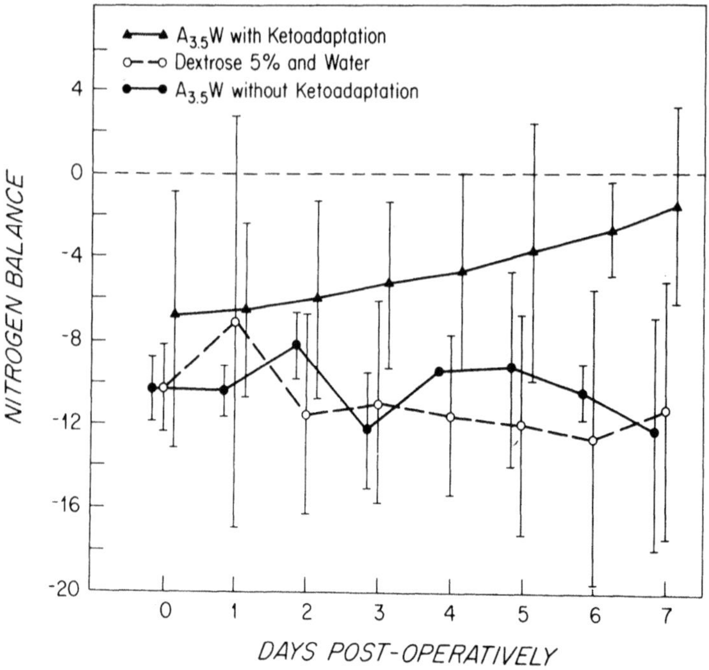

Figure 8.5 Nitrogen balance in patients who did not develop ketonuria. Those patients on amino acids who did not develop ketonuria had nitrogen balances similar to patients receiving dextrose who also did not develop ketonuria

DISCUSSION

The renewed interest and abundance of investigators studying post-operative management has given rise to nearly an equal number of opinions concerning the appropriate electrolyte, fluid, and nutritional support[15]. However, many investigators tend to base results on nitrogen balance and fail to recognize the underlying principles that determine what is appropriate or just merely adequate for most patients[16].

The supply of energy is pre-eminent among cellular wants. Those who advocate the administration of carbohydrate and amino acids together in hypocaloric amounts deprive the patient the use of endogenous fat and the hormonal substrate environment which will allow redistribution of body cell mass. The release of insulin, a necessary consequence of infusing glucose, inhibits muscle amino acid release, ketone production and fat mobilization, thereby depriving tissues of amino acids and a readily usable form of energy. Reducing the supply of fat-derived energy beyond that replaced by glucose (3–4 kcal/g hydrous glucose) requires the body to increase the oxidation of amino acids, either directly as in muscle, or through gluconeogenesis. If nutritional support is restricted to a dextrose-free regimen, fat is mobilized much as it is during starvation and amino acid oxidation is reduced to the minimum of 12–16% of total energy expenditure which can easily be provided by isotonic amino acid infusions.

Greenberg *et al.*[17] have concluded that nitrogen intake is the most important variable affecting nitrogen balance post-operatively. These studies however limit themselves to the 3 days following elective surgery and do not take into consideration the need for redistribution of body cell mass. The addition of glucose to amino acid solutions did not improve nitrogen equilibrium, an observation best understood by the decrease in FFA and ketone body availability to meet the energy requirement.

Elwyn *et al.*[18] has demonstrated an improvement in nitrogen balance in the first 4 days following operation when glucose is added to amino acid solutions, prior to starvation adaptation; however during the period between 4 and 8 days after operation, when adaptation has occurred, there is no difference between the two populations of patients, one receiving amino acids, the other receiving amino acid with added glucose. These results are at variance with those submitted by Greenberg. Our data would emphasize the need for 5–7 days' time to maximize dietary nitrogen utilization and starvation adaptation.

Freeman and colleagues[19] have evaluated the protein-sparing effect of amino acid infusions and conclude the nitrogen-sparing effect depends upon the mobilization and use of body fat as the major source of calories. An improved nitrogen balance correlated with increased FFA and ketone body levels. They do not attribute the nitrogen-sparing effect to the patient's adaptation to partial starvation, however. Yet adaptation to the semi-starved state metabolism, both protein and energy, is crucial to nitrogen sparing in terms of protein turnover and appropriate support of visceral tissues. Time to switch body fuels from carbohydrate to fat and slow protein turnover is necessary in reaching this goal. Any administration of dextrose after adaptation has occurred will immediately throw back the metabolic fuel cycle to a dependence upon carbohydrate. Similar nitrogen balance is not an observation that would allow one to refute the argument that nitrogen sparing using amino acids alone is benefited by starvation adaptation. Rather it is an observation in favour of the argument since similar nitrogen balance is less reflective of nitrogen uptake in muscle.

Hoover *et al.*[20] arrive at the same conclusion as Greenberg *et al.*, that nitrogen intake is the key factor in nitrogen sparing. Nitrogen intake has been emphasized by us since the original manuscripts[4,5]. The efficacy of amino acid administration in supporting visceral function, particularly host defence and the mechanisms for this protein-sparing effect have yet to be definitively determined. Skillman[21] has shown an increase in albumin synthesis in patients receiving amino acids compared with those receiving dextrose. He reports a 51% increase or ($P < 0.05$) 140 mg/kg/day above the normal albumin synthesis rate in those receiving amino acids. This supports the concept that albumin synthesis depends upon the availability of substrate, viz. amino acids and starvation modified by dextrose-free amino acid infusion. The effect of adding glucose to the amino acids is not likely to improve this response as glucose lowers the amount of amino acids available to the liver that can be used for synthesis, which has the potential to affect the albumin synthesis rate.

O'Keefe's[22] data corroborate Skillman's work. O'Keefe measured protein breakdown and synthesis rates on the 2nd and 3rd post-operative day in patients receiving either 100 g of dextrose or 90 g of amino acids. Breakdown rates were comparable for the two groups but synthesis rates in the amino acid group were significantly higher ($P < 0.001$).

Miller *et al.*[14] have shown that those patients receiving amino acids for whom fat utilization is diminished are in negative nitrogen balance similar to those patients receiving simply dextrose. We concluded that nitrogen intake is not sufficient to insure the goals of optimal protein sparing. What is crucial is the presence of non-protein fuel substrate and a hormonal setting that will redistribute the body cell mass. If carbohydrate is to supply the majority of caloric needs it must be delivered in a hyperosmolar solution, a procedure that is indicated in moderately hypermetabolic and nutrionally depleted patients. If 5% glucose is added to amino acid solutions, the osmolarity

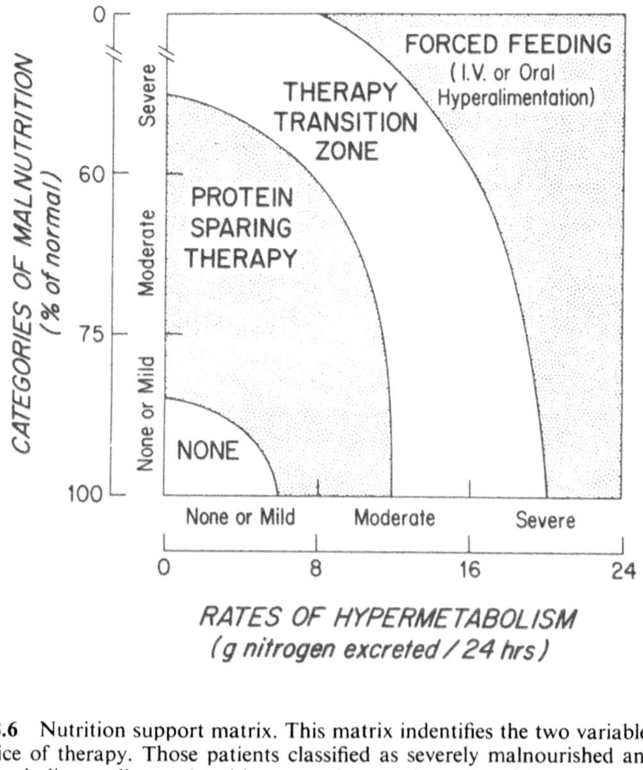

Figure 8.6 Nutrition support matrix. This matrix indentifies the two variables influencing the choice of therapy. Those patients classified as severely malnourished and/or severely hypermetabolic usually require either enteral or total parenteral hyperalimentation

(600 mOsm) exceeds the threshold which peripheral veins can tolerate. The addition of glucose reduces the utilization of endogenous fat. High insulin levels and a relative scarcity of non-protein fuel substrates will lead to greater amino acid oxidation. The use of hypercaloric glucose changes the amino acid pattern in the blood as well. High insulin levels resulting from glucose infusions enhance muscle uptake of amino acids, depriving the liver and other visceral tissue of a source of protein needed for synthesis. BCAA are retained by muscle which results in the preservation of that tissue mass.

In the absence of alternative fuels oxidation of BCAA lowers the total amount of amino acids that can be used for synthesis. BCAA levels below the 2 h post-prandial level reflect depleted free amino acid concentrations which produces amino acid imbalances that can cause the oxidation of non-essential amino acids in the liver. The factors important in promoting the optimal response to injury include the hormonal/enzyme setting, the supply of non-protein calories, and the size of the free amino acid pool which itself depends upon protein breakdown, dietary intake, and adaptation to starvation.

Figure 8.6 illustrates the two variables that determine nutritional support. The rate of hypermetabolism is estimated by the daily rate of urinary urea nitrogen excretion. The presence or degree of malnutrition is determined by the patient's weight: height ratio compared to standards. Clearly hypocaloric feedings are reserved for preservation of visceral protein mass and the prevention of protein malnutrition.

CONCLUSIONS

The metabolic response to injury is characterized by an increase in protein catabolism so that amino acids might be provided for synthesis of acute phase proteins, immune function, and repair of breeched tissue. Energy is provided by glucose and fat. After 48 h the contribution to energy expenditure by glucose derived from glycogen stores does not exceed 100 cal because the supply is exhausted. Fat and its derivatives supply over 80% of the energy needed. The point at which the body begins to depend almost exclusively upon fat for energy is termed adaptation to semi-starvation. It is manifested by urinary ketones and low insulin and blood sugar levels. After most surgery, the body reaches an adaptive state by the 3rd or 4th day[23]. Initially, there is in muscle an obligatory oxidation of BCAA, presumably so that the remaining amino acids may be used for gluconeogenesis and visceral protein synthesis[24]. This has been termed the functional redistribution of body protein—the transfer of amino acids to tissue where the need is more acute to survival.

Metabolic adaptation to injury is similar to adaptation to short-term starvation: fuel comes from stored fat, amino acids from gut, collagenous tissue, and skeletal muscle. Administering amino acids alone only enhances what is already a normal, teleologic response. The addition of small amounts of glucose to the amino acid solution is a metabolically contradictory signal.

Force feeding routines of total parenteral nutrition are required for resuscitation from sepsis, shock and treatment of protein calorie malnutrition. The addition of lipid to the solution would not affect the overall protein sparing of amino acids as most patients have an adequate supply of fat. Given the osmotic limitations of peripheral veins, isotonic amino acid solution with electrolytes is the appropriate therapy, one which takes advantage of a protein-sparing mechanism that has evolved to deal most effectively with injury[10].

Recovery from injury depends upon the status of the body cell mass. If malnutrition and infection are superimposed on injury, the morbidity is greater and the effects of stress are exaggerated[25]. To evaluate protein sparing in terms of nitrogen balance is to ignore the relative importance of certain tissue compared to others. Visceral tissues, including liver and heart, are arguably more important in restoring the injured body to health. Consideration should therefore be given to what tissue is being spared. Carbohydrate infusions enhance muscle retention of amino acids, but for what purpose? The reapportionment of muscle protein on the other hand to the viscera can provide amino acids to organs vital for survival. The infusion of near isotonic amino acids is a therapy that efficiently provides substrates necessary for recovery from injury.

References

1. Blackburn, G. L. and Flatt, J. P. (1972). A new concept of metabolic fuel cycle. *Proceedings of Eighth Midwest conference on Endocrinology and Metabolism.* (Columbia: University of Missouri), p. 115
2. Blackburn, G. L. and Flatt, J. P. (1974). Substrate profile in protein wasting states. In H. Brown (ed.). *Protein Nutrition*, p. 201. (Springfield, Ill.: Charles C. Thomas)
3. Blackburn, G. L. (1973). A new concept and its application for protein-sparing therapies during semi-starvation. Ph.D. Thesis. Mass. Inst. Tech.
4. Blackburn, G. L., Flatt, J. P., Clowes, G. H. A. and O'Donnell, T. F. (1973). Peripheral intravenous feeding with isotonic amino acid solutions. *Am. J. Surg.*, **125**, 447
5. Blackburn, G. L., Flatt, J. P., Clowes, G. H. A., O'Donnell, T. F. and Hensle, T. E. (1973). Protein-sparing therapy during periods of starvation with sepsis or trauma. *Ann. Surg.*, **177**, 588
6. Flatt, J. P. and Blackburn, G. L. (1974). The metabolic fuel regulatory system: Implications for protein-sparing therapy during caloric deprivation or disease. *Am. J. Clin. Nutr.*, **27**, 175
7. Ryan, N. T., Blackburn, G. L. and Clowes, G. H. A. (1974). Differential tissue sensitivity to elevated endogenous insulin levels during experimental peritonitis in rats. *Metabolism*, **23**, 1081
8. Kusaka, M. and Vi, M. (1977). Activation of the Cori cycle by epinephrine. *Am. J. Physiol.*, **232** (2), E145
9. O'Donnell, T. F., Blackburn, G. L., Ryan, N. T. and Miller, J. D. B. (1976). Proteolysis associated with a deficit of peripheral energy fuel substrate in septic man. *Surgery*, **80**, 192
10. Blackburn, G. L. (1977). Nitrogen metabolism after surgical injury. In Physiology of Medicine. *N. Engl. J. Med.* (In press)
11. Blackburn, G. L. and Bistrian, B. R. (1976). Nutritional care of the injured and/or septic patient. In G. H. A. Clowes, Jr. (ed.). *Symposium on Response to Infection and Injury II. Surg. Clin. N. Am.*, **56**, 1195

12. Cahill, G. F. (1971). Physiology of insulin in man. *Diabetes*, **20**, 785
13. Miller, J. D. G., Bistrian, B. R., Blackburn, G. L., Rienhoff, H. Y., Jr. *et al.* (1977). Failure of post-operative infection to increase nitrogen excretion in patients maintained on peripheral amino acids. *Am. J. Clin. Nutr.*, **30,** 1523–1527
14. Miller, J. D. B., Bistrian, B. R., Blackburn, G. L., Rienhoff, H. Y., Jr. *et al.* (1977). Effect of deep surgical sepsis on protein-sparing therapies and nitrogen balance. *Am. J. Clin. Nutr.*, **30,** 1493–1497
15. Editorial, *Lancet*, August 9, 1975, p. 263.
16. Moldawer, L. L., Nakano, Y., Etter, G. *et al.* (1977). The ability of fat to preserve cell-mediated immunity in the rat. *Surg. For.*, **28** (In press)
17. Greenberg, G. R., Marliss, E. B., Anderson, G. H. *et al.* (1976). Protein-sparing therapies in post-operative patients: Effect of added hypocaloric glucose or lipid. *N. Engl. J. Med.*, **294**, 1411
18. Elwyn, D. H., Long, C. L., Iles, M. *et al.* (1977). Energy and nitrogen-sparing of 5% glucose added to peripheral infusions of amino acids in post-operative patients (abstract). *J. Parenteral and Enteral Nutrition* (C. B. Slack, pub.) **1**, 8A
19. Freeman, J. B., Stegink, L. D., Whittine, M. F. *et al.* (1977). Current status of protein sparing. *Surg. Gynecol. Obstet.*, **144**, 843–849
20. Hoover, H. C., Grant, J. P., Gorschboth, C. *et al.* (1975). Nitrogen-sparing intravenous fluids in post-operative patients. *N. Engl. J. Med.*, **293**, 172
21. Skillman, J. J., Rosenoer, V. M., Smith, P. C. *et al.* (1976). Improved albumin synthesis in post-operative patients by amino acid infusions. *N. Engl. J. Med.*, **295**, 1037
22. O'Keefe, S. J. D., Sender, P. M., Clark, G. C. *et al.* (1974). The effect of varying the post-operative parenteral regime on the dynamics of protein metabolism following operative trauma. *Proceedings, International Conference on Parenteral Nutrition.* Montpelier, France, p. 133
23. Blackburn, G. L., Flatt, J. P. and Heddle, T. E. (1976). Peripheral amino acid infusions. In J. Fischer (ed.). *Total Parenteral Nutrition*, Chap. 19, pp. 363–394 (Boston: Little, Brown & Co.)
24. Benotti, P. N., Blackburn, G. L., Miller, J. D. B. *et al.* (1976). Role of branched-chain amino acids (BCAA) intake in preventing muscle proteolysis. *Surg. For.*, **27**, 7
25. Bistrian, B. R., Blackburn, G. L., Scrimshaw, N. S. and Flatt, J. P. (1975). Cellular immunity in semi-starved states in hospitalized adults. *Am. J. Clin. Nutr.*, **28**, 1147

Discussion

H. N. Munro: (USA) Questions might focus on four points:

1. The metabolic background and its quantitation.
2. The actual result of administering amino acid solutions with glucose or without.
3. The appropriate type of patient on which this can be practised—how does one select suitable cases for this therapy and how short-term and long-term is it?
4. The payoff to be expected in planned and unplanned injuries in terms of long-term function, returning to work, and long-term effects of the injury.

H. F. Woods: (UK) Dr Blackburn showed two slides that indicate clearly how, on his regimen, infusing amino acids, the ketone body concentrations in blood are higher. How much of the amino acid nitrogen that he infuses is actually used to generate ketone bodies from ketogenic amino acid such as phenylalanine?

G. L. Blackburn: (USA) We are not sure we know how to quantitate that. When we use the amino acid infusion-free state as in the physiological electrolyte solution, we do see about the same amount of ketone bodies as we do with the amino acids. About 50% of the amino acids infused after this adaptation at 5–7 days is retained as nitrogen, and 50% lost. The contribution of the ketogenic amino acids in the diet is small (approximately 20%).

In answer to the question, ketogenesis from the infused amino acids will be a very small fraction, but I cannot specify the contribution. This is one reason we are developing branched-chain amino acid supplements to be used when insulin levels block ketogenesis from fat (i.e. the non-ketone adapted state of sepsis and injury).

Woods: Secondly, when the patients are provided with amino acids, what is the fuel that is providing energy for hepatic protein synthesis, rather than muscle protein synthesis?

Blackburn: A number of *in vitro* liver *perfusion* studies would suggest that the fuel is partially fat plus complete oxidation to ketones which is energy yielding oxidation of fat to CO_2 and water. Net protein utilization is about 50%. Many of the amino acids are lost through urea excretion by the liver, the carbon skeleton providing fuel for liver work. There is also the availability of amino acids—those being broken down in peripheral tissues and recirculated.

It would be a combination of amino acids and free fatty acids.

P. Vinay: (Canada) Would Dr Blackburn say more about the apparent relationship between inadequate fat mobilization and muscle breaking down its own protein as a source of energy. Is this more or less circumstantial? The fact that the free fatty acids drop in concentration in the plasma does not necessarily mean that they are not available for muscle oxidation, or does Dr Blackburn feel that it does?

Blackburn: Clearly the forearm studies show that there is much regional fat oxidation. There is fat in muscle that could be burned and we would never be able to reflect that in the general circulation substrate measurements. There is also fat mobilized in the limb and consumed in the limb that we could not measure. We have carried out forearm studies in which we have looked at superficial-vein and deep-vein contribution to confirm that point. I can only agree with Dr Vinay that the evidence is circumstantial. I do believe that much data support the hypothesis. Issenkutz and others[1] report remarkable correlation between plasma concentrations and rates of oxidation. In the ranges that we are discussing (0.2–1.0 mM free fatty acid levels), their flux and their turnover are correlated. We cannot go beyond that. We are leaning heavily on these relationships, free fatty acid concentrations, and their contribution to a respiratory quotient and their turnover rate[2,3].

E. M. Copeland: (USA) Would Dr Blackburn put protein sparing in the clinical setting? When exactly does he use it, and where does IVH fit into that system?

Secondly, in his immune rat studies, Dr Blackburn did not use a protein diet; he had a fat diet and a carbohydrate diet. In our own studies with a protein diet immune competence was not maintained. Is he saying that it was not maintained because of lack of fat in the annular and the inability to mobilize ketone bodies, which might have maintained immune competence?

Blackburn: To take the second question first. We have not been able to get the rats to drink crystalline amino acids in adequate amounts. Since the rats are without adequate non-protein calorie reserves they become catabolic. Thus no effect of a protein only, hypocaloric diet can be studied in rats other than for a few days. We believe the observations of Dr Copeland's group can be explained by this lack of energy reserve in the rat[4]. In Moldawer's experiments the feeding of hypocaloric amounts of fat, without protein, does retain cell-mediated immunity similar to control rats with the exception of weight gain. Detailed tissue analysis reveals that the protein content of the visceral tissue particularly the liver is maintained by hypocaloric feeding of fat with 20% of the calories provided as protein but carbohydrate free!

We conclude that if rat experiments are to be used for studying nutritional support the energy state will have to be controlled. This will make it necessary to survive more than a few days. The figures provided emphasize that as free fatty acid and ketone levels fall nitrogen excretion increases (Figure 1). Further the provision of non-protein calories as fat will significantly decrease nitrogen loss in a rat (Figure 2). Dr Jim Long, in personal communication, has told me he has observed similar findings with his experiments.

We were encouraged along these lines because at MIT we have fed volunteers amino acids alone for as long as 330 days, and the work has been published in the *American Journal of Clinical Nutrition* (**28**, 1147; 1975). Immune competence is maintained. Therefore man clearly can maintain his immune competence, his creatinine height index, his ^{40}K and his body composition for as long as 330 days on a protein carbohydrate-free diet.

The clinical indications for protein sparing are not worked out. We have spent the past 5 years trying to work out the metabolism of this area, and the appropriate clinical trials are not yet complete. Our indications for hyperalimentation are patients with: (1) deteriorating visceral protein function, e.g. albumin and transferrin: and (2) falling immune competence. We do 'protein-spare' those patients in whom we can project that they will get into moderate or severe malnutrition based on serum albumin levels in the range 3.0 or 3.2 as being only mildly malnourished. When, however, transferrin levels fall below

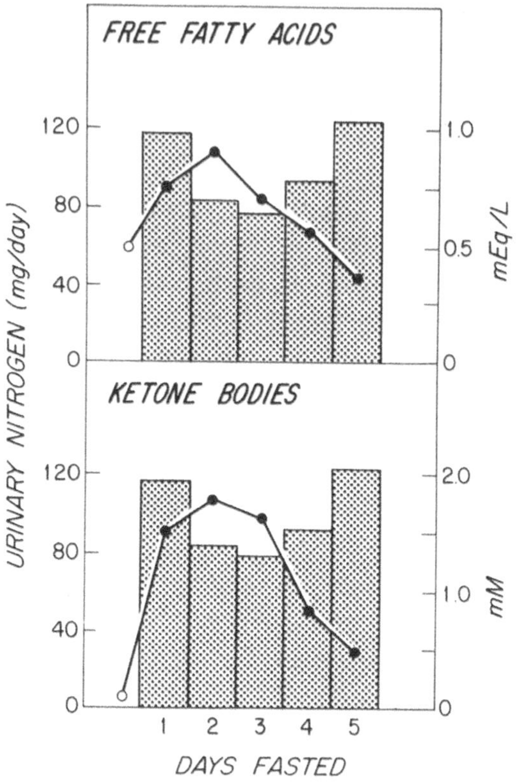

Figure 1 Free fatty acids, ketone bodies and urinary nitrogen during fasting in rats

170 mg%, or in patients whose skin tests convert from positive to negatives, these patients are immediately put onto intravenous hyperalimentation.

We have seen work at the MGH on patients getting 4500 rads and a total cystectomy and ileal loop who were given dextrose and water. Half of the patients who were malnourished had to go to hyperalimentation, whereas none of twenty-nine patients given isotonic amino acids had to have hyperalimentation.

When does one start? Clearly there is no need to start any well-nourished patient who is only to be starved for a short (1–3 day) period of time. However either in anticipation, or for patients who are moderately depleted, we would use near-isotonic amino acid infusion. Those indices for us are anthropometric measurements 15–20% below normal in weight for height, weight loss, skin-fold thickness or arm muscle circumference. These indices are easy to identify. There are a remarkable number of young women, particularly, who are underweight as far as fat reserves are concerned and they may be ill-advised to have elective surgery without some protein/amino acid nutritional support. We believe that many of them can be supported adequately by a protein-sparing regimen. There are a variety of geriatric patients who have moderate to severe malnutrition by the indices that have been stated, and they clearly must have hyperalimentation.

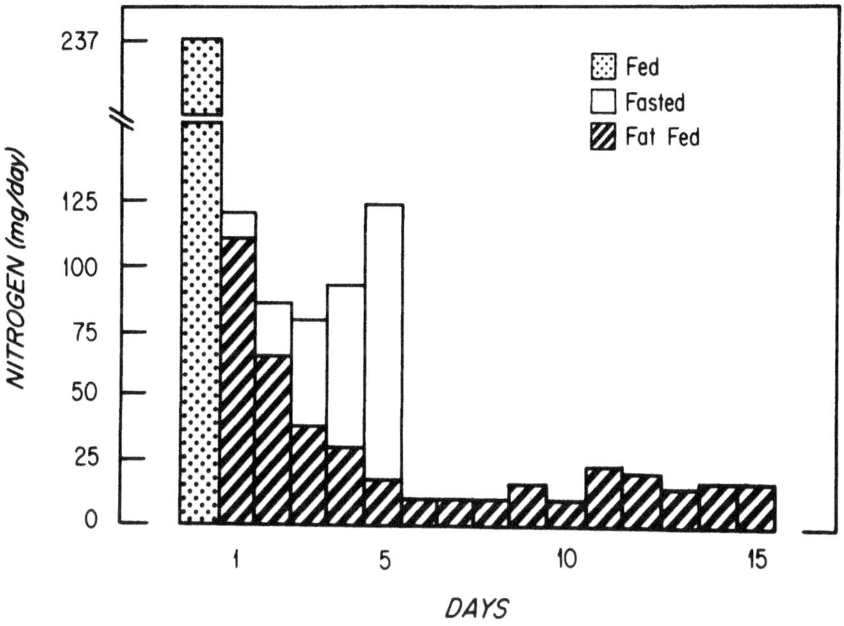

Figure 2 Urinary nitrogen excretion during different feeding programmes in rats

These are our guidelines obtained from prospective studies and we shall have to see what the cost-benefit/risk–benefit of this practice is. Anybody who thinks that protein-sparing is a substitute for hyperalimentation is mistaken.

Vinay: At the beginning of his presentation, Dr Blackburn referred to the state of gluconeogenesis during fasting with usage of oxaloacetate which would not impair the TCA cycle, and would not be a disadvantage, since oxaloacetate is also synthesized in a similar and proportional manner.

Blackburn: I am not quite sure that oxaloacetate can be generated from a resting TCA during the process of gluconeogenesis in the same way that oxaloacetate can be generated from a resting TCA. I am calling on the work of Hansen showing that the PEP CK activity goes on outside the mitochondria. This may indeed be the rate-limiting step. It is primarily an NAD/NADH ratio that will control entrance in the TCA cycle. Perhaps we should discuss whether in the process of gluconeogenesis there can be simultaneous TCA energy regeneration.

A. B. Jones: (Canada) The corollary to 'a man is not a rat' is that a child is not a man. We should include in the contra-indications for amino acids alone young children who have a much higher metabolic rate and who can ill afford to lose any of their fat stores.

Blackburn: Not only that, but they evidently have an enormous dependence on exogenous glucose to maintain glucose homeostasis, so I would subscribe to that.

Fürst: What is Dr Blackburn's opinion of glycogen stores? There is both direct and indirect evidence that liver glycogen stores will be exhausted within 3 days of carbohydrate deprivation. In this condition practically all infused amino acids should go primarily to glyconeogenesis, to restore glycogen.

Blackburn: This clearly does not happen because the nitrogen balance is improved and protein synthesis is improved. Further, not all of the glycogen is depleted. It appears to be only about 50% by tissue analysis in this protein-sparing state.

Fürst: Muscle glycogen is not critical. I agree that this takes a long time to deplete. However, liver glycogen is very sensitive to carbohydrate deprivation. There is evidence that liver glycogen stores, from direct measurements in biopsy material in healthy subjects, are practically empty after 3 days.

Dr Blackburn's protein effect is surely an adaptation to a lower protein intake—in reality.

Blackburn: The protein intake is twice the recommended daily allowance. It is 1.5–2 g/kg/day and so it is not a low-protein diet at all. It is clearly protein-sparing and is associated with reduced, but not depleted, liver glycogen stores.

D. W. Wilmore: (USA) It is important for all of us to work on categorizing and characterizing patients. Now it is apparent that certain patients will respond to certain kinds of therapy, and others will not. This may be contingent on whether patients can make ketone bodies, so that those patients who can keto-adapt will be responsive to fat in their diet, and can nitrogen-spare depending on the amount of energy, and they will be responsive to amino acid inputs over a period of time.

We know the ends of the spectrum of these critical illnesses. What we need to do is to think about how to fill in that spectrum. At one end of the spectrum is starved man who can make a lot of ketones. At the other end of the spectrum is man who is quite critically ill, and who has a very high mortality rate.

Can Dr Blackburn help us by describing his patients. Can he say something about them? Dr Shizgal and others have the ability to characterize some of these patients so that we shall know when to use these different kinds of therapy.

Blackburn: We have looked at our results and although we do not have burn patients we know that 85% of the hospitalized patients can benefit by protein therapy as we describe it. The septic population is in the remaining 15% and is a small fraction of hospital admissions. These septic patients' proper therapy has yet to be worked out. However, the criteria will be more than the measurement of nitrogen balance. We feel that our branch chain amino acid studies and [^{14}C]leucine turnover studies will help produce the answer. Certainly the patient who cannot keto-adapt will have to have alternate non-protein fuel. While glucose is certainly effective in producing nitrogen balance it should not be substituted for large infusions of protein in the neighbourhood of $1\frac{1}{2}$–$2\frac{1}{2}$ g/kg/day.

We would emphasize that in resuscitation of critically ill traumatized patients, particularly those who are hyperdynamic and have renal failure, will benefit by early aggressive use of 2% amino acid and 25% glucose. We prefer to see this effect as pharmacological and not necessarily nutritional or protein-sparing. An increased carbohydrate flux, subsequent lactate production and oxidation in heart and skeletal muscle appear to be most beneficial during these hypermetabolic stress states.

However during convalescence after this stress state, protein-sparing therapies may be utilized effectively, providing the patient does not become malnourished.

In summary the resuscitated group, the hypermetabolic septic group and the burn group are examples in which presently available crystalline amino acids should not be infused alone without further investigation.

These patients are treated with crystalline amino acids and 25–35%

glucose depending upon fluid tolerance. This includes patients with fevers of 102–103 °F, positive blood culture, deep wound infections, subphrenic abscesses, etc. However, patients with mild infections such as pneumonitis, urinary tract infection, limited superficial wound infections who will produce ketones can be effectively 'protein-spared'.

The long-term hypermetabolic patients with a pulse of 110–120 and low-grade fever of 100–101 °F are being investigated using high doses of protein ($1\frac{1}{2}$–$2\frac{1}{2}$ g/kg/day) with or without glucose. I again would emphasize that nitrogen balance is not the criterion which will decide the nutritional effect.

A. Goode: (UK) In peripheral infusion of isotonic amino acid solutions, what is the incidence of thrombophlebitis for Dr Blackburn's patients?

Blackburn: We currently have a study under way to get data on this. It is no different in our hands to the incidence of vein intolerance with 5% dextrose. These peripheral intravenous catheters can be kept open for several days.

The exception has been with solutions which are too high in potassium, beyond the requirements needed in protein-sparing, and which have damaged the veins. We have found individuals who have a particular intolerance to intravenous feeding. The phlebitis incidence with pH-6 non-buffered dextrose and water has been higher than in the 3.5% amino-acid group with only 15–20 mg K and an osmolality of 880 mOsm.

Clearly there is a substantial intolerance to certain factors such as electrolyte additives to the amino acids in certain individuals.

R. K. Ausman: (USA) Some 2–3 years ago a paper by Schulte *et al.*[5] described protein-sparing. They achieved nitrogen balance in accordance with the postulates set forth by Dr Blackburn, but, curiously, they found no keto-adaptation. Dr Schumer and I were curious, and repeated the work. We measured nitrogen balance and got the results suggested by Dr Blackburn, but we failed to see keto-adaptation. There were no differences in the levels of ketone bodies in either group, the control or the experimental. Would Dr Blackburn comment[2].

Blackburn: Using $1\frac{1}{2}$ g of protein/kg/day, I don't believe that we have seen good nitrogen balance using protein-sparing therapy that is glucose free in which we do not see ketosis or ketonuria. I believe Schulte *et al.* used considerably higher concentrations of protein which may have produced enough glyconeogenesis, hyperglycaemia and insulin stimulation to reduce ketogenesis. Further if the monitoring used is only ketonuria, the renal threshold and/or muscle consumption of the ketones may preclude identification of a state of ketosis.

The important role of ketones in protein sparing has been reported by Smith and Alberti[6], who observed the effect of ketones on protein-sparing in patients receiving dextrose solutions. Ketones is a key factor influencing preservation of body cell mass, particularly visceral protein during hypocaloric feedings, and has been reviewed extensively in the recent AMA symposium on nutrition: *Amino Acids* (H. Green, ed.). Buse[7] and Sherwin *et al.*[8] are but a few of the numerous references to support the role of ketone bodies in protein-sparing therapy.

References

1. Issekutz, B. (1967). *Metabolism*, **16,** 1001
2. O'Donnel *et al.* (1976). *Surgery*, **80,** 192
3. Imamara *et al.* (1975). *Surgery*, **77,** 868
4. Moldawer, Linc, *et al.* (1977). *Surg. For.* (in press)
5. Schulte, W. J., Condon, R. E. and Kraus, M. A. (1975). *Arch. Surg.* **110,** 914
6. Smith, R., Fuller, D. J., Wedge, J. H., Williamson, D. H. and Alberti, K. G. G. M.

Initial effect of injury on ketone bodies and other blood metabolites. (1975). *Lancet*, **1,** 1
7. Bone, M. G. and Reid, S. S. A possible regulator of protein turnover in muscle. (1975). *J. Clin. Invest.*, **56,** 1250
8. Sherwin, R. S., Herdler, R. G. and Felig, P. Effect of ketone infusions on amino acid and nitrogen metabolism in man. (1975). *J. Clin. Invest.*, **55,** 1382

9
The protein-sparing effect of isotonic amino acids: metabolic considerations

K. J. FOSTER, K. G. M. M. ALBERTI AND S. J. KARRAN

INTRODUCTION

Ideas change in medicine, as in other fields, for a variety of reasons. The use of isotonic amino acid solutions as protein sparing therapy has appeared to be contrary to established ideas on parenteral nutrition, and has illustrated recent advances in our knowledge of metabolism.

Traditionally, it was believed that glucose infusions were valuable both in reducing the nitrogen loss and in limiting the ketosis which usually accompany starvation (as well as supplying water without a sodium load). It is now recognized that in starvation ketosis is self-limiting and both ketone bodies and precursor non-esterified fatty acids (NEFA) provide valuable fuel from fat stores. The brain adapts to use ketones as fuel during starvation[1], thus decreasing the total body glucose requirements and the use of amino acids for gluconeogenesis.

During parenteral nutrition it has been established that the most efficient use of infused amino acids is obtained only when adequate calories are supplied simultaneously[2]. At least 40 non-protein calories should be given per kg body weight daily to obtain positive nitrogen balance, together with appropriate amino acids and other essential nutrients.

Insulin, too, is recognized as having valuable anabolic actions. Though it is well known that there may be severe resistance to some of the actions of insulin after injury, increasing with the severity of the injury, Allison and his colleagues[3] noted improved nitrogen balance during glucose and insulin therapy in patients with severe burns. Some workers have reported improved healing of experimental wounds in non-diabetic animals during insulin therapy[4,5].

In contrast to these views, Blackburn[6] and his colleagues found that infusions of a 3% amino acid solution, without additional calories, produced greater nitrogen sparing than 5% glucose infusion in surgical patients. They noted raised ketone body and NEFA concentrations during amino acid therapy and this was associated with lower insulin levels. They suggested the lower insulin levels during amino acid infusion permitted release of lipid fuels from fat stores more readily, thus decreasing the need for muscle breakdown to provide substrates for gluconeogenesis.

Conventional parenteral nutrition demands administration of highly concentrated solutions of nutrients through central venous catheters. The technique is sometimes hazardous. The 3% amino acid solutions are isotonic with plasma and can theoretically be administered safely through a peripheral vein. It is likely that isotonic amino acid infusions are safer than conventional parenteral nutrition, and it is for this reason that there has been so much interest in a form of therapy which is not quite so effective in preserving nitrogen balance.

We believed there was a need to explore the reasons for the nitrogen sparing action of isotonic amino acid solutions, particularly with reference to patients with sepsis. Adipose tissue is more sensitive to insulin than muscle and lipolysis is readily inhibited by insulin. The use of infusions of isotonic amino acids is said to depend on the development of the adaptation of metabolism usually seen in prolonged starvation. During periods of infection insulin levels are elevated and NEFA concentrations decreased[7]. Thus it is necessary to account for the metabolic effects of isotonic amino acid infusions in terms not only of the changes seen during starvation but also of those found after the stress of operation or infection.

Patients and methods

We have studied 35 patients from the first to the fourth day after laparotomy to test the influence of various solutions upon metabolism before oral feeding was restarted. The period from operation until 9 a.m. the following morning was used to adjust fluid balance as required and to allow the patient to enter the flow phase of the metabolic response to operation: the period during which we expected the greatest nitrogen loss. In this initial pre-study period most patients received glucose or saline infusions containing a total of 80–120 g of glucose. Five volunteers were also studied. They fasted for a similar period. To make them really comparable they received 50 g glucose orally on the evening of the first day of the fast (corresponding to operation day) and a further 50 g orally the next morning (the first 'post-operative' day) 2 h before blood samples were taken. These subjects therefore form a control group to test the effect of starvation alone on metabolism.

The test infusion was given for 72 h from 9 a.m. on the first post-operative day. Urine and venous blood collections were made during this period. Blood glucose, lactate, pyruvate, glycerol, acetoacetate, 3-hydroxybutyrate,

Table 9.1 Details of infusion solutions used with amounts given per 24 h, and of subjects studied with each solution

Infusion	*No.*	*Mean age (range)*	*Mean wt. % (range)*
Fasting volunteers	5	27 (21–35)	108 (96–111)
Elective Operation			
0.9% saline + 2 g KCl/l (2–3 l/day)	6	58 (41–73)	104 (86–126)
4.3% glucose: 0.18% saline + 2 g KCl/l (1.5 g glucose/kg)	8	59 (47–65)	103 (86–125)
4.3% glucose: 0.18% saline + 2 g KCl/l (1.5 g glucose/kg) + 16 Sol. Insulin/l	6	67 (59–75)	101 (88–110)
3.5% Synthamin (Na 35 mmol/l) (K 30 mmol/l) (Mg 25 mmol/l) (PO_4 15 mmol/l) (1.5 g amino acids/kg)	6	61 (52–75)	107 (98–117)
Peritonitis			
4.3% glucose: 0.18% saline + 2 g KCl/l (1.5 g glucose/kg)	5	51 (32–74)	95 (84–110)
3.5% Synthamin (1.5 g amino acids/kg)	5	50 (37–70)	109 (98–140)

Weight is shown as a percentage of Ideal Body Weight (Metropolitan Life Insurance Co., 1959).

glycerol and alanine, and plasma NEFA, urea and insulin were determined as previously described[8]. Urinary nitrogen excretion was estimated from urinary urea, with allowances for changes in blood urea, as described by Lee[9].

Table 9.1 shows details of patients and infusions. None of the subjects had significant hepatic, renal, cardiorespiratory or endocrine dysfunction, and none were on medication likely to disturb metabolism significantly before operation. All subjects took their own regular diet until the day before operation, although some had experienced anorexia and weight loss until this time. The fasting volunteers were all healthy, and apart from the initial glucose, consumed only water. There were four groups of patients undergoing elective operation and two groups of patients undergoing emergency operation because of a perforated viscus and peritonitis. Both glucose and isotonic amino acid infusions were given at a rate calculated to supply 1.5 g glucose or amino acids per kg body weight per day.

Starvation

Figures 9.1 and 9.2 show results obtained for a fasting volunteer. Several of the features of the metabolic adaptations to starvation are shown. On the equivalent of the first post-operative day there was, not surprisingly, a rise in glucose after the glucose load and this was accompanied by a rise of serum insulin. After 12 h, both glucose and insulin levels have fallen substantially, and a further slow decline is seen over the next 3 days. Blood lactate levels rise after the glucose load, more so in the group as a whole than in this particular subject, and subsequently remain fairly constant.

Alanine levels in the group as a whole declined slightly during the 96 h of the fast. Alanine is a key gluconeogenic substrate. During the period of study it is known that rates of gluconeogenesis will fall markedly, from an estimated 147 g/24 h after an overnight fast to 99 g/24 h on the 3rd or 4th day[10]. A further slight fall in gluconeogenesis may occur subsequently during a period of several weeks of starvation. Decrease in gluconeogenesis from alanine may well account for a large part of this fall. Oxidation of amino acids in muscle yields both pyruvate and NH_2 groups for transamination forming alanine, which is released from muscle in quantities much exceeding its content. In starvation, muscle provides a reservoir of amino acids and these may serve as gluconeogenic substrates. Other tissue protein is less labile.

As glycogen reserves in liver and gluconeogenesis fall in the first few days of a fast, lipid mobilization increases. Our subject (Figure 10.2) shows a steady rise in NEFA and a marked rise in ketone body (3-hydroxybutyrate plus acetoacetate) concentrations. At this stage ketone bodies are probably the more important source of fuel, at least for resting skeletal muscle[11]. Ketone bodies also have an important regulatory role in metabolism. High levels inhibit lipolysis directly and stimulate insulin secretion which in turn inhibits lypolysis and ketone body formation from NEFA in the liver[10].

Raised ketone levels may also inhibit muscle breakdown, after a prolonged fast at least[12], and raised levels of both NEFA and ketone bodies inhibit glucose oxidation in several[10] tissues.

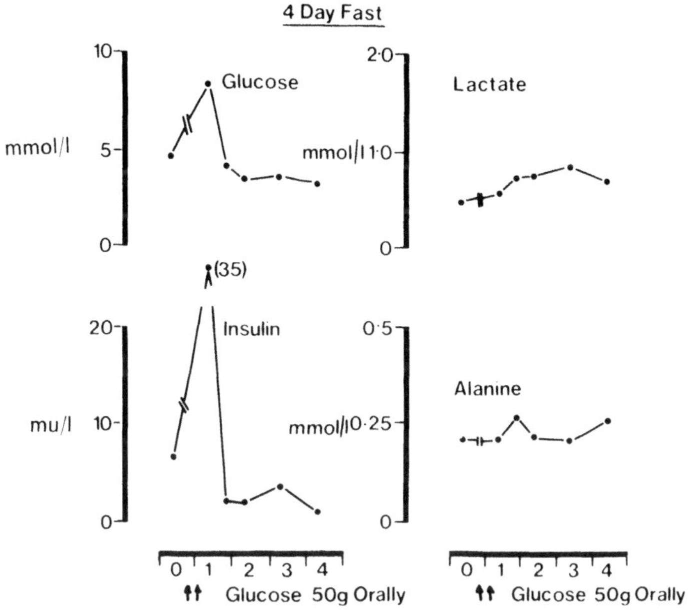

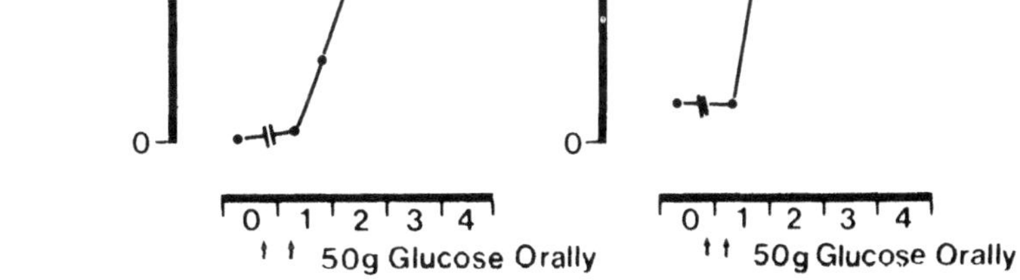

Figures 9.1 and 9.2 R.K. male: 21 years, 81 kg. Metabolite changes observed during a 96 h fast. At 9.00 p.m. on the evening of Day 0 (corresponding to Operation Day) the subject took 50 g glucose. A similar amount was taken at 7.00 a.m. the following morning so that he was comparable with patients undergoing laparotomy

Post-operative metabolic changes

The fasting data should be compared with metabolite concentrations observed during a saline infusion in a post-operative patient (Figures 9.3 and

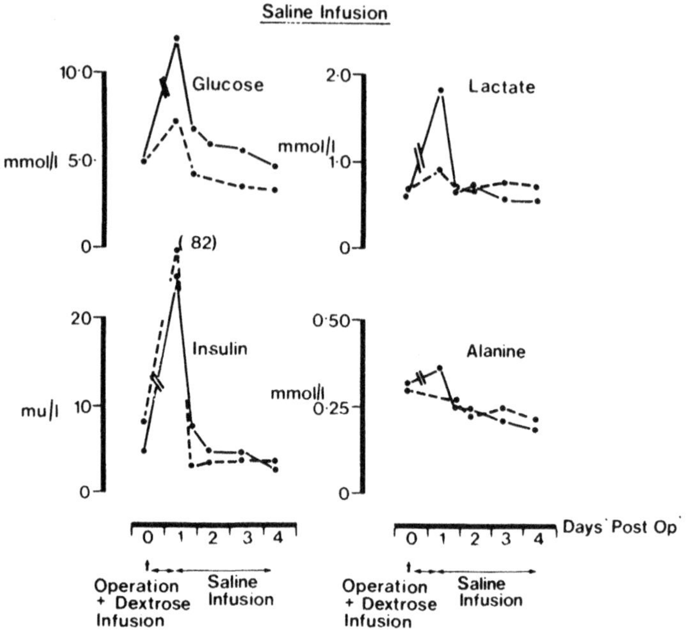

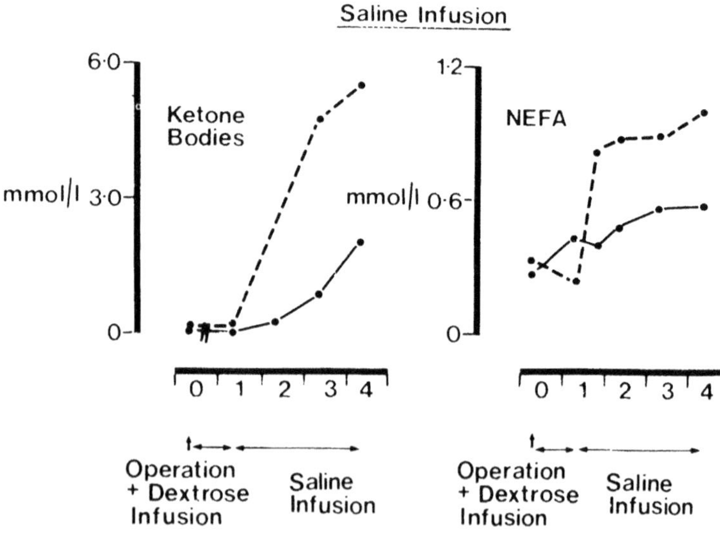

Figures 9.3 and 9.4 C.S. male: 53 years, 85 kg. Metabolite changes after operation during a period of normal saline infusion after right hemicolectomy for carcinoma of the caecum (mean results for five fasting volunteers shown thus – – •– –)

9.4). The subject, C.S., underwent right hemicolectomy for a carcinoma of the caecum. The disturbance of metabolism arising from the stress of operation may be deduced by comparison with the levels observed during fasting. There is clearly an elevation in blood glucose though insulin levels are comparable 36 h after operation. There was a more marked rise in insulin in the fasting volunteers after their glucose load. This may be accounted for by three mechanisms: the time course of administration is different, oral glucose is known to produce a greater rise in insulin than an equal amount given intravenously[13] and the mechanisms which impair insulin release during surgery may still be active[14].

Lactate levels also rose more after operation and glucose but not subsequently. During the next 3 days there was a steady rise in the lactate:pyruvate ratio. A rise in intracellular NADH with respect to NAD favours lactate formation:

$$\text{Lactate} + \text{NAD} \rightleftharpoons \text{Pyruvate} + \text{NADH}_2$$

Factors other than tissue anoxia such as acidaemia can increase the ratio. During saline infusion after operation there was a rise in ketone bodies and a fall in plasma bicarbonate from 26 to 22 mmol/l. These changes were not as marked as were found during fasting when greater rises of the lactate:pyruvate ratio were seen.

Alanine levels fell more quickly after operation. Since urea excretion was also greater this implies increased gluconeogenesis from alanine derived presumably from muscle catabolism.

It is notable that both NEFA and ketone body levels (Figure 9.4) rise later and more slowly than in simple starvation. This cannot be explained by higher insulin levels (Figure 9.3). One possibility is the release of prostaglandins during surgery, some of which inhibit lipolysis. Increased utilization cannot be ruled out, but resting metabolic rate is only slightly altered by elective operation[15].

Metabolic effects of glucose infusion post-operatively

Patient C.T. received a glucose infusion during the test period (Figures 9.5 and 9.6). The infusion provided 1.5 g glucose/kg body weight/day or 136 g glucose in this patient. Amounts of glucose of similar quantity are known to inhibit gluconeogenesis markedly during fasting[16] but may not prevent the adaptations which limit nitrogen loss in more prolonged starvation[17]. For the first 24 h after 100 g glucose our fasting volunteers excreted 3.2 mmol urea/kg body weight whereas for the last 24 h of the fast they excreted 5.4 mmol urea/kg. The carbon skeletons derived from the amino acids, which are broken down to form this urea, are mostly converted to gluconeogenic substrates.

Figure 9.5 shows how glucose and insulin levels declined for this patient

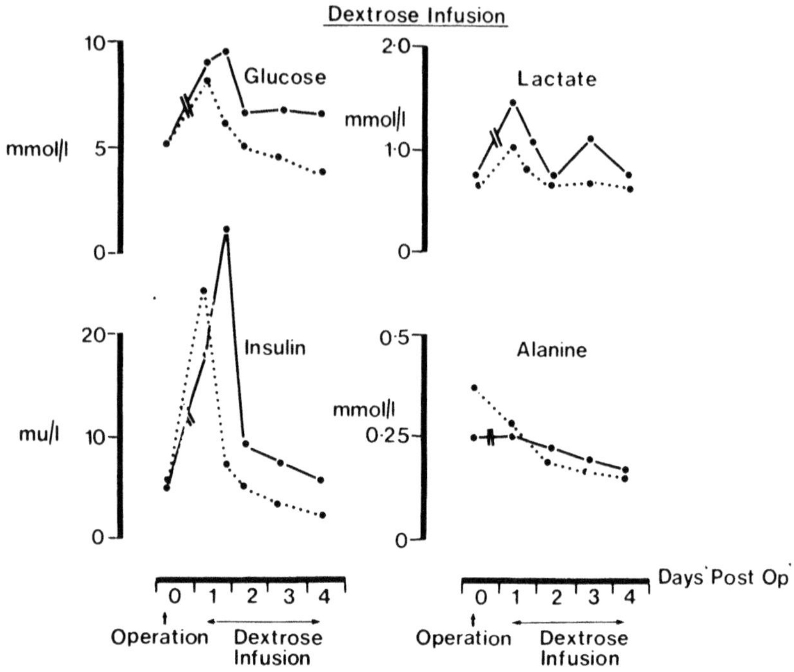

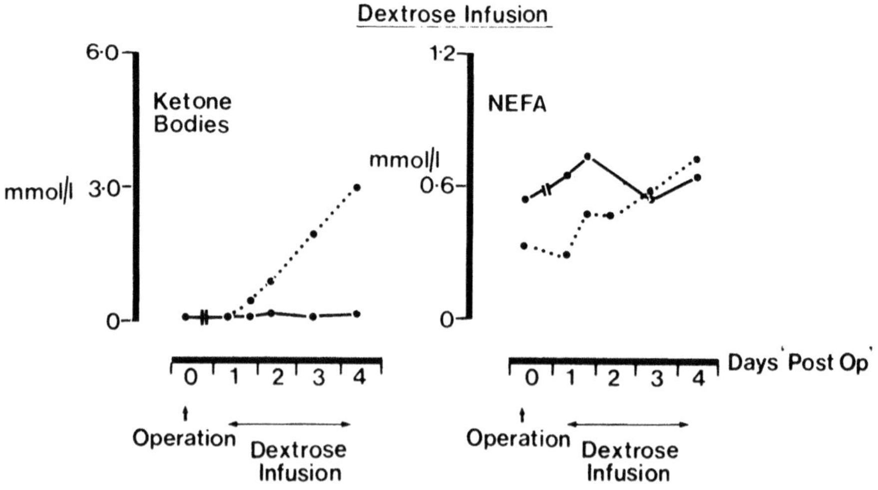

Figures 9.5 and 9.6 C.T. male: 57 years, 91 kg, undergoing partial gastrectomy for benign gastric ulcer. Metabolite concentrations observed during dextrose infusion of 1.5 g/kg/24 h. (Compared with means of results for patients receiving saline, . . ● . . . ● . .)

over the 4 days of the study. The levels were higher than those seen during a saline infusion. Concentrations of the gluconeogenic substrates lactate and alanine were also higher and nitrogen excretion lower. This suggests that the protein sparing effect of dextrose infusions is mediated by decreased hepatic uptake of alanine for gluconeogenesis, which results in a raised blood alanine concentration. This in turn may shift the equilibrium of amino acid metabolism in muscles away from catabolism (compared with saline infusions). The comparatively raised levels of insulin might also decrease muscle breakdown directly, but this would tend to lower blood alanine concentrations so that a direct effect of insulin at these concentrations appears to be of secondary importance in the nitrogen sparing effects of glucose infusions.

NEFA release and ketone body formation (Figure 9.5) was markedly inhibited by glucose infusion, although insulin levels were falling. Clearly if raised concentrations of ketone bodies do have a direct inhibitory action on muscle catabolism at this time during starvation, it is less effective than that exerted by a small amount of exogenous glucose which caused a marked fall in urinary nitrogen loss. Despite the lower blood NEFA and ketone body levels during dextrose infusion, it is likely that endogenous fat remained the major source of energy[15].

Peritonitis—metabolic changes

Serious infection is well known to increase the metabolic disturbances which follow injury. Figure 9.7 contains observations made on F.S. while recovering from laparotomy for peritonitis consequent upon perforation of a jejunal carcinoma. He also received 1.5 g glucose/kg body weight as a continuous infusion.

Compared with glucose infusions after elective laparotomy, glucose and insulin levels were higher. This presumably represents greater insulin resistance. It is likely that these changes follow increased protein breakdown. Blood alanine (and lactate) levels were raised and since urea excretion was also increased, this must have been due to increased release from peripheral protein stores.

It has previously been noted that in times of serious infection, hepatic gluconeogenesis from alanine is not so readily inhibited by glucose and insulin[16]. Inhibition of gluconeogenesis is usually a major feature of insulin action upon carbohydrate metabolism. It is clear that after major injury there is not only increased muscle catabolism but also failure of inhibition of gluconeogenesis by insulin. This may account for the difficulty in maintaining nitrogen balance after a major limb fracture even when protein and calories are supplied orally in excess of usual requirements while resting metabolic rates are only modestly elevated[18]. The mechanism of this insulin resistance is not entirely understood but levels of gluconeogenic hormones such as cortisol, glucagon and catecholamines are increased after injury. Batstone

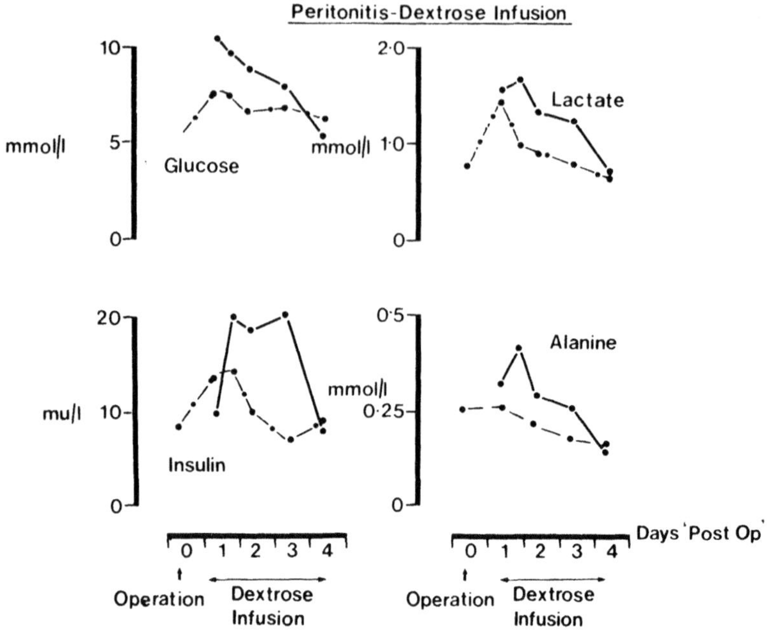

Figure 9.7 F. S. male: 74 years, 61 kg. Influence of serious infection (peritonitis arising from perforation of a carcinoma of the jejunum) upon metabolite concentrations during dextrose infusion (1.5 g/kg/24 h) after operation (compared with means for patients receiving dextrose after elective operation, – – • – – • – –)

et al.[19] have recently presented evidence that blood cortisol levels correlate best with metabolite levels after severe burns. In this context it is interesting to note that F.S. showed very high plasma cortisol levels for the first 3 mornings after operation (3311, 2836 and 1528 μmol/l respectively) but that this had fallen to 811 μmol/l by the fourth morning by which time metabolite levels were more comparable to those observed after elective operation.

Despite the lipolytic actions of several hormones released after injury, there was no increase in NEFA or ketone body concentration. Insulin appears to suppress lipolysis despite resistance to other actions of this hormone. It has now been clearly shown that glucagon and cortisol stimulate lipolysis and ketogenesis only when there is co-existent insulin deficiency. NEFA and ketone body levels in these infected patients were similar to those in patients receiving dextrose after elective operation, though nitrogen loss was quite dissimilar.

Glucose and insulin infusion after operation

Operations not complicated by serious infection are associated with less insulin resistance. After an exploratory laparotomy and cholecystojejunostomy for carcinoma of the pancreas, K.H. (53 kg) received an infusion of

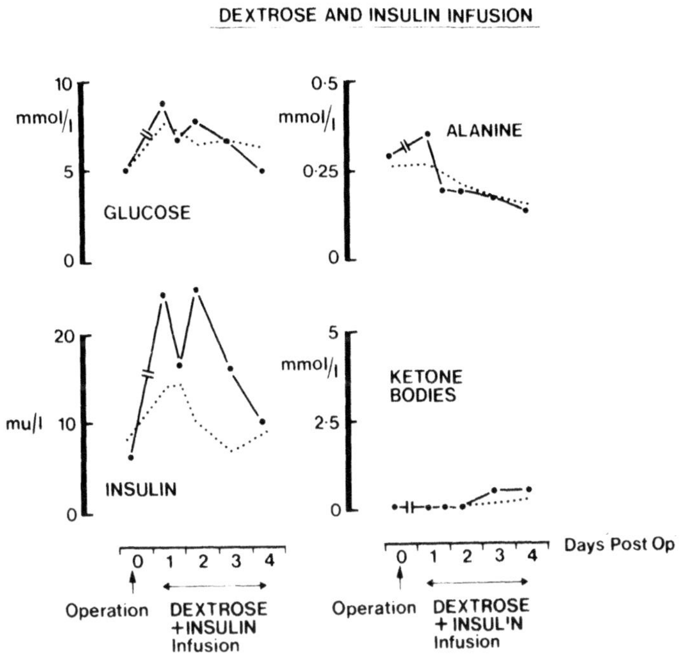

Figure 9.8 Additional insulin was given in this case, K.H. Female, 68 years, 53 kg, after cholecystojejunostomy for carcinoma of the pancreas. The infusion gave 80 g of glucose and 30 u soluble insulin per day. Comparison is with means for patients receiving glucose alone (. . . . . . .)

80 g glucose with 30 units soluble insulin daily. Figure 9.8 shows there was a moderate depression of blood glucose (significant for the group as a whole) and raised blood insulin levels compared with infusion of glucose alone. The latter are close to those seen in the patient with peritonitis. At higher levels, insulin clearly has a direct anabolic action. There was less nitrogen loss and lower blood alanine concentrations early in the test period which suggests decreased release of amino acid from muscle. Compared with F.S., K.H. had much lower cortisol levels (626, 789, 811 and 618 μmol/l for each post-operative morning). Excess of such hormones with a catabolic action on muscle presumably is the cause of increased alanine levels in F.S. despite insulin levels which are high relative to those found after elective surgery.

Despite a constant infusion of insulin based upon body weight, there is considerable variation in the levels achieved in different patients: this has been noted previously[19]. Lactate levels were similar to those during infusions of dextrose alone and ketone body levels remained low.

Isotonic amino acid infusion

The metabolic profile during isotonic amino acid infusions is quite distinct from that seen during saline and dextrose infusions. The appropriate

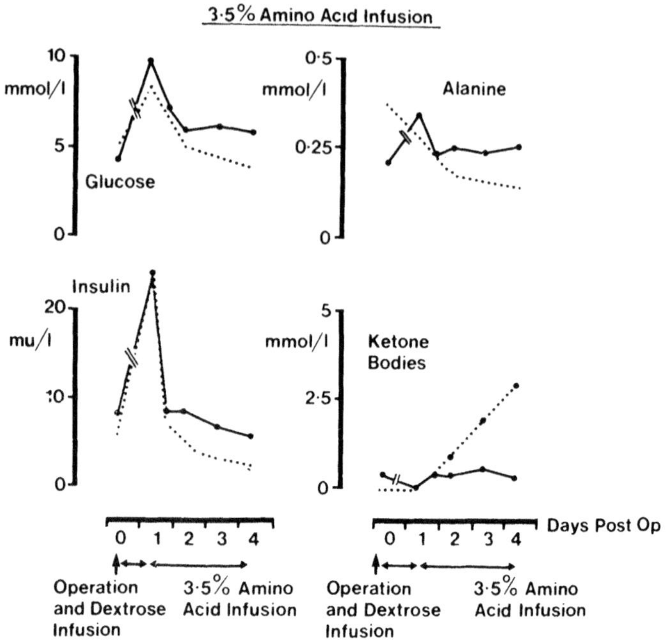

Figure 9.9 A.G. Male: 57 years, 74 kg, received 1.5 g/kg Synthamin amino acids after sigmoid colectomy for carcinoma. Metabolite levels are compared with means for patients receiving saline infusions (........)

comparison is with saline infusion since that is metabolically inert. Figure 9.9 shows observations made on a patient after sigmoid colectomy, compared with those found during saline infusions. Glucose and insulin concentrations were higher than after saline. Alanine levels were sustained. The infusion supplies 82 mmol/l alanine plus that alanine derived from catabolism of other amino acids. The raised glucose levels probably reflect increased gluconeogenesis from amino acids, urea production being much increased. Gluconeogenesis from amino acids depends not only on their concentration but also upon hormonal activity. It is well recognized that amino acids stimulate glucagon release[20]. Net nitrogen loss however, was reduced (Figure 9.11), being lower in this group than with any other therapy.

Ketone bodies showed only a modest elevation and the levels achieved after 72 h were close to those reported after 3 and 7 days in the accompanying paper. The levels were much closer to those seen during dextrose infusions than during saline infusions. In this patient NEFA levels on the 4th morning were actually lower than before operation. NEFA availability is only one factor governing ketogenesis, the actual rates of ketogenesis being greater (relative to NEFA concentration) in starved animals. A small proportion of the infused amino acids yield ketones on catabolism. These factors may explain the disparity between NEFA and ketone bodies in these patients.

Lactate concentrations and the lactate:pyruvate ratios were similar to those seen during dextrose infusions.

Elevation of insulin (relative to saline infusions) in these subjects may result from three mechanisms: raised glucose concentrations, lower ketone body levels and a direct stimulatory effect of the amino acid infusion. It is clear that there is no rise in ketone body formation compared with saline infusion. Indeed, the reverse appears to be true. Therefore, raised ketone body and NEFA concentrations cannot be the major nitrogen sparing mechanism of amino acid infusions.

Peritonitis—metabolic changes during isotonic amino acid infusion

Following operation associated with serious infection, isotonic amino acid administration does not mask the changes noted above. D.J. (Figure 9.10)

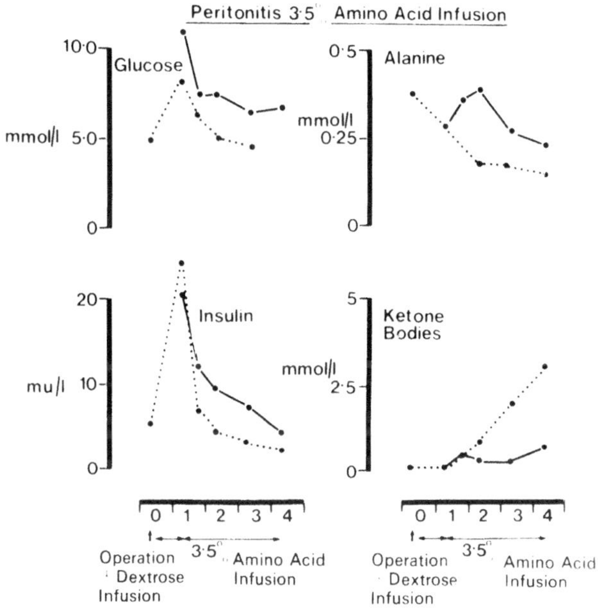

Figure 9.10 D.J. Female: 70 years, 61 kg, suffered from peritonitis as a result of perforation of a carcinoma of the transverse colon. After colectomy she received 3.5% Synthamin amino acids, 1.5 g/kg/day. Metabolite values are compared with values during saline infusions after elective operation (.......)

underwent laparotomy for perforation of a carcinoma of the transverse colon. Glucose levels tended to be higher than during amino acid therapy after elective operation, maintained presumably by increased gluconeogenesis from the amino acids. Hence alanine levels were lower than for the group receiving the isotonic amino acid solution after elective operation, and urea production was greater. Insulin and ketone body concentrations were similar in both groups.

Comparative nitrogen excretion

Figure 9.11 shows the mean estimated nitrogen excretion per kg body weight per day for all the groups studied. For the groups who received amino

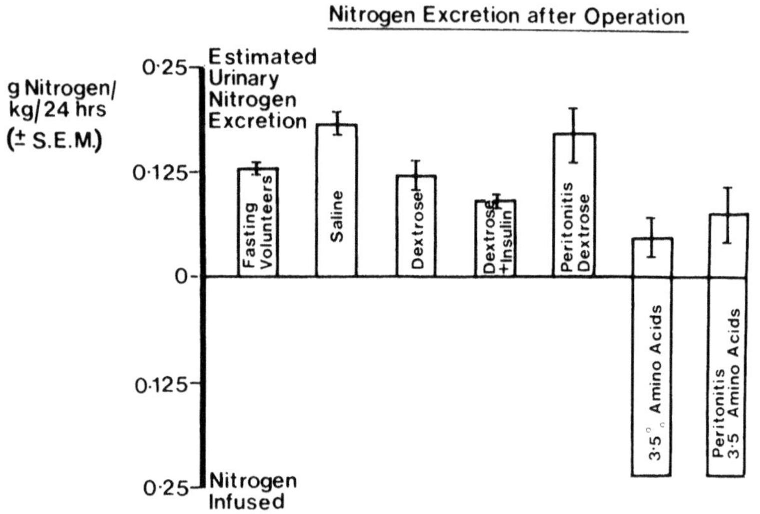

Figure 9.11 Mean urinary nitrogen excretion (estimated from urinary urea) ± SEM for the groups investigated. For those groups who received amino acid infusion, nitrogen excretion equal to the infused nitrogen is shown below the line, leaving net nitrogen excretion above the line

acid infusions nitrogen excreted equal to that infused is shown below the line, leaving net nitrogen excretion above the line. There were no faecal losses, and as losses from drain sites and cutaneous losses are small they have been disregarded. Dextrose and insulin and isotonic amino acid infusions had the best nitrogen sparing effect. Dextrose and isotonic amino acid infusions resulted in significantly less nitrogen loss than saline ($P < 0.05$ and < 0.001 respectively). There was significantly less nitrogen loss during amino acid infusion than during dextrose infusion ($P < 0.05$). The differences between dextrose infusion after elective operation and dextrose infusion after peritonitis were not significant ($P > 0.05$).

Conclusions

Several conclusions may be drawn. Operation increased the loss of nitrogen compared with a similar period of fasting ($P < 0.02$). Glucose infusion reduces this loss by stimulating a decrease in gluconeogenesis from amino acids. Additional insulin, however, appears to decrease nitrogen loss still further, perhaps by inhibiting protein breakdown directly. However, the best nitrogen balance was obtained during isotonic amino acid therapy. The amino acid solution also exerts a nitrogen sparing effect during infection and its efficiency may possibly be less affected by the presence of infection than that of isocaloric amounts of dextrose.

Glucose and amino acids have definite but distinct effects on metabolism in our study. Since the mechanism of nitrogen sparing with each appears different, it is clear that direct assessment of the method by which nitrogen sparing is achieved can only be valid for comparisons made with saline infusions.

Raised ketone body and NEFA concentrations are not the mechanisms of nitrogen sparing seen in these subjects. As a consequence we should not presume and do not find that low insulin levels are necessarily advantageous. Glucose (100 g/day) probably exerts its protein sparing effect indirectly by reducing gluconeogenesis from alanine as a consequence of increasing portal vein insulin delivery to the liver. After operation, and especially in the event of infection, there is increased muscle catabolism with increased release of alanine and greater gluconeogenesis leading to greater urea production.

Mechanism of nitrogen sparing by amino acid infusion

Infusion of amino acids in amounts isocaloric with dextrose increases urea excretion. The infused amino acids enter the amino acid pools, including those in muscle and liver, disturbing the equilibrium in the direction of reduced net release of amino acid from peripheral stores (though protein turnover may be increased[21]) and toward increased metabolism of the carbon skeletons and production of urea from amino acids in the liver. The normal turnover of protein may be increased after injury[21,22] and this would ensure sensitivity to such a mechanism of action by amino acid infusions. Equicaloric amounts of amino acids may be more effective than glucose in nitrogen sparing because they raise amino acid levels more directly than the indirect effect of glucose infusions:

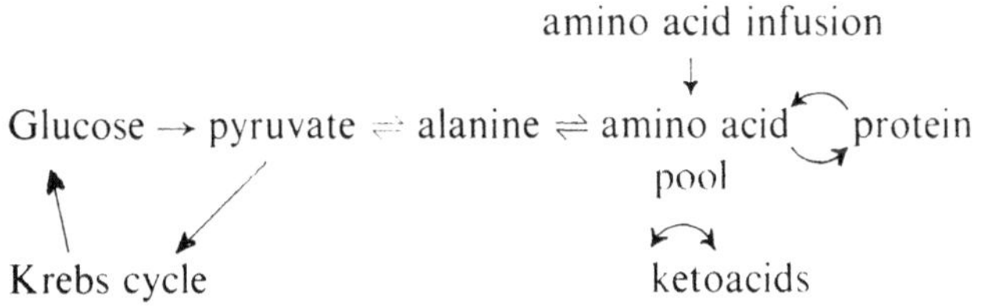

Alpha keto acids result from transamination of amino acids. Infusion of a mixture of keto acids, which can themselves be involved in transamination from other amino acids to form new amino acids, is an effective way of maintaining nitrogen balance[23]. Presumably a keto acid infusions spare nitrogen in the same way as isotonic amino acids do by maintaining amino acid concentrations, but without imposing a nitrogen load which might be undesirable in hepatic or renal failure.

From the mean nitrogen excretion noted in Figure 9.11 we can calculate the net urinary nitrogen excretion after operation for a 70 kg man to be 8.5 g/day during glucose infusions but 3.4 g/day during amino acid therapy.

Table 9.2 Comparison of nitrogen sparing effect of synthetic amino acid mixtures with glucose observed by various authors

First author	*Dose of infused amino acid*	*Nitrogen balance (g/24 h) glucose*	*: amino acid*	*Comment*
Early Post-op.				
Heller 1969[28]	50 g	−7.9	−4	
Freeman 1975[24]	1 g/kg	−9	−1	Phlebitis
	1.7 g/kg		1	Dose related
Hoover 1975[29]	90 g	−12.5	−7	
Schulte 1975[30]	1.5 g/kg	−10	−2	'No ketosis'
Greenberg 1976[25]	1.5 g/kg	−8	−5	Added lipid, carbohydrate no effect
Rowlands 1976[31]	1.44 g/kg	−0.17 g/kg	−0.13 g/kg	
Skillman 1976[21]	75 g	−3	0	4th day estimate
Foster 1977	1.5 g/kg	−8.5	−3.4	Balance on intravenous saline −13 g N (approx. for 70 kg patient)
Late Post-op.				
Blackburn 1973[6]	90 g	−8.5	−0.4	
Tweedle 1975[32]	85 g	−6.2	0.1	

Table 9.2 compares our results with those of other authors. The study by Freeman[24] suggested the nitrogen sparing effect was dose related. This implies a mechanism relating to mass, such as is outlined above. Greenberg and his colleagues[25] found that the raised insulin levels observed during concurrent glucose and amino acid infusion did not impair nitrogen balance and again suggested that the nitrogen sparing effect of isotonic amino acid infusions was due to provision of substrate. The additional glucose calories these authors provided with amino acids have no benefit when compared with amino acids alone. The nitrogen sparing effect of the two substrates is quite different and there may be adverse interactions between the two and their metabolites. Thus increased availability of pyruvate (an a keto acid) secondary to glucose oxidation in muscle results in increased alanine release from muscle. These authors also noted a slight (but not statistically significant) improvement in nitrogen balance when lipid was added to the amino

acid infusion. Exogenous lipid has a poor nitrogen sparing potential in the absence of carbohydrate, perhaps because there are large reserves of fat and the pathways of degradation of most amino acids are widely divergent from those of lipids, although leucine, of all amino acids, is both strongly ketogenic and may be particularly important in promoting muscle protein synthesis[26]. In any case it is likely that endogenous or exogenous lipid was the major fuel in all these patients. The conclusions of both these sets of authors are valid since comparisons are made between different infusions of amino acids.

Skillman *et al.*[21] noted increased albumin synthesis during isotonic amino acid therapy compared with that during dextrose infusion. There was however a fall in serum albumin concentration in both patients receiving glucose and those receiving amino acids after operation in that study. Possibly there is increased protein turnover during isotonic amino acid therapy.

Amino acid therapy after prolonged starvation

It will be noted that Blackburn[6] has studied patients in the late post-operative period after the development of complications. This may be more relevant than the standardized post-operative period we and most other investigators have used. Though the catabolic stimulus of operation might have been distant in time in some of Blackburn's patients, some of them did have serious infections. Very good nitrogen sparing was obtained probably because there was more complete adaptation to starvation. It should be noted that while ketone bodies are an important fuel source for resting muscle for 2–3 days of starvation, they become less important (and NEFA become more important) after 2–3 weeks of starvation[11]. At the same time ketone bodies reach concentrations of about 8 mmol/l in blood though they appear to be cleared more slowly[12]. At this time ketone bodies may have a direct nitrogen sparing effect[12] but at concentrations far higher than obtained during amino acid therapy. In obese subjects fasted for prolonged periods insulin appears to have less effect in inhibiting lipolysis and to more readily inhibit release of amino acids from peripheral stores[27]. If such a mechanism were even partially operative in Blackburn's patients then the nitrogen sparing effect of amino acids must relate to the mass of infused amino acids rather than increased lipolysis due to lower insulin levels seen during amino acid therapy compared with glucose infusions.

Since the benefits of isotonic amino acid infusions appear related to their mass it is not surprising that they are effective during periods of hyperinsulinism such as occur during periods of severe infection or corticosteroid therapy.

Isotonic amino acid therapy has a logical basis and does not contradict the established ideas on metabolism in total parenteral nutrition. The two therapies are just not comparable in metabolic terms, since achieving nitrogen balance in one depends on obtaining and using adaptations which occur in starvation and, in the other, on providing completely every need for nutrients.

Acknowledgements

We would like to thank Mrs. B. Lloyd, Miss P. Smythe and Miss L. Hinks, for expert technical assistance.

We gratefully acknowledge financial support from Travenol Laboratories Ltd., and the British Diabetic Association.

References

1. Owen, O. E., Morgan, A., Kemp, H., Sullivan, J., Herrera, M. and Cahill, G. (1967) Brain metabolism during fasting. *J. Clin. Invest.*, **46,** 1589
2. McNair, R., O'Donnell, D. and Quigley, W. (1954). Protein nutrition in surgical patients. *Arch. Surg.*, **68,** 76
3. Hinton, P., Allison, S., Littlejohn, S. and Lloyd, J. (1971). Insulin and glucose to reduce catabolic response to injury in burned patients. *Lancet*, **i,** 767
4. Rosenthal, S. P. (1968). Acceleration of primary wound healing by insulin. *Arch. Surg.*, **96,** 53
5. Udupa, K. N. and Chansouria, J. P. (1971). The role of protamine zinc insulin in accelerating wound healing in the rat. *Brit. J. Surg.*, **58,** 673
6. Blackburn, G., Flatt, J., Clowes, G., O'Donnell, T. and Hensale, T. (1973). Protein sparing therapy during periods of starvation with sepsis or trauma. *Ann. Surg.*, **177,** 588
7. O'Donnell, T., Clowes, G., Blackburn, G., Ryan, N. T., Benotti, P. and Miller, J. (1976). Proteolysis associated with a deficit of peripheral energy fuel substrates in septic man. *Surgery*, **80,** 192
8. Batstone, G. F., Alberti, K. G. M. M., Hinks, L., Smythe, P., Laing, J., Ward, C., Ely, D. W. and Bloom, S. R. (1976). Metabolic studies in subjects following thermal injury. *Burns*, **2,** 207
9. Lee, H. A. (1974). *Parenteral Nutrition in Acute Metabolic Illness*, p. 315. (London and New York: Publ. Academic Press)
10. Newsholme, E. (1976). Carbohydrate metabolism *in vivo*. Regulation of the blood glucose level. *Clin. Endocrinol. Metab.*, **5,** 543
11. Owen, O. and Reichard, G. (1971). Human forearm metabolism during progressive starvation. *J. Clin. Invest.*, **50,** 1536
12. Sherwin, R., Hendler, R. and Felig, P. (1975). Effect of ketone infusion on amino acid and nitrogen metabolism in man. *J. Clin. Invest.*, **55,** 1382
13. Unger, R. and Eisentraut, A. (1969). Entero-insular axis. *Arch. Int. Med.*, **123,** 261
14. Allison, S. P., Prowse, K. and Chamberlain, M. J. (1967). Failure of insulin response to glucose load during operation and after myocardial infarction. *Lancet*, **i,** 478
15. Tweedle, D. and Johnston, I. D. A. (1971). Factors affecting the metabolic expenditure of surgical patients. *Brit. J. Surg.*, **58,** 771
16. Long, C., Kinney, J. and Geiger, J. (1976). Non suppressibility of gluconeogenesis by glucose in septic patients. *Metabolism*, **25,** 193
17. O'Connell, R., Morgan, A., Aoki, T., Ball, M. and Moore, F. D. (1974). Nitrogen conservation in starvation graded responses to intravenous glucose. *J. Clin. Endocrinol. Metab.*, **39,** 555
18. Cuthbertson, D. P. (1936). Further observations on the disturbance of metabolism caused by injury, with particular reference to the dietary requirements of fracture cases. *Brit. J. Surg.*, **23,** 505
19. Page, M., Alberti, K. G. M. M., Greenwood, R., Cumea, K., Hockaday, T., Lowy, C., Nabarro, J., Pyke, D. A., Sonksen, P. H., Watkins, P. J. and West, T. E. T. (1974). Treatment of diabetic coma with continuous low dose infusion of insulin. *Brit. Med. J.*, **2,** 687

20. Unger, R. (1974). α and β cell interrelationship in health and disease. *Metabolism*, **23**, 581
21. Skillman, J., Rosenoer, V., Smith, C. and Fang, M. (1976). Improved albumen synthesis in post-operative patients by amino acid infusion. *N. Engl. J. Med.*, **295**, 1037
22. O'Keefe, S. J., Sender, P. M. and James, W. P. (1974). Catabolic loss of body nitrogen in response to surgery. *Lancet*, **ii**, 1035
23. Sapir, D., Owen, O., Pojefsky, T. and Walser, M. (1974). Nitrogen sparing induced by a mixture of essential amino acids given chiefly as their keto analogues during prolonged starvation in obese subjects. *J. Clin. Invest.*, **54**, 974
24. Freeman, J., Stegink, L., Meyer, P., Thompson, R. and Den Besten, L. (1975). Metabolic effects of amino acid versus dextrose infusion in surgical patients. *Arch. Surg.*, **110**, 916
25. Greenberg, G., Marliss, E., Anderson, G., Langer, B., Spence, W., Toves, B. and Jeejeebhoy, R. N. (1976). Protein sparing therapy in post-operative patients. Effect of added hypocaloric glucose or lipid. *N. Engl. J. Med.*, **294**, 1411
26. Buse, M. and Reid, S. (1974). Regulation of protein synthesis in muscles by leucine. *Clin. Res.*, **22**, 58a
27. Cahill, G. F. (1971). Physiology of insulin in man. *Diabetes*, **20**, 785
28. Heller, L. (1969). Clinical and experimental studies as complete parenteral nutrition. *Scand. J. Gastroenterol.*, **4**, (Suppl. 3), 7
29. Hoover, H., Grant, J., Gorschboth, C. and Ketcham, A. S. (1975). Nitrogen sparing intravenous fluids in post-operative patients. *N. Engl. J. Med.*, **293**, 172
30. Schulte, W., Condon, R. and Kraus, M. (1975). Positive nitrogen balance using isotonic crystalline amino acid solution. *Arch. Surg.*, **110**, 914
31. Rowlands, B. J. and Clark, R. G. (1976). Amino acid infusion following surgery. *Brit. J. Surg.*, **63**, 161
32. Tweedle, D., Brennan, M., Fitzpatrick, G., Ball, M. and Moore, F. D. (1975). Protein conservation with peripheral isotonic amino acid solutions. *Surg. Forum*, **26**, 32

Discussion

D. E. F. Tweedle: (UK) No one doubts that if tissue can be persuaded to use ketone bodies as an energy source then there will be nitrogen sparing, particularly during starvation. Our concern is to find out in which patients we can actually use this therapy, and I was interested to see Dr Foster's results of ketone body levels during the amino acid infusion.

We have looked at patients after vagotomy and pyloroplasty, and found no difference between the ketone body levels in a group receiving an electrolyte solution and an Intralipid group; but there was also no difference between a glucose-fed group and an amino acid fed group, and the ketone bodies are very low in both groups. One reason for these findings is that there was no difference in the glucose levels or in the insulin levels between these groups.

G. L. Blackburn: (USA) What was the nitrogen balance in the various groups?

Tweedle: The nitrogen balances in the amino acid group were much better than the nitrogen balances in the dextrose group. What concerns me is that when I infuse amino acids, I find that I am lowering the blood ketones. I cannot get the ketone levels that Dr Blackburn gets when he infuses amino acids.

Blackburn: Most investigators agree that the physiological factor that influences ketone body levels is the rate of production, which in turn is tightly controlled by insulin. Therefore, it is important to know the insulin level between various study groups in order to interpret these data. Secondary, various amino acids have different insulinogenic effects which can be further enhanced by altered flow rates and the amount of the amino acid infusion. Time also is a key factor, to allow adaptation. Short-term studies of 3 or 4 days are not likely to be adequate to demonstrate these points. Most of the studies which have explored the effect of providing carbohydrate-free protein have seen rises in free fatty acids and ketone bodies, both in control volunteers and in post-operative patients. It would appear that blood samples from hepatic veins are an easy way to obtain helpful data in the understanding of the mechanism of protein sparing therapy.

I would challenge any effort to minimize the key role of keto acid metabolism during hypocaloric feeding in which the goal is to allow redistribution of body cell mass in order to support key tissue anabolism in generating host defence. The criteria of efficacy is not nitrogen balance but is protein synthesis; particularly in visceral tissues such as liver, bone marrow, mesentery lymph nodes etc. The goal of protein-sparing therapy is to infuse crystalline amino acids to supplement amino acid requirements, while maintaining the physiological state best able to shuttle reserves of calories and protein toward the viscera. In the hypocaloric state this appears to be dependent upon the effort of catecholamines, glucocorticoids, growth hormone, and glucagon (cf. Clowes, G. H. A. Jr., Symposium on the response to infection in injury. *Surg. Clin. of N. Amer.* **56,** No. 5, October 1976).

I have not seen Dr Foster's data before. How would he rule out the ketones? If the ketones have no effect, then why not try infusions of ketones, and show that they will not improve the nitrogen balance?

K. Foster: (UK) That is a reasonable suggestion. Our data showed improved nitrogen balance in some patients, or groups of patients at least, with reduced levels of ketones. One is always in a slight difficulty here. One knows that ketones are being used by both groups in this hypocaloric type of feeding. Nevertheless, the evidence suggests that ketone body levels themselves are not necessarily as powerful a protein-sparing mechanism as the mass of either dextrose or of amino acids.

We have looked at ketone body levels during a constant infusion of amino acids for as much as 7 days after operation, and the ketone body levels are virtually the same as we reported *here*, yet by the seventh day we see a reduced nitrogen loss, presumably an effect both of physiological adaptation to near starvation and also an increased time interval from the catabolic stimulus of operation.

P. Vinay: (Canada) A comment on the interesting idea of infusing ketones to reproduce the keto-adaptation. It is well known in several species that infusion of ketone bodies acutely increases the insulin level. One might therefore observe something other than a pure keto-adaptation.

I am not sure about the reaction of the pancreas of man to ketone infusion.

H. N. Munro: (USA) Were insulin levels measured?

Foster: Insulin levels were measured in our patients, but we have not done a ketone infusion.

S. J. Karran: (UK) Dr Blackburn mentioned the figures produced with physiological saline. Would he comment on the very large differences that we found with the starvation patients. In fact, we found almost an inhibition of ketosis with the dextrose group.

Blackburn: We have looked at physiological electrolyte solution against dextrose and against amino acids. At the sixth to seventh day we found between 0.5 and 0.7 millimolar levels, which is what we were seeing in our physiological electrolyte solution. Many investigators have confirmed these observations.

D. W. Wilmore: (USA) We seem to be struggling with the role of ketones versus mass action etc. If a man who is starvation-adapted is infused with ketones, or ketones are administered to him, will he further spare nitrogen?

Munro: Without any amino acids being administered? I would not think so. It is known that feeding fat to starving people does not reduce nitrogen output.

Foster: Ketones have been infused into starved man in other studies and they have been reported to have an effect.

Wilmore: I know that if keto-adaptation had not taken place they would have an effect in normal man.

Section IV
Fat Emulsions in Parenteral Nutrition

10
The use of fat emulsions in parenteral nutrition

D. E. F. TWEEDLE

In 1869 subcutaneous injections of fat were given to an emaciated patient suffering from Pott's disease[1] but the first investigations into intravenous infusion of fat emulsions were performed in Japan during the 1920s. Research into this and other aspects of intravenous feeding was hampered by the Second World War, but following this, an intravenous fat emulsion, Lipomul, was developed in the United States of America and the early clinical and experimental studies were reported at the Brook Lodge Symposium[2]. Although the early results appeared very encouraging, further extensive studies showed the emulsion to be toxic in routine clinical use and manufacture was discontinued. The emphasis on development and research then switched to Europe with the introduction of the commercial fat emulsion Intralipid (Kabivitrum, Sweden). This solution was followed quickly on the commercial market by the introduction of Infonutril (Astra, Sweden), Lipofundin (Braun, Germany) and Lipiphysan (Egic, France). Infonutril has since been withdrawn from the market and the most recent development has been the production of Lipofundin-S.

Although the basic ingredients of these solutions are very similar as each contains a vegetable oil, an emulsifier and a polyhydric alcohol to render the solution isotonic, differences within these basic ingredients produce marked differences in their composition (Table 10.1). This difference in composition appears to be of considerable importance. The vegetable oil in Intralipid and Lipofundin-S is derived from the soya bean and the vegetable oil in Lipiphysan and Lipofundin is derived from the cotton seed. The problem of toxicity of fat emulsions will be dealt with in greater detail by Dr Darby. Toxicity studies in man and experimental animals have demonstrated that emulsions of soya bean oil are safer than preparations containing cotton seed oil[3-5].

Table 10.1 The composition of intravenous fat emulsions (g/l)

	Lipiphysan	*Lipofundin*	*Intralipid*	*Lipofundin-S*
Vegetable oil				
Cotton seed	150	100		
Soya bean			100 or 200	100 or 200
Emulsifier				
Soya bean lecithin	20			
Soya bean phosphatide		7.5		7.5 or 15
Egg-yolk phosphatide			12	
Polyol				
Sorbitol	50	50		
Xylitol				50
Glycerol			25	

However, unlike Intralipid, Lipofundin-S induced haemorrhage and death in dogs so that other possible explanations for the differing toxicity of fat emulsions might lie in differences in their emulsifying agents, polyhydric alcohols, or in their particle size. My experience of fat emulsions is confined to Intralipid and all subsequent references to fat emulsions will be to that solution. However, this is the only fat emulsion that can be used in North America and it is the most frequently used emulsion in Europe.

Whenever it is appropriate I use large quantities of fat emulsion during intravenous feeding to avoid overloading my patient with solute. The initial solute load induced by 1 litre of Intralipid 10% and 20% compared with approximately equicalorific and equivolaemic quantities of glucose is shown in Table 10.2. The difference in initial solute load and concentration is obvious. Of course, complete utilization of either substrate results in the production of energy and the excretion of the carbon atoms as carbon dioxide and the hydrogen atoms as water without any change in osmolarity. But utilization may not be rapid so that problems may be encountered with hyperosmolar syndromes provoked by hypertonic solutions of glucose[6]. Although these hyperosmolar syndromes can be modified to some extent by the use of insulin,

Table 10.2 The energy and solute content of intravenous carbohydrate and fat solutions

Energy content (kcal)	*Substrate*	*Concentration* (%)	*Volume* (ml)	*Solute load* (mOsm)
1000	Intralipid	10	1000	280
1140	Glucose	30	1000	2100
2000	Intralipid	20	1000	330
1900	Glucose	50	1000	3800

this expertise is not available in every hospital. The ability to handle a large intravenous solute load differs from patient to patient and in health and disease, being particularly affected by renal function. The neonate has particular difficulty in excreting a large solute load[7]. When we first began to feed neonates intravenously in Newcastle, we had considerable trouble with fluid retention. Data typifying this problem are shown in Figure 10.1 Fluid

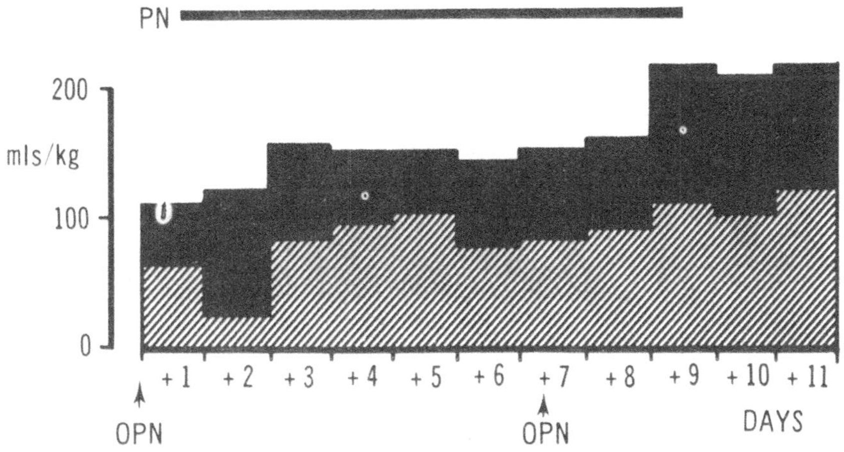

Figure 10.1 Fluid balance during intravenous feeding in a neonate

excretion from the kidneys, naso-gastric and peritoneal drains has been subtracted from fluid intake. Allowing for insensible loss, this child had still retained a considerable volume of fluid. Measurement of urinary solute excretion (Figure 10.2) emphasizes this point. This neonate excreted a very small quantity of urinary solute compared with the large intravenous solute load that he had received. If similar studies are performed in adults it is found that the quantity of solute excreted is much greater. It is unlikely that all the intravenous solute infused was utilized in tissue formation or oxidized to water and carbon dioxide and consequently this small rise in plasma osmolality indicates that the neonate's primary homeostatic response to a solute load is to dilute the load by fluid retention. Certainly many of them did develop severe oedema. Because of these findings, our initial neonatal regimen contained 5 g fat emulsion/kg body weight/24 h[8] to reduce the osmolarity as much as possible. Recently, this regimen has been modified and the fat content reduced to 4 g/kg body weight/24 h[9].

There are still some questions that remain to be answered concerning the utilization of Intralipid. The results of studies of energy utilization performed by indirect calorimetry are shown in Figure 10.3[10]. Studies were performed before and after surgery and the elective abdominal procedures performed are shown in Table 10.3. Normograms indicate the mean values for the protein,

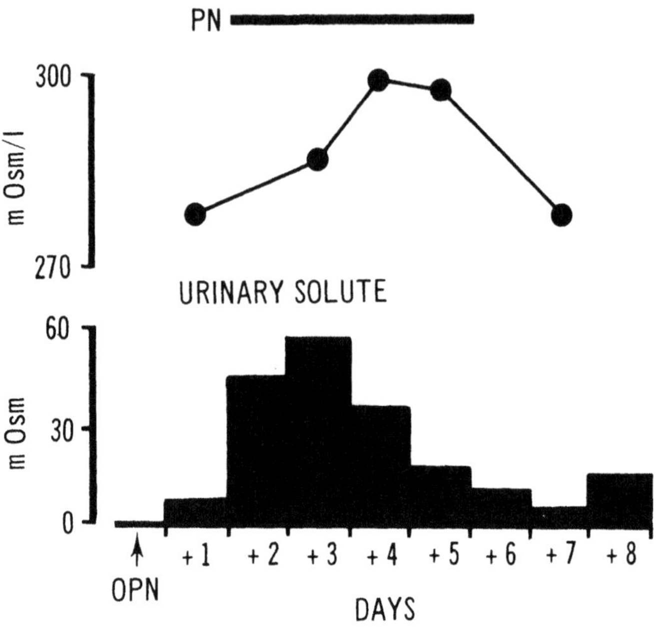

Figure 10.2 Plasma osmolality and urinary solute excretion during intravenous feeding in a neonate

carbohydrate and fat energy contribution to total energy intake and resting energy expenditure. The dots represent the individual values for total energy intake and resting energy expenditure. Physical activity was assessed by activity charts and the additional energy expenditure in excess of resting expenditure was found to be extremely small. All patients received a normal intake up to and including their evening meal and they were in positive balance on the day preceding operation. For technical reasons it was impossible to perform indirect calorimetric studies on the day of operation. Following operation the patients received quantities of amino acids, carbohydrate and fat emulsion that should have been in excess of that required to cover energy requirement. It is interesting to note that the nitrogen and in particular the urea excretion of these patients was greater than that in a similar group who did not receive intravenous feeding during this time, indicating that some of the infused amino acids were broken down. However,

Table 10.3 Operations performed

Truncal vagotomy and pyloroplasty (three patients)
Truncal vagotomy and gastroenterostomy
Partial gastrectomy
Conversion of partial gastrectomy to Roux-en-Y anastomosis

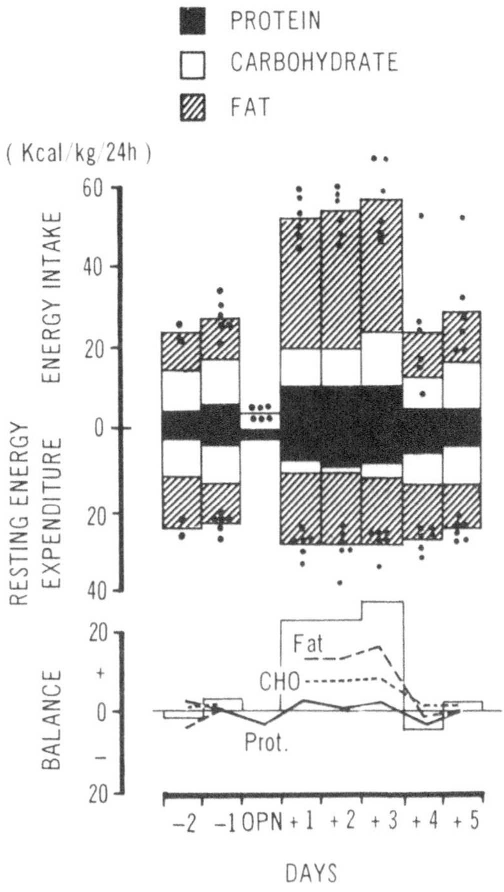

Figure 10.3 Resting metabolic expenditure during intravenous feeding after elective abdominal operations

sufficient quantities were retained to abolish the usual postoperative negative nitrogen balance. Due to the usual postoperative carbohydrate intolerance, the carbohydrate intake did not appear to be utilized and the major source of energy during this period was from fat catabolism. It is impossible from these studies to ascertain whether the source of fat was the infused emulsion or the patient's depot fat. Studies of fat clearance[11,12] indicate increased clearance of Intralipid following operation but clearance is not synonymous with utilization. Isotopic studies of Intralipid utilization[13] suggest that only 30% of the infused Intralipid was catabolized in the first 24 h after operation.

Another method of studying the relative efficacy of fat emulsions as an energy source is to study their effect upon nitrogen balance. Although infusion of Intralipid as a sole energy source at two levels of intake did produce some protein conservation in healthy subjects, the degree of conservation was far less than might be expected when related to the total energy intake[14]. It was concluded from this and a subsequent study[15] that the protein conservation was due to the short carbon chain of the free and esterified glycerol. The results of similar protein conservation studies performed after elective truncal vagotomy and pyloroplasty[16] are shown in Table 10.4. On the day

Table 10.4 Total negative nitrogen balance (g/4 days)

Electrolyte group	53
Fat emulsion group	52
Carbohydrate group	38
Amino acid group	13

of operation and the subsequent 3 days the patients received the same electrolyte and fluid intake. The control group received no energy and the other three treatment groups received equicalorific quantities of either carbohydrate, amino acids or fats.

The groups receiving amino acids and carbohydrates showed a significant improvement in nitrogen balance when compared with the control group but when given as a sole substrate Intralipid had virtually no protein sparing effect. Of course the infusion of Intralipid as a sole substrate is not to be recommended. What we require to ascertain is the ideal combination of non-protein energy substrates to infuse with amino acid solutions. The ideal contribution of carbohydrate and fat emulsion is likely to vary with different clinical situations.

The fatty acid composition of triglycerides was not thought to have any great significance for human nutrition until it was demonstrated that certain fatty acids (the so-called essential fatty acids) were required in the diet of a rat[17]. Subsequently, much work has been done on essential fatty acid deficiency in experimental animals but less is known about its occurrence in man. Nevertheless, with the more frequent use of long-term fat-free intravenous feeding, essential fatty acid deficiency has become more frequent[18,19].

Why are some fatty acids essential? Some such as stearic acid are completely saturated with hydrogen and some such as oleic acid are monounsaturated, that is to say they contain a single double bond carbon linkage (Figure 10.4). These acids can be synthesized by animals. Other fatty acids, such as linoleic acid and linolenic acid, are polyunsaturated. That is to say they have more than one double bond carbon linkage in their chain and in the case of the essential fatty acids these double bonds are situated at the end furthest away from the carboxyl group. Animals cannot manufacture double bonds at sites proximal to the ninth carbon atom in the chain. Thus not only are animals unable to synthesize linoleic and linolenic acid they are also unable to synthesize linolenic acid from linoleic acid. The distribution of these two groups of fatty acids in the human body are very different, adipose fat containing mainly saturated sixteen to eighteen carbon chain

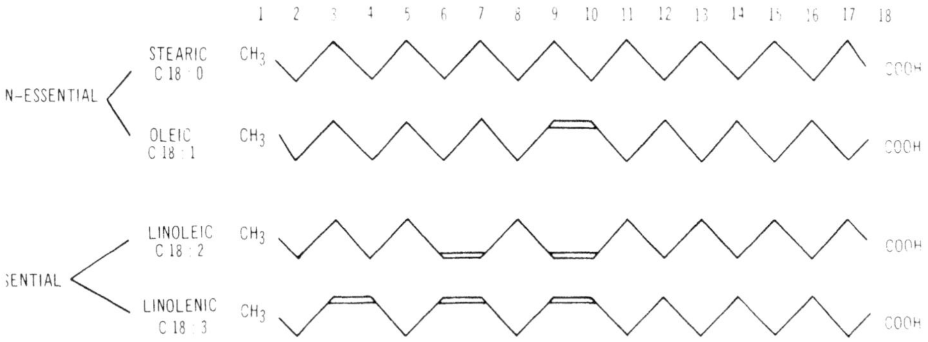

Figure 10.4 The structure of fatty acids

fatty acids, but the structural fats such as the grey matter of the brain may contain as much as 20% of its fats as polyunsaturated essential fatty acids with eighteen to twenty-two carbon chains[20,21].

There are two major families derived from linoleic and linolenic acids, further chain elongation and desaturation producing arachidonic and docosahexaenoic acid respectively (Figure 10.5). It has been suggested that

LINOLEIC (C 18 : 2) ⟶ ARACHIDONIC (C 20 : 4)

LINOLENIC (C 18 : 3) ⟶ DOCOSAHEXAENOIC (C 22 : 6)

Figure 10.5 Chain elongation and desaturation of essential fatty acids

these higher homologues are the most significant of the polyunsaturated constituents of cell membrane lipids in the brain, reproductive organs, endocrine glands and vascular endothelium, and doubts have been expressed about the ability of animal systems to carry out this chain elongation and desaturation, such a process being slow and rate limiting in the rat and perhaps not occurring at all in the cat[22].

The fatty acid composition of Intralipid is shown in Table 10.5. It is apparent that the solution only contains a small quantity of linolenic acid. Cotton seed oil emulsion does not contain any linolenic acid and neither it nor the soya bean oil contain arachidonic or docosahexaenoic acid. The egg yolk phospholipid emulsifying agent contains a negligible quantity of arachidonic acid. It is now apparent that the clinical features of essential fatty

Table 10.5 Fatty acid composition of Intralipid (%)

Palmitic acid	(C16)	9
Stearic acid	(C18)	3
Oleic acid	(C18:1)	26
Linoleic acid	(C18:2)	54
Linolenic acid	(C18.3)	8

acid deficiency are preceded by a fall in plasma linoleic acid concentration and the appearance of an abnormal fatty acid (eicosatrienoic) which can occur within 3 days of starting a fat free intravenous diet[18]. The concentration of arachidonic acid usually falls a few days later. Infusions of Intralipid have cured the dermatological manifestation of essential fatty acid deficiency, restored the depleted phospholipid content of erythrocyte membranes and restored the depressed plasma concentrations of arachidonic acid[19,23]. These clinical studies in man would suggest that chain elongation and desaturation can occur and are at variance with the conclusions from studies on experimental animals. Further work is required to establish essential fatty acid requirement in man.

Until recently, it has been recommended that nothing should be added to the fat emulsion as this might affect the particle size which may be essential for its safe use. The specific gravities at room temperature of Intralipid 10% and 20% are shown in Table 10.6 and compared with some amino acid

Table 10.6 The specific gravities of Intralipid emulsions and amino acid solutions (room temperature)

Intralipid 10%	0.996
Intralipid 20%	0.989
Synthamin 9%	1.025
Synthamin 14%	1.035
Synthamin 17%	1.039
Vamin-glucose	1.06
Vamin-fructose	1.06

solutions. The fat emulsion has a lower specific gravity than the amino acid solutions, and if there is an insufficient pressure and insufficient flow rate in the amino acid infusion set the fat will float up into the amino acid solution bottle as shown in Figure 10.6. To avoid this and the possible consequence of mixing the two solutions outside the body for any length of time, the solutions should be infused through separate infusion sets and mixed with a Y giving set with a short common arm (Travenol Labs. Ltd., England. Code: FKC 0055) immediately before infusion into the vein. Recently dual and triple infusion sets have been developed for parenteral nutrition which join immediately proximal to the Luer-lock adaptor (Travenol Labs. Ltd., England. Codes: FKC0180 and FKC0181.).

A recent development has been the deliberate mixing of fat emulsions with amino acid, carbohydrate and electrolyte solutions[24]. The Montpelier group have not noted any untoward reactions following infusion of such combined solutions which have been stored in the pharmacy, thus casting doubt on the necessity for keeping the fat emulsions separate from the other solutions. These findings require confirmation. A multivitamin preparation, Vitalipid (Kabivitrum, Sweden), containing the fat soluble vitamins which can be

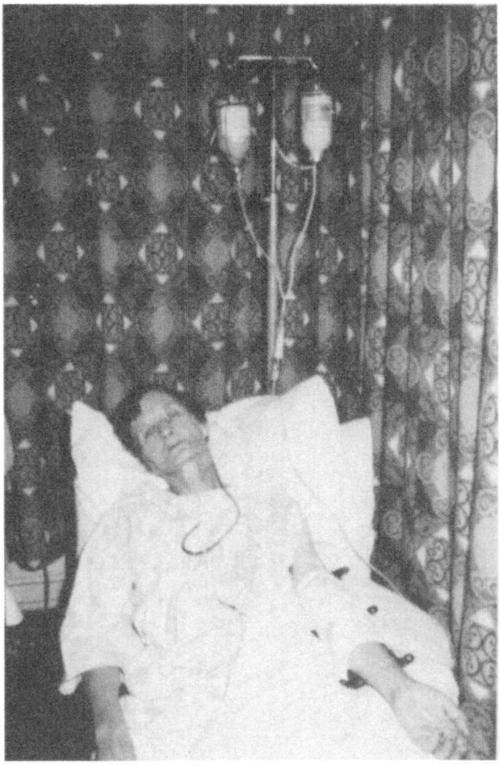

Figure 10.6 Simultaneous infusion of fat emulsion and amino acid solution—the incorrect method

added to Intralipid, has been developed and the constituents are shown in Table 10.7. I have used this preparation without observing any effect upon the emulsion or untoward reaction in the patients. However, I cannot comment upon its efficacy as a vitamin supplement.

It has been said than when isotonic fat emulsions are used as the major energy source, peripheral infusion can be used particularly if the infusion sites are changed every 24 h. However, Intralipid is irritant to the subcutaneous tissues. The consequences of subcutaneous extravasation of Intralipid in a neonate fed through a scalp vein are shown in Figure 10.7. This child subsequently died from unrelated events and post mortem examination revealed that a plaque of soap had been formed due to saponification of the fatty acids. Although the use of central catheters is associated with occasional serious complication, it is doubtful whether most patients would appreciate having their infusion sites changed every day.

The clearance of the fat emulsions from the serum can be used as an index of utilization. A severe example of incomplete clearance is shown in one of

Table 10.7 The composition of Vitalipid

Vitamin A	750 μg	(2500 I.U.)
Vitamin D_2	3 μg	(120 I.U.)
Vitamin K_1	150 μg	
10 ml daily		

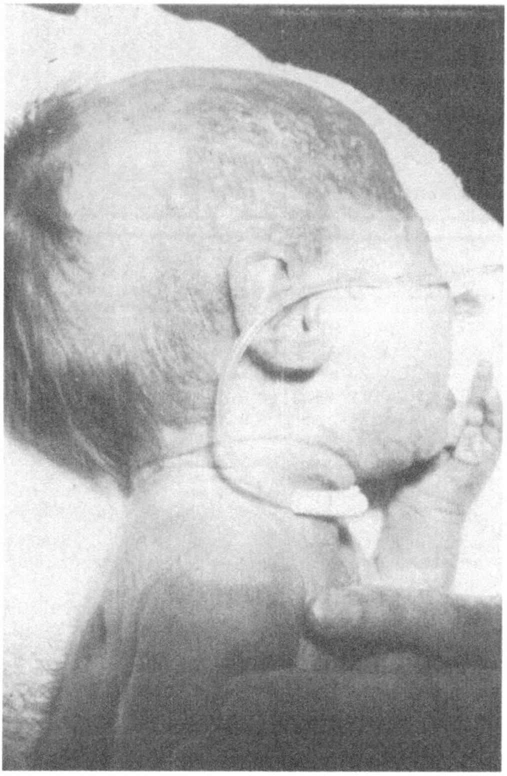

Figure 10.7 Subcutaneous extravasation of fat emulsion in a neonate

the samples in Figure 10.8 and compared with a normal sample. The manufacturers suggest that Intralipid should be infused initially at a dose of 2 g/kg body weight/day and if the serum is completely cleared of Intralipid then this dose can be increased to a maximum of 4 g/kg body weight/day with complete clearance in the serum. Others have infused as much as 12 g/kg body weight/day[25]. In general, patients who have been starving for prolonged periods of time clear the fat emulsion very rapidly and I sometimes give them as much as 70% of their non-protein requirements in the form of fat emulsion. In contrast, patients with sepsis do not appear to clear the fat quickly.

Although there have been occasional disturbing and usually unconfirmed reports of complications attributed to infusion of Intralipid[26], the majority of 'adverse reactions' reported in the literature are in the nature of febrile responses. Intralipid should be stored at 4 °C, but on the ward it is frequently kept in the refrigerator. The infusion of chilled saline will induce a typical febrile reaction and if Intralipid is temporarily stored in the ward refrigerator, it should be removed at least 1 h prior to infusion. Although I have not kept accurate records, I estimate that I have infused 6000–10 000

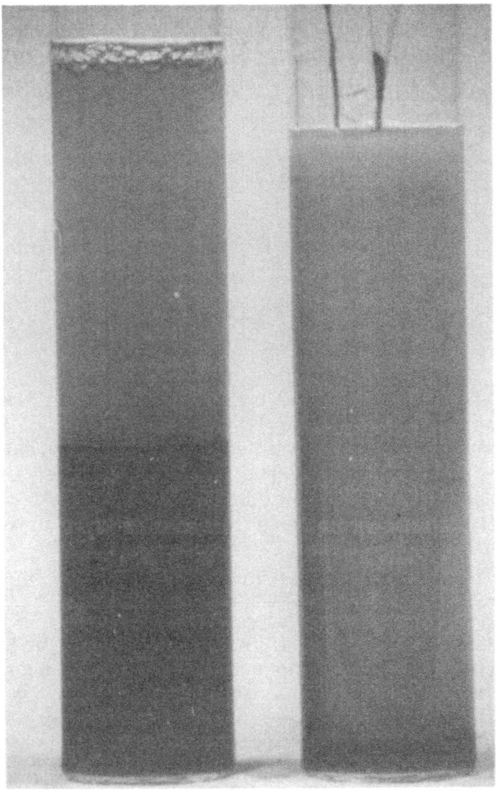

Figure 10.8 Incomplete clearance of fat emulsion from the serum

units (500 ml) of Intralipid 10% or 20% since 1969 and I have not witnessed any untoward clinical reaction (other than that shown in Figure 10.7) that I could definitely attribute to the infusion of the fat emulsion.

Fat in the serum can also interfere with biochemical and haematological estimations. Major aberrations involve colorimetric methods and the values for serum calcium, magnesium and phosphate are particularly affected but haemoglobin and plasma protein levels may also be artificially elevated by mild lipaemia. In order to reduce this problem to a minimum it is advisable to plan the intravenous feeding regimen so that no intravenous fat is given during the early hours of the morning and the routine blood samples should then be clear of fat.

CONCLUSION

Intravenous fat emulsions have been used in Europe for more than a decade. Soya bean oil emulsions appear to be very safe and their isotonicity avoids the hyperosmolar syndromes associated with equicalorific and equivolaemic quantities of carbohydrate. Further investigation is required into the relative utilization of fat emulsions and carbohydrates in patients suffering from different diseases and the fatty acids which are essential in man require to be defined.

ACKNOWLEDGEMENT

I am very grateful to Mr J. Waggett for allowing me to study neonates under his care.

References

1. Menzel, A. and Perco, H. (1869). Uber die resorption von Nahrungsmitteln vom Unterhautzellgewebe aus. *Wien. Med. Wschr.* **19,** 517
2. Report of a conference on intravenous fatty acids (1957). Metabolism 6
3. Hallberg, D., Schuberth, O. and Wretlind, A. (1966). Experimental and clinical studies with fat emulsion for intravenous nutrition. *Nutr. Dieta.*, **8,** 245
4. Hakansson, I. (1968). Experience in long-term studies on nine intravenous fat emulsions in dogs. *Nutr. Dieta*, **10,** 54
5. Jacobson, S. (1970). Complete parenteral nutrition in man for seven months. In Berg, G. (ed.). "Advances in Parenteral Nutrition" p. 6. *Symp. Int. Soc. Parenteral Nutrition.* (Stuttgart: Georg Thieme Verlag)
6. Dudrick, S. J., Steiger, E., Long, J. M., Ruberg, R. L., Allen, T. R., Vars, H. M. and Rhoads, J. E. (1972). General principles and technique of administration in complete parenteral nutrition. In A. W. Wilkinson (ed.). *Parenteral Nutrition.* p. 222. (Edinburgh and London: Churchill Livingstone)
7. Wilkinson, A. W. (1966). Surgical aspects of neonatal metabolism. *Ann. Roy. Coll. Surg.*, **39,** 84
8. Tweedle, D. E. F., Wagget, J., Flear, C. T. G. and Dale, G. (1973). Parenteral nutrition in newborn surgical patients. *I.R.C.S.* (73–4) 31–0–2
9. Dale, G., Panter-Brick, M., Wagget, J. and Young, G. (1976). Plasma amino acid changes in the postsurgical newborn during intravenous nutrition with a synthetic amino acid solution. *J. Paed. Surg.*, **11,** 17
10. Tweedle, D. E. F. and Johnston, I. D. A. (1971). Factors affecting the metabolic expenditure of surgical patients. *Brit. J. Surg.*, **58,** 771
11. Hallberg, D. (1965). Studies on the elimination of exogenous lipids from the blood stream. The effect of fasting and surgical trauma in man on the elimination rate of a fat emulsion injected intravenously. *Acta Physiol. Scand.*, **65,** 153 (1965)
12. Fegetter, J. G. W., Tweedle, D. E. F. and Wright, P. D. (1974). Energy requirements after surgery. *E.U.S.R.B.M.*, (Suppl. 1.), 110
13. Eckart, J., Tempel, G., Kaul, A., Witzke, G., Schurnbrand, P. and Schaaf, H. (1973). Metabolism of radioactive-labelled fat emulsions in the postoperative and post traumatic period. *Am. J. Clin. Nutr.*, **26,** 578
14. Brennan, M. F. and Moore, F. D. (1973). An intravenous fat emulsion as a nitrogen sparer: comparison with glucose. *J. Surg. Res.*, **14,** 501

15. Brennan, M. F., Fitzpatrick, G. F., Cohen, K. H., Ball, A. B. and Moore, F. D. (1975). Glycerol: major contributor to the short term protein sparing effect of fat emulsions in normal man. *Ann. Surg.*, **182**, 386
16. Craig, R. P., Davidson, H. A., Tweedle, D. E. F. and Johnston, I. D. A. (1977). Intravenous glucose, amino acids and fat in the postoperative period: a controlled evaluation of each substrate. *Lancet*, **ii**, 8
17. Burr, G. O. and Burr, M. M. (1930). On the nature and role of the fatty acids essential in nutrition. *J. Biol. Chem.*, **86**, 587
18. Wene, J. D., Connor, W. E. and Den Besten (1975). The development of essential fatty acid deficiency in healthy man fed fat-free diets intravenously and orally. *J. Clin. Invest.*, **56**, 127
19. Riella, M. C., Broviac, J. W., Wells, M. and Scribner, B. H. (1975). Essential fatty acid deficiency in human adults during total parenteral nutrition. *Ann. Int. Med.*, **83**, 786
20. O'Brien, J. S., Fillerup, D. L. and Mead, J. F. (1964). Quantification and fatty acid and fatty aldehyde composition of ethanolamine, choline and serine glycerophosphatides in human cerebral grey and white matter. *J. Lipid Res.*, **5**, 329
21. Whitting, L. A., Harvery, C. C. and Horwitt, M. K. (1963). Dietary alterations of fatty acids of erythrocytes and mitochondria of brain and liver. *J. Lipid Res.*, **2**, 412
22. Crawford, M. A. and Hassam, A. G. (1976). Intravenous fat and E.F.A. *Lancet*, **ii**, 94
23. Wilmore, D. W., Moylan, J. A., Helmkamp, G. M. and Pruitt, B. A. (1973). Essential fatty acid deficiency in the red cell membrane following thermal injury: Correction with parenteral fat emulsion. *Surg. For.*, **23**, 499
24. Solassol, C., Joyeux, H., Serrou, B., Pujol, H. and Romieu, C. (1973). Nouvelles techniques de nutrition parenterale a long terme pour suppleance intestinale. *Chirurgie*, **105**, 15
25. Hadifeld, J. I. H. (1966). High calorie intravenous feeding in surgical patients. *Clin. Med.*, **73**, 25
26. Jellinek, E. H. (1976). Dangers of intravenous fat infusions. *Lancet*, **ii**, 967

Discussion

N. Zöllner: (Germany) With respect to the comparison of man with animals there are few aspects of metabolism where differences in turnover are so marked as with polyunsaturated fatty acids. For example, in the rat, arachidonic acid is the main polyunsaturated acid in the serum and if polyunsaturated acids are withdrawn from the diet it disappears very rapidly. If man is fed arachidonic acid, he gets very high serum levels; and if it is then withdrawn, it is weeks before it falls to normal levels. The turnover related to energy metabolism in man is on the level of linoleic acid, with arachidonic acid in a side shuttle, which is very sensitive. In the rat, by contrast, arachidonic is included in the total turnover.

G. L. Blackburn: (USA) I should like to ask about the advisablility of not using Intralipid during sepsis.

D. E. F. Tweedle: (UK) I have no actual figures on sepsis and starvation. It is something that has become apparent to me over a number of years. If Intralipid is used in a septic patient, then utilization problems are more common, whereas starving patients seem to be particularly avid users of fat, and they have been able to tolerate as much as 6 g/kg/day.

Y. A. Carpentier: (USA) There is a study comparing intravenous fat tolerance in animals infected with Gram-negative and Gram-positive germs. An impairment of the removal of the fat emulsion was observed only with the Gram-negative infection.

Tweedle: Gram-negative or coliform-infection is of course the usual type of septicaemia found in gastroenterological problems.

J. T. Harries: (UK) We tend to avoid using Intralipid in children with liver disease. Would Mr Tweedle comment on his experience in adults with liver disease?

Tweedle: I have used Intralipid on occasions in patients who have had obstructive jaundice and have had no problems. I have never used it in patients with hepatocellular disease.

11
Lipid metabolism in stress

R. L. HOLLIDAY, T. VIIDIK AND B. JENNINGS

INTRODUCTION

'I hope that when the metabolic pattern of shock has been outlined as completely as possible, it will be possible to discern patterns which indicate what metabolic alterations may prove critical' (F. Engel, 1969).

The body's response to stress and injury has been the subject of much investigation over the past half-century. Pioneers such as Cuthbertson, Bywaters, Moore, etc. have led clinical investigators to search out the patterns of altered metabolism in stressful states, to understand their implications and hence to test and prove the usefulness of therapeutic modalities. Clinical research into surgical stress must also pay respect to the groundwork of Cahill, Felig, Unger and others.

This paper will review lipid metabolism. A brief background of basic knowledge will be presented, followed by a review of current knowledge of altered lipid metabolism in stress, and from this, therapeutic implications will be derived.

BASIC FAT METABOLISM

The chemical-free energy contained in food is the single form of energy man can use. 'The inability of the body to utilize any energy source other than food is an unfortunate oversight in these times of high cost electrical energy and high food prices'[1].

Lipids constitute approximately 40% of our daily caloric intake. Two-thirds of all dietary fats arise from animal sources; the other one-third originates from vegetable sources. Almost all ingested lipid is in the form of triglyceride.

Evolution has been kind to man. Survival is partially due to man's ability to store most of his excess calories as triglyceride in adipose tissue. As a fuel, fat yields 9.0 calories per gram, twice that of an equal dry weight of carbohydrate or protein. Also, carbohydrate and fat are stored in water-soluble body tissue, thus decreasing their weight efficiency.

It is estimated that resting man requires 1500–1800 cal/day to maintain basal energy needs. The 15 kg of triglyceride in fat in the average 70 kg male thus can provide energy for 1–3 months' survival (Figure 11.1).

	Glycogen or glucose		*'Mobilizable' protein*		*Triglyceride*	
	(g)	(cal)	(g)	(cal)	(g)	(cal)
Blood	15	60	0	0	5	45
Liver	100	400	100	400	50	450
Brain	2	8	0	0	0	0
Muscle	300	1200	6000	24 000	50	450
Adipose	20	80	10	40	15 000	135 000

Figure 11.1 Cahill, G. F.[3]. Available fuel resources in man

Fat also provides insulation, padding protection and a source of fat soluble substances such as vitamins as well as structural components of cell membranes.

Fat is stored as adipose tissue. Deposition and mobilization are substrate- and hormone-dependent. In the fed state, lipoprotein lipase acts to convert triglyceride to free fatty acids and glycerol. The fatty acids combine to form fatty acetyl Co-A and under the influence of insulin and with glucose available are reconstituted as new triglycerides and stored in the fat cell[1].

During fasting, the plasma glucose and insulin falls and there is an associated decrease in glucose and insulin in adipose tissue. This results in free fatty acid mobilization. There is also a concomitant humoral response of increased catecholamines, glucagon and growth hormone in the circulation. Glucocorticoids appear to be necessary as 'permissive' hormones.

ROLE OF LIVER IN FAT METABOLISM

The liver is important in intermediary metabolism. It is suggested that stress[2], i.e. shock and sepsis, alters liver function, and this situation may be partially responsible for altered energy kinetics.

With normal liver function, and in the post-absorptive state, the liver takes up dietary chylomicrons, free fatty acids and dietary carbohydrate and produces very low density lipoproteins. These lipoproteins are released and stored in adipose tissue or used as fuel in peripheral tissues.

The liver can also release ketone bodies under appropriate circumstances. Most extrahepatic tissues can utilize ketone bodies as energy sources. In the much studied starvation state[3], by the third day, there is increased keto acid production—acetone, acetoacetate and β-hydroxybutyrate. The heart and brain are especially efficient at keto adaptation, the heart acquiring as much as three-quarters of its energy from keto acids. Keto acid levels plateau after two weeks of starvation. All of this altered metabolism serves to decrease gluconeogenesis and hence preserve muscle mass. The protective mechanism is grossly abnormal for many reasons in stressful situations.

The hormonal pattern consists of decreasing insulin levels with increased glucagon. At a molecular level, there is increased activity of hormone sensitive lipase with less glucose available for conversion to L-α glycerophosphate, a necessary step in triglyceride formation[3]. These hormonal and molecular enzyme patterns are also disturbed in stress.

LIPID METABOLISM DURING EXERCISE

Knowledge of altered metabolism of fat has been achieved by studying man during exercise and starvation. Felig and Wahren[4] have reviewed recently fuel metabolism in exercise. Exercise results in great increases in glucose uptake but, more important, fatty acid utilization continues to increase, especially with prolonged exercise. This does not appear to be the case in other stressful situations. It appears that fatty acid uptake is regulated not by the muscle itself, but by external factors. This may not occur in certain states such as sepsis.

There is also one further relationship discovered in exercising and starving man which may have implications for stressed man. There appears to be a unique inter-relationship among keto acids, fatty acids and the metabolism of branched chain amino acids[4]. As has been seen, keto acids are a major fuel source. Late in starvation, however, keto acid oxidation in muscle ceases, teleologically sparing them for the brain. There is increased oxidation of fatty acids and decreased deamination of the branched chain amino acids resulting in protein conservation. This may occur because leucine, isoleucine and valine share the same co-factors for metabolism with keto and fatty acids (Figure 11.2).

Again, there is evidence that this may not be the situation in stress.

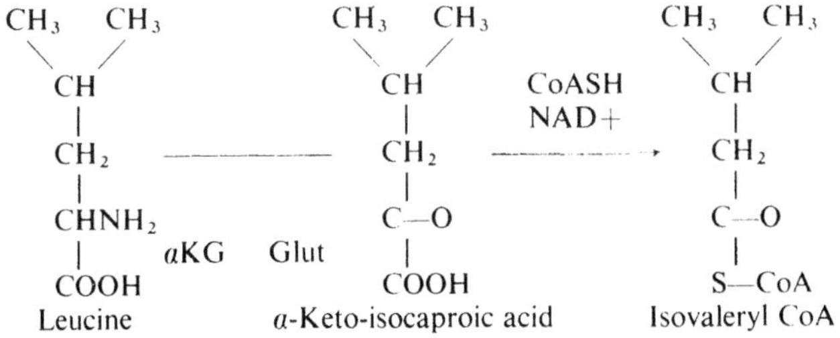

Figure 11.2 Cahill, G. F.[3]. Leucine catabolism in muscle

ALTERED LIPID METABOLISM IN 'STRESS'

Compared with the amount of data available concerning substrate metabolism in fasting, exercising and normal man, there is little data concerning stressed man.

More has been written on glucose and protein homeostasis during stress, i.e. haemorrhage[5], burns[6], sepsis[7], than on lipid homeostasis.

Animal and a few human studies have demonstrated hormonal patterns in various stress states to be much different from fasting man. It appears that the finely tuned mechanism resulting in preservation of body cell mass, especially muscle mass, is altered.

Gluconeogenesis continues; there is failure of ketone adaptation and increasing ureagenesis. It is remarkable that severely ill, especially septic patients, die without apparently calling on the fat reserves of their bodies. The reasons for this are many and a pattern is emerging, but the critical substrate abnormality or humoral aberration has yet to be elucidated.

Hanson *et al.*[5] examined the lipid response to a 15% haemorrhage and norepinephrine infusion in healthy young males. Free fatty acids rose significantly during norepinephrine infusion before and after haemorrhage. They suggested that this occurs secondary to sympathetic nervous stimulation. No attempts were made to ascertain the role of fatty acids as an energy source during haemorrhage or norepinephrine infusion.

Lipid metabolism in burned individuals has been studied by Birke *et al.*[6] Free fatty acids increased in relation to the size of the burns, either due to caloric requirement or sympathetic stimulation. Excess mobilization of free fatty acid may be detrimental, producing fatty infiltration and inducing thrombogenesis. They also correlated norepinephrine with free fatty acid levels[6]. Levels of other hormones, such as insulin and glucagon, were not measured. Excessive lipolysis may diminish organ function (Kjekshus and Mjos[8] and Rowe *et al.*[9]). Increased free fatty acids secondary to catecholamine release in myocardial infarction increased the effect of experimental injury. Inhibition of lipolysis lessened the effect.

Rowe's work[9] demonstrates that antilipolytic treatment with a nicotinic-acid analogue decreases the frequency of arrhythmias after myocardial infarction in humans. Again, the elevated free fatty acid levels are presumed secondary to catecholamine release.

While it appears that stimulation of lipid metabolism may be detrimental in certain stress states, other stress states such as sepsis may be associated with a lack of stimulation of lipid metabolism.

The hormonal and substrate patterns of sepsis are currently undergoing much review[10]. This is because patients surviving the initial insults of burns or major injury then die of multiple organ failure, often associated with sepsis. Many of the problems may be related to an inadequate or inappropriate utilization of the body's energy stores.

Recent studies[7,11] suggest that in sepsis fat utilization is essentially zero. Continued protein breakdown to make up for this fat deficit leads to further complications and death. O'Donnell *et al.*[11] have expanded their original observations in septic man. Using haemodynamic studies to divide sepsis into high and low flow states, they distinguished two substrate and hormone profiles which differ markedly from fasting. Patients with high flow sepsis demonstrate increased blood glucose and insulin. FFA levels were low, ketone levels decreased, while alanine and lactate were higher than in fasting individuals. Low flow sepsis was associated with net release of fat from limbs and again, no ketone uptake; alanine and lactate were again greatly increased. Our studies confirm and extend this work.

Fatty acids and glycerol are important substrates in gluconeogenesis, but cannot be utilized without energy. Furthermore, these substrates are regulated by important metabolic hormones[12,13]. Ketone and lactate are linked integrally to both protein and fat metabolism. Ketones reduce substrate availability for gluconeogenesis[14]. Keto acid infusions result in hypoalaninaemia and in nitrogen conservation in starvation. Ketones inhibit lipolysis either directly or indirectly by stimulating insulin. Lactate infusions can increase leg blood flow, stimulate oxidative metabolism and cause a fall in arterial FFA due to an augmental removal of FFA from the plasma pool, but without any effect on mobilization of FFA from adipose tissue[15]. This implies, at least in the resting state, that skeletal muscle is quantitatively more important than the liver in the disposal of lactate[7]. However, these key substrates have yet to be fully evaluated in the septic state.

The adaptive response to prolonged fasting includes a decrease in breakdown of muscle protein, as a source of carbohydrate intermediates for intermediary metabolic pathways. This protective phenomenon does not occur in sepsis. Rather, accelerated protein catabolism continues as shown by the disappearance of muscle mass. Patterns of metabolism in sepsis are different from exercise unless we postulate that there is lactate inhibition of lipolysis[16]. If the septic patient is viewed as a man during prolonged exercise, then the usual 90% of oxidative metabolism supplied by FFA must be replaced by proteolysis[4].

MATERIALS AND METHODS

Protocol

Seventeen patients treated at Victoria Hospital, London, Ontario for septic shock were studied. The patients were investigated for patterns of lipid metabolism and were compared to fasting post-operative non-septic controls.

Criteria for sepsis included: (1) clinical history and physical findings; (2) documented septic focus at surgery or at post-mortem; (3) positive cultures of septic sites and/or blood. These patients were then divided into two groups based on their insulin levels at the time of blood sampling. O'Donnell *et al.*[11] have demonstrated that this differentiation correlated both with the haemodynamic response and prognosis.

All patients were studied within the initial 72 h of their septic course. All patients were receiving 5% dextrose crystalloid infusions, but no parenteral nutrition. The entire group had no pre-existing diabetic or metabolic disease, and there had been no previous malnutrition or steroid therapy.

Substrate measurements from the leg included the arteriovenous differences (AVD) for free fatty acids, glycerol and betahydroxybutyrate (ketones). Femoral arterial blood was also sampled for insulin, glucagon, glucose, lactate and catecholamines.

The control patients were elective post-operative surgical patients who had fasted up to 72 h, but had been maintained on 5% dextrose infusions according to conventional intravenous therapy. These patients too had no metabolic derangements, malignant disease, and were in normal nutritional balance.

Biochemical analysis

Plasma glucagon was assayed radioimmunologically with antiserum (30K) specific for pancreatic glucagon[17]. Serum insulin was measured by the double antibody direct precipitation method (Amersham Searle, Des Plaines, Ill.). Blood glucose was measured by the glucose oxidase method employed in the Beckman glucose analyser. After deproteinization with perchloric acid, lactate was enzymatically calculated by methods adapted from Bergmeyer[18]. Ketones were also measured microfluorimetrically as described by Williamson[19]. FFA determination was by the method of Dole and Meinertz[20]. Glycerol was measured by a technique used by Calbiochem Laboratories.

Catecholamines were analysed using the method of Griffiths and Leung[21].

RESULTS

Table 11.1 represents the patient groups. Peritonitis was the most common septic process. Blood cultures and cultures from the septic sites were primarily Gram-negative organisms. *Pseudomonas* and *E. coli* were the most frequent and consistent organisms found. Patients with pneumonia had *Staphylococcus aureus*, *Klebsiella* and *Monilia*. Both insulin groups had Gram-positive and Gram-negative septicaemias, although the latter predominated. In twelve of the patients sepsis developed as a complication. The remainder were medical patients who in their septic state displayed rampant pneumonias.

Tables 11.2 and 11.3 illustrate the lipid metabolic profile of the two septic groups as well as the control group. The control group demonstrates an uptake of FFA and glycerol across the leg. Conversely, the septic groups showed a release of these lipids from the leg.

The FFA and ketone levels in the normal insulin and control groups are

Table 11.1 Septic patients

	Normal insulin levels	*High insulin levels*
	7	10
Septic process		
Pneumonia	2	3
Peritonitis	4	5
Septic burn	1	1
Amnionitis	0	1
Positive cultures		
Blood	6	8
Abscess	3	4
Sputum	2	3
Abdominal cavity	4	5
Burn eschar	1	1
Survival	1/7	4/10

Table 11.2 Lipid metabolism

	FFA (mM/l)			*Glycerol* (mg%)			*Ketones* (mM/l)			*Lactate* (mM/l)
	Art.	*Ven.*	△*	*Art.*	*Ven.*	△*	*Art.*	*Ven.*	△*	*Art.*
CONTROL GROUP Mean ($n = 6$)	.50	.43	.07	.90	.78	.12	.38	.32	.06	.93
HIGH INSULIN Mean ($n = 10$)	.21	.28	−.07	1.10	1.59	−.49	.18	.18	.00	

△*—refers to AVD (arteriovenous difference)

Table 11.3 Lipid metabolism

	FFA (mM/l)			*Glycerol* (mg%)			*Ketones* (mM/l)			*Lactate* (mM/l)
	Art.	*Ven.*	△*	*Art.*	*Ven.*	△*	*Art.*	*Ven.*	△*	*Art.*
CONTROL GROUP Mean ($n = 6$)	.50	.43	.07	.90	.78	.12	.38	.32	.06	.93
NORMAL INSULIN Mean ($n = 7$)	.50	.59	−.09	1.60	2.13	−.53	.31	.33	−.01	

△*—refers to AVD (arteriovenous difference)

almost identical. The high insulin group had lower levels of circulating FFA and ketones. Arteriovenous differences of ketone levels in all three groups are virtually immeasurable. However, circulating arterial levels in the normal insulin and control groups are higher than for non-fasting man.

Table 11.4 deals with the hormonal and energy substrate responses using the data of Finley[10] for control insulin, glucagon, catecholamines and glucose

Table 11.4 Comparison of patterns of response

	Controls	*Normal insulin*	*High insulin*
Insulin (μU/ml)	13*	10	52
Glucagon (pg/ml)	119*	522	700
I/G	2.7*	.44	2.4
Lactate (art.) (mM/l)	.93	3.16	2.35
FFA (mMole/l)			
Art.	.50	.50	.21
△A-V	.07	−.09	−.07
Glycerol (mg%)			
Art.	.90	1.60	1.10
△A-V	.12	−.53	−.49
Ketones (mM/l)			
Art.	.38	.31	.18
△A-V	.06	−.01	0
Glucose (mg%) Art.	154*	148	153
Catecholamines (ng/ml)			
Total	1.02*	1.92	1.75
Norepinephrine	.64	1.38	1.18
Epinephrine	.38	.54	.57

* Finley, R. J.[10]

values. Extremely high insulin levels were seen in both septic groups, but a significantly low I/G ratio in the normal insulin group, while the high insulin group matches the control group. All three groups maintain normal arterial glucose levels.

Plasma catecholamine levels were elevated in both the normal insulin and high insulin groups. Norepinephrine increase was greater than epinephrine in both groups. There was no remarkable difference between the insulin groups (Table 11.5).

The normal insulin group had the highest lactate values, while the high insulin group was intermediate in value.

The patterns of metabolic response are depicted in graphic form in Figures 11.3 and 11.4.

Table 11.5 Catecholamine levels in septic patients

	Normal insulin group		*High insulin group*	
	Norepinephrine (ng/ml)	*Epinephrine* (ng/ml)	*Norepinephrine* (ng/ml)	*Epinephrine* (ng/ml)
Patient No.				
1	—	—	2.04	.91
2	.22	.003	.30	.07
3	5.49	1.55	1.18	.62
4	.06	.09	.48	.91
5	1.69	.46	5.09	1.70
6	.43	.57	.93	.28
7	.41	.54	.004	.04
8	—	—	.31	.27
9	—	—	.56	.30
10	—	—	.88	.57
Mean	1.38	.53	1.18	.57

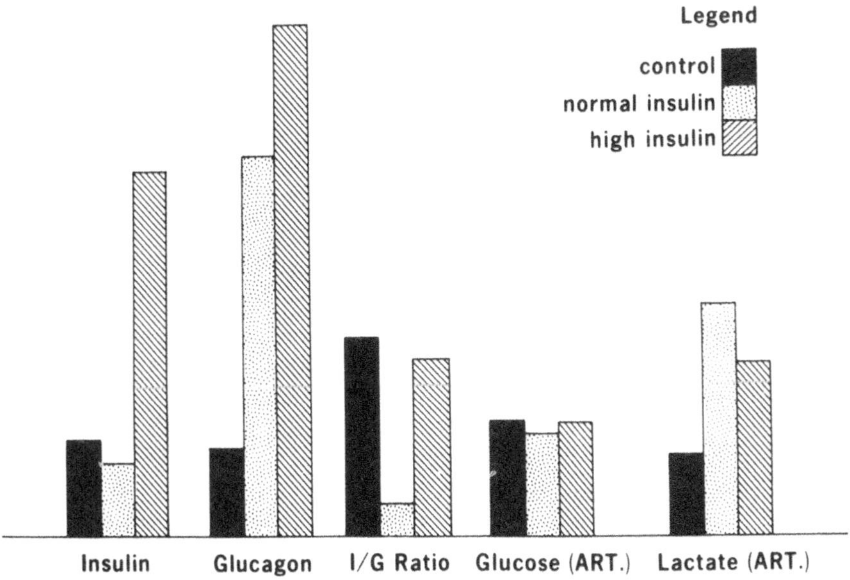

Figure 11.3 Hormonal, glucose and lactate values

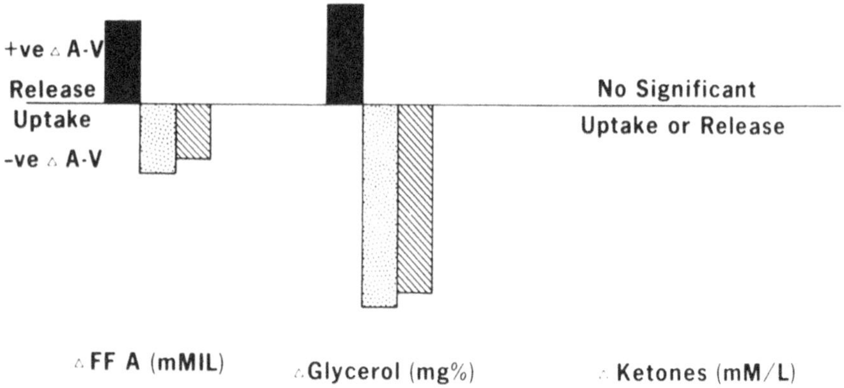

Figure 11.4 Fat response of hind limb

DISCUSSION

Septic patients in this study demonstrate markedly elevated catecholamine levels. This is predominantly norepinephrine, especially in the normal insulin or so-called low flow state. There appears to be no significant difference between the septic groups with respect to catecholamine production. This differs from previous findings[22,23]. However, catecholamines, as previously demonstrated[24,25] are important mediators of the abnormal substrate hormonal environment demonstrated here.

Normal post-operative patients (controls) showed an antilipolytic response, which was small perhaps due to the short period of starvation, the minimal stress and the infusion of glucose. Both septic groups released free fatty acids and glycerol from the hind limb. This has been demonstrated previously and suggests a central, or liver fuel, deficit. There would appear to be little lipid available for peripheral utilization.

Septic patients demonstrate hyperlacticacidaemia. This is particularly noticeable in the 'normal' insulin group, suggesting an increase in anaerobic metabolism or impairment of lactate clearance by a failing liver. Also in this anaerobic environment, available lipids would not be used efficiently.

The insulin:glucagon ratio may be important in catabolic illness[12]. The high insulin group of septic patients demonstrates an insulin:glucagon ratio (I/G) not unlike normal individuals. This suggests that they are in a metabolically compensated state. The 'normal' insulin group demonstrates a very low I/G ratio suggestive of overwhelming stress, a fact borne out by the high mortality in this group.

Ketone metabolism is abnormal in both groups of septic patients. Ketones are essentially not utilized across the hind limb.

Circulating free fatty acids and glycerol are higher in the 'normal' insulin group of patients. The free fatty acid turnover is rapid and similar in both groups, but the increasing lipid is presented to a compromised liver[10]. These changes, combined with increased lactic acid, could impair alanine uptake by the liver, and cause failure of gluconeogenesis resulting in increased protein breakdown, thus continuing the vicious cycle[26]. Continued delivery of lipid to the liver could also result in fatty infiltration, which has been well demonstrated[2].

CLINICAL IMPLICATIONS

The altered hormonal and substrate profiles in stress situations suggest the need for treatment.

Attempts to provide non-protein caloric intake with glucose often lead to further hyperglycaemia and its associated problems. These can be managed by increasing insulin uptake, but this situation can become very difficult. Blackburn *et al.*[27] have suggested the use of amino acid infusion alone to spare protein breakdown. Their studies suggest that nitrogen equilibrium can be achieved with this method and they postulate that avoiding glucose intake will result in fatty acid mobilization and ketone production and utilization similar to prolonged fasting. Problems with keto-acidosis are not encountered, presumably because ketones will stimulate insulin production in the non-diabetic individual[7]. Greenberg *et al.*[29] disagree with this hypothesis and suggest that nitrogen equilibrium is achieved partially by nitrogen breakdown to glucose. If enough nitrogen is infused, some will be available for protein synthesis.

The use of fats as a non-protein caloric source has been studied for many years in Europe and these solutions are now available in North America. The safety of fat infusions is appealing, but how fats are utilized in catabolic situations remains debatable[30]. Our data and that of others suggest that in sepsis, fatty acids may not be utilized and in some situations, could be detrimental[8,9].

What then is available in the catabolic patient? It has been suggested that branched chain amino acids (BCAAs) are oxidized in muscle to provide energy[31]. Infusions of BCAAs in an attempt to decrease proteolysis are presently being carried out[11].

The infusion of ketones in catabolic man also require study. There is preliminary evidence that keto analogues may decrease proteolytic changes of disease[32]. These areas are the source of much future clinical research.

SUMMARY

The efficient use of lipids has enabled man to evolve through the ages. We are now at a stage in evolution when afflicted man suffers from metabolic abnormalities not previously described or understood. By applying the knowledge from fasting normal man and documenting the abnormalities in 'stressed' man, the problem of the most effective parenteral formulation to aid survival will be solved.

References

1. Ruch, T. C. and Patton, H. D. (eds.) (1973). *Physiology and Biophysics*, 20th ed., Vol. 3, p. 89. (Philadelphia: W. B. Saunders Co.)
2. Champion, H. R. and Jones, R. T. (1976). A clinicopathologic study of hepatic dysfunction following shock. *Surg. Gynecol. Obstet.*, **142,** 657
3. Cahill, G. F., Jr. (1976). Starvation in man. *Clin. in Endocrinol. Metab.*, **5,** 397
4. Felig, P. and Wahren, J. (1975). Fuel homeostasis in exercise. *N. Engl. J. Med.*, **293,** 1078
5. Hanson, E. L., Brennan, M. E., O'Connell, R. C. and Moore, F. D. (1973). Response of glucose, insulin free fatty acid and human growth hormone to nor-epinephrine and hemorrhage in normal man. *Ann. Surg.*, **177,** 453
6. Birke, G., Carlson, A., VonEuler, U. S., Liljedayl, S. O. and Planten, L. O. (1972). Studies on burns. *Acta Chir. Scand.*, **138,** 321
7. Clowes, G. H., O'Donnel, T. F., Ryan, N. T. and Blackburn, G. L. (1974). Energy metabolism in sepsis. *Ann. Surg.*, **179,** 684
8. Kjekshus, J. K. and Mjos, O. D. (1973). Effect of inhibition of lipolysis on infarct size after experimental coronary artery disease. *J. Clin. Invest.*, **52,** 1770
9. Rowe, M. J., Neilson, J. M. M. and Oliver, M. F. (1975). Control of ventricular arrhythmias during myocardial infarction by antilipolytic treatment using a nicotinic acid analogue. *Lancet*, **295,** (Feb. 8)
10. Finley, R. J. (1976). The metabolic basis of severe sepsis in man. *Ann. R. Coll. Surg. Can.*, **9,** 133
11. O'Donnell, T. F., Clowes, G. G. Jr., Blackburn, G. L., Ryan, N. T., Benotti, P. N. and Miller, J. D. B. (1976). Proteolysis associated with a deficit of peripheral energy fuel substrates in septic man. *Surgery*, **80,** 191
12. Unger, R. H. (1971). Glucagon and insulin:glucagon ratio in diabetes and other catabolic illnesses. *Diabetes*, **20,** 834
13. Bondy, P. K. and Felig, P. (1974). *Disorders of Carbohydrate Metabolism—Duncan's Diseases of Metabolism*, 7th ed., p. 234. (Philadelphia: W. B. Saunders Co.)
14. Sherwin, R. S., Hendler, R. G. and Felig, P. (1975). Effect of ketone infusions on amino acid and nitrogen metabolism in man. *J. Clin. Invest.*, **55,** 1382
15. Ahlborg, G., Hagenfeldt, L. and Wahren, J. (1976). Influence of lactate infusion on glucose and free fatty acid metabolism in man. *Scand. J. Clin. Lab. Invest.*, **36,** 193
16. Boyd, A. E. III, Giauber, S. R., Mager, M. and Lesovitz, H. E. (1974). Lactate inhibition of lipolysis in exercising man. *Metabolism*, **23,** 531
17. Aguitor-Parada, E., Eisentraut, A. M. and Unger, R. H. (1969). Pancreatic glucagon secretion in normal and diabetic subjects. *Am. J. Med. Sci.*, **257,** 415
18. Passonneau, J. V. (1970). Lactate. In H. U. Gergmeyer (ed.). *Methoden der Enzymatichem Analyse*. (Weinheim, W. Germany: Verlag Chic)
19. Mellanlz, J. and Williamson, D. H. (1972). Beta-hydroxy butyrate. In H. U. Gergmeyer (ed.). *Methoden der Enzymatischem Analyse*. (Weinheim, W. Germany: Verlag Chic)
20. Dole, V. P. and Meinertz, M. (1960). Microdetermination of long chain fatty acids in plasma and tissues. *J. Biol. Chem.*, **235,** 2595
21. Griffiths, J. D. and Leung, F. Y. T. (1970). Fluorometric determination of plasma catecholamines—normal human epinephrine and nor-epinephrine values. *Clin. Chir. Acta*, **30,** 395
22. O'Donnell, T. F., Jr., Clowes, G. H. A. *et al.* (1974). Relationship of hind limb energy fuel metabolism to the circulatory responses in severe sepsis. *J. Surg. Res.*, **16,** 112
23. Clowes, G. H. A., Jr. (1971). *Septic Shock in Man*. S. G. Hershev, L. R. M. DelGuercie and R. McCann, (eds.). (Boston: Little Brown and Co.)

24. Wilmore, D. W., Long, J. M., Mason, A. D., Skreen, R. W. and Pruitt, B. A. (1974). Catecholamines: mediators of the hypermetabolic response to thermal injury. *Ann. Surg.*, **180,** 653
25. Wilmore, D. W., Long, J. M., Mason, A. D. and Pruitt, B. A. (1976). Stress in surgical patients as a neurophysiologic reflex response. *Surg. Gynecol. Obstet.*, **142,** 257
26. Marliss, E. B., Aoki, T. T., Toews, C. J., Felig, P., Cannon, J. J., Kyner, J., Huckabee, W. E. and Cahill, G. R. (1972). Amino acid metabolism in lactic acidosis. *Am. J. Med.*, **52,** 474
27. Blackburn, G. L., Flatt, J. P., Clowes, G. H. A., Jr., O'Donnell, T. F. and Hensle, T. E. (1973). Protein sparing therapy during periods of starvation with sepsis or trauma. *Ann. Surg.*, **177,** 588
28. Sherwin, R. S., Hendler, R. G. and Felig, P. (1975). Effect of ketone infusions on amino acid and nitrogen metabolism in man. *J. Clin. Invest.*, **55,** 1382
29. Greenberg, G. R., Marliss, E. B., Anderson, G. H., Langer, G., Spence, W., Tovee, E. B. and Jeejeebhoy, K. N. (1976). Protein sparing therapy in post-operative patients. *N. Engl. J. Med.*, **294,** 1411
30. Long, J. M. III, Wilmore, D. W., Mason, A. D., Jr. and Pruitt, B. A. (1977). Effect of, carbohydrate and fat intake on nitrogen excretion during total intravenous nutrition. *Ann. Surg.*, **185,** 417
31. Odessey, R., Khairallah, E. A. and Goldberg, A. L. (1974). Origin and possible significance of alanine production by skeletal muscle. *J. Biol. Chem.*, **249,** 7623
32. Close, J. H. (1974). The use of amino acid precursors in nitrogen accumulation diseases. *N. Engl. J. Med.*, **290,** 663

Discussion

N. Zöllner: (Germany) I should like to add a further observation in severely stressed patients, by showing some results.

Figure 1 shows what happens to essential fatty acids after a major operation in a patient with carcinoma of the stomach. We analysed his values before the operation and they were low, but still within the normal range. Within 3 days of the operation they went down to very

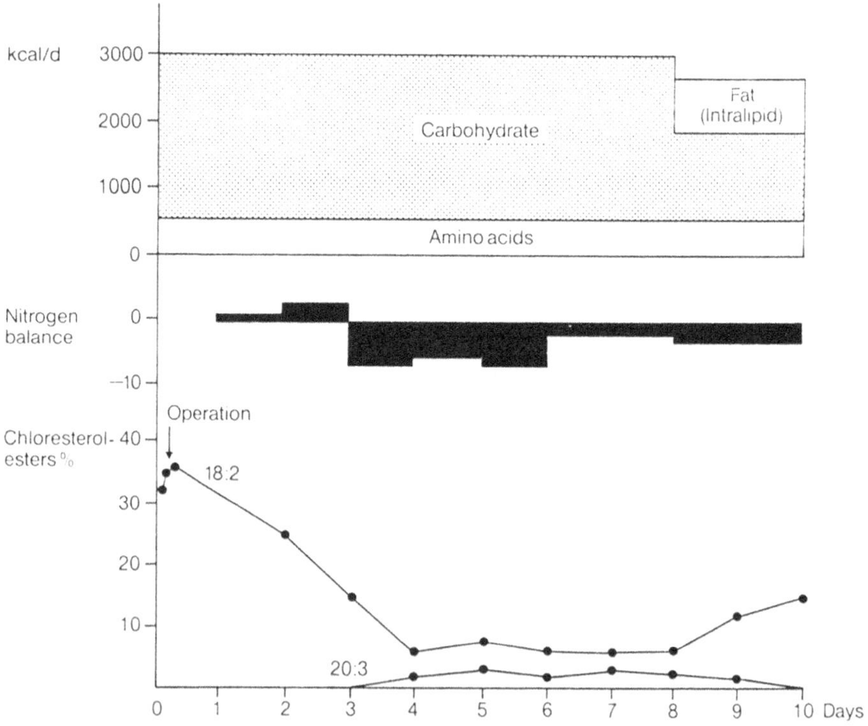

Figure 1 Cholesterol esters of 18:2 – and 20:3 – fatty acids following the operation of a carcinoma of the stomach in a 66-year-old male. Parental nutrition was administered as indicated and consisted of amino acids, carbohydrate and fat (Intralipid). Nitrogen balance was negative

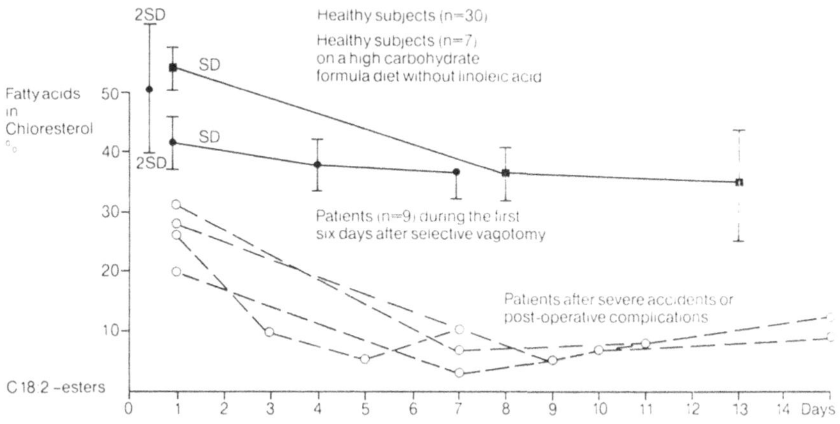

Figure 2 Linoleic acid in cholesterol esters of serum in healthy subjects after moderate surgery and during severe illness (Wolfram *et al.*, 1977)

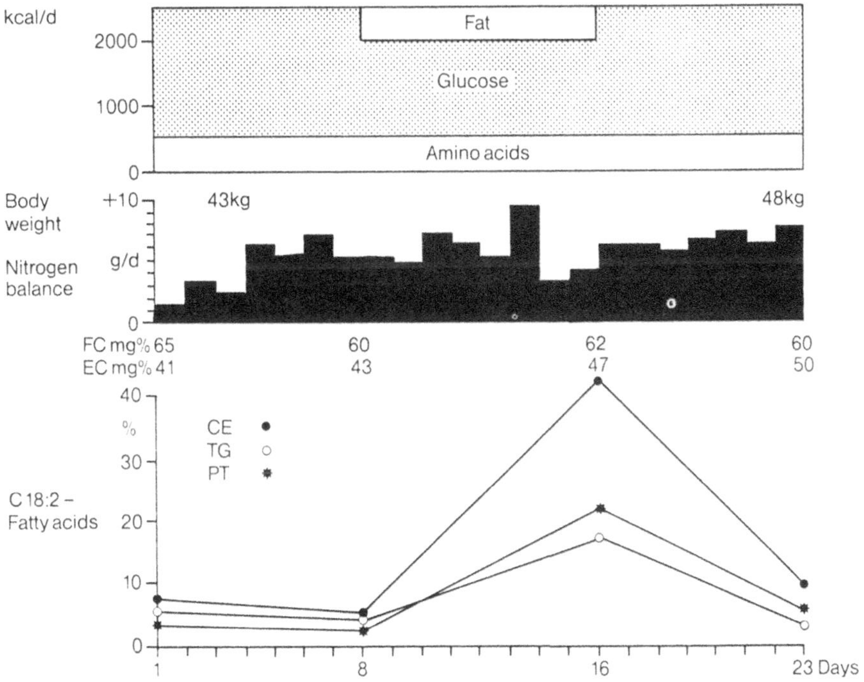

Figure 3 Influence of parental soy bean triglycerides (Infonutrol) on linoleic acid in cholesterol esters (CE), triglycerides (TG) and phospholipids (PT) after major surgery (pancreatectomy and splenectomy) in a 37-year-old male. FC is free cholesterol, EC esterified cholesterol

low levels, and at the same time three unsaturated fatty acids appeared, which are the signs of essential fatty acids deficiency. The amount of fat that had to be given to the patient to start correction was comparatively large.

Figure 2 shows that it certainly depends on the severity of the trauma. The upper line shows the level of linoleic acid in the serum of a normal person fed an iso-cabric diet without linoleic acid; then, after moderate surgery—selective vagotomy for ulcer. On the other hand, patients after severe accidents, or with severe post-operative septic complications, show dramatic falls in linoleic acid levels.

Figure 3 shows the amount of linoleic acid necessary to correct the deficiency which appears. The minimum amount needed is about 25 g, and in some cases it is up to 50 g, if the situation is to be corrected. This compares with the German Nutrition Society's recommended dietary allowance of 10 g/day.[2] The requirement is from 2½ to 5 times greater.

A. B. Jones: (Canada) We often use peripheral veins for intravenous feeding in babies, and they often get a little white plaque if extravasation occurs and stays for some time afterwards. However, we have seen nothing that looked like Mr. Tweedle's example of fat in the tissues.

We have had two episodes of candida septicaemia in seven years of parenteral feeding in peripheral veins and central veins in babies. In one of the candida septicaemias, the baby did get quite a marked problem with Intralipid, and became very hyperlipaemic.

D. W. Wilmore: (USA) I have one question about Dr. Holliday's conclusion that there is little ketone utilization in the limb. Does he want to leave us with the understanding that the muscle does not take up ketones, or that ketones are not produced, and consequently they are not available as a fuel from muscle?

R. L. Holliday: (Canada) I think that they are not produced and therefore are not available.

References

1. Wolfram, G., Zumtobel, V., and Zöllner N.; (1977). Anaesthesiology and Resuscitation. In A. Wretlind, R. Frey, K. Eyrich, H. Makowski (eds). *Fettemulsionen in der parenteralen Ernährung*, vol. 103, p. 81 (Berlin: Springer)
2. Deutsche Gesellschaft Für Ernahrung. (1975). (Frankfurt am Main: Umschau Verlag)

12
Role of lipid as a source of nonprotein calories

D. W. WILMORE

Lipids are organic chemicals which are relatively insoluble in water but may be extracted by nonpolar substances or 'fat solvents'. As a fuel, fats are densely packed with unoxidized carbon atoms and yield 9 calories/g of lipid; twice the quantity of heat produced by an equal dry weight of carbohydrate or protein. Because lipid is stored in the body in an intracellular yet extra-aqueous environment, 1 g of metabolized adipose tissue yields very close to the 9 calories obtained by combustion in a bomb calorimeter. In contrast, however, carbohydrate and protein are stored as hydrated fuels, which yield only 1 or 2 calories/g as water-soluble body tissue. Thus, fat is the critical lightweight high-energy fuel which is essential to mobile species carrying their endogenous energy supply.

Fat forms the largest source of available calories in the body, and lipid stores are related to age, sex, and weight of the individual. Fat accounts for approximately 15 kg of body weight in the average man, which represents about 135 000 calories of stored energy. In addition to providing a lightweight available body fuel, lipid serves as endogenous thermal underwear, insulating against cold ambient environments; stabilizes, supports, and protects vital structures; providing fat-soluble substances, such as vitamins essential to body metabolism; and contributes structural components to biologic membranes which partition and protect the intracellular or subcellular milieu from the surrounding environment.

The role of fat calories on energy balance

Nonprotein energy is utilized by the body for three general purposes: (1) mechanical work, (2) transport work, and (3) synthetic processes. The energy provided by the conversion of food to heat, work, or growth can be measured, and dietary energy provided in excess of these demands results in fuel storage. When the intake of food energy equals energy expenditure, a steady state is achieved (energy intake = energy expenditure), and body weight remains stable. When energy expenditure exceeds food intake, weight loss results. This relationship can be expressed as:

$$\text{Energy balance (kcal/day)} = \text{food intake (kcal/day)} - \text{energy expenditure (kcal/day)}$$

Positive energy balance is characteristic of weight gain, and negative energy balance predictive of weight loss.

Because fat is relatively anhydrous in its biologic storage state, each gram of fat yields only slightly less energy than when oxidized in a bomb calorimeter. This value is about 8 kcal/g. Thus, the positive or negative energy balance of approximately 8000 calories accounts for the gain or loss of approximately 1 kg body fat (3500 calories $\simeq$ 1 pound)[1,2]. While acute changes in body weight in critically ill patients usually reflect alterations in total body water, long term alterations in body weight reflect positive or negative energy balance. Kinney has emphasized that critically ill patients may gain up to 250 g of tissue per day, but, an increase of body weight in excess of this amount usually reflects positive fluid balance and not positive energy balance[3].

From the standpoint of bioenergetics, more body fat should be stored when administering diets rich in fat when compared with isocaloric diets high in carbohydrate or protein. This is because the heat generated with the ingestion or administration of fat, known as specific dynamic action, is much lower when compared with the other nutrients. Protein exerts the greatest increase in heat production following ingestion; if an individual is placed in a warm room, approximately 15% of the fed protein is dissipated as heat in the next 4 h following ingestion of the foodstuff. Studies in normals demonstrate that the specific dynamic effect of carbohydrate is approximately 6% of the ingested foodstuff, 2% for fat, 12% for protein rich foods, and only 6% for a mixed diet[4]. Thus, in theory, fat storage is more efficient with the administration of extra calories as fat, not protein or carbohydrate. However, in practice, the difference may be quite small. The increased heat production following food ingestion is minimal in patients with infectious disease[5], critically ill individuals, and obese females[6].

Using the energy balance equation, and measuring or estimating metabolic rate, alterations in body weight can be predicted while the patient receives specific dietary support. Thus, both fat-free and fat-containing diets have been administered to a variety of patients, including infants[7], severely burned patients[8,9], and patients with gastrointestinal dysfunction[10], and weight stabilization or weight gain has been observed regardless of the nonprotein calorie source utilized. Alterations in body weight can be accounted for in all subjects by the energy balance equation regardless of the infused energy source. If isocaloric, isonitrogenous diets are provided and the nonprotein caloric source varied, the observed alterations in body weight are comparable. The marked difference between the high fat and the high carbohydrate infusion is that the fat-containing parenteral diets can be administered by peripheral vein, while a comparable calorie load derived from glucose must be infused into a central vein because of the hypertonicity of the solution.

The role of fat calories in nitrogen balance

To evaluate the impact of nonprotein calories on nitrogen retention, nitrogen intake is held constant and nonprotein energy intake varied in a group of subjects with similar metabolic expenditure. Such data have been collected in young healthy men receiving oral diets[11]. If exogenous energy is administered to young healthy individuals without dietary nitrogen, urinary nitrogen excretion decreases (nitrogen balance becomes less negative). However, the negative nitrogen balance is maximally reduced by supplying only about 700 nonprotein calories; no further significant protein sparing is achieved by intakes as high as 2800 calories in the absence of protein.

When nitrogen is added to the diet, calories and nitrogen interact to

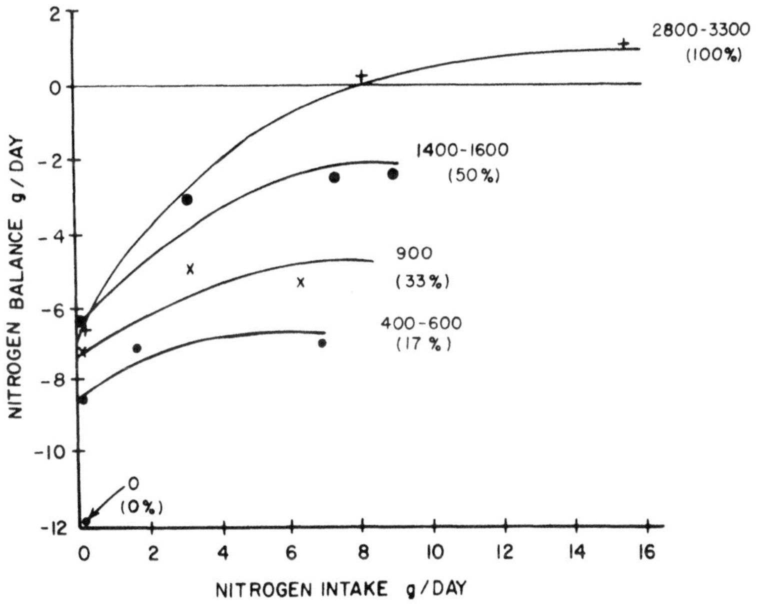

Figure 12.1 At any level of nitrogen intake, increasing calorie intake improves nitrogen balance, and at any level of calorie intake, increasing nitrogen intake improves balance. The range of calorie intake in these active young men is listed to the right of each isobar. The number in parentheses below each calorie intake expresses total calorie intake as a percentage of total daily metabolic expenditure. (Data collected by Calloway and Spector.)

improve balance (Figure 12.1). At any level of nitrogen intake, increasing the calorie intake moves balance toward the zero balance line. This interaction between nitrogen and energy intake resulted in the Calloway–Spector thesis that '. . . on a fixed adequate protein intake, energy level is the deciding factor in nitrogen balance and that with a fixed adequate calorie intake, protein level is the determinant.'

Exogenous nonprotein energy decreases nitrogen excretion when no protein intake is provided, and this effect is the result of administering a mixed energy source—both fat and carbohydrate. Several studies in man and animals have evaluated the impact of each caloric source individually when no dietary protein is given. These investigations demonstrate a prompt decrease in urinary nitrogen excretion with administration of carbohydrate[12]. As noted by Gamble, this response is curvilinear with maximum retention approached in normal man with administration of 100 g of carbohydrate[13]. Fat administration alone does not affect excretion of nitrogen in fasting man. Alterations in nitrogen excretion which occur with time have been attributed to adjustments in nitrogen loss secondary to starvation adaptation[14]. The effect of administering fat emulsion alone on protein loss is mimicked by infusing only the glycerol (carbohydrate) component of soybean oil emulsions[15].

When fat and carbohydrate calories are administered with dietary nitrogen to normal men or adult animals, they interact with the protein component of the diet to improve nitrogen retention. Excess or surfeit feeding studies of either carbohydrate or fat to normal men yield approximately comparable nitrogen retention when these extra calories are added to an adequate mixed diet[16]. Isocaloric exchange of fat and carbohydrate at lower levels of energy intake has been evaluated in studies utilizing a variety of experimental designs in a wide range of experimental species. Several apparent conclusions emerge from this information. When carbohydrate is removed from the diet, there is a period of several days when increased urinary nitrogen loss occurs, followed by a readjustment in urinary nitrogen excretion to near pre-exchange levels[17]. This transient rise in nitrogen excretion accounts for the results of many short-term studies which find less protein sparing efficiency with fat when compared to carbohydrate. If long-term study periods are allowed, adequate transition time is provided between dietary exchanges, and isocaloric switch-back studies made using diets adequate in protein and energy content, the impact of fat and carbohydrate on nitrogen balance in normal adults appears equal[18].

Few studies in normals or stable patients are available to assess the dose response to protein and energy intake during parenteral administration of nutrients. However, data are emerging to confirm the comparability of fat and carbohydrate as a caloric source in the stable patient in resting starvation. If patients without a hypermetabolic disease process are analysed with the scanty data from studies in normals, a relationship emerges which is similar to that observed during the oral feeding studies (Figure 12.2). Patients with severe weight loss can store nitrogen and increase nitrogen balance in a linear manner above the zero balance line as energy and nitrogen are increased in the parenteral diet. This dose response relationship in depleted patients and the single nutrient parenteral infusion studies in normals suggest that the interaction between energy and nitrogen and the impact of non-protein energy administered on nitrogen balance are quite similar when intravenous infusions are compared to continuously administered enteral feedings.

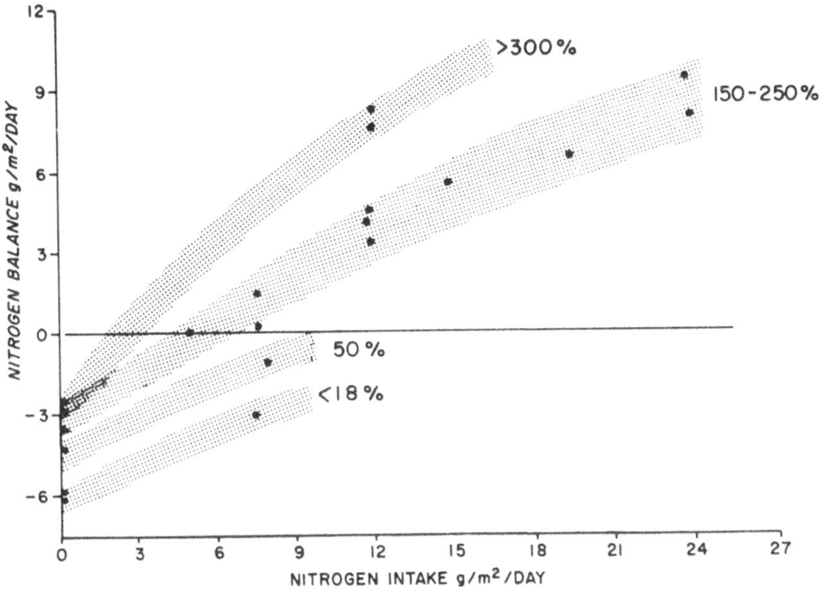

Figure 12.2 The effect of intravenous amino acid and calorie intake appears similar to oral dietary intake in normals and nonstressed patients (compare with Figure 12.1). Each stippled bar includes data points from subjects receiving comparable total calorie intakes by the intravenous route as related to the metabolic rate of the individual. The number to the right of each stippled bar is the total calorie intake as related to the metabolic rate of the individual expressed as a percentage (100% would provide all energy requirements and maintain body weight)

Moreover, there is little question that a similar response occurs in normals or depleted starved patients receiving amino acids when comparing intravenous fat with carbohydrate as an energy source. For example, Wolf and associates compared a near isotonic diet containing fat emulsion with isocaloric–isonitrogenous infusion of hypertonic glucose and amino acids (approximately 6 g nitrogen/m^2/day) administered to normal subjects[19]. Nitrogen equilibrium was maintained in each study group over the 8-day period, and no significant difference in nitrogen balance was found when comparing the two calorie sources. Jeejeebhoy *et al.* compared the two different calorie sources in the same patient, evaluating each diet during a 1-week study period and then switching to the other diet[10]. The patients studied were markedly depleted because of severe gastrointestinal disease. No difference in nitrogen balance was observed when comparing the lipid-rich intravenous diet with the isocaloric carbohydrate infusion, both calorie sources administered with the same dose of amino acid nitrogen. These studies evaluated fat and carbohydrate calories in normals and depleted patients. Nitrogen equilibrium or positive nitrogen balance was associated with the quantity of nitrogen and energy administered, regardless of the energy source[19]. In both studies, nitrogen balance was not dependent upon the hormonal milieu (I/G ratio) or substrate profile (appearance of ketone bodies, serum fatty acid levels, blood glucose concentrations). These hormonal and substrate variables were altered depending upon the type of fuel administered and did not appear to be set or fixed in regulating metabolism, as occurs in association with hypercatabolic disease processes.

In contrast to these studies, there are variations on the general theme which suggest that fat and carbohydrate calories are not always comparable. A specific nitrogen sparing action of carbohydrate on protein metabolism does appear in some studies of subjects given sub-maximal diets[16]. This impact of carbohydrate addition on nitrogen sparing in subjects receiving inadequate dietary intake is much more pronounced than the effects of isocaloric quantities of fat. Moreover, several studies on human subjects receiving approximately 20 g protein per day show increases in nitrogen excretion when fat is replaced by carbohydrate.

The impact of carbohydrate on nitrogen retention during hypermetabolic disease processes appears to be greater than the effect of equal caloric quantities of fat. Studies of oral diets in patients with typhoid fever demonstrated that nitrogen balance could be improved by increasing the quantity of dietary protein and carbohydrate, but not fat[20]. These investigators suggested that greater efficiency in nitrogen retention could be achieved by supplementing high quantities of dietary carbohydrate, which exerted a specific effect on the sparing of body protein.

In long-term oral dietary studies in hypermetabolic thermally injured patients, various proportions of fat and carbohydrate energy were administered at constant doses for 7–14 days while nitrogen intake was fixed for all subjects at 15 $g/m^2/day$[21]. The impact of the nonprotein calorie source demonstrated a good correlation between carbohydrate intake as related to metabolic expenditure of the patients. Nitrogen retention was achieved when dietary carbohydrate plus nitrogen calories approximately equalled daily total metabolic expenditure. At no time in these studies could dietary fat intake be related to the nitrogen balance.

To evaluate the impact of fat and carbohydrate calories in the parenteral diets of severely burned patients, a constant dose of nitrogen was infused (11.7 $g/nitrogen/m^2/day$) to six critically-ill patients, and the effect of varying doses of two nonprotein caloric sources on nitrogen excretion assessed[22]. Nitrogen excretion decreased steadily as carbohydrate intake increased. Administration of fat emulsions over the broad range of doses utilized (0–1108 kcal/m^2/day) exerted minimal influences on the excretion of urinary nitrogen. In a second study, McDougal and associates evaluated the impact of near-isotonic diets containing amino acid, glucose, and fat emulsions administered by peripheral vein to thermally injured patients[23]. Nitrogen balance improved in a dose-related manner with the administration of amino acids and glucose. One to two units of fat emulsion infused per day exerted an effect indistinguishable from 60 g of glucose, and this nitrogen sparing effect could be accounted for by the free glycerol content of the fat emulsion, which exerts metabolic effects similar to that of carbohydrate. No alteration in nitrogen balance was observed with time (up to 2 weeks), demonstrating that adaptation to the fat emulsion did not occur.

In all of the studies cited comparing the effects of fat and carbohydrate on nitrogen balance in critically ill patients, carbohydrate intake exerted a dominant effect on nitrogen balance. Similar results in the framework of varying experimental design have been reported by Halmagyi[24], Heller[25], Beisbarth[26], and Allison[27]. The carbohydrate effect appears to be mediated through the insulin mechanism: additional nitrogen sparing may be achieved by the administration of exogenous insulin with high carbohydrate diets.

Added information, describing the post-traumatic metabolic abnormalities which are associated with inflammatory disease processes, allow formulation of a general hypothesis about the body's response to injury and infection and the specific impact of carbohydrate calories on nitrogen balance during hypermetabolic disease processes. First, it has recently been demonstrated that infected animals[28] and critically ill patients[29] do not or cannot initiate the keto-adaptive mechanisms which are essential to minimize protein loss following starvation. Although restricting dietary carbohydrate results in a marked decrease in insulin, ketone production is far below levels observed in fasting man. Second, it has been noted that inflammatory tissue—fibroblasts, macrophages, epithelial cells, and neutrophils—are glycolytic, and demonstrate a major capacity for anaerobic metabolism. Studies in our laboratory over the past year have determined substrate flux across injured and uninjured extremities of severely burned patients. These investigations demonstrate that the peripheral utilization of the large quantity of glucose produced by the liver is confined principally to the wound[30]. Net glucose flux across uninjured extremities is low, suggesting that fat, not glucose, is the primary fuel for skeletal muscle, a finding similar to that observed in normal man (Table 12.1). While the quantity of oxygen utilized by the extensively injured extremity is sufficient to account for oxidation of the quantity of glucose in the burned extremity, a large quantity of lactate is produced in the traumatized leg. Calculated on a weight basis, the lactate produced accounts for a major portion of the glucose consumed by the extensively injured limb. The data suggest that little or no oxygen is utilized for glucose metabolism in the extensively injured limbs. The oxygen consumed must be utilized to oxidize fat, which occurs primarily in skeletal muscle.

Table 12.1 Substrate utilization in patients with small and large leg burns (Mean and range of SEM)

	Small leg burns	*Large leg burns*
Patient characteristics		
Number of subjects	8	7
Number of studies	9	7
Age (years)	28 (17–50)	27 (18–50)
Weight (kg)	73.2 (57.5–89.4)	70.1 (58.6–83.7)
Body surface area (m^2)	1.89 (1.63–2.10)	1.88 (1.70–2.07)
Percentage total body surface burn	40.5 (12–57.5)	42 (12–61.5)
Percentage total leg burn	9.5 (0–17.5)	58.0 (37.5–82.5)
Postburn day studied	12 (8–19)	14 (7–22)
Systemic responses		
Cardiac index (L/m^2 min)	7.82 ± 0.70	7.46 ± 0.81
Oxygen consumption (ml/m^2 min)	204 ± 12	241 ± 22
Rectal temperature (°C)	38.5 ± 0.3	38.3 ± 0.3
Mean skin temperature (°C)	36.1 ± 0.2	36.1 ± 0.2
Peripheral responses		
Mean leg skin temperature (°C)	35.2 ± 0.3	35.5 ± 0.3
Leg blood flow (ml/100 ml leg min)	4.22 ± 0.43	8.02 ± 0.51***
Leg oxygen consumption (ml/100 ml leg min)	0.187 ± 0.037	0.240 ± 0.010
Leg glucose uptake (mg/100 ml leg min)	0.037 ± 0.033	0.336 ± 0.077**
Leg lactate release (mg/100 ml leg min)	0.060 ± 0.055	0.299 ± 0.075*

* $P < 0.05$; ** $P < 0.01$; *** $P < 0.001$

Glucose serves as the primary fuel for granulation tissue and is not utilized by the uninjured limb. The glucose which is converted to lactate in the wound is recycled by the liver to new glucose; what glucose is oxidized is replaced by amino acids, which arise from skeletal muscle, and are transported to the liver to serve as additional gluconeogenic precursors (Figure 12.3). The energy required to support hepatic gluconeogenesis is derived from fat. Provision of exogenous fat to hypermetabolic patients stabilizes body fat mass, and serves as an exogenous fuel for this system, but does not exert a major impact on nitrogen balance. In contrast, exogenous glucose stimulates insulin which signals skeletal muscle to reduce proteolysis, thus diminishing nitrogen excretion.

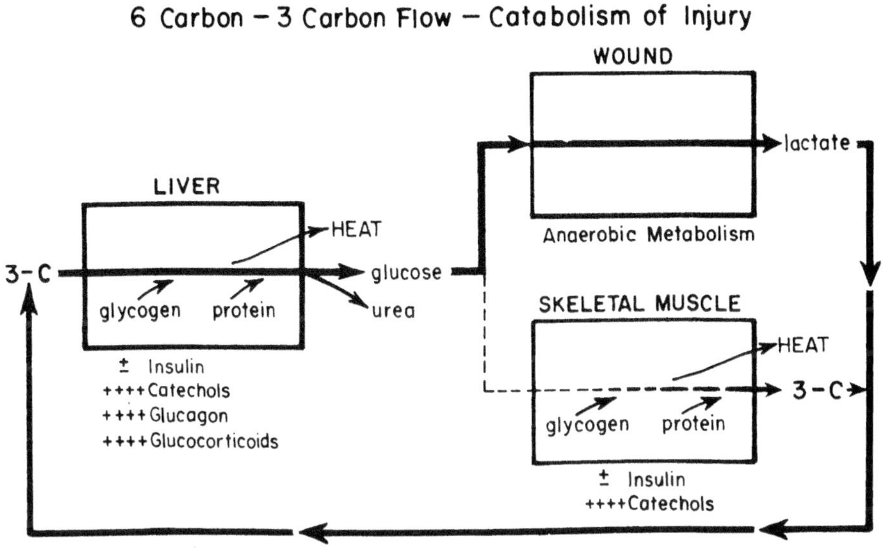

Figure 12.3 Increased gluconeogenesis occurs following major injury and infection. The glucose is converted to three-carbon intermediates and recycled to the liver for reconversion to new glucose. In noninfected burn patients, the major portion of peripheral glucose metabolism occurs by anaerobic mechanisms in the wound, producing lactate. The glucose which is oxidized is replaced by gluconeogenic amino acids which arise from the skeletal muscle

The role of fat in essential fatty acid deficiency

While the major portion of fat stores may arise from *de novo* synthesis, an essential quantity of polyunsaturated fat cannot be synthesized in the body but is necessary for optimal body nutrition. When fat is excluded from the diet, carbohydrate may be readily converted to fatty acids and stored as triglyceride. In 1927, Evans and Burr revealed that exclusion of fat from the diet of rats prevented satisfactory growth and development[31]. Subsequent studies demonstrated that fat-free diets in animals resulted in scaling of the skin, loss of hair, emaciation, impaired reproductive capacity, increased intake of food and water, increased metabolic rate, and early death. These symptoms could be reversed by providing a small amount of fat in the diet, and it was later determined that linoleic acid was the essential fatty acid dietary component.

Many early studies in human beings attempted to establish a relationship between low-fat or fat-free diets, and most of these observations were in newborn infants receiving feeding formulas. These observations suggested that diets low in fat deleteriously affected growth, increased susceptibility to infection, and were associated with the appearance of skin eruptions. However, it was generally believed that human beings could subsist on a fat-free diet with no deleterious effects.

Hansen and co-workers fed healthy infants five proprietary milk mixtures, adequate in protein, minerals, and vitamins but with varying fat and linoleic acid content[32]. Two diets were found inadequate in linoleic acid, and a high proportion of babies fed these mixtures developed dry, thickened, desquamated skin. The skin lesions rapidly disappeared with the addition of linoleic acid to the formula. In 1971, Collins and his associates described essential fatty acid deficiency in an adult male who had undergone massive intestinal resection and was maintained solely by fat-free intravenous nutrition therapy for 100 days[33]. This patient developed a skin rash in association with biochemical features of polyunsaturated fatty acid deficiency. The signs of the deficiency were reversed with the intravenous administration of a soybean emulsion containing linoleic acid. These and other studies[34] suggest that linoleic acid should constitute approximately 4% of the calories of the diet to prevent the development of the deficiency state. The biochemical characteristics of essential fatty acid deficiency may occur after as little as 3 weeks in infants who receive fat-free parenteral nutrition[35]. However, the clinical features of the deficiency state, particularly the skin rash, are rarely seen until after several months or more of a fat-deficient diet. Thrombocytopenia, increased haemolysis[36], and impaired wound healing are associated clinical features which occur with the skin lesions.

Deficiencies of polyunsaturated fatty acid may occur in patients with major injury who receive inadequate fat in their diets[9]. Examination of the red cell membrane in five critically ill burn patients demonstrated an essential fatty acid deficiency with marked decrease in linoleic, arachidonic, and decosahexanoic acids, all members of the polyunsaturated fatty acid series which cannot be synthesized *de novo*. All patients studied had extensive burns, and most had received fat-free parenteral diets for a prolonged period before the essential fatty acid deficiency occurred. Delay in wound healing occurred in one patient and haemolytic anaemia requiring massive blood transfusion was present in a second. The deficiency, which appeared to be related both to the stress of thermal injury and to nutritional inadequacies, could be corrected by intravenous administration of soybean emulsion containing polyunsaturated fat or administration of tube feedings containing essential fatty acids.

The biochemical manifestations of essential fatty acid deficiency are accentuated by increased metabolic demands, associated with growth in children or hypermetabolism following injury or infection in adults. The chemical findings are characterized by abnormally low levels of essential polyunsaturated fats in the serum or red cell membrane, associated with a compensatory increase of saturated fatty acids. These alterations may be expressed as an absolute level or a ratio of the triene and tetra-enoic fatty acids present. The ratio rises during the deficiency state, and may be used as a guide to follow the response to polyunsaturated fatty acid replacement therapy. In addition, one fatty acid (5,8,11-eicosatrienoic acid) is virtually absent from normal tissue, but appears during essential fatty acid deficiency. Its presence in serum or red cell membrane is diagnostic of the polyunsaturated fatty acid deficiency state.

Most hospital diets, tube feedings, and chemically defined or synthetic formulae contain an adequate quantity of polyunsaturated fat for stable resting man. Deficiency can be prevented by supplying approximately 4% of the caloric requirements as polyunsaturated fat. This quantity of fat can be included in the diet in patients receiving long-term parenteral nutrition by administering an intravenous fat emulsion rich in polyunsaturated fatty acids, such as soybean emulsion, or by providing small amounts of polyunsaturated fat (safflower oil) daily by the enteric route. This may be accomplished in patients with gastrointestinal dysfunction by instilling the oil twice a day through a nasogastric tube and clamping the tube for 1 h or by infusing the material through a small, soft, feeding catheter placed in a fistulous tract into distal small bowel. Provision of this essential nutritional requirement is especially important in newborn infants, depleted–starved patients, and hypercatabolic injured or septic adults in whom biochemical abnormalities have been identified.

References

1. Bortz, W. M. (1968). Predictability of weight loss. *J. Am. Med. Assoc.*, **204,** 101
2. Antonetti, V. M. (1973). The equations governing weight change in human beings. *Am. J. Clin. Nutr.*, **26,** 64
3. Kinney, J. M., Long, C. L., Gump, F. E. and Duke, J. H., Jr. (1968). Tissue composition of weight loss in surgical patients. *Ann. Surg.*, **168,** 459
4. Benedict, F. G. and Carpenter, T. M. (1918). Food ingestion and energy transformations with special reference to the stimulating effects of nutrients. Carnegie Institute of Washington, Publication No. **361,** p. 355
5. Coleman, W. and DuBois, E. F. (1915). Calorimetric observations on the metabolism of typhoid patients with and without food. *Arch. Int. Med.*, **15,** 887
6. Bradfield, R. B. and Jourdan, M. H. (1973). Relative importance of specific dynamic action in weight-reduction diets. *Lancet*, **ii,** 640
7. Heird, W. C., MacMillan, R. W. and Winters, R. W. (1976). Total parenteral nutrition in the pediatric patient. In J. E. Fisher (ed.). *Total Parenteral Nutrition*, pp. 253–284. (Boston: Little, Brown & Co.)
8. Wilmore, D. W., Currcri, P. W., Spitzer, K. W., Spitzer, M. E. and Pruitt, B. A., Jr. (1971). Supranormal diet in thermally injured patients. *Surg. Gynecol. Obstet.*, **132,** 881
9. Wilmore, D. W., Moylan, J. A., Jr., Helmkamp, G. M., Jr. and Pruitt, B. A., Jr. (1973). Clinical use of a 10% intravenous fat emulsion in thermally injured patients. *Ann. Surg.*, **178,** 503
10. Jeejeebhoy, K. N., Marliss, E. B., Anderson, G. H., Greenberg, G. R., Kuksis, A. and Breckenridge, C. (1975). Lipid in parenteral nutrition: Studies of clinical and metabolic features. In H. C. Meng and D. W. Wilmore (eds.). *Fat Emulsions in Parenteral Nutrition*, pp. 35–54. (Chicago: American Medical Association)
11. Calloway, D. H. and Spector, H. (1954). Nitrogen balance as related to calorie and protein intake in active young men. *Am. J. Clin. Nutr.*, **2,** 405
12. O'Connell, R. C., Morgan, A. P., Aoki, T. T., Ball, M. R. and Moore, F. D. (1974). Nitrogen conservation in starvation: Graded responses to intravenous glucose. *J. Clin. Endocrinol. Metab.*, **39,** 555
13. Gamble, J. L. (1947). *Chemical Anatomy, Physiology and Pathology of Extracellular Fluid: A Lecture Syllabus*. 5th ed. (Cambridge, Mass: Harvard University Press)

14. Cathcart, E. P. (1909). The influence of carbohydrates and fats on protein metabolism. *J. Physiol. (Lond.)*, **39,** 311
15. Brennan, M. F., Fitzpatrick, G. F., Cohen, K. H. and Moore, F. D. (1975). Glycerol: major contributor to the short term protein sparing effect of fat emulsions in normal man. *Ann. Surg.*, **182,** 386
16. Munro, H. N. (1964). General aspects of the regulation of protein metabolism by diet and hormones. In H. N. Munro and J. B. Allison (eds.). *Mammalian Protein Metabolism* pp. 382–468. (New York: Academic Press)
17. Silweb, H. (1937). Studien uber Die N-Ausscheidung im Harn bei Einschrankung des Kohlehydratgehaltes der Nahrung ohne wesentliche Veranderung des Energiengehaltes derselben. *Acta Med. Scand.*, 79–81 (Suppl.), 1
18. Munro, H. N. (1951). Carbohydrate and fat as factors in protein utilization and metabolism. *Physiol. Rev.*, **31,** 449
19. Wolf, B. M., Culebras, J. M., Sim, A. J. W., Ball, M. R. and Moore, F. D. (1977). Substrate interaction in intravenous feeding. *Ann. Surg.* (In press)
20. Shaffer, P. A. and Coleman, W. (1909). Protein metabolism in typhoid fever. *Arch. Int. Med.*, **4,** 538
21. Wilmore, D. W. (1977). Energy requirements for maximum nitrogen retention. In *Proceedings of the Amino Acid Symposium*, (Chicago: American Medical Association) (In press)
22. Long, J. M., Wilmore, D. W., Mason, A. D., Jr. and Pruitt, B. A., Jr. (1977). Effect of carbohydrate and fat intake on nitrogen excretion during total intravenous feeding. *Ann. Surg.*, **185,** 417
23. McDougal, W. S., Wilmore, D. W. and Pruitt, B. A., Jr. (1977). Effect of near-isosmotic intravenous nutrient infusions on nitrogen balance in critically ill injured patients. *Surg. Gynecol. Obstet.*, **145,** 408
24. Halmagyi, M. (1974). Well-balanced replacement therapy by infusion of electrolytes, amino acids and energy carriers in severely ill traumatized patients. *Infusionstheropie*, **1,** 473
25. Heller, L. (1972). The effect of fat in complete parenteral nutrition on the nitrogen balance. Presented at the *Ninth International Congress of Nutrition*, September, Mexico City.
26. Beisbarth, H. (1976). Influence of stress on intravenous fat requirements. In H. C. Meng and D. W. Wilmore (eds.). *Fat Emulsions in Parenteral Nutrition*, pp. 79–81. (Chicago: American Medical Association)
27. Allison, S. P. (1975). Modifying nitrogen loss after injury. Presented at the *Conference on the Current Aspects of the Metabolic Response to Injury Including Nutritional Implications*, Glasgow, Scotland
28. Neufeld, H. A., Pace, J. and White, L. (1976). The effect of bacterial infections on ketone concentrations in rat liver and blood and on free fatty acid concentrations in rat blood. *Metabolism*, **25,** 887
29. Border, J. R., Chemier, R., McMenamy, R. H., LaDuca, J., Seibel, R. W., Birkhahn, R. and Yu, L. (1976). Multiple systems organ failure: Muscle fuel deficit with visceral protein malnutrition. In E. H. Clowes (ed.). *The Surgical Clinics of North America*, **56,** 1147
30. Wilmore, D. W., Aulick, L. H., Mason, A. D., Jr. and Pruitt, B. A., Jr. (1977). Influence of the burn wound on local and systemic responses to injury. *Ann. Surg.* (In press)
31. Evans, H. M. and Burr, G. O. (1927). New dietary deficiency with highly purified diets. *Proc. Soc. Exp. Biol. Med.*, **24,** 740
32. Hansen, A. E., Stewart, H. A., Hughes, C. and Soderhjelm, L. (1962). The relation of linoleic acid to infant feeding. *Acta Pediat.*, **51,** 31; *Acta Pediat.*, **51** (Suppl.), 137
33. Collins, F. D., Sinclair, A. J., Boyle, J. P., Coats, D. A., Maynard, A. T. and Leonard, R. F. (1971). Plasma lipids in human linoleic acid deficiency. *Nutr. Metab.*, **13,** 150
34. Holman, R. T. (1976). Function and biological activities of essential fatty acids in man. In H. C. Meng and D. W. Wilmore (eds.). *Fat Emulsion in Parenteral Nutrition*, pp. 5–14. (Chicago: American Medical Association)

35. Caldwell, M. D. (1976). Human essential fatty acid deficiency: A review. In H. C. Meng and D. W. Wilmore (eds.). *Fat Emulsion in Parenteral Nutrition*, pp. 14–18. (Chicago: American Medical Association)
36. Terry, B. E. and Wixon, R. L. (1976). Hemolytic anemia associated with essential fatty acid deficiency in a normal man on long-term total parenteral nutrition. In H. C. Meng and D. W. Wilmore (eds.). *Fat Emulsion in Parenteral Nutrition*, pp. 18–21. (Chicago: American Medical Association)

Discussion

P. Vinay: (Canada) The level of ketone bodies in plasma is not only a function of ketone body production, but also of removal of ketone bodies. When we speak of the absence of ketosis in the hypermetabolic state, as in burn patients, is that because of lack of production? Or is it because of increased utilization of ketone bodies?

D. W. Wilmore: (USA) We have only looked at concentration levels, and they are quite low. Turnover has been done (by Dr John Border[1]) by looking at ketone body production across the liver and a production rate has been measured. Those data were in the *Surgical Clinics of North America*, autumn 1976. It was done in patients with infection following severe injury, and those patients did not produce ketones at satisfactory rates.

Vinay: Were the studies done when the patient was already catabolic and had no more fat with which to produce ketones?

Wilmore: These patients were not depleted of their fat mass. The studies were done early in the catabolic course.

Neufold[2], working in animals, has used labelled ketone in infected animals and has not seen rates of ketogenesis comparable to simple starvation (*Metabolism*, December 1976).

H. F. Woods: (UK) Looking at the metabolic balance on the small leg burn, and the glucose uptake and lactate production, there would seem to be the expected 2:1 ratio. This is roughly accounting for all the glucose utilization in terms of lactate production. That does not seem to be the case for the large leg burn. Could Dr Wilmore suggest where that extra glucose is going?

Wilmore: If granulation tissue is put into a Warburg flask and its rate of metabolism measured using labelled glucose, some of that glucose is oxidized, but there is a high rate of lactate production. About half or two-thirds of the glucose can be accounted for within the range of errors of these studies. There is no contention that all of the glucose in inflammatory tissue has to go to anaerobic metabolism, but many studies of inflammatory and granulation tissue point out that a good deal of the glucose does go there.

Woods: If all the glucose utilized could be converted to lactate, there would be no increased need for the breakdown of amino acids. It is fascinating that there is a situation where as soon as tissue damage is increased not all the glucose utilization can be accounted for.

Glucose is obviously not going straight down the glycolytic pathway and must be channelled off elsewhere.

J. M. Kinney: (USA) Are there any further thoughts about the correlation between the increased heat production and the increase in the so-called glucose turnover or flow?

If I understand correctly, there is an increased metabolism, presumably oxidizing free fatty acids, taking place in many sites throughout the body, in the injured and the non-injured part. Is that true?

DISCUSSION

Wilmore: That is our interpretation; skeletal muscle is oxidizing free fatty acid and the liver is oxidizing free fatty acid. The energy derived from free fatty acid oxidation is the energy used for this conversion process.

Kinney: Then would these chemical reactions account for the increase in the resting energy expenditure?

Wilmore: Not for all of it. But they account for a major portion of it. If gluconeogenesis is blocked in these patients, with the infusion of ethanol, the hypermetabolic response can be reduced significantly, but some still remains. There are of course synthetic processes which are heat producing and heat requiring, and a good deal of mechanical work is going on.

References

1. Border, J. R., Chemier, R., McMewamy, R. H., LaDuca, J., Seibel, R. W., Birkhahn, R., and Yu, L. (1976). Multiple systems organ failure: Muscle fuel deficit with visceral protein malnutrition. *Surg. Clin. North Amer.*, **56,** 1147
2. Neufeld, H. A., Pace, J. and White, L. (1976). The effects of bacterial infections on ketone concentrations in rat liver and blood and on free fatty acid concentrations in rat blood. *Metabolism*, **25,** 887

13
Effect of long-term administration of fat emulsion on lipid deposition in the reticuloendothelial system in man

U. FREUND, A. L. DURST, Y. KRAUSZ, I. S. LEVIJ AND M. ELIAKIM

The use of fat emulsions for parenteral nutrition started more than 30 years ago. They are now available for use in total parenteral nutrition (TPN), and they meet the need for a high calorie intravenous solution in a relatively small volume. Fat emulsions have no effect on the osmolar balance of the body fluids, since the solutions are essentially iso-osmolar and the oxidation of fatty acids does not exert an osmolar load.

The early use of fat emulsions was followed by adverse effects including changes in blood pressure, respiration and heart rate, and pyrexia. The major problem was the 'fat overloading syndrome' or the so-called 'long-term reaction'. It was characterized by fever, anorexia, vague abdominal discomfort, bleeding phenomena, anaemia, jaundice and hepatosplenomegaly. The syndrome occurred in patients who received multiple infusions of fat emulsions. Little is still known about the cause of this syndrome. Clinical studies indicated a combination of coagulation defects, liver dysfunction, anaemia, lipaemia and tissue lipidosis.

The modern fat emulsions differ in their toxicity, bloodstream elimination rate, uptake by reticuloendothelial system (RES) and effect on endotoxin resistance[1]. Since their introduction the previously mentioned complications have been losing their clinical significance. The egg-yolk phospholipid soyabean oil emulsion (Intralipid) seems to have a low toxicity and its clearance from plasma resembles chylomicrons[2].

Chronic toxicity tests of Intralipid in dogs showed no significant liver damage and only minimal 'intravenous fat pigment' deposited in the reticuendothelial cells of the liver, spleen and bone marrow[3]. However, autopsy findings in dogs given 6 g fat/kg/day as Intralipid during 10 weeks showed 'intravenous fat pigment' in the liver, lung and spleen and a proliferation of reticuloendothelial cells containing lipids were found in the liver[4]. In addition to 'intravenous fat pigment', micrograrulomas composed of small aggregated lipid-laden epithelial cells were found within the hepatic parenchyma[5]. Electron microscopy showed intravenous fat pigment deposited in the lysosomes, mitochondrial swelling, central core formation and dilatation of profiles of rough endoplasmic reticulum with dislocation of ribosomes[6]. In the same study there were no changes in liver function tests despite the presence of those histopathological changes. This makes the value of liver function tests questionable for detecting minute structural changes.

The accumulation of fat from fat emulsions in the cells of the RES occurs both in man and experimental animals. Various fat emulsions differ in the extent of accumulation observed[7]. Fat particles of Intralipid were taken up by the RES much less than fat particles from Lipofundin (soya bean phosphatide–cottonseed-oil emulsion). Lemperle showed that this was due to reticuloendothelial cell phagocytosis[8]. It was also shown that when the RES is blocked by fat, antibody production is reduced significantly. The phagocytic capability of many individual cells was impaired. However, uptake studies with radioactive colloidal gold were not affected[6]. The endotoxin clearance rate and RES organ uptake in rabbits were not reduced after Intralipid administration despite the deposition of 'intravenous fat pigment' in reticuloendothelial cells[9].

The endothelial cells of the lung vessels in man can also take up fat particles following an infusion of soya bean oil emulsion[10]. Greene[11] showed a significant decrease in pulmonary membrane diffusion following administration of Intralipid. Electron microscopic findings showed that in the liver the lipid is transported into the spaces of Disse and taken up by the Kupffer cells. In the lungs a large amount of the lipid was localized at the periphery of the vessel. Greene speculated that lipid particles surrounding the red cells in the lung capillary interfere with gas exchange mechanism. Meng *et al.*[12] studied the long-term effect of intravenous administration of Intralipid (6 g/kg) in rats and demonstrated the accumulation of reticuloendothelial cells with foamy cytoplasm in the liver. It was also shown[5] that a significant percentage of the intravenously infused lipid is taken up by the reticuloendothelial cells, the amount depending on the type of emulsion.

The clinical experience accummulated thus far with Intralipid is satisfactory and major complications have been rare. However, the experimental data have shown that the RES plays a significant role in the clearance of fat emulsions. It is possible that the harmful side-effects of the first generation fat emulsions were related, at least in part, to their uptake by the RES. It was suggested therefore that only those fat emulsions which, like the natural chylomicrons, are not taken up by the RES, should be used[7].

A patient was observed recently at our institution, where massive fat involvement of the RES was documented at autopsy. A study of this case gives some insight into the risks which may accompany the use of even the modern fat emulsions.

The patient died during prolonged TPN in which Intralipid was the main caloric source. It was found at autopsy that the patient had developed a hitherto undescribed complication which could be described as 'iatrogenic lipidosis'[13]. We believe that a detailed description of the findings in this case may improve the understanding of some undesirable long-term effects of intravenous fat emulsions.

A 44-year-old male had an operation for a leiomyoma of the lower esophagus. He weighed 60 kg before surgery. The post-operative course was uneventful. Three months later he developed postprandial epigastric pain, anorexia, aversion to food and vomiting. He lost 15 kg during a period of 9 months. The finding of stones in the gall bladder justified a reoperation when a detailed exploration of the abdominal cavity was carried out. After cholecystectomy and otherwise negative exploration the previous complaints persisted and the patient's weight fell further to 39 kg. The patient had extensive laboratory investigations and the main findings were that the liver function tests (including lipase and serum cholesterol) were normal, the blood serum was not lipaemic and the serum proteins were normal.

It was thought that his complaints were due to depression and anxiety related to the first operation. The patient did not tolerate nasogastric feeding and a trial of medical therapy combined with psychiatric support failed entirely. Two months after the second operation TPN was instituted. At this stage the patient weighed 37 kg. The TPN regimen consisted of 500 ml 20% Intralipid, 1000–2500 ml Amigen (5 g dextrose and 5 g hydrolysate, USP casein/100 ml) and 450 ml glucose 50% fluids; vitamins and trace elements were added as required.

During the first 70 days the patient gained 10 kg in weight. He was transferred to the Department of Psychiatry on the 60th day, where the intravenous caloric intake was reduced gradually and stopped after 10 days. It was hoped that the patient would be able to take food by mouth. However, the patient refused to eat and lost all the weight he had gained during the TPN period. Intravenous feeding was reinstituted on the 105th day. The liver was noted to be enlarged, the SGOT was 460 mu/ml (normal 50), and the alkaline phosphatase was 300 mu/ml (normal = 85) and the prothrombin time fell to 34% of the normal. Following reinstitution of TPN the patient's condition improved and the liver function tests returned to normal. On the 124th day the patient developed sepsis and died in shock on the same day.

At autopsy there was no mechanical obstruction or narrowing throughout the gastrointestinal tract. The kidneys and the myocardium had multiple abscesses containing coagulase-positive staphylococci. The liver weighed 2100 g and the spleen was pale, pink and weighed 270 g. There were two unexpected histological features: (1) Small fat droplets were found in the renal glomeruli, the lung capillaries, the intramural cardiac vessels and in the sinusoids of the liver and spleen. These gave a positive stain with Sudan III and were morphologically identical to fat emboli. They were also found in smaller quantities in several other organs (Figures 13.1, 13.2). (2) All the examined organs contained large macrophages with foamy, lipid-laden cytoplasm. They were of reticuloendothelial origin because they were particularly numerous in the Kupffer cells of the liver and the sinusoids of the spleen (Figures 13.3–13.6). Another striking finding was the presence of large foamy cells in the lumina of capillaries and some medium-sized arteries.

COMMENT

The widespread lipidosis found at autopsy was striking and unexpected.

The marked enlargement of the spleen and the liver, the presence of fat droplets in blood vessels, the very severe and widespread storage of lipid material in the cells of the reticuloendothelial system and the foamy cells in blood vessels were obviously the result of the long-term administration of the fat emulsion. These findings demonstrate that Intralipid may give rise to 'iatrogenic lipidosis'. The dosage recommended for the use of Intralipid is 1.5–2.0 g/kg/day for adults. For children the dosage may be as high as 3–4 g/kg/day[14]. Our patient received 2.0–2.5 g/kg fat daily for a total of 90 days.

The type of lipidosis described in this report is not observed even when very high doses of fat are given orally. This characteristic distinguishes intravenous fat emulsions from dietary chylomicrons. It seems that despite the improvement of modern fat emulsions, the reticuloendothelial cells may respond to foreign fat particles as objects for phagocytosis. We do not know why this phenomenon occurred so extensively in this patient. The possibility that, to a limited extent, similar phenomena exist in most patients on long-term administration of fat emulsions suggests the need for further investigation. The mild anaemia, thrombocytopenia and changes in liver function described with long-term use of fat emulsions, may all relate to the RES involvement. However, when the involvement of the RES is not massive it is generally not detected by routine clinical and laboratory tests. Increased susceptibility to sepsis may also be due to blockage of the RES by fat accumulation. These observations call for more caution in the use of fat emulsions in TPN.

References

1. Wretlind, A. (1972). Modern principles of the use of fat emulsions in parenteral nutrition. *Z. Ernachrungswiss*, **13** (Suppl.), 27
2. Hallberg, D. (1965). Studies on the elimination of exogenous lipids from the blood stream. *Acta Physiol. Scand.*, **64**, 306
3. Edgren, B., Hallberg, D., Håkansson, I., Meng, H. C. and Wretlind, A. (1964). Long-term tolerance study of two fat emulsions for intravenous nutrition in dogs. *Am. J. Clin. Nutr.*, **14**, 28

Figures 13.1, 13.2 Fat embolization

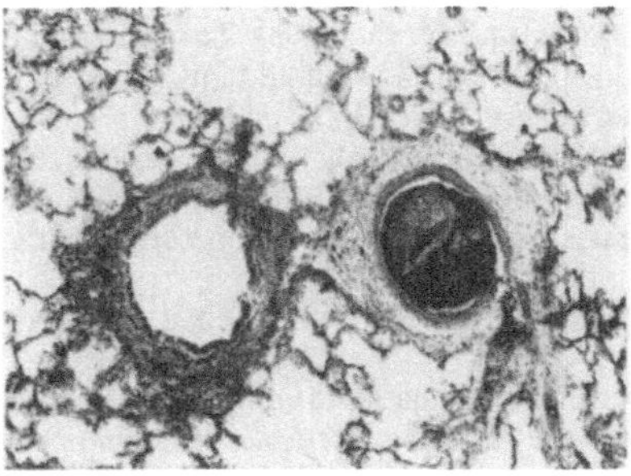

Figure 13.1 Lung—fat in a medium-sized artery (Sudan III)

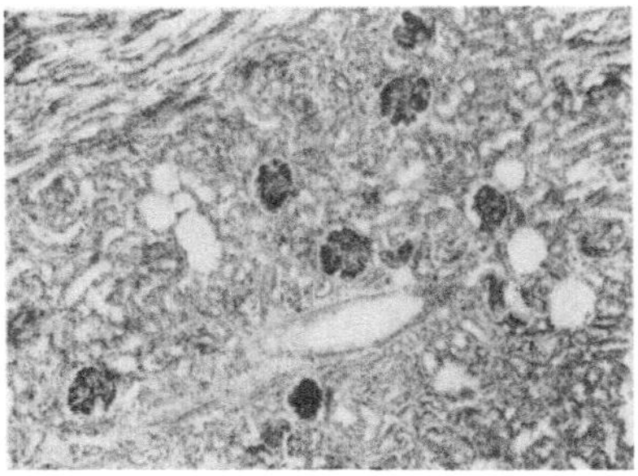

Figure 13.2 Kidney—fat in glomerular capillaries (Sudan III)

Figures 13.3–13.6 Reticuloendothelial involvement

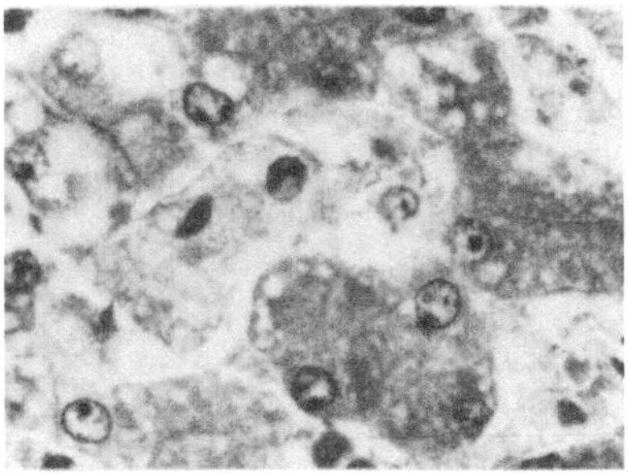

Figure 13.3 Liver—foamy cytoplasm of the Kupffer cells (Hematoxylin and eosin)

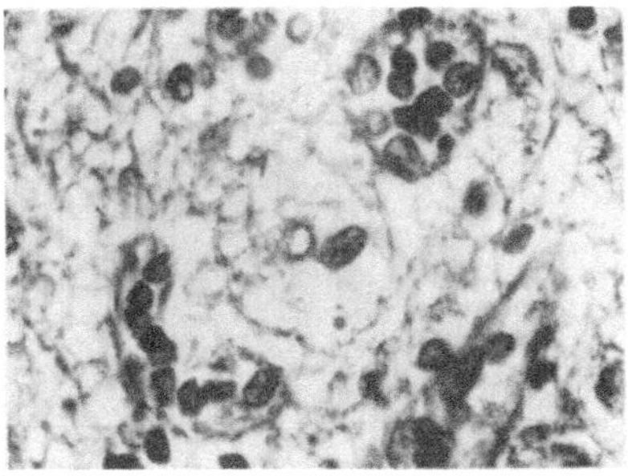

Figure 13.4 Spleen—macrophages with lipid-laden cytoplasm lining the sinusoids (Masson)

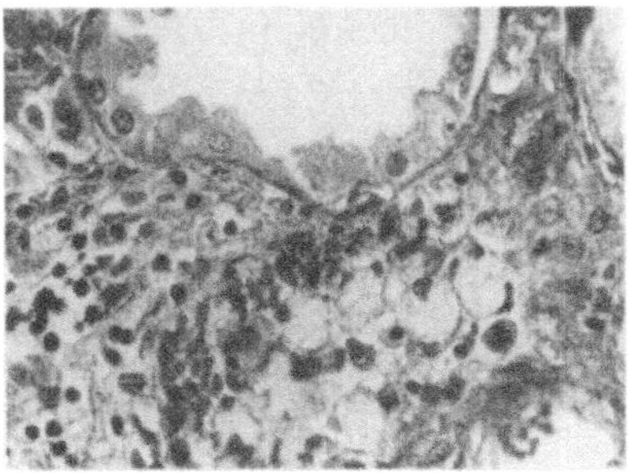

Figure 13.5 Kidney—artery containing macrophages with foamy cytoplasm (Hematoxylin and eosin)

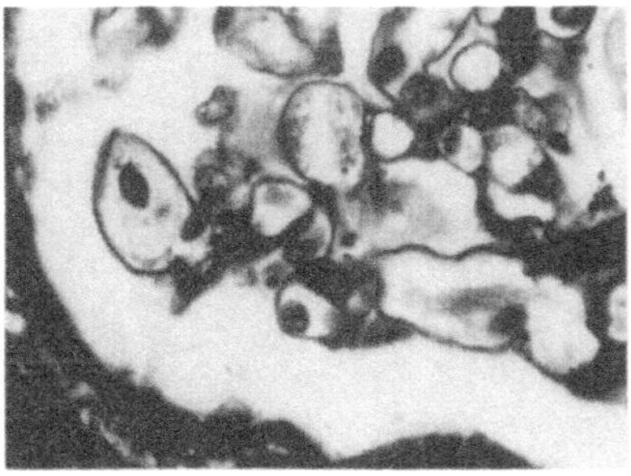

Figure 13.6 Kidney—Glomerular capillary containing macrophage with foamy, lipid laden cytoplasm (Silver—methenamine)

4. Edgren, B. and Wretlind, A. (1967). Ernährungsphysiologische und pharmakologische gesichtspunkte der verwendung von aminosäuren und fett in der intravenösen. *Ernährung. Wien. Med. Wschr.*, **117**, 32
5. Sasaki, H., Schoffner, F., Thompson, S. W. and Hunt, R. D. (1965). Toxicity testing of fat emulsions II. Ultrastructural changes in the liver following administration of a new intravenous fat emulsion (Intralipid). *Am. J. Clin. Nutr.*, **16**, 37–42
6. Thompson, S. H., Jones, L. D., Ferrell, J. F., Hurt, R. D., Meng, H. C., Kuyama, T., Sasaki, H., Schaffner, F., Singleton, W. S. and Cohn, I. (1965). Testing of fat emulsions for toxicity. III. Toxicity studies with new fat emulsions and emulsion components. *Am. J. Clin. Nutr.*, **16**, 43–61
7. Sholler, K. L. (1968). Transport und speicherung von fettemulsionsteilchen. *Z. Prakt. Anasthesie Wiederbelebung*, **3**, 193
8. Lemperle, G., Reichelt, M. and Denk, S. (1970). The evaluation of phagocytic activity in men by means of a lipid-clearing test. Abstr. *6th Int. Meet. Reticuloendothelial Soc.*
9. Tovar, J. A., Mahour, G. H., Miller, S. W., Isaacs, H. Jr. and Smith, C. N. (1976). Endotoxin clearance after Intralipid infusion. *J. Paed. Surg.*, **11**, 23
10. Gigon, J. P., Enderlein, F. and Scheidegger, S. (1966). Uber das Schicksal infundierter fettemulsioner un der menschlichen lung. *Schweiz. Med. Wschr.*, **96**, 71
11. Greene, H. L. (1972). *Total Parenteral Nutrition.* pp. 241–256. (Acton, Mass.: Publishing Sciences Group, Inc.)
12. Meng, H. C., Kuyama, T., Thompson, S. W. and Ferrell, J. F. (1965). Toxicity testing of fat emulsions. Tolerance study of long term intravenous administration of Intralipid in rats. *Am. J. Clin. Nutr.*, **16**, 29–36
13. Freund, U., Krausz, Y., Levij, I. S. and Eliakim, M. (1975). Iatrogenic lipidosis following prolonged intravenous hyperalimentation. *Am. J. Clin. Nutr.*, **28**, 1156
14. Coran, A. G. (1972). The intravenous use of fat for the total parenteral nutrition of the infant. *Lipids*, **7**, 455–458

Discussion

D. E. F. Tweedle: (UK) It appears that all the fat was taken up by the reticuloendothelial system. This has been used as a test of effectiveness of the reticuloendothelial system.

It has been suggested by some that Intralipid is not taken up by the reticuloendothelial system but Dr Freund has shown that this is not the case. How much Intralipid was used in the treatment regimens?

U. Freund: (Israel) We used 10% and 20% Intralipid alternately.

Tweedle: It would require therefore about 150 g/day in patients weighing roughly 50 kg, or 3 g/kg/day to produce the effects described.

D. W. Wilmore: (USA) What was the other calorie input?

Freund: Glucose and amino acids, providing an average of 2500 cal/day. Shaul recommended that only those fat emulsions which did not enter the reticuloendothelial system in significant amounts should be used in patients. In retrospect most of the problems with the first generation of fat emulsions were related to uptake by the reticuloendothelial system.

However, we were surprised that Intralipid could produce the same problem in certain situations. We do not know why. It may be that sepsis has something to do with it, but the sepsis was of very short duration, and the process that I demonstrated in the histology is a long-term process and not produced in a day or two.

M. Ste Marie: (Canada) Maybe the pediatricians have seen some of these complications in neonates, and particularly in premature babies. We have had at least five premature babies given Intralipid, glucose and amino acid solutions, who died of intracerebral haemorrhage or severe hyaline membrane disease, in whom we found a picture such as Dr Freund showed, with fat emboli in the lung vessels. These babies had not developed any signs of toxicity to Intralipid while they were on parenteral nutrition, which was a somewhat unusual finding.

E. M. Copeland: (USA) Is it possible that the patient actually had a disease of his reticuloendothelial system and we are looking at malfunction of that system with excessive uptake of fat? Did the post-mortem examination show anything else?

Freund: There was nothing to suggest hepatomegaly or changes in the spleen. We looked at every single organ in this patient and we found nothing abnormal. The patient was very healthy before he was operated on and there is no reason to believe that he had any disease of his reticuloendothelial system. I believe that the Intralipid was the cause of the pathology in the reticuloendothelial system.

A. B. Jones: (Canada) When we first started to use Intralipid for long periods we carried out biopsies on some babies and occasionally found the so-called intravenous fat pigment in the Kupffer cells. Whether the pigment is released from reticuloendothelial cells which have taken up fat or in some other way is uncertain.

At autopsy in neonates who have been on Intralipid and who have died from respiratory distress, the pathologist has not noted pigmentation in the reticuloendothelial cells.

We control our plasma lipid levels very carefully because of other reasons in relation to albumin binding capacity and serum bilirubin levels. It may of course be that one of the associated problems was the acute sepsis.

Has Dr Freund any evidence to show that it was a long-term problem and not an acute problem associated with the metabolism of Intralipid?

Freund: There is something to suggest it. We noticed the enlargement of the liver about 2–3 weeks before death, and there was some degree of splenomegaly as well. There was some jaundice with elevation of the alkaline phosphatase for about a week, but everything came back to normal and we did not change the regimen.

14
Toxicity of lipids

T. D. DARBY AND R. F. WALLIN

While the title of this paper is 'Toxicity of Lipids', I assume our interest is in the safe and effective use of a product which contains utilizable lipid substrate. If this is so, then safety and effectiveness are dependent upon factors associated with manufacture, distribution and therapeutic use of the product. Good manufacturing practices require selection of a suitable raw material, and production of a stable emulsion in a clean environment[1]. This is necessary to prevent the presence of endotoxin concentrations in the final product which are capable of causing adverse clinical reactions. The emulsion must remain stable *in vitro* during shipment and storage. There are several problems associated with the therapeutic use of the product and these include: (1) *in vivo* stability of the emulsion; (2) potential for drug interactions; (3) potential for sepsis from the addition of other substances; and (4) possible interactions with plastic containers and administration sets when these items are used in lipid administration.

Fat emulsions provide 9 cal/g; therefore an emulsion containing 15% fat and 5% carbohydrate furnishes approximately 1550 cal/l. The fat contributes little to osmotic pressure, and administration of large quantities of fat parenterally results in small urinary losses. Patients receiving soya bean oil emulsions clear the fat from their plasma and remain free of either acute or chronic adverse reactions[2]. Skin lesions which are attributed to essential fatty acid deficiency occur during long periods of intravenous feeding. This condition is treated successfully by fat emulsion administration. Munro states that nitrogen sparing by parenteral feeding requires an essential amount of carbohydrate and others suggest that insulin administration elicits a specific additive effect on nitrogen conservation[2,3].

TOXICITY ASSOCIATED WITH INTRAVENOUS FAT ADMINISTRATION

Frequently, reports of parenteral nutrition show an association between intravenous administration of fat in large quantities and signs of toxicity. At high dose levels, fat may cause alterations in metabolism through simple overloading of normal metabolic mechanisms, or by causing changes in usual metabolic pathways. This may be associated with alterations in the plasma clearance of injected fat. In this regard the ratio of carbohydrate to fat in the infusion may be important.

The liver does play a role in fat clearance and metabolism. Investigators of fat emulsion therapy report evidence of a decrease in liver function[4]. This evidence includes: measured bromsulphaphthalein retention, cephalin flocculation test data, and elevated alkaline phosphatase activity. Edgren (1960) reports that marked fatty degeneration of the liver and icterus occur with administration of lethal doses of fat[5]. Baxter/Travenol studies involving dogs receiving 6 g of emulsified fat per kg of body weight each day, show rapid clearance of fat from the blood following the first few days of treatment; however, as the number of treatment days increase, the fat clearance slowly decreases. Concomitant with the failure to clear fat, histological examination reveals fat accumulation in the liver. The Kupffer cells are always laden with fat and the parenchymal cells frequently show similar involvement. Other organs containing reticuloendothelial system (RES) cells are always fat-laden. A yellowish-brown pigment occurs in the liver following fat emulsion administration.

While the exact mechanism of fat toxicity awaits elucidation, it is evident that this process involves the RES in many tissues. Fat overload or coating of the fat particles by abnormal protein leads to uptake by the RES. Apparently, parenchymal cell involvement and liver engorgement follow saturation of the RES. Fat uptake by bone marrow and anaemia are reported in fat toxicity. There is some question about haemolytic activity and Levenson[4] observes a reticulocytosis.

Fat toxicity involves the lungs where macrophage activity occurs. These cells take up particulate matter and migrate into the alveolar space. Respiratory distress syndrome occurs with acute administration of particulate fat. Death during fat infusion may be related to pulmonary and liver dysfunction, as well as anaemia.

MANUFACTURING FACTORS WHICH CAN AFFECT SAFETY

Selection of raw materials is extremely important. While soya bean oil emulsion is reported to be safe, other oils such as cottonseed oil are associated with a number of clinical problems[4]. The contribution of various chain length fatty acids to the make up of the oil is quite different for different oil sources[4].

The type of emulsifier is also very important, and toxicity associated with the emulsifier is reported[4]. Since fat is insoluble in water it exists in solution as liquid micelles. These emulsified oil droplets exist in a variety of sizes. There are no conclusive data reported as to optimal particle size distribution in such emulsions either from concern for physiological use or adverse reactions. The stability of the emulsion may be affected by particle size. The value of 1 μm in diameter is frequently referred to as acceptable. Most likely, the particle sizes change over time. One investigator finds an average particle size of 3 μm[4].

Endotoxin reactions

Reports state that a moderate incidence of pyrogenic reactions occurs during clinical use of fat emulsions. Other reactions associated with endotoxins occur, such as nausea and vomiting, flushing, dyspnoea, apprehension, cyanosis, and hypotension[4]. While a number of reasons have been suggested for these reactions, it is obvious that a patient given material from one batch can have a reaction, but subsequent administration of material of the same composition and ingredients from a different batch does not cause a response. There is a requirement to test each batch for the presence of pyrogens, but there is still a strong possibility that rabbit pyrogen tests miss endotoxin contained in fat emulsion products.

Endotoxin levels in medical products present some interesting detection problems. The *U.S. Pharmacopeia* rabbit test is designed to detect endotoxin using the average rise in rabbit temperatures as an endpoint for a positive response. Therefore, the term 'pyrogen' has become synonymous with endotoxin. The rabbit responds, and one would expect that man also responds to a specific dose of endotoxin and not a concentration of endotoxin. For this reason, different volumes are required for each product dosage quantity. For example, large volume parenteral solutions are tested using a dose of 10 ml/kg, whereas 1 ml dosage forms require only 1 ml/kg dosage. The rabbit test will detect a concentration of purified *E. coli* endotoxin as low as 0.1 ng/ml when the 10 ml/kg dose is used, but will detect a concentration of only 1 ng/ml when the 1 ml/kg dosage is used. In each instance the rabbit test detects 1 ng/kg. Thus, one would expect a 3 kg rabbit to detect a total amount of endotoxin equal to 3 ng of purified *E. coli* endotoxin regardless of the concentration of endotoxin administered.

A look at the biological variation inherent in the rabbit test and the basic design of the USP pyrogen test is interesting. Table 14.1 illustrates individual results from seven USP eight-rabbit pyrogen tests where the solution tested yielded a positive test. When the individual temperature changes for the eight rabbits are arranged from lowest to highest temperature change, the variation in individual rabbit responses to the same quantity of endotoxin is obvious. The number of false negative three-rabbit tests which can be obtained by selection of three of the eight rabbits in a single test is shown in Table 14.2. There are fifty-six possible three-rabbit tests. The proportion of false negative tests can be as high as 20%. It should be remembered that the product must fail the three-rabbit screen in order for the additional five rabbits to be injected. Thus, false positive tests can be ruled out, but false negative tests will not.

With these data in mind, it is apparent that a fat emulsion product containing sufficient endotoxin to fail an eight-rabbit pyrogen test could be released as often as at least five times out of 100 batches. This may help to explain some of the problems associated with fat emulsion.

Currently, 'Good Manufacturing Practices', which include screening of raw materials and production of the product in a clean environment prevent accumulation of endotoxin in medical products. Thus the rabbit test is

Table 14.1 Percentage of all possible combinations of ranked rabbit responses passing three rabbit test (56 possible)

Test	*Total increase*	*Combinations of ranks rabbit responses*	*Percentage passing*
A	3.70	(1, 2, 3) (1, 2, 4) (1, 2, 5) (1, 2, 6) (2, 3, 4) (2, 3, 5) (2, 3, 6) (3, 4, 5) (3, 4, 6)	16.07
B	3.80	(1, 2, 3) (1, 2, 4) (1, 2, 5) (1, 2, 6) (2, 3, 4) (2, 3, 5) (2, 3, 6) (3, 4, 5) (3, 4, 6) (4, 5, 6)	17.86
C	4.55	(1, 2, 3) (1, 2, 4) (2, 3, 4)	5.36
D	4.15	(1, 2, 3) (1, 2, 4) (1, 2, 5) (2, 3, 4) (2, 3, 5)	8.93
E	4.45	(1, 2, 3) (1, 2, 4) (2, 3, 4)	5.36
F	3.75	(1, 2, 3) (1, 2, 4) (1, 2, 5) (1, 2, 6) (1, 2, 7) (2, 3, 4) (2, 3, 5) (2, 3, 6) (2, 3, 7) (3, 4, 5) (3, 4, 6)	19.64
G	4.40	(1, 2, 3) (1, 2, 4) (2, 3, 4)	5.36

Table 14.2 Results of seven eight-rabbit tests with failing total temperature increases

Rank of rabbit response	*Eight-rabbit test*						
	A	*B*	*C*	*D*	*E*	*F*	*G*
1	0.25	0.35	0.20	0.40	0.30	0.35	0.10
2	0.35	0.35	0.20	0.40	0.30	0.40	0.35
3	0.35	0.40	0.30	0.40	0.50	0.40	0.40
4	0.40	0.40	0.40	0.50	0.55	0.45	0.55
5	0.45	0.45	0.60	0.50	0.60	0.50	0.60
6	0.55	0.50	0.60	0.60	0.65	0.50	0.65
7	0.65	0.65	1.10	0.65	0.70	0.55	0.85
8	0.70	0.70	1.15	0.70	0.85	0.60	0.90
SUM	3.70	3.80	4.55	4.15	4.45	3.75	4.40
AVERAGE	0.46	0.48	0.57	0.52	0.56	0.47	0.55

presented with few if any opportunities to miss pyrogenic materials. The Limulus Amebocyte Lysate Test is a much more convenient test system for detection of endotoxin[6].

INTERACTION OF FAT EMULSIONS WITH PLASTIC CONTAINERS AND ADMINISTRATION SETS

Emulsions of fat in aqueous solutions are composed of at least two phases, a micellar-phase of oil and a water continuous-phase. This type of product presents solubility problems which do not exist with solutions of amino acid, electrolytes and carbohydrate which can be made into true solutions. Understanding of the adverse effects of immiscible lipid liquid in aqueous solutions depends upon an appreciation of the solubility effects on total body distribution and subsequently elimination. The RES is largely responsible for removal of the large insoluble fat micelles. This leads to engorgement of the liver, spleen, lungs and to some extent the kidney. These points are covered in the section titled 'Toxicity Associated with Intravenous Fat Administrations'.

Plastic containers and administration sets are usually manufactured from polyvinyl chloride (PVC), a rigid material. Di-2-ethylhexyl phthalate (DEHP) is an oil-like liquid that is added to PVC to make the material flexible. Like fat, DEHP is insoluble in water. Therefore, an emulsifying agent is needed to provide a suitable injectable form to study toxicity of this material. Solutions stored in PVC containers such as normal saline, glucose, Ringer's lactate, etc. that do not contain lipid, contain very little DEHP. In fact, the level seems to be at or near the level of chemical analytical detection. Accumulation of DEHP in a lipid-containing solution is related to the rate of removal of surface DEHP at the liquid/plastic interface. The initial uptake into blood or other lipid-containing solutions is determined by the quantity of DEHP on the surface of the plastic. After this removal of surface accumulation the rate of uptake is determined by the migration rate of DEHP in the plastic matrix. For blood this rate has been determined to be 0.25 mg/day/100 ml of blood. Thus short periods of storage of fat emulsions in PVC would not allow significant quantities of DEHP to accumulate in the fat micelles. Administration sets do not present a problem, but implanted catheters do present a potential problem from several points of view. When these catheters are made of PVC which has been plasticized with DEHP, long-term contact with the cells of the blood vessels will allow migration of DEHP into the cells. The catheter becomes rigid and causes cellular damage. The DEHP accumulation may cause focal tissue necrosis. Therefore, PVC plasticized catheters should be allowed to remain in the vessel only for short periods.

The reactions described for catheters are quite different from potential reactions associated with the leaching of DEHP from plastic containers into lipid-containing solutions. The primary concerns with both DEHP and fat emulsion in regard to toxicity are the effects caused by particulate substances.

Table 14.3 Kinetics of DEHP disappearance from rat blood after administration in different vehicles

Vehicle	*Half life*		*Vd* (± *SD*)
	Initial phase	*Slow phase*	
Tween-80	5.6	263	28.0 ± 2.2
Plasma added in:			
Tween-80	4.4	83	57.6 ± 0.5
Ethanol	5.9	181	65.0 ± 1.5
Plasma: diffusion from polyvinyl	4.2	31	100.2 ± 1.9

Table 14.3 gives the values for rate of distribution, volume of distribution, and elimination rate for several forms of DEHP. Notice that both the Tween and alcohol micellar forms give different rate and volume values for distribution and elimination. When DEHP is leached slowly into plasma and accumulates in the plasma lipid DEHP is undetected in plasma water. Therefore, the distribution is controlled by lipoprotein distribution; whereas with emulsions of DEHP where the micelles are distributed in plasma water the values for rate and volume of distribution are considerably different. Of course considerably more DEHP can be administered in the emulsified form. The leaching rate determines both the dose and the dose form; the liquid micelles of both fat and DEHP are taken up by the RES and by lung macrophages. It is not surprising that 300–400 mg/kg of DEHP administered in a particulate dose form can give both pulmonary and liver effects. Death after acute injection is due to respiratory distress syndrome.

Studies by Waddell *et al.* demonstrate DEHP distribution in the mouse using ^{14}C-labelled DEHP[7]. They find the uptake of the plasma-leached form to be largely by the liver. Studies show that the permeability of the liver sinuses and fenestrated capillaries is greater than that of continuous capillary beds of most other organ systems[8,9]. The kidney and the intestine show rapid uptake of labelled DEHP. Both the kidney and the intestinal mucosa contain fenestrated capillaries. One expects an increase in DEHP concentration in the lymph, and this appears to be the case for the first hour after injection. However, rapid clearance by the liver and the elimination of unchanged DEHP is reported in several studies. The metabolites are more water-soluble and are eliminated by the kidney. The rate of elimination is determined by the rate of production of the metabolites, therefore, accumulation of metabolites is not expected. In the Waddell *et al.* studies, the dose administered is 4–5 mg/kg, that amount equal to a total body transfusion of 21-day-old blood stored in plastic, and total clearance of the ^{14}C label on DEHP occurs in 24 h. Similar distribution and excretion patterns occur in the pregnant rat, which shows yolk sac distribution of DEHP; otherwise the distribution and clearance is similar to that found in the non-pregnant animal. Thomas has reviewed the toxicity of DEHP recently[10].

POTENTIAL ADVERSE EFFECTS ASSOCIATED WITH CLINICAL USE OF FAT EMULSIONS

We discussed the consequence of administration of endotoxin and the possible accumulation of DEHP in lipid solutions. However, the metabolic changes which may occur with fat emulsions have not been discussed. It is well known that free fatty acids are utilized by cardiac muscle when adequate oxygen is present to support the metabolic demand. During ischaemia or during periods of catecholamine stimulation, the heart prefers glucose as a substrate. Glycogen stores are broken down and lactate excretion occurs. The basic biochemical lesion occurring in shock remains elusive.

However, the shock syndrome is characterized by a marked depression of oxidative metabolism. Jones ascribes this state to an attenuation of essential translocation of metabolites across the inner mitochondrial membrane in target organs. Jones suggests a sequence of events leading to esterification with CoA to give long-chain fatty acyl thioesters which cause competitive inhibition of adenine nucleotide translocase[11]. This same type of inhibition might occur by overloading the system with long chain fatty acids from certain oil sources used in preparation of fat emulsions. Treatment with palmitoyl-CoA (Sigma) inhibited the enzyme function by 85–90%. Morel

Table 14.4 Interactions with plasma proteins

Albumin	α_1	β_2, β_1, α_2
Ca^{2+}, Cu^{2+}, Zn^{2+}	Steroid hormones	Zn^{2+}, lipids
Bilirubin	(Transcortin)	Cholesterol
Uric acid	Vitamin B_{12}	Vitamins A, K, D, E
Vitamin C	Sialic acid	
Adenosine	Thyroxine	
Tetracyclines		
Chloramphenicol	α_2	β_1
Digitonin	Cu^{2+} (Caeruloplasmin)	Fe^{2+}
Fatty acids	Lithium carmine	(Transferrin)
Suramin	Haemoglobin	
Quinacrine	(Haptoglobin)	
Penicillin		
Salicylate		
Para-aminosalicylate		
Sulphonamides		
Streptomycin		
Acid dyes		
Phenol red		
Histamine		
Triiodothyronine		
Thyroxine		
Barbiturates		

et al. reported that K_1 values of long chain fatty acyl thioesters vary considerably depending on the chemical nature of the fatty acyl residue. In shock, soluble intracellular enzymes essential to the functioning of the malate–aspartate shuttle escape into the blood stream. While the importance of these biochemical changes associated with shock awaits further elucidation, they certainly raise questions about the effects of free fatty acid administration, particularly of long chain lengths, on oxidative metabolism.

Table 14.4 illustrates potential drug interactions with the plasma proteins. Many substances compete for binding sites on these proteins[12]. This is particularly true for albumin binding sites. Free fatty acid binds to albumin. Recently Brodeau and his collaborators published a series of articles describing the potential interactions between concentrations of plasma-free fatty acids and coumarin or indanedione anticoagulants[13–15]. They report that fasting and stress enhance the anticoagulant response to warfarin and suggest that this might be due to an interference of endogenous free fatty acids with binding of warfarin to plasma protein. They also report that addition of free fatty acids to plasma containing warfarin *in vitro* causes an elevation of free warfarin levels. Such competition for binding sites on plasma protein can cause increased responses to administered drugs as well as promoting elimination of the free drug component thus reducing duration of drug action.

OSMOTIC PROBLEMS ASSOCIATED WITH USE OF HYPERTONIC SOLUTIONS

There is a serious problem associated with hyperosmolarity of plasma. Elevated glucose levels cause changes in brain enzyme activity. Aldoreductase activation causes conversion of glucose to sorbitol and then fructose is formed. Both fructose and sorbitol accumulate in the brain cells, thus increasing intracellular osmolarity. This results in cerebral oedema. The glial cells are initially involved, but subsequently the grey matter shows vacuolization on histological examination. These changes are well documented in diabetic coma[16–20]. Marked cellular changes in the brain were found in normal dogs given rapid administration of hypertonic solutions. Therefore, hypertonic solutions should be administered cautiously to prevent hyperosmolarity of plasma. The clinical picture of hyperosmolarity is characterized by lethargy coma, convulsions and death. Restoration of plasma osmolality with albumin could be helpful.

SUMMARY

Fat emulsion therapy must be practised with caution. A stable emulsion dosage form, low in endotoxin concentration, is desirable. The rate and total dose administered must be controlled. This is also true with concentrated glucose solutions. Here insulin used judiciously may be advisable.

While DEHP will leach into fat emulsions from plasticized PVC containers, the short period of time that emulsions should be held in plastic containers and the transmission time of fat through PVC administration sets should prevent the complication.

Concern for potential drug interaction with fat emulsion is necessary and further study is required to elucidate potential problem areas. This is also true with the use of fat emulsions in states such as shock.

References

1. Alexander, S. F., Farage, D. J. and Hassan, W. E. (1971). R. D. Martin (assoc. ed.) *Hazards of Medication.* (Philadelphia and Toronto: J. B. Lippincott, Co.)
2. Long, J. M., III, Wilmore, D. W., Mason, A. D. and Pruitt, B. A. (1977). Effect of carbohydrate and fat intake on nitrogen excretion during total intravenous feeding. *Ann. Surg.*, **185** (4), 417
3. Munro, H. N. (1951). Carbohydrate and fat as factors in protein utilization and metabolism. *Physiol. Rev.*, **31**, 149
4. Geyer, R. P. (1960). Parenteral nutrition. *Physiol. Rev.*, **40**, 150
5. Edgren, B. (1960). Tolerance of the dog to intravenous fat emulsion. *Pharmacol. Toxicol.*, **16**, 260
6. Weary, M. and Baker, B. (1977). Utilization of the Limulus Amebocyte test for pyrogen testing of large volume parenteral solutions, administration sets, and medical devices. Parenteral Drug Association (In press)
7. Waddell, W. J., Marlowe, C., Miripol, J. E. and Garvin, P. J. (1977). The distribution in mice of intravenously administered plasma solution of ^{14}C di-2-ethylhexyl phthalate determined by wholebody autoradiography. *Toxicol. Appl. Pharmacol.*, **39**, 339
8. Mayerson, H. S., Wolfram, C. G. and Shirley, H. H. (1960). Regional differences in capillary permeability. *Am. J. Physiol.*, **198**, 155
9. Karnovsky, M. J. (1968). The ultrastructural basis of transcapillary exchanges. *J. Gen. Physiol.*, **52**, 641
10. Thomas, J. A. (1977). Toxicity of di-2-ethylhexyl phthalate (DEHP). *Toxicol. Appl. Pharmacol.* (In press)
11. Jones, C. R. N. (1977). The basic biochemical lesion in shock. *Biochem. Soc. Trans.*, **5**, 213–214
12. Goldstein, A., Aronow, L. and Kalman, S. M. (1974). *Principles of Drug Action.* (New York and London: John Wiley & Sons)
13. Laliberte, R., Chakrabarti, S. and Brodeau, J. (1976). The influence of fasting and stress on the response of rats to warfarin. *J. Pharmacol. Exp. Ther.*, **196**, 194
14. Chakrabarti, S. K., Laliberte, R. and Brodeau, J. (1976). Influence of long-chain free fatty acids on the binding of warfarin to bovine serum albumin. *Biochem. Pharmacol.*, **25**, 2515
15. Laliberte, R., Chakrabarti, S. K. and Brodeau, J. (1977). The influence of fasting on the disposition of warfarin in rats. *J. Pharmacol. Exp. Ther.*, **200**, 44
16. Clements, R. S., Jr., Prockop, L. D. and Winegrad, A. I. (1968). Acute cerebral edema during treatment of hyperglycemia. *Lancet*, **ii**, 384
17. Clements, R. S., Jr., Blumenthal, S. A., Morrison, A. D. and Winegrad, A. I. (1971). Increased cerebrospinal-fluid pressure during treatment of diabetic ketosis. *Lancet*, **ii**, 671
18. Garbay, K. H. (1973). The sorbitol pathway and the complications of diabetes. *N. Engl. J. Med.*, **288**, 831
19. Raja, R. M., Moros, J. G., Kramer, M. S. and Rosenbaum, J. L. (1970). Hyperosmotic coma complicating peritoneal dialysis with sorbitol dialysate. *Ann. Int. Med.*, **73**, 993
20. Bischel, M. D. and Barbour, B. H. (1974). Peritoneal dialysis with sorbitol versus dextrose dialysate. *Nephron*, **12**, 449

Discussion

R. E. Dolkart: (Belgium) Apparently the only way that a fat emulsion can be utilized is by being broken down by the appropriate enzyme system. The infrequency of occurrence of what Dr Freund described would make one wonder if something took place with the appropriate enzyme system which has to do with the control of the use of fat under the particular circumstances in which it was being used.

T. D. Darby: (USA) Often, during studies of toxicity, mechanisms become very apparent that one should have known about previously but their importance was overlooked. We were studying a polyol F-38 sold by BASF Wyandotte Corporation and observed vacuolization in tissues. The vacuolization was seen in the kidney with dilation of the tubules and the glomerular space. The lungs were filled with the polyol material. The liver had a spongy-looking appearance. Electron microscopy showed that many of the vacuoles one sees on light microscopy are really lysosomal vacuoles. F-38 was well encapsulated in a membrane that contained lysosomal enzymes. However, the lysosomal enzymes could not act on the material to break it down, so it merely accumulated in the tissues. Within 15 min following the intravenous administration one could see good clearance of F-38 from blood. However, F-38 remained in the tissue for a long time. The K value for uptake was very large compared to the K value of release from tissues. After 7 days minimal vacuolization was present. The kidney, the liver and other organs looked essentially normal after 14 days. This was compared to the marked vacuolization of the tissues within 15 min after the injection. We were shocked at the potential for toxicity evident in the light microscopy changes one sees early in the course of F-38 administration. Following uptake into lysosomal vacuoles, the rate at which substances can be removed is usually enzyme-dependent. But in the case of F-38 the accumulation in tissue occurred and the materials remained in the tissue for several days. Since the material was resistant to metabolism by lysosomal enzymes it remained in cytoplasm vacuoles for several days. With large doses of lipid, intravenous fat particles could certainly exist in cytoplasm vacuoles like the F-38 experience. The presence of fat in the cytoplasm could have a deleterious effect on certain enzyme reactions. This is particularly true of translocase.

U. Freund: (Israel) The rate of elimination from the blood stream of the substance has nothing to do with utilization. It was shown many times that the elimination rate of the fat emulsions, especially Intralipid, is very similar to what is happening with chylomicrons. But the conclusions that this is the rate of utilization and that this is identical with chylomicrons have still to be proven.

N. J. Kartinos: (USA) Years ago, when we were interested in intravenous fat emulsions, the Upjohn product Lipomol was being used, and there was frequently a delayed pyrogenic response with the Lipomol in the clinical situation, which could not be called a pyrogenic reaction because the fat emulsion had passed the USP rabbit test.

This suggests to me that there was a different clearance of fat in the rabbit, which masked a pyrogenic response, whereas in man the same was not experienced. That would lead me to the view that with lipid there is altered pharmacokinetics. I believe that a sustained release may occur with endotoxin and we have the additional experience that in the presence of phthalate a sustained or prolonged increase in hexobarbitol sleeping time can occur, demonstrating that there is sustained release and altered pharmacokinetics of drugs or hormones with fat emulsions. This may explain some of the experiences in the septic patient.

Darby: I think that that is very true. The presence of any substance in the vascular system, particularly if it is different in nature from plasma, will change distribution of drugs in plasma and in the body. The accumulation in the lungs, leading to phagocytosis, some degree of capillary blockade, release of endogenous pyrogen, and other substances may take time to occur, but will present an entirely different picture than we associate with aqueous solutions.

P. Vinay: (Canada) It is obvious that 10% Travasol* has an osmolarity of around 1260, and yet when mixed with dextrose 33% it gives a final solution of nearly 1600 mOsm/l. Nevertheless from what we experience, this is not an osmotic charge. As the amino acids are utilized and the glucose is utilized, the water is left behind. What we see when we measure water clearances and water excretion in these patients during hyperalimentation is a rapid increase in free water clearance. If one considers the fact that plasma osmolarity measured before and during TPN never changes, I believe that we can challenge the fact that TPN is an osmolar load.

D. W. Wilmore: (USA) For the pediatricians I should re-emphasize a slide of Dr Darby's that had to do with binding of fat to albumin. We are all, I am sure, concerned with bilirubin transport and kernicterus and how to influence this by nutritional inputs; not only by fat, but by carbohydrate which will change the mobilization of free fatty acids from the periphery.

* Synthamin 17

Section V
Trace Elements in Parenteral Nutrition

15
Trace element formulations in intravenous feeding

N. J. KARTINOS

INTRODUCTION

Total parenteral nutrition as pioneered by Dudrick *et al.*[1], is employed to reverse negative nitrogen balance in the malnourished patient. Weight gain and restoration of lean body mass are accompanied by enhanced wound healing and improved morbidity and mortality.

The main objective of total parenteral nutrition is to provide the necessary nutrients in sufficient quantity to stimulate cellular and tissue growth. These nutrients must be provided at appropriate levels to support the growth, development, repair and the recovery process.

Mixtures of essential and non-essential amino acids with adequate calories

Table 15.1 Trace elements in blood, plasma*, and plasma fractions†

Element	*Whole blood* (μg/l)	*Plasma* (μg/l)	*Plasma fraction*, 5%* (mg/l)	*Plasma fraction*, 20%* (mg/l)
Co	0.35	0.29		
Cr		(27–180)‡	20 ± 5 μg	40 ± 5 μg
Cu	(720–1060)‡	(980–1200)‡	0.47	0.89
Fe	(440–560 mg)‡	(580–2100)‡	1.1	4.8
Mn	200	(1.8–3.1)‡	40 ± 5 μg	150 ± 5 μg
Se	(20–220)‡			
Zn	(8.84–16.0 mg)‡	(1.1–3.0 mg)‡	1.48	3.27
F	(40–360)‡	(140–190)‡		
I	—	(38–60)‡		

* Compiled from literature sources.

† Buminate, Hyland Laboratories, analyses by G. Fell, Glasgow.

‡ ( ) range of various means reported.

(fats and/or carbohydrates), vitamins, and electrolytes are administered over extended periods of time. Electrolytes (macro elements) are provided with amino acid mixtures or introduced as additives. It was clear that trace elements (micro elements) were also required and these have been provided in the form of whole blood, plasma, and plasma fractions (Table 15.1).

TRACE ELEMENTS IN HUMAN NUTRITION

Some eleven elements constitute the bulk of living matter. Approximately seventeen others have been classified as trace elements in that their biological significance in animals has been demonstrated. Chromium, cobalt, copper, iron, manganese, molybdenum, selenium, zinc, fluorine, and iodide are believed to be important in human nutrition. The minimum daily requirements for some of these trace elements have been established[2].

Studies in human and animal nutrition, biochemistry and intermediary metabolism have established a pharmacologic basis for the essential nature of several trace elements.

Iron is essential to haemoglobin synthesis. *Copper* is an important trace element for the maturation of red cells and occurs in coenzyme A dehydrogenase, which is associated with the conversion of lower fatty acids and in phospholipid synthesis. *Iodide* is required for thyroxine synthesis. *Zinc* is an essential constituent of many enzymes—carbonic anhydrase, carboxy peptidase, several dehydrogenases, and phosphatases. *Manganese* is prominent with a variety of phosphatases and carboxylases which are important in the total energy cycle (reproduction, growth, calcium and phosphorus metabolism). *Chromium* is thought to be a cofactor with insulin for normal glucose utilization and is believed to be an important trace element in intravenous feeding when large amounts of glucose are infused. The minimum daily requirements for selenium have not been established, but it is known to be a component of the glutathione peroxidase system and required for efficient oxidation of sulphydryl groups.

Trace element deficiencies in patients

Trace element levels are not normally monitored in patients. The analytical procedures are complex, require special instrumentation, and are not routinely available.

However, trace element deficiencies in humans have been reported. Vallee *et al.*[3] have reported low serum concentrations of zinc in patients with severe cirrhosis. Decreased serum zinc levels and increased zincuria have occurred in burned patients and after extensive abdominal operations[4]. Apparent iron deficiency anaemias have been associated with copper[5] and zinc[6] deficiencies. Zinc deficiencies have also been reported in patients on prolonged total parenteral nutrition[7,8].

It cannot be predicted when a trace element deficiency may occur or whether it will be apparent clinically. It is most likely to be associated with the duration of total parenteral nutrition and the severity of the malnutrition.

Trace elements in commercial parenteral products

Intravenous fluids and intravenous additives may contain variable amounts of trace elements[9-11]. The water and drug substances employed in the manufacture of these parenterals are controlled rigorously for their heavy metal content but specific trace element analyses are not required nor performed. The rubber stopper has been implicated as a source of zinc. It is known that zinc accelerator salts are employed in the vulcanization process. Some plastic polyvinyl chloride containers may contain low levels of zinc as a result of the additives employed. Trace element deficiencies may not be more prevalent as a result of these variations in the trace element content of intravenous fluids. However, present commercial parenteral products can not be relied upon to provide a consistent and uniform level of trace elements (Tables 15.2a, 15.2b). Variations have been reported between different manufacturers, and batches. Zinc concentrations in commercial dextrose injections (5–50% concentrations) can range from not detectable to 270 μg/l. Manganese levels are reported to range from 0.5 to 5.5 μg/l. Copper was detected in the range of 15–80 μg/l. These ranges are not concentration dependent.

TRACE ELEMENT FORMULATIONS

From the minimum daily requirements (oral) and from an estimation of the percentage of absorption, Shils[12] has estimated the parenteral requirements of trace elements for child and adult. Because of the forced metabolism associated with total parenteral nutrition the requirements of the malnourished adult may more likely approximate the requirements of a child (Table 15.3).

Several trace element formulations as additives for hyperalimentation have been proposed[12-14]. The ones presented have been used clinically. They have been prepared in the hospital pharmacy or are available commercially as an investigational drug (Table 15.4).

These formulae differ both in qualitative and quantitative character. Formulae are not represented uniformly in the literature. Concentrations of the ions are presented as milligrams (micrograms) or micromoles. Further, concentrations may be presented as concentration per unit volume or total volume per dose. They have been recalculated as μg/ml to facilitate ready comparisons.

In formulating these preparations the hydrate forms of the various salts should be specified to avoid errors and confusion.

Table 15.2a Trace elements in crystalline amino acid injections (μg/l)

Ion	5.5% *Travasol**	10% *Travasol**	7% *Vamin with fructose*†	8.5% *FreAmine*‡
Co	40, 50	40, 50	400	
Cu	400	300, 700	600	70, 85
Fe	560, 1020	1560, 1640	1240	
Mn	<60, <100	<60, 70	<60	
Mo	<500	<500	<500	
Zn	150, 250	1060, 1370	280	1220, 1850
F	20, 150	20	20	
I	10, 20	10	<10	

* Travenol Laboratories (Synthamin).

† Vitrum AG.

‡ McGraw Laboratories.

F by ion selective electrode. Limits of detection 10 ppb.

I colorimetrically (Cr IV Redox). Limits of detection 10 ppb.

Cations by atomic absorption spectrophotometry. Limits of detection (ppm): Co, 0.04; Cu, 0.1; Fe, 0.12; Mn, 0.06; Mo, 0.5; Zn, 0.02.

Compiled from literature sources and Pharmacy Dept., Travenol Laboratories.

Table 15.2b Trace elements in protein hydrolysates

Ion	5% *Amigen** *D5W*	5% *Amigen**	5% *Aminosol*† *D5W*	5% *Aminosol*†	7% *Polynute*‡	5% *Hyprotigen*§ *D5W*
Zn	1438	3700	40	240	2490	3200
Cu	78	50	99	40	150	0–23.3
Mn		220		56	240	56–82
Se						22–25

* Casein hydrolysate, Travenol.

† Fibrin hydrolysate, Abbott.

‡ Casein hydrolysate, Cutter.

§ Casein hydrolysate, McGraw.

Compiled from literature sources.

Figure 15.3 Suggested *daily* intravenous requirements for trace elements

	Infants and young children	*Adults*
Fe	1 mg*	1 mg†
I	5 μg/kg	1–2 μg/kg
Cu	15 μg/kg	1 mg
F	1 μg/kg	1–2 mg
Z	20–40 μg/kg	2–4 mg
Mn	12–20 μg/kg	1–12 mg
Cr	0.5 μg/kg	15 μg

* To be given daily or weekly.

† Monthly or bimonthly to adults. Double level for menstruation.

Adapted from M. E. Shils.

Table 15.4 Proposed trace mineral formulation

	MW	Human plasma (μg/ml)	Addam* (per ml) (μmoles)	(μg)	Shil:† (μg/ml)	Jeejeebhoy‡ (μg/ml)
Cu	63.5	1.1	0.5	31.75	400	200
Zn	65.4	1.1	2	130.8	2000	400
Mn	54.9	0.03	4	219.6	200	200
I	126.9	0.05	0.1	12.7	60	24
Cr	52.0	0.03–0.20	—	—	—	0.4
F	9	0.14	5	45	—	—

* Vitrum AB, Stockholm. Also contains macro minerals. In 10 ml vials. As recommended by Wretlind and Jacobson.

† Adult dose 5 ml/day.

‡ In 5 ml vials.

In the clinical use of these preparations it would be well to specify the concentration per unit volume plus total volume administered or total dose and the administered volume. The total volume administered may be varied as appropriate for a particular patient.

Travenol trace element formulations and stability

The Travenol trace element formula has been adopted from Jeejeebhoy *et al.*[14]. This formula has been used with success in Canada, particularly in Toronto and Vancouver (Table 15.5).

Only the halogen salts of the trace minerals are employed in the commercial approach. The Virtum product is similarly formulated. This is necessary to achieve a stable, autoclavable product. Formulations containing some trace minerals as sulphate salts have been described and have been employed. These, however, have been formulated in hospital pharmacies and were sterilized by membrane filtration. Their shelf life may be limited, and they are not stable to steam sterilization.

The Travenol product is designed as a unit dose. By employing increments

Table 15.5 Travenol trace mineral formula

Ion	MW	Salt	MW	Salt (mg/5 ml)	Ion conc. in 5 ml	Ion conc. (μg/ml)
Zn	65.4	$ZnCl_2$	136.3	4.170	2 mg	400
Cu	63.5	$CuCl_2.2H_2O$	170.4	2.683	1 mg	200
Mn	54.9	$MnCl_2.4H_2O$	197.9	3.602	1 mg	200
Cr	52.0	$CrCl_2.6H_2O$	266.5	0.0102	2 μg	0.4
I	126.9	KI	166.	0.157	120 μg	24

* HCl for pH adjustment, pH 3.0–3.5.

† 9 mg NaCl/ml for tonicity.

‡ Packaged in 5 ml vials.

of 1 ml, flexibility is provided to accommodate both child and adult. The product is presently undergoing shelf life tests at controlled room temperature (22 °C) and 45 °C. All at 6 months are stable and compatible. These studies are continuing with the objective of establishing an expiration date. Analyses of the cations are performed by a carbon rod atomic absorption spectrophotometer. The trace anion (iodide) is analysed by ion selective electrode.

Stability and compatibility of admixtures

The physical and chemical stability of the Travenol trace element intravenous additive, after combining it with the injections typically employed in total parenteral nutrition, was also assessed.

Admixtures were prepared by adding 5 ml of the trace element preparation to each of the following large volume parenterals:

(a) 5.5% Travasol* with electrolytes, 500 ml
(b) 8.5% Travasol with electrolytes, 500 ml
(c) 10% Travasol with electrolytes, 250 ml
(d) 3.5% Travasol M with electrolyte 45, 500 ml
(e) 0.9% NaCl, 500 ml
(f) 5% dextrose, 500 ml
(g) 50% dextrose, 500 ml
(h) $33\frac{1}{3}$% dextrose, 750 ml
(i) 50:50 mixture of (a) and (g), 1000 ml
(j) 50:50 mixture of (b) and (g), 1000 ml
(k) 1:3 mixture of (c) and (h), 1000 ml

* Synthamin.

Table 15.6 Admixture 50% dextrose injection (500 ml) and trace mineral additive (5 ml)

	Storage conditions	*Initial* (mg/l)	6 *h* (mg/l)	6 *h* Δ%	24 *h* (mg/l)	24 *h* Δ%
Zn	5 °C	4.26	4.28	+0.47	4.36	+2.35
	RT	4.27	4.36	+2.11	4.40	+3.04
Mn	5 °C	2.29	2.40	+4.80	2.26	−1.31
	RT	2.37	2.46	+3.80	2.36	−0.42
Cu	5 °C	2.18	2.15	−1.38	2.06	−5.50
	RT	2.25	2.23	−0.89	2.11	−6.22
I	5 °C	(0.24)	(0.23)	−2.90	(0.22)	−7.30
	RT	(0.24)	(0.24)	−1.80	(0.23)	−2.50
Cr	5 °C	(0.004)	(0.004)	−0.98)	(0.004)	−0.46
	RT	(0.004)	(0.004)	−5.10	(0.04)	−2.90
Visual examination	5 °C	Clear	Clear		Clear	
	RT	Clear	Clear		Clear	
pH	5 °C	3.8	3.8		3.8	
	RT	3.8	3.8		3.8	

Units were stored at controlled room temperature (22 °C) or refrigerator temperature (4 °C) and sampled at 0, 6, and 24 h. After visual examination for physical compatibility, pH values and trace element contents were determined. Analyses were performed as described above, except for chromium and iodine which were determined by isotope dilution. All admixtures were demonstrated to be stable and compatible under these experimental conditions. Representative data are presented in Tables 15.6–15.8 for admixtures (b), (g) and (j).

Table 15.7 Admixture 8.5% Travasol injection (500 ml) and trace mineral additives (5 ml)

	Storage conditions	(mg/l)	6 *h* (mg/l)	△%	24 *h* (mg/l)	△%
Zn	5 °C	4.28	4.32	+0.93	4.46	+4.21
	RT	4.14	4.25	+2.65	4.19	+1.21
Mn	5 °C	2.08	2.17	+4.33	2.18	+4.81
	RT	2.14	2.21	+3.27	2.21	+3.27
Cu	5 °C	2.00	1.89	−5.50	1.85	−7.50
	RT	1.96	1.91	−2.55	1.83	−6.63
I	5 °C	(0.24)	(0.24)	−0.40	(0.23)	−3.00
	RT	(0.24)	(0.24)	+1.60	(0.24)	+0.70
Cr	5 °C	(0.004)	(0.004)	+0.54	(0.004)	−0.21
	RT	(0.004)	(0.004)	+1.50	(0.004)	+3.10
Visual examination	5 °C	Clear	Clear		Clear	
	RT	Clear	Clear		Clear	
pH	5 °C	5.9	5.9		5.9	
	RT	5.9	5.9		5.9	

Table 15.8 Admixture 8.5% Travasol injection (500 ml) and 50% dextrose injection (500 ml) and trace mineral additive (5 ml)

	Storage conditions	*Initial* (mg/l)	6 *h* (mg/l)	△%	24 *h* (mg/l)	△%
Zn	5 °C	1.96	1.90	−3.06	1.96	0
	RT	2.10	1.90	−9.25	2.00	2.86
Mn	5 °C	1.13	1.20	+6.19	1.17	+3.54
	RT	1.17	1.24	+5.98	1.21	+1.03
Cu	5 °C	1.18	1.18	0	1.20	+1.70
	RT	1.22	1.20	−1.64	1.23	+0.82
I	5 °C	(0.12)	(0.12)	−0.3%	(0.12)	−0.5%
	RT	(0.12)	(0.12)	−2.0%	(0.12)	+1.8%
Cr	5 °C	(0.002)	(0.002)	−0.93	(0.002)	−1.60
	RT	(0.002)	(0.002)	+0.90	(0.002)	+0.63
Visual examination	5 °C	Clear	Clear		Clear	
	RT	Clear	Clear		Clear	
pH	5 °C	5.8	5.8		5.8	
	RT	5.8	5.8		5.8	

Data of this type are necessary for a new intravenous additive so as to provide adequate directions for use. Further studies of this nature are required increasingly in support of product registrations.

CONCLUSION

A Travenol trace element intravenous additive under development is described. It has been demonstrated to be stable after 6 months' ageing and further shelf life studies are continuing. Admixtures of the intravenous additives with large volume intravenous fluids employed in total parenteral nutrition were found to be physically and chemically compatible.

ACKNOWLEDGEMENTS

I acknowledge with appreciation A. N. Mather, Biochemistry Department, R. L. Nedich and W. E. Brochu, Pharmacy Department, and J. D. Lueck, Analytical Department of Travenol Laboratories for the analytical data on the trace element contents of large volume parenterals and the admixture studies.

References

1. Dudrick, S. J., *et al.* (1974). Long term parenteral nutrition with growth, development, and positive nitrogen balance. *Surgery*, **64,** 134
2. Recommended dietary allowances. Food and Nutrition Board (1974). *National Research Council, 8th Edition*
3. Vallee, B. L., *et al.* (1956, 1957). Zinc metabolism in hepatic dysfunction. *N. Engl. J. Med.*, **255,** 403; Correlation of metabolic patterns with biochemical findings. *N. Engl. J. Med.*, **257,** 22, 1055
4. Henzel, *et al.* (1967). Significance of magnesium and zinc metabolism in the surgical patient. *Arch. Surg.*, **95,** 991
5. Karpel, J. and Peden, V. (1972). Copper deficiency in long-term parenteral nutrition. *J. Pediat.*, **80,** 32
6. Prasad, A. D., *et al.* (1963). Zinc metabolism in patients with zinc syndrome of iron deficiency anaemia, hepatosplenomegaly, dwarfism, and hypogonadism. *J. Lab. Clin. Med.*, **61,** 537
7. Tucker, S. B., *et al.* (1976). Acquired zinc deficiency. *J. Am. Med. Assoc.*, **235,** 2399
8. Okada, A., *et al.* (1976). Skin lesions during intravenous hyperalimentation. Zinc deficiency. *Surgery*, **80,** 629
9. Hoffmann, R. P. and Ashby, D. M. (1976). Trace element concentrations in commercially available solutions. *Drug. Intell. Clin. Pharm.*, **10,** 75
10. Bozian, R. C. and Shearer, C. (1976). Copper, zinc and manganese content of four amino acid and protein hydrolysate preparations. *Am. J. Clin. Nutr.*, **29,** 1331
11. Jetton, M. M., *et al.* (1976). Trace element contamination of intravenous solutions. *Arch. Int. Med.*, **136,** 782
12. Shils, M. E. (1972). Minerals in total parenteral nutrition. *Drug. Intell. Clin. Pharm.*, **6,** 385
13. Hull, R. L. (1974). Use of trace elements in intravenous hyperalimentation solutions. *Am. J. Hosp. Pharm.*, **31,** 759
14. Jeejeebhoy, K. N., *et al.* (1973). Total parenteral nutrition at home. A study of technical and metabolic features. *Gastroenterology*, **65,** 811

16
Zinc and other trace elements

G. S. FELL AND R. R. BURNS

INTRODUCTION

At least fourteen trace elements (Cr, Co, Cu, F, I, Fe, Mn, Mo, Ni, Se, Si, Sn, V and Zn) are known to be required for the normal growth and development of one or more animal species[1]. Many of these elements have only recently been considered as essential, from evidence provided by animal growth experiments conducted by Schwarz and his colleagues[2].

All of these elements must play some part in the regulation of biochemical pathways. Numerous metalloenzymes are known and trace elements activate or inhibit many intracellular biochemical processes.

It has been customary to consider only seven of these elements (Co, Cu, Fe, F, I, Mn and Zn) as important in human nutrition, and deficiencies of most of these cause signs and symptoms in man similar to those reported in experimental animals. To some extent, the prolonged use of total parenteral nutrition (TPN) has alerted clinicians to the necessity of providing an adequate range and quantity of the essential inorganic micronutrients. Clinical effects attributed to acute deficiency of Cu and Zn are now well established[1], and there is some evidence that Cr and Mn deficiency can occur during prolonged intravenous feeding[3,4]. The provision of *complete* parenteral nutrition, as defined by Shenkin and Wretlind[5], does require the clinician to supply *all* known nutrients present in the normal diet. Furthermore, they should be provided in the same quantity and chemical form as that absorbed from the gastrointestinal tract and taken up by the portal circulation.

Present knowledge of many aspects of nutrition is inadequate to allow the formulation of intravenous feeding regimes on this basis, and in particular data on trace element metabolism is lacking.

It is often assumed that the trace metal content of whole blood, blood products and other intravenous fluids, such as protein hydrolysates, will supply most requirements. The trace element content of the purified solutions often employed is rather low[6], and insufficient to meet the requirements in clinical situations where TPN is required for weeks or months. Various trace element mixtures are now used intravenously and although they vary widely in the range and quantity of the elements provided[7,8], they do prevent the overt signs of deficiency. Whether the available formulations are fully adequate in all clinical circumstances is less certain and it is useful to consider the type of information which would be required to design appropriate mixtures of the known essential trace elements.

DIETARY CONTENT AND INTESTINAL ABSORPTION

As a first step to the estimation of intravenous dosage, some knowledge is needed of the normal dietary content of each essential trace element and its absorption across the intestinal mucosa. Recommended dietary levels for seven essential elements are proposed, although these vary widely for each element[9]. One such example is shown in Table 16.1

Table 16.1 Recommended daily dietary allowance, for seven trace metals*

Element	*mg/day*
Co (as Vit B_{12})	0.00013
Cu	2
F	3
Fe	10
I	0.1–0.15
Mn	2–3
Zn	15

* Taken from National Research Council (1974), *Recommended Dietary Allowances*, 8th ed. (Washington, Nat. Acad. Sci. and WHO (1973). *Tech. Rep. Ser. Wld Hlth Org.* no. 532)

There are no recommendations as to the dietary content of the remaining essential elements (Cr, Mo, Ni, Se, Si, Sn and V). The variable nature of the intestinal uptake of essential trace elements is a considerable problem, and little is known of the mechanism of intestinal mucosal transport, of the various inter-element competitive effects and of the blocking effects of other substances in the diet[10]. The use of a single percentage uptake figure for each element to convert oral dietary intake to intravenous dosage is not recommended.

Most elements occur in foodstuffs as organo-complexes. Some of these may be absorbed preferentially from the gut and some such as Co in the cobalamines or Cr in the 'glucose tolerance factor' of yeast[11], have a biological potency much greater than inorganic salts of the element. It may be desirable therefore to infuse the appropriate form of an essential trace element as well as the correct total amount.

BLOOD TRANSPORT AND TISSUE DISTRIBUTION

Once absorbed, each element is carried in portal blood to the liver where redistribution amongst various transport proteins may occur, and allow the element to be conveyed in the peripheral circulation in a form suitable for cellular absorption. It is useful to recognize these processes for each element given intravenously, since this may allow the selection of a laboratory test able to detect early signs of deficiency and help to give guidance about the effectiveness of therapy.

The pattern of tissue distribution differs considerably amongst the various elements. Some, for example iron, exist in a reserve or storage form as haemosiderin in bone marrow. Whether equivalent reserves are present for other elements is less certain, and many may require regular daily intake to maintain optimal tissue concentrations.

ROUTES OF EXCRETION

The maintenance of intracellular concentrations of the essential elements at an appropriate level, in spite of a very variable dietary supply, requires efficient homeostatic mechanisms to regulate excretion and absorption. The routes of excretion differ for the various elements. Many are excreted via the gastrointestinal tract into the faeces. A proportion of the absorbed elements is secreted into the gut in bile, pancreatic juice or other intestinal fluids. For some elements urinary excretion is of importance and the homeostatic control of renal output is a primary mechanism for conservation. Thus the early stages of Mg deficiency are best detected by finding a low urine magnesium output. Significant losses of certain elements occur in sweat[9] and even excretion in expired air is said to take place in selenium metabolism[9]. Knowledge of the various methods of excretion is obviously important when attempting metabolic balance studies.

ALTERATIONS TO TRACE ELEMENT METABOLISM

Even if the 'normal' or basal requirements were known for most trace elements, it is certain that for the ill patient, substantially different and often increased requirements exist. Trace element metabolism is altered by the response to injury, disease and infection.

Metabolic response to injury

The endocrine events following trauma produce a complex series of biochemical and physiological changes. Prominent amongst these is a reduction in the lean body mass, caused by the degradation of intracellular proteins.

D. P. Cuthbertson[12] noted the inappropriately high urine phosphorus excretion relative to that of Ca following long-bone injury. This led him to suspect protein catabolism of lean tissue as the origin of the phosphorus and not bone. Nitrogen balances demonstrate the extent of protein catabolism after trauma. More recently, atomic absorption spectrophotometry has allowed an extension of D. P. Cuthbertson's original observations to include other elements. Thus in Figure 16.1 it is seen that in a severely catabolic patient, some 3–5 weeks after a 55% burn injury, there is a greatly increased urinary zinc excretion which closely parallels that of N, K, Mg and creatine, and doubtless other end-products of protein breakdown. Similar studies on children show increases in copper[13] and chromium[14] excretion in urine.

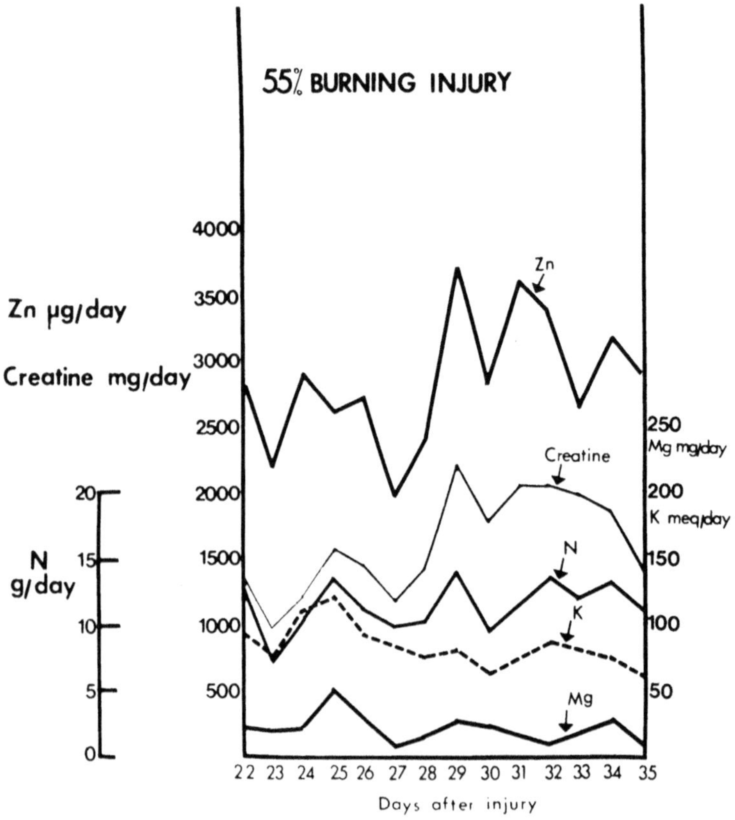

Figure 16.1 Increased urine excretion of Zn (normal output about 500 µg/day), following burn injury, showing relationship to other products of skeletal muscle catabolism

Such changes in trace element metabolism are of interest as a guide to the nature of the response to injury and may be an index of patient recovery. Where such losses of essential inorganic nutrients are prolonged and input is inadequate, an acquired deficiency will result.

Effect of disease and infection

Changes in the whole blood or serum levels of various trace metals occur in a wide range of diseases. Few such changes are specific, and may instead be secondary alterations caused by a redistribution of the given element amongst the various body compartments or by changes in the plasma transport proteins. The central role of the liver in the metabolism of many elements is demonstrated by changes in serum iron, copper and zinc, and by alterations of the urinary excretion of these elements in various liver diseases.

Marked changes in trace element metabolism occur in infectious disease. A rapid drop in plasma iron and zinc and a rise in copper concentrations are induced in the early stages of experimental infections in animals and man. These observations are part of a series of reactions apparently designed to redistribute nutrients to the liver and allow the elaboration of acute phase reactants as part of the immune response[15]. The abrupt removal of some inorganic micronutrients from circulating blood plasma may also confer a degree of 'nutritional immunity' by denying invading pathogens these essential trace metals[16].

DIAGNOSIS OF TRACE ELEMENT DEFICIENCY

Although modern analytical methods allow the determination of many trace elements with good sensitivity, not all can be determined directly in biological material due to serious and variable interference effects.

As methodology improves, the reported 'normal values' change. Thus much of the earlier literature records high results for some elements. For example, the concentration of chromium in blood has changed from 35 μg Cr/l in 1948 to 0.72 μg/l in 1974 with a wide range of estimates being made in the intervening years[17].

Even where reliable analytical methods are available and contamination can be avoided during sample collection and storage, there remains the considerable problem of the interpretation of results. Most essential elements are intracellular, but blood plasma or serum is the usual material submitted for analysis. Variations in the circulating levels of the element which occur secondarily to the effects of injury, disease and infection must therefore be allowed for when attempting to assess a possible tissue depletion of the element based upon its measurement in such extracellular fluids.

Since a wide range of intracellular biochemical reactions are trace-element-dependent, it is possible to examine enzyme activities and metabolite concentrations with a view to the detection of changes in advance of the clinical presentation of deficiency.

For example, the importance of iron supply for haemoglobin synthesis is well recognized. Yet serum iron concentration is a poor guide to the iron status of an individual since this is affected by numerous factors unrelated to the body reserves of iron. The development of a low haemoglobin concentration is a late stage in iron deficiency which could, however, be diagnosed at a pre-clinical stage by measurement of red cell protoporphyrin, a metabolite which increases in concentration when the synthesis of haem is limited by iron availability. Other laboratory tests may be designed to measure the effects of stressing biochemical pathways known to be dependent upon a particular trace element. Thus it is proposed that marginal deficiency of Cr may be revealed by glucose loading. A failure of increase in plasma and urinary Cr in response to a glucose tolerance test is thought to be suggestive of sub-clinical Cr deficiency, although interpretation of this test is still questionable.

Further examples of such biochemical investigations are known, but all depend on detailed understanding of biochemical pathways involving the trace element. For many essential elements such as Mn, Ni, V, Sn, Si, Mo and Se, very little indeed is understood of their role in human biochemistry.

ASPECTS OF ZINC METABOLISM

To illustrate some of the general observations made in the preceding sections, a more detailed account is now given of zinc metabolism. Within the last 10 years there has been a rapid increase in knowledge of zinc biochemistry in human medicine. Useful reviews are by Prasad 1976[18], Halsted *et al.* 1974[19], and Underwood 1977[1].

Clinical importance

Zinc is known to be essential for the normal growth and development of micro-organisms, plants, animals and man. Clinical interest was first stimulated by reports that zinc deficiency was a complicating factor in growth defects of certain populations in Middle Eastern countries. Addition of zinc supplements to the diet reversed many of the clinical signs and symptoms reported.

Use of oral zinc therapy at high dosage is said to improve wound healing in surgical patients, and this treatment is used effectively in the management of varicose ulcers.

The prolonged use of TPN without the addition of zinc to the intravenous fluids may result in skin rash, hair loss and intestinal disorders in susceptible patients, many of these symptoms being relieved by the addition of zinc. The clinical presentation of the condition acrodermatitis enteropathica is similar and it is thought that this serious condition of early childhood is an inborn error of intestinal zinc absorption[20]. Dramatic improvements in the skin rash, intestinal symptoms and the regrowth of hair are observed after zinc therapy. An important observation in such zinc-deficient children is an impairment of immune response with increased susceptibility to opportunistic bacterial infection.

Loss of appetite in experimental animals is an early sign of zinc deficiency and an impairment of taste and smell in zinc-deficient patients is reported. Zinc deficiency may therefore contribute to the anorexia which complicates the management of seriously undernourished patients.

Dietary intake of zinc and intestinal absorption

Zinc is present in most foodstuffs, and normal mixed diets provide an adequate supply. Since first-class protein, in particular animal protein, is considered the best source of readily absorbed zinc, there is a possibility that certain deprived populations may not receive the recommended intake of some 15–20 mg zinc/day. A survey of hospital diets showed them to be marginally deficient in some cases[21]. The intestinal absorption of zinc is affected by the nature of the diet consumed. Plant fibre and phytic acid from cereal foodstuffs inhibit the absorption of zinc and this is thought to be an important cause of the nutritional deficiencies reported in the Middle Eastern populations. The amount of dietary zinc absorbed varies considerably, and earlier reports of figures of 10–15% for intestinal uptake are now considered low, and values of around 35% considered more representative[9].

In our own experimental work, using ^{65}Zn chloride, values of from 8% to 85% absorption were recorded. Little change in an individual patient's blood level was seen after 3 months of oral zinc sulphate (220 mg zinc sulphate/tid) was given[22]. This did not suggest any feedback control of zinc absorption, which has been proposed[10]. In effect little is known of the absorption of zinc from the gut and therefore it is difficult to recommend confidently a basal intravenous requirement. In practice, clinical experience seems to suggest that about 3 mg zinc/day is required in intravenous fluids to avoid the development of a negative zinc balance[5].

Body distribution

Use of ^{65}Zn has shown that zinc given orally or intravenously concentrates initially in the liver, and then is distributed to muscle, bone and other tissues (Figure 16.2). Equilibration is rapid with organs such as the liver, kidney and pancreas; it is slower with muscle, red cells and bone. As long as 3–4 months is required for full equilibration of ^{65}Zn, and the rate-limiting factor is bone uptake. In man, about 2–4 g of zinc is present in the whole body. In terms of percentage content, skeletal muscle has 60%, bone and skin around 20%

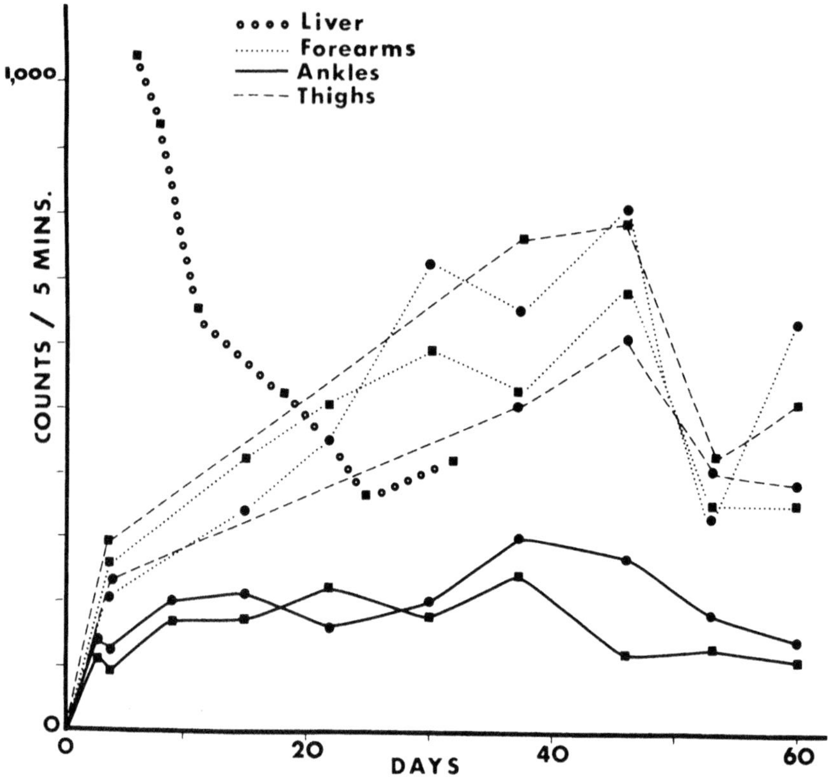

Figure 16.2 Distribution of radioactive counts following oral dosage with 5 μCi of $^{65}Zn\,Cl_2$. After some 30 days the activities over liver and muscle (thighs and forearms) are about equal

each, and the remainder is distributed in various organs and in blood. Schroeder[23], has noted the high proportion of zinc present in skeletal muscle. He also noted that in muscle cells zinc concentration is greater than that of calcium; therefore in this tissue zinc may be thought of as a bulk element. Almost all zinc (98%) is intracellular, having the third highest concentration of the divalent cations inside cells.

Subcellular location of zinc

Detailed studies of the location of zinc in liver, mammary and muscle cells are reported[24]. The metal is found in all cell fractions but is in highest concentration in the supernatant or cytoplasmic fractions following ultra-centrifuge separations.

We have studied ^{65}Zn distribution in rat skeletal muscle and some results are shown in Table 16.2. The cytoplasmic zinc (40K supernatant) was further investigated by gel chromatography and electrophoresis and shown to consist of at least seven proteins of unknown structure.

Table 16.2 Subcellular fractionation of rat muscle, by ultracentrifugation. (Two rats, given 100 μCi ^{65}Zn by intubation, 2 weeks prior to sacrifice)

	^{65}Zn (cpm)	*Percentage activity*	*Percentage DNA*
Total homogenate	17 400	100	100
3K pellet	5260	30	86.5
40K pellet	600	3	6.6
40K supernatant	12 150	70	nil

Blood content and zinc transport

The total amount of extracellular zinc is less than 2%, but zinc content of circulating blood plasma is important in terms of intestinal absorption and transport to tissue cells. Early studies by Vallee and Gibson[25] show that of whole blood zinc, some 75–88% is in red cells, probably as the zinc metalloenzyme carbonic anhydrase. Plasma zinc forms from 12% to 22% of the whole blood zinc content and the white cells have 3%, although each individual white cell has a high intracellular concentration. The total plasma zinc concentration of about 100 μg zinc/100 ml is similar to that of iron and copper. With the availability of atomic absorption spectrophotometry, numerous studies of plasma zinc in health and disease have been published[19]. Many physiological factors such as age, sex, diet, circadian variation, as well as the method of analysis, affect the reference values. Most disease processes lower the total plasma zinc, and this is a non-specific response to any 'stress' such as acute infection or injury. Zinc in plasma is distributed into three main fractions. Fraction 1 (20–30%) is an α_2 macroglobulin and does not alter significantly as total plasma zinc decreases. The zinc in this molecule is very firmly bound, and it is not therefore likely that it is an important transport protein. Fraction 2 (50–60%) is zinc associated with plasma albumin, and this is the labile fraction of plasma zinc which does decrease markedly in disease and in response to infusions of ACTH[26]. A much smaller fraction (fraction 3, approximately 10%) is probably in equilibrium with fraction 2. This consists of low molecular weight compounds of zinc (less than 10 000 daltons), probably mainly zinc amino acid complexes.

By a combination of selective protein precipitation and an ultrafiltration technique we have estimated the distribution of zinc in normal plasma and the results are shown in Table 16.3.

Table 16.3 Distribution of Zn between the main plasma fractions, in ten healthy persons

Total Zn μg/100 ml)	*Fraction I* α_2 *macroglobulin Zn*	*Fraction II albumin Zn*	*Fraction III ultrafilterable Zn*
83.6 ± 11.7	24.1 ± 13.1	50.3 ± 13.7	9.1 ± 7.8
% of total	28.8%	65.8%	10.8%

Intracellular biochemical functions of zinc and effects of deficiency

About seventy metalloenzymes have now been characterized and zinc may also activate or inhibit numerous other biochemical pathways. Most stages of both nucleic acid and protein synthesis are zinc-dependent, and therefore normal cellular functions and cell replication are affected by zinc deficiency. In zinc-deficient animals' tissue zinc, RNA, DNA and total protein are all lowered, whereas ribonuclease activity and the concentration of free amino acids are increased[27]. Hsu has clearly shown an impairment of amino acid incorporation into skin protein of zinc-deficient animals[28].

Numerous other biochemical changes in zinc-deficient animals are reported, but few such changes are clearly described for man. One consistent finding in severe human zinc deficiency is a reduction in serum alkaline phosphatase and its restoration to normal activity by zinc therapy[29]. Persistent hypoproteinaemia is reported by Fodor *et al.*[30] in a severely zinc-deficient patient, and is only improved when substantial zinc replacement therapy is given (Figure 16.3).

Determination of specific plasma proteins such as retinol-binding protein, synthesis of which is zinc-dependent, may give an early indication of diminished hepatic protein synthesis in malnourished patients with marginal zinc deficiency[31].

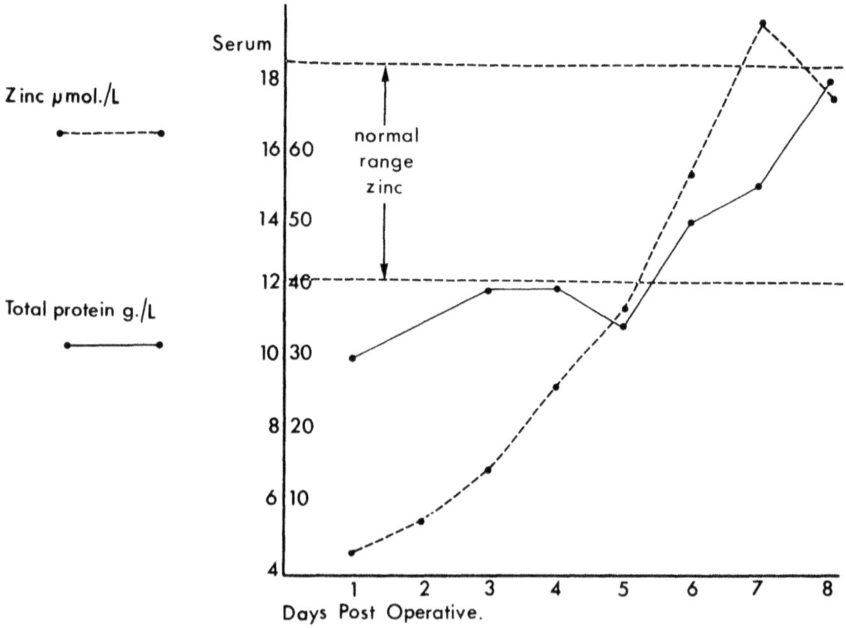

Figure 16.3 Improvement in total protein levels as serum Zn concentration increases during intravenous Zn therapy (80 mg Zn aspartate/day). ('Normal range' for serum Zn equivalent to 78–119 μg Zn/100 ml). (Redrawn from Fodor *et al.*[30])

Excretion of zinc

The main route of excretion of zinc is in the faeces. The faecal output consists both of unabsorbed dietary zinc and a smaller proportion as zinc secreted into the gut in various intestinal fluids such as pancreatic juice and bile. Using oral doses of ^{65}Zn, Spencer *et al.*[32] have shown that after 21 days 70% of the dose is excreted in faeces, and only 2% in urine, with 28% tissue retention. Urinary zinc excretion is normally less than 0.5 mg/day and is independent of dietary intake. Calculations suggest that to maintain this low urinary output at least 99% of the plasma zinc (fraction 3) filtered at the renal glomerulus must be re-absorbed. Any increase in the diffusible or ultra-filterable fractions in plasma will therefore exceed the tubular re-absorptive capacity and result in zincuria. By a similar mechanism diffusion of zinc across the intestinal mucosa into the gut may also increase losses of endogenous zinc in the faeces, although this is much more difficult to prove due to the variable amounts of unabsorbed dietary zinc normally present.

Significant loss of zinc in sweat also occurs and up to 5 mg zinc/day could be lost in this manner. It is apparent that the determination of a zinc balance for a critically ill patient, while technically feasible, is practically very difficult. Losses in fistula fluid, wound exudate, shed skin and hair would have to be measured to provide an accurate zinc balance.

Metabolic response to injury and zinc metabolism

The complex series of endocrine events associated with physiological and biochemical changes after injury alter zinc metabolism along with other biochemical pathways. Typical changes observed in the plasma and urine following elective orthopaedic surgery are illustrated in Figure 16.4. The net catabolism of skeletal muscle protein is a consistent feature of the response to injury and involves the degradation of zinc metalloproteins along with other protein molecules of muscle. Several zinc metalloproteins are located in the soluble cell fraction of rat muscle so that the degradation products could be released as zinc amino acid or zinc peptide complexes into the circulating blood plasma. In this way fraction 3 of plasma is increased, the re-absorptive capacity of the renal tubules exceeded and zincuria occurs. This mechanism can occur in spite of the apparent lowering of the total plasma zinc, since it appears that the stress of surgery, or infection, can lower the albumin zinc fraction in plasma possibly under the influence of ACTH[26]. In effect this means that there has been a redistribution of zinc among the plasma fractions as a response to injury.

The increased urinary zinc excretion does originate from endogenous tissue, most probably muscle, as demonstrated by giving oral ^{65}Zn to patients some 3–5 weeks prior to surgery. This is sufficient time to allow equilibration of ^{65}Zn with skeletal muscle (Figure 16.2). When measurements of

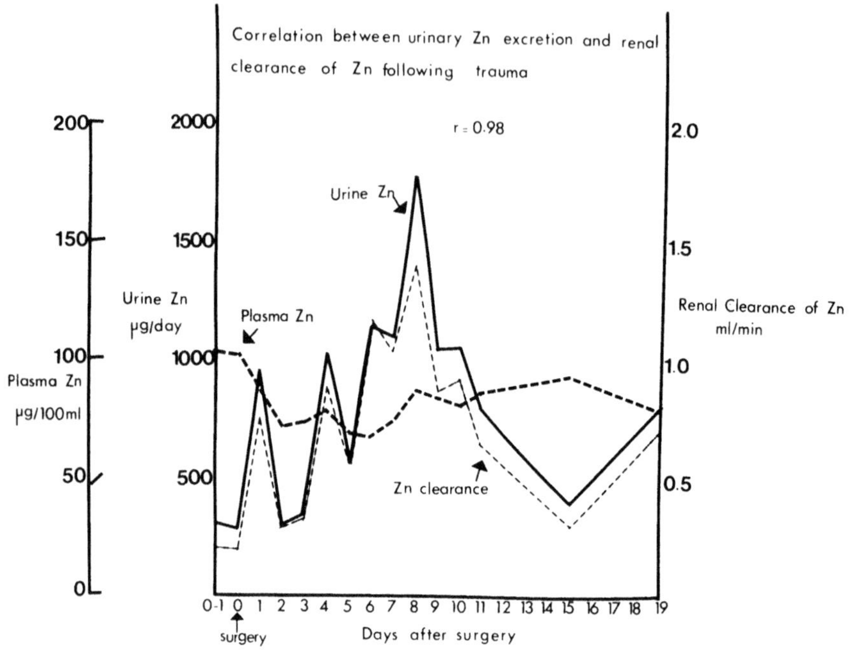

Figure 16.4 Changes in plasma Zn concentration and urinary Zn excretion following total hip replacement. The increase in urine Zn is greatest at about 5–10 days after operation while the plasma Zn remains below the initial pre-operative levels for at least 14 days

^{65}Zn and stable zinc in urine are made (Figure 16.5) there is a close correlation, suggesting a common tissue origin. In other studies it has been shown that the extent and duration of the zincuria is proportional to the severity of the injury[33]. When this urinary zinc loss is translated into the equivalent of muscle tissue broken down, a reasonable agreement with similar calculations based upon urinary nitrogen is observed (Figure 16.6), although calculations based on nitrogen and zinc do give a lower estimate than those based upon potassium.

There is a sustained increase in urinary zinc during total starvation of obese subjects. Yet during many months of such zinc loss (approximately 5 mg/day) total plasma zinc does not decrease but may even increase[34]. When semi-starvation (600 kcal/day) was used following hip fracture in an obese patient, we also found an increased urinary zinc loss which lasted until resumption of normal diet (Figure 16.7). The dissociation of urinary zinc and urinary creatine excretion after the first few weeks of the study does suggest that in this case muscle zinc is not the only source of urinary zinc output. It seems possible that the keto acids, produced in starvation as a consequence of increased fat mobilization, could form stable zinc chelates and increase the proportion of zinc in fraction 3 which is then available for urinary excretion.

Yet another mechanism for increasing the diffusible proportion of zinc in

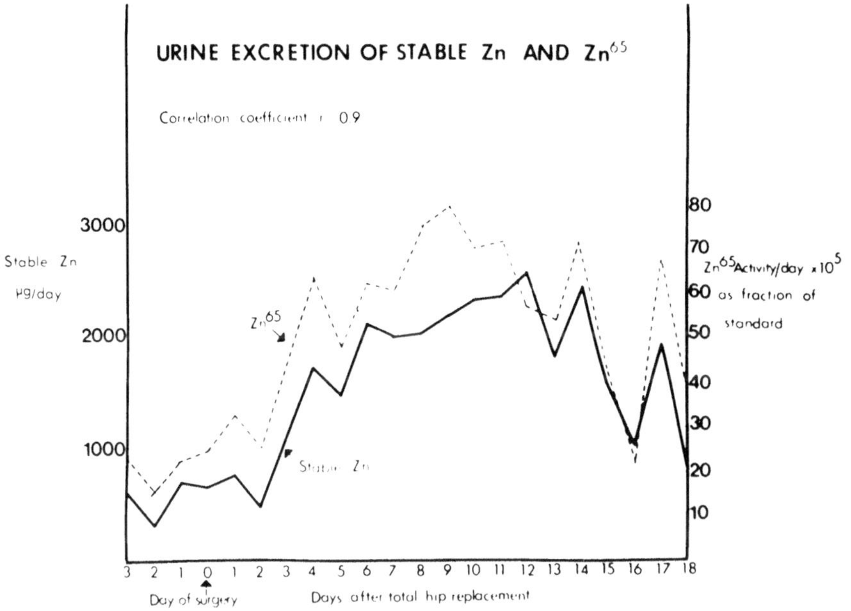

Figure 16.5 Measurement of ^{65}Zn and total Zn content of urine following surgery. 5 μCi of ^{65}Zn Cl_2 given 4 weeks prior to operation. Parallel excretion of ^{65}Zn and stable Zn suggest a common tissue origin, namely skeletal muscle

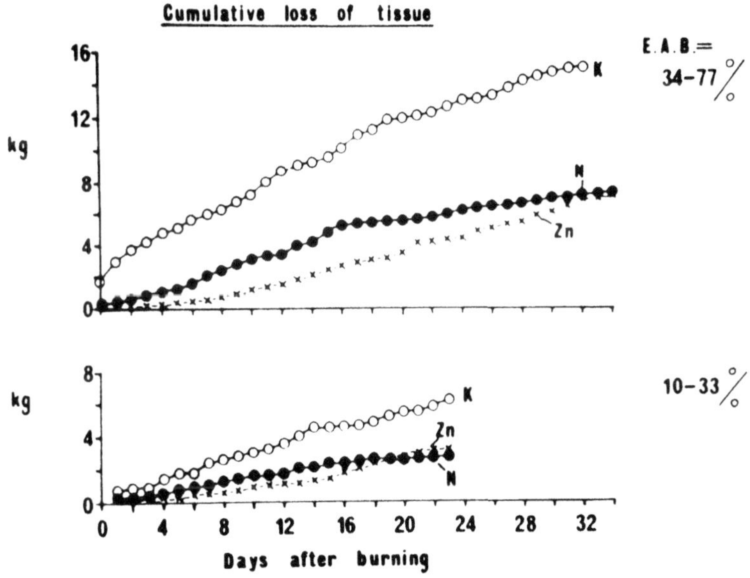

Figure 16.6 Cumulative loss of body tissue calculated from the urinary excretion of Zn, N and K, for two groups of patients with differing estimated area of burns (EAB)

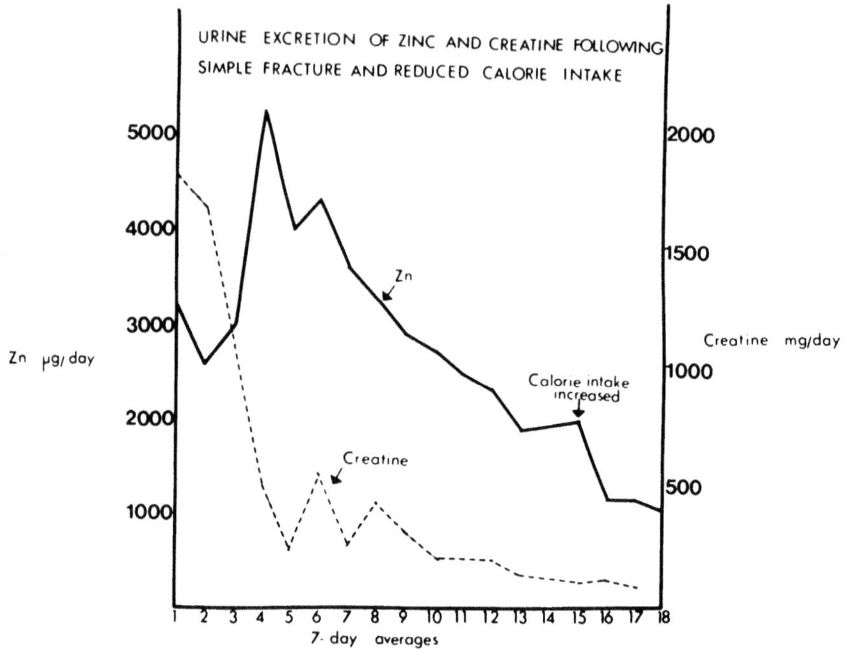

Figure 16.7 Increased urine zinc (normal <500 μg/day) persisting until normal food intake is resumed

plasma is the therapeutic use of certain drugs which can form highly stable chelation complexes with zinc. Experimental studies by Tarui, 1959[35] established that known chelating agents such as EDTA, BAL, 8-hydroxyquinoline and others did increase urinary zinc loss. Drugs which also have this effect include penicillamine, ethanbutol and certain antibiotics. Quite dramatic zinc deficiency in a young man taking penicillamine for treatment of Wilson's disease has been described by Klinberg, Prasad and Oberleas[36]. Hair loss and severe skin changes were greatly improved when oral zinc therapy was given.

Immediately following the inoculation of experimental animals with various pathogens there is a rapid drop in plasma zinc concentration as well as a decline in those of iron and free amino acids. These substances are taken up by the liver and used for the elaboration of acute phase reactants, such as caeruloplasmin and other glycoproteins. The whole process may be initiated by a substance released from leucocytes known as leucocyte endogenous mediator, or LEM. Active extracts can be prepared from white cells of infected animals and these are assayed by the extent of the decrease in plasma zinc following injections of the extract into other experimental animals[15]. It is thus apparent that total plasma zinc is low during periods of infection and will not reflect tissue zinc content.

Zinc deficiency during Total Parenteral Nutrition

Zinc deficiency is now recognized as a potential complication of prolonged TPN when inadequate zinc is present in the intravenous fluids. The majority of patients have a previous history of gastrointestinal disease, often with severe post-operative complications[37-39]. After several weeks of successful management the patients can exhibit variable degrees of dermatitis, which often starts in the nasolabial areas and spreads to the rest of the face, the perianal area and the other parts of the body. Bacterial and fungal invasions of the lesions are common and are often resistant to antibiotic or other therapy. Typical skin changes are shown in Figures 16.8 and 16.9.

Other clinical effects noted include moderate or severe abdominal pain, with increased bowel frequency. In many patients mental depression and personality changes are reported. A late stage in the deficiency disease is the partial or complete loss of head hair. There is a complete reversal of most of these signs and symptoms within a few days or weeks of giving zinc intravenously. Regrowth of hair is the last stage of complete recovery and may take weeks or months to complete.

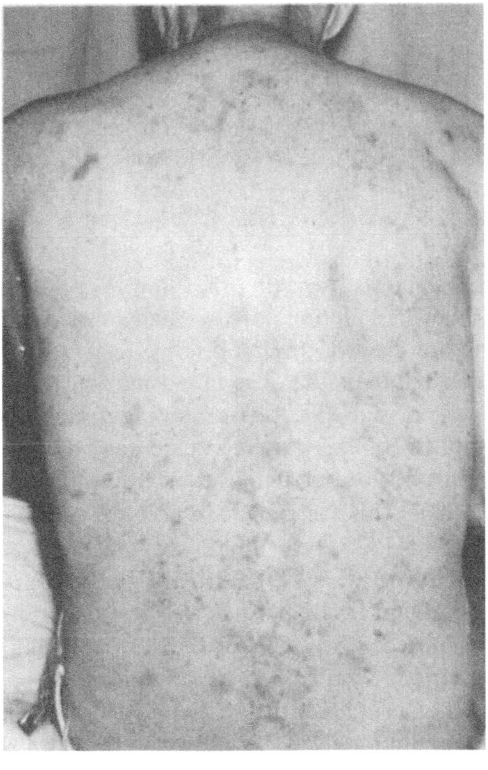

Figure 16.8

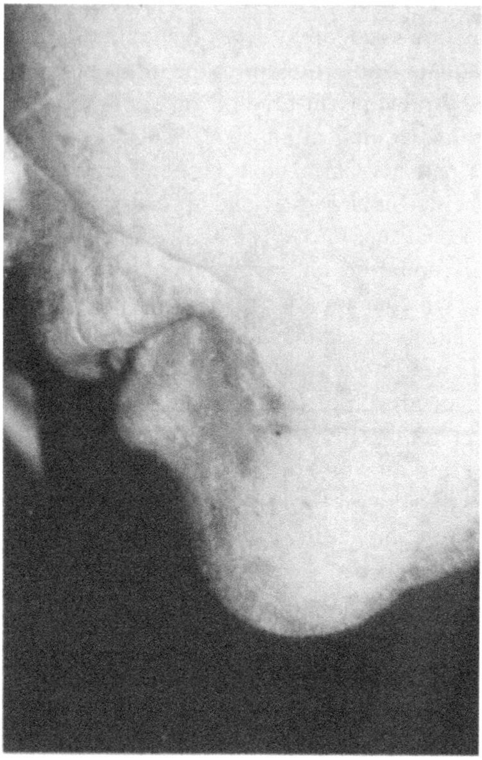

Figure 16.9

The biochemical changes preceding the clinical development of deficiency are of interest. Good descriptions of the changes in zinc concentrations in plasma and urine are given in the reports by Kay *et al.*[37,38]. One of their cases demonstrates well the rapid drop in plasma zinc to below half 'normal' during the recovery or anabolic phase of weight gain. These changes are illustrated in Figure 16.10. This particular case was a 42-year-old woman with a long history of post-operative complications following total protocolectomy for ulcerative colitis. This patient had become severely emaciated and responded well to TPN (5000 kcal, 28 g N/day), with a weight gain of up to 7 kg in under 2 weeks. Although the urinary zinc excretion was somewhat elevated (around 5 mg/day) the plasma zinc remained almost normal until body weight gain started, when it fell within 14 days from 79 to 16 μg zinc/100 ml. Two days prior to intravenous zinc sulphate therapy (80 mg/day) the patient complained of a sore mouth and 'wind burned skin'. These symptoms cleared completely within 3 days of being given the extra zinc.

It is now apparent that some patients are at risk of developing degrees of zinc deficiency. Usually they will have a prior history of intestinal disease

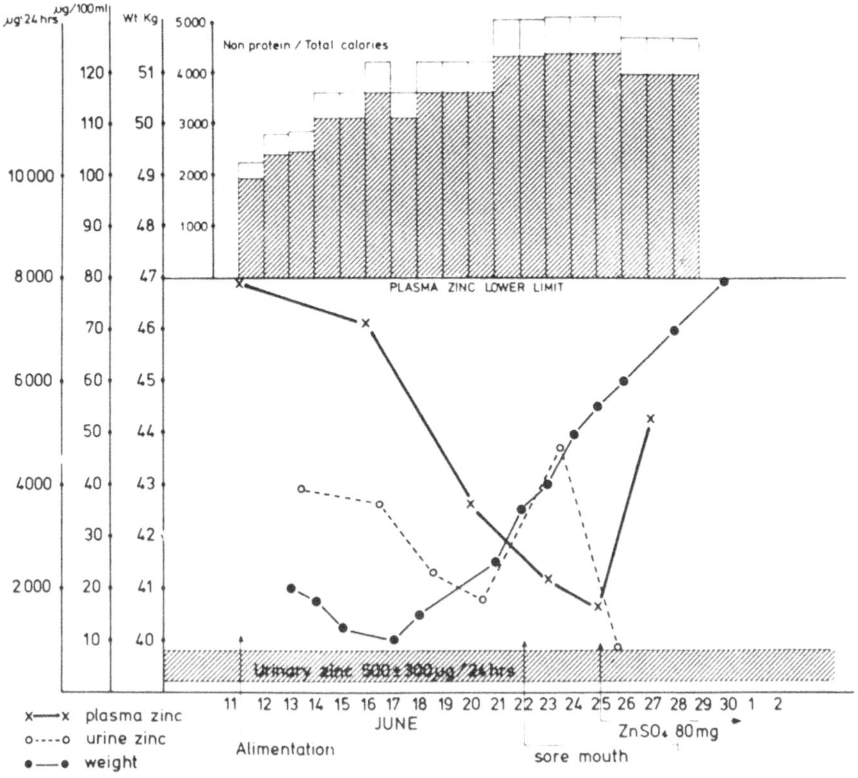

Figure 16.10 Changes in plasma and urine zinc in relation to body weight during prolonged TPN. As body weight increases plasma zinc concentration falls (Reproduced with permission)

which itself may have resulted in marginal zinc deficiency through malabsorption. In addition, the increased faecal and fistula fluid losses of zinc will have occurred over a period of many weeks prior to the institution of TPN. The fluid regimes given may not only lack sufficient zinc to make good such deficiencies but may also actively promote zinc loss. Freeman *et al.*[40] have noted that amino sugar complexes formed during the heat sterilization of certain intravenous nutrient mixtures can form stable zinc chelates and cause increased urinary zinc excretion.

The overt clinical signs of tissue zinc deficiency may not appear until there is an expansion of the body cell mass in the anabolic phase of recovery.

Diagnosis of zinc deficiency

The specific reversal of clinical signs and symptoms by zinc therapy remains the only unequivocal proof of the existence of clinical zinc deficiency. However, useful indications as to the potential development of such deficiency can be obtained from the following:

(*a*) *Zinc balance studies*
Even limited or partial estimation of the input and output of zinc may well reveal a negative zinc balance. If this persists then zinc deficiency will develop eventually.

(*b*) *Radioisotope studies*
^{65}Zn can be used to demonstrate a reduced 'exchangeable' zinc pool or, after full equilibration (3–4 months), be used to derive the total body zinc content by whole-body counting and isotope dilution calculations. However, since ^{65}Zn has a half-life of almost 300 days sequential patient studies are not possible.

(*c*) *Estimation of zinc concentrations in biological material*
The reliable determination of zinc in whole blood, blood plasma, red cells, leucocytes, skin, hair, faeces and urine are all now possible, providing appropriate care is taken with the analytical procedures.

The interpretation of such results, however, remains difficult at least until severe deficiency is already well established. The measurement of the zinc content of the various plasma zinc transport fractions[41], may well provide more useful information than simple determination of total plasma zinc. For example, a rapid drop in the albumin zinc fraction could precede any other measurable changes.

(*d*) *Biochemical consequences of zinc deficiency*
Various procedures designed to assess protein synthesis should be of value in revealing incipient zinc deficiency. Assay of specific plasma proteins such as albumin and retinol-binding protein are useful, and studies using labelled amino acids could well be considered. A cystine loading test has been proposed[19] with estimation of urinary sulphate as an index of cystine incorporation into protein.

The levels of zinc-dependent enzymes in tissue and circulating blood should also be of use but results are extremely variable in marginal deficiency. However, as noted above, persistently low levels of serum alkaline phosphatase remain the most consistent enzyme finding in fairly severe zinc deficiency.

CONCLUSIONS

Basic knowledge of the metabolism of all of the known essential trace elements is certainly insufficient to allow a fully scientific assessment of the intravenous requirements in common clinical circumstances. One of the most detailed proposals yet published[5] for nine of the trace elements is shown in

Table 16.4 Some allowance has been made for the moderate and high requirements which may be needed in different patients. The simpler mixtures used at present, of about seven trace elements, are largely based upon empirical clinical experience. If they are used early enough they may well avoid the development of frank deficiency and do not appear to cause adverse clinical side-effects.

Table 16.4 Suggested daily intravenous requirements for some essential trace elements for a 70 kg man[5]

Trace element	*Basal requirement*	*Moderate requirement* (mg)	*High requirement* (mg)
Fe	1.17 mg	1.95	3.91
Mn	0.38 mg	0.77	1.92
Zn	3.2 mg	6.4	6.9–13.7
Cu	0.31 mg	1.3	1.8–4.4
Cr	54.6 μg	—	—
Se	33.3 μg	—	—
Mo	20.1 μg	—	—
F	0.9 mg	—	—
I	133 μg	—	—

However, further detailed investigation of the full range of the essential trace elements is needed, and balance studies[9] should be conducted in a wide range of clinical conditions.

In view of the uncertainty as to the intravenous dosage, consideration should be given to using *oral* supplementation wherever at all practicable.

The need for nutritional supplementation with trace elements will be most evident during the recovery period when there is renewed growth in children and weight gain in adults.

Potential contra-indications to the intravenous use of substantial doses of certain essential elements may well be the presence of an active septicaemia or marked abnormalities of plasma protein concentration when the binding capacity of the various transport proteins could be impaired.

References

1. Underwood, E. J. (1977). *Trace Elements in Human and Animal Nutrition.* 4th Ed. (New York: Academic Press)
2. Schwarz, K. (1970). Control of environmental conditions in trace element research: an experimental approach to unrecognized trace element requirements. In C. F. Mills (ed.). *Trace Element Metabolism in Animals. Proceedings of WAAP/IBP International Symposium,* July 1969, Aberdeen
3. Jeejeebhoy, K. N., Chu, R., Marliss, E. B., Greenberg, G. R. and Bruce-Robertson, A. (1975). Chromium deficiency, diabetes and neuropathy, reversed by chromium infusion in a patient on total parenteral nutrition (TPN) for 3½ years. *Clin. Res.,* **23,** 636A
4. Doisy, Jr. E. A. (1972). Micronutrient control or biosynthesis of clotting protein and

cholesterol. In D. D. Hemphill (ed.). *Trace Substances in Environmental Health.* Vol. VI, p. 193. (Columbia: University of Missouri)

5. Shenkin, A. and Wretlind, A. (1977). Complete intravenous nutrition including amino acids, glucose and lipids. In *Nutritional Aspects of the Care of the Critically Ill* (In press). (London: Churchill-Livingstone)
6. James, B. E. and MacMahon, R. A. (1970). Trace elements in intravenous fluids. *Med. J. Aust.*, **1**, 1161
7. Hull, R. L. (1974). Use of trace elements in intravenous hyperalimentation solutions. *Am. J. Hosp. Pharm.*, **31**, 759
8. Shils, M. E., Wright, W. L., Turnbull, A. and Brescia, F. (1970). Longterm parenteral nutrition through an external arteriovenous shunt. *N. Engl. J. Med.*, **283**, 341
9. Jacobsen, S. and Wester, P. O. (1977). Balance studies of twenty trace elements during total parenteral nutrition in man. *Br. J. Nutr.*, **37**, 107
10. Evans, G. W. (1976). Zinc absorption and transport. In A. S. Prasad and D. Oberleas (eds.). *Trace Elements in Human Health and Disease* Vol. I, p. 186. (New York: Academic Press)
11. Doisy, R. J., Streeten, D. H. P., Freiberg, J. M. and Schreider, A. J. (1976). Chromium metabolism in man. In A. S. Prasad and D. Oberleas (eds.). *Trace Elements in Human Health and Disease*, Vol. II, p. 80. (New York: Academic Press)
12. Cuthbertson, D. P. (1930). The disturbance of metabolism produced by bony and non-bony injury, with notes on certain abnormal conditions of bone. *Biochem. J.*, **24**, 1244
13. Carr, G. and Wilkinson, A. W. (1975). Zinc and copper urinary excretion in children with burns and scalds. *Clin. Chim. Acta*, **61**, 199
14. Barlow, D. (1976). Institute of Child Health, London. Private communication
15. Beisel, W. R., Pekarek, R. S. and Waunemacher, R. W. (1976). Homeostatic mechanisms affecting plasma zinc levels in acute stress. In A. S. Prasad and D. Oberleas (eds.). *Trace Elements in Human Health and Disease*, Vol. I, p. 87. (New York: Academic Press)
16. Dixon, B. (1975). God's neglected handiwork. *World Medicine*, **10**, 23
17. Mertz, W. (1975). Trace-element nutrition in health and disease: contributions and problems of analysis. *Clin. Chem.*, **21**, 468
18. Prasad, A. S. and Oberleas, D. (eds.). (1976). *Trace Elements in Human Health and Disease*, Vol. III. (New York: Academic Press)
19. Halsted, J. A., Smith, Jr. J. C. and Irwin, M. J. (1974). A conspectus of research on zinc requirements of man. *J. Nutr.*, **104**, 345
20. Acrodermatitis enteropathica—a hereditary zinc deficiency. (1975). *Nutrition Reviews*, **31**, 327
21. Osis, D., Kramer, L., Wiatrouski, E. and Spencer, H. (1972). Dietary zinc intake in man. *Am. J. Clin. Nutr.*, **25**, 582
22. Husain, L. (1973). *The Metabolism of Zinc in some Human Skin Diseases.* Ph.D. Thesis, Glasgow University
23. Schroeder, H. A., Nason, A. P., Tipton, I. H. and Balassa, J. J. (1967). Essential trace metals in man: zinc in relation to environmental cadmium. *J. Chron. Dis.*, **20**, 179
24. Underwood, E. J. (1977). *Trace Elements in Human and Animal Nutrition.* 4th Ed. p. 197. (New York: Academic Press)
25. Vallee, B. L. and Gibson, J. G. (1948). The zinc content of normal human blood, plasma, leucocytes and erythrocytes. *J. Biol. Chem.*, **176**, 445
26. Falchuk, K. (1977). Effect of acute disease and ACTH on serum zinc proteins. *N. Engl. J. Med.*, **296**, 1129
27. Underwood, E. J. (1977). *Trace Elements in Human and Animal Nutrition.* 4th Ed. p. 220. (New York: Academic Press)
28. Hsu, J. M. (1974). Metabolic studies in rat skin during zinc deficiency. In W. J. Pories, W. H. Strain, J. M. Hsu, and R. L. Woosley. (eds.). *Clinical Applications of Zinc Metabolism.* pp. 43–56. (Springfield, Ill.: Charles C. Thomas)
29. Neldner, K. H. and Hambridge, K. M. (1975). Zinc therapy of acrodermatitis enteropathica. *N. Engl. J. Med.*, **292**, 879
30. Fodor, L., Eschner, J., Dick, W. and Ahnefeld, F. W. (1972). The clinical significance of the zinc deficiency syndrome. Relationships between zinc deficiency and hypoproteinaemia. *Anaesthetist*, **21**, 456

31. Smith, Jr. J. C., McDaniel, E. G., Fan, F. F. and Halsted, J. A. (1973). Zinc—a trace element essential in vitamin A metabolism. *Science*, **181**, 954
32. Spencer, H., Rossof, B., Fieldstain, A., Colin, S. H. and Gusamano, E., (1965). Metabolism of zinc^{65} in man. *Radiation Res.*, **24**, 432
33. Davies, J. W. L. and Fell, G. S. (1974). Tissue catabolism in patients with burns. *Clin. Chim. Acta*, **51**, 83
34. Spencer, H. and Samachson. J. (1970). Studies of zinc metabolism in man. In C. F. Mills (Ed.). *Trace Element Metabolism in Animals. Proceedings of WAAP/IBP International Symposium*, July 1969, Aberdeen
35. Tarui, S. (1959). Studies on zinc metabolism. The influences of chelating agents on urinary excretion of metals. *Med. J. Osaka Univ.*, **10**, 499
36. Klinberg, W. G., Prasad, A. S. and Oberleas, D. (1976). Zinc deficiency following penicillamine therapy. In *Trace Elements in Human Health and Disease*. Vol. I, p. 51. (New York: Academic Press)
37. Kay, R. G., Tasman-Jones, C., Pybus, J., Whiting, R. and Block, H. (1976). A syndrome of acute zinc deficiency during total parenteral alimentation in man. *Ann. Surg.*, **183**, 331
38. Kay, R. G. and Tasman-Jones, C. (1975). Acute zinc deficiency in man during IV alimentation. *Aust. N.Z. J. Surg.*, **45**, 325
39. Tucker, B. T., Schroter, A. L., Brown, P. W. and McCall, J. T. (1976). Acquired zinc deficiency, *J. Am. Med. Assoc.*, **235**, 2399
40. Freeman, J. B., Stegink, L. P., Meyer, P. D., Fry, L. K. and Denbesten, L. (1975). Excessive urinary zinc losses during parenteral alimentation. *J. Surg. Res.*, **18**, 463
41. Fell, G. S. and Burns, R. R. (1976). Zinc. *Proc. Roy. Soc. Med.*, **69**, 474

Panel Discussion

D. B. Allardyce: (Canada) It appeared that the fairly large amount of zinc in Travasol* did not appear to be sufficient to prevent clinical zinc deficiency in a patient who is rapidly anabolizing and gaining weight. That 1000 or 1200 μg in Travasol is obviously insufficient. As Dr Fell pointed out, the patients did gradually better for 3–4, or 5 weeks, and as soon as they got into a rapidly anabolizing phase, gained weight, and became ambulant, with returning muscle mass, the whole thing was spoiled at this point by the appearance of dermatitis.

Dr Fell's picture showed typical facial effects. All that I can add is that there is quite a severe scrotal component in the males which is extremely distressing. I have noticed that previously healed incisions break down, as one might expect in scurvy, with secondary infection.

Dr Kartinos showed that Amigen contains a lot of zinc. We thought initially that Travasol must be causing the dermatitis, but whether we withdrew Travasol or Amigen or gave the patient dextrose and water, and dextrose and saline a cure was effected. In other words, we did not have to give zinc, but we had to take away the high protein intake which caused the anabolism. Presumably the patients' muscle mass was increasing and they were using up zinc, causing the deficiency manifestation to appear in the skin with this very distressing dermatitis.

We understood that zinc was bound to low molecular weight compounds, and appeared in the urine in large amounts in patients who were anabolizing. I wonder if Travasol, or the amino acid components of Travasol, chelate or bind zinc in some way and increase the urinary excretion.

G. S. Fell: (UK) I am not sure that I have a specific answer. I would say that on theoretical grounds it would be very unwise to give trace metal mixtures together with amino acids, since this would simply form stable complexes of zinc/amino acids which would filter through into the low molecular fraction and out into the urine. This is difficult to prove in controlled conditions in man, but in the rat when we gave orally ^{65}Zn histidine complex it appeared immediately in the urine quantitatively. In other words, it was passing straight through the animal, and not having any biological function whatsoever. I have no doubt that the giving of trace metal mixtures together with other nutrients has to be studied to see whether the nutrient one is giving is actually available.

H. M. Shizgal: (Canada) Where is most of the total body zinc located?

Fell: 60% of the total body content is in muscle and 20% is in skin. There is a significant amount in the other organs, with active metabolic processes, and some in bone.

*Synthamin

Shizgal: In the skin is the zinc in the collagen or in the cytoplasm?

Fell: It is almost always in the cytoplasm.

P. Vinay: (Canada) If it is true that zinc follows creatine, then zinc excretion is independent of urinary volume. If zinc clearance follows urinary concentration, then it cannot be independent of urinary volume. Can some one resolve this?

Fell: The expression of zinc excretion as a clearance was only a device to show that there was a relationship—we thought an inverse relationship—between total plasma concentration and the increase in urinary concentration. It probably is not correct to talk about zinc clearances.

A. B. Jones: (Canada) We have been making up a trace metal solution in our hospital for addition to amino acids, and we have shown sequentially that low zinc levels and low copper levels have both returned to normal in the plasma, suggesting an effect on plasma levels of zinc and copper which may be to the patient's advantage.

R. K. Ausman: (USA) After the experience reported by Dr Allardyce and the further note by Dr Kartinos that Amigen has substantially more zinc than any of the crystalline amino acids, I adopted the practice of giving 1 l of Amigen every other day as a source of trace elements. Later Dr Hardy had the idea that perhaps it would be a good idea to see if albumin—one of the products of the Cohn fractionation—contained any zinc and Dr Kartinos has reported the results in his paper. It would certainly be easier to give albumin.

Fell: It would seem logical to supply the zinc as an albumin complex, if that is the main circulating form. But that is not even agreed by everyone.

It is perhaps a safer way to supply these ions as protein complexes—provided that the formation constant is not too great for cellular uptake—rather than allowing the possibility of increasing the free ionic form in circulating plasma, which may well be toxic.

Ausman: Can Dr Kartinos give us the comparison between albumin and Amigen solutions?

N. J. Kartinos: (USA) Dr Fell has shown that 20% Buminate contains 3.27 mg/l zinc, 4.8 mg/l iron; 0.89% mg/l copper and many other trace elements. As a comparison we have shown that Amigen contains 3.7 mg/l zinc. So on a per-litre basis they would be equivalent.

Ausman: I am not sure that one would want to give a litre of albumin to a patient, but we have now found a different answer with a source that is human, and which has no risk of hepatitis. There are some further studies that I know about that suggest that the oncotic characteristics of the albumin, even on a short-term basis, in patients with severe malnutrition, could be helpful as well.

Vinay: It certainly could help in a number of clinical manifestations. The point is how much zinc would one want to give. If 1 l of Amigen is all right, then it should be about 3 mg zinc. If that is done every other day, huge quantities of albumin could be given, at quite a considerable cost, because albumin is much more expensive than Amigen. Maybe it would be better to give the zinc as a supplement.

Ausman: I have heard of several people who give single donor source plasma to their patients to supply trace elements, and it has been given empirically. The pediatricians give blood, which must be doing the same thing.

Section VI
Parenteral Nutrition in Paediatrics

17
Aspects of intravenous feeding in childhood

J. T. HARRIES

In 1966 Dudrick[1] demonstrated that beagle puppies receiving nutrients only by the intravenous route grew and developed normally for several months. These experiments represented a major breakthrough in the field of intravenous feeding, and provided the basis for the subsequent application of this therapy in patients of all ages[2-9]. There is no doubt that intravenous feeding can be a life-saving procedure but, as with all major therapeutic advances, many questions remain unanswered, and a wide variety of complications are becoming increasingly recognized. This paper will consider some of the more important aspects of intravenous feeding in childhood, emphasizing the different problems which this form of treatment poses to the child compared with the adult patient.

SPECIAL CONSIDERATIONS OF INTRAVENOUS FEEDING IN CHILDHOOD

Table 17.1 lists some of the important factors which must be considered when applying an intravenous feeding programme in the child, and these factors are of particular importance in the young infant. In this context it is relevant to bear in mind that the indications for intravenous feeding apply much more to the young infant compared with the older child.

Table 17.1 Special considerations of intravenous feeding in childhood

Starvation and duration of survival
Nutritional requirements
Brain development
Brain injury
Organ immaturity

Starvation and duration of survival

During starvation 'survival energy' is derived from endogenous body stores of carbohydrate, fat and protein. Such energy is derived by sequential catabolism of hepatic glycogen, adipose tissue and protein. Hepatic glycogen is rapidly depleted, and it is the body content of fat and protein which ultimately determines the duration of survival during periods of starvation. The body composition of premature and full-term newborns, older children and adults differs markedly[10–12]. For example, a very small premature infant (1 kg) contains only 1% fat and 8.5% protein compared with the full-term infant (3.5 kg) which contains 16% fat and 11% protein. Both fat and protein content increase up to late childhood when some fat is replaced by protein. The adult contains more protein and less fat than the 1-year-old child. Heird *et al.*[6] have estimated the expected duration of survival during starvation at different age groups: the small premature infant (1 kg), the large premature infant (2 kg), the full-term infant (3.5 kg), the 1-year-old child and the adult will survive for approximately 4, 12, 32, 44 and 90 days respectively. Thus, the young child is at a major disadvantage when faced with nutritional deprivation, compared with the adult.

Nutrient requirements

Table 17.2 lists the approximate daily intravenous maintenance requirements for water, electrolytes, protein, fat, carbohydrate and calories for different age groups ranging from birth to adulthood. It can be seen that there are marked differences particularly for the requirements of water, protein,

Table 17.2 Approximate maintenance daily intravenous requirements

Age (years)	*Water* (ml/kg)	*Sodium* (mEq/kg)	*Potassium* (mEq/kg)	*Protein* (g/kg)	*Fat* (g/kg)	*Carbo-hydrate* (g/kg)	*Calories* (per kg)
0–1	150	2.5	2.5	4.4	4	13	100–120
1–3	100	2.5	2.5	3.5	4	10	90
3–6	90	2.0	2.0	3.0	4	8	80
7–12	70	1.5	1.5	2.5	3	8	70
Adult	35	1.0	1.0	1.0	2	2	35

carbohydrate and calories; these differences will be accentuated during periods of nutritional deprivation in the young infant compared with the adult, and present formidable technical problems in the intravenous delivery of adequate amounts of nutrients to sustain growth and tissue repair in the infant.

Table 17.3 compares the amino acids which are essential to the young growing infant and to the adult. In addition to the eight amino acids known to be essential to adults[13], histidine is also essential to the growing infant[14]. During periods of rapid growth and/or tissue repair, demands for certain 'non-essential' amino acids may exceed endogenous synthesis so that they become 'essential' or 'semi-essential'. Recent evidence suggests that proline[15], alanine[16], and cystine and/or cysteine[17] may also be 'essential' or 'semi-essential' to the young infant. Histidine, proline, alanine, cystine and cysteine should therefore be included in amino acid solutions used in infancy. The absolute and relative optimal amounts of amino acids contained in such solutions have not been defined clearly.

Table 17.3 Essential amino acids in man

Infants	*Adults*
Valine	Valine
Leucine	Leucine
Isoleucine	Isoleucine
Threonine	Threonine
Methionine	Methionine
Lysine	Lysine
Phenylalanine	Phenylalanine
Tryptophan	Tryptophan
Histidine	
?Proline	
?Cystine and/or Cysteine	
?Alanine	

The administration of vitamins and trace metals is integral to any intravenous feeding programme. The role of trace metal deficiency in human disease is currently attracting increased attention, and studies directed towards trace metal requirements during intravenous feeding deserve high priority in this field.

Brain development

Brain cell replication continues after birth, and periods of malnutrition in infancy may arrest this process, resulting in permanent intellectual deficits[19,20]. In infants who are malnourished, and in whom nutritional deficits cannot be corrected by the oral route, intravenous feeding presents the possibility of preventing long-term impairment of intellectual function.

Brain injury

There is an urgent need to define the intravenous requirements of amino acids, particularly in the newborn infant; the amino acid content of the infusate should resemble that of human plasma as closely as possible. Low and high circulating concentrations of various amino acids have been reported in newborns receiving intravenous feeding[6–8,18,21,22]. High plasma and/or cerebrospinal fluid levels of some amino acids may induce irreversible brain damage in young infants resulting in a paradox: preservation of life but impairment of intellectual function. Plasma amino acid concentrations should be carefully monitored in newborns receiving intravenous feeding.

High circulating levels of blood ammonia have been reported in infants receiving intravenous feeding[23], and this is also a potential cause of brain injury.

Organ immaturity

The functional capacity of a variety of organs is immature at birth, and does not reach maturity until several weeks or months after birth. For example, the renal excretion of inorganic solutes and H^+ ions does not mature until about the age of 9 months, and is a predisposing factor to the development of metabolic acidosis in infants receiving intravenous feeding[24].

INDICATIONS FOR INTRAVENOUS FEEDING

Table 17.4 lists the indications for intravenous feeding in childhood.

The need for intravenous feeding in childhood is greatest in early infancy, and in our experience protracted infantile diarrhoea[25] and major alimentary tract surgery in the newborn are the most important indications.

Table 17.4 Some indications for intravenous feeding in childhood

Protracted infantile diarrhoea
Major alimentary tract surgery in newborns
'Prematurity'
Extensive burns
Severe trauma
Crohn's disease

In carefully selected older patients, however, the effects of this form of treatment may be dramatic, as for example in Crohn's disease.

Case report (Figure 17.1)

D.C. presented at the age of 14.5 years with Crohn's disease involving the entire small intestine. Despite treatment with high doses of prednisolone, metronidazole and azathioprine, he lost 9.4 kg in body weight during the subsequent 16 months. At this stage he was emaciated, very depressed, and sufficiently weak as to be unable to climb stairs. The parents were convinced that he would not survive. Intravenous feeding was started (10% glucose Vamin*, 20% Intralipid* and 15% glucose) and continued for a period of

* Manufactured by Vitrum, Sweden

2 months during which time there was a dramatic weight gain of 8.5 kg; this was accompanied by a marked improvement in mood and well-being. Since stopping intravenous feeding he has continued to gain weight on a maintenance dose of azathioprine with minimal gastrointestinal symptoms.

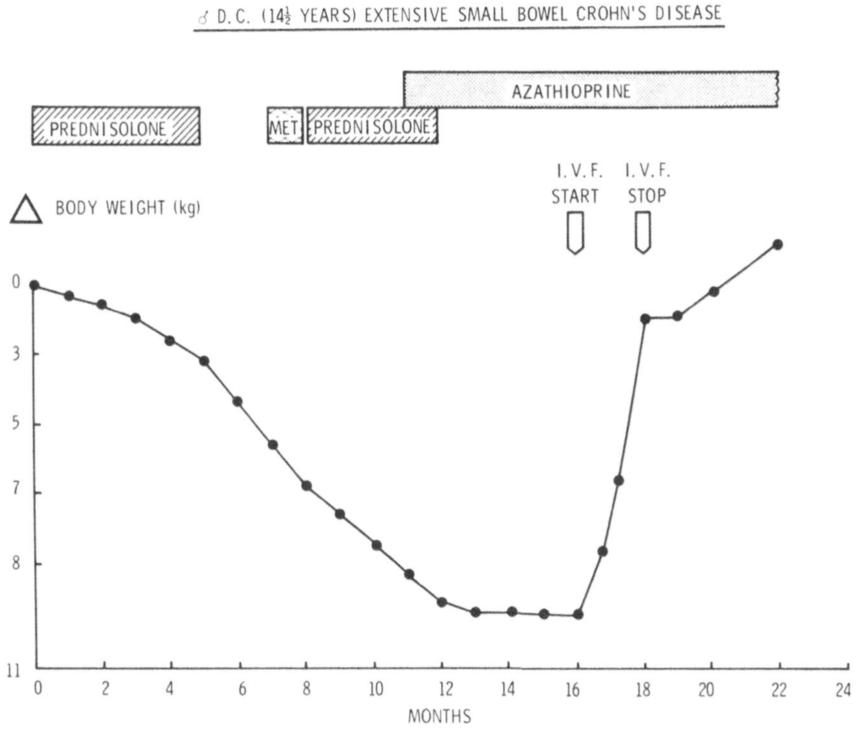

Figure 17.1 Effect of intravenous feeding in a 14½-year-old boy with extensive small bowel Crohn's disease

Abbreviations:
MET = Metronidazole
I.V.F. = Intravenous feeding
△ = Increment change in body weight

COMPLICATIONS

The protean complications which may accompany intravenous feeding are formidable[5,26], infection being one of the most prominent. A number of allied metabolic complications are becoming apparent, as shown in Table 17.5.

Electrolyte disturbances are common, and frequent determinations of plasma electrolyte concentrations are essential in any child receiving intravenous feeding.

Table 17.5 Metabolic complications of intravenous feeding in childhood

Electrolyte disturbances
Metabolic acidosis
Hypophosphataemia
Anaemia
Hypoxia
Thrombocyte and neutrophil dysfunction
Hypo- and hyperglycaemia
Trace metal deficiencies
Hyperammonaemia
Hyper- and hypocalcaemia
Essential fatty acid deficiency
Hepatic dysfunction
Activation of infection

Metabolic acidosis may occur, particularly in young infants in whom renal excretion of inorganic solutes and H^+ ions is immature[24]. The factors involved in the pathogenesis of the acidosis are shown in Table 17.6. Infusion of fructose- or sorbitol-containing solutions may result in a lactic acidosis, which may be aggravated by the inclusion of ethanol in such solutions, by hepatic dysfunction, or by hypoxia[24,27–29]. The load of titratable acid administered[30,31], the load of certain cationic amino acids such as arginine, lysine and histidine[9], and the hypertonicity of infusates[32] are other factors which must be considered in the pathogenesis of metabolic acidosis. The acid–base status must be carefully monitored during intravenous feeding.

Table 17.6 Pathogenesis of metabolic acidosis during intravenous feeding in childhood

Fructose → Lactic acid
Hypoxia
Ethanol
Hepatic dysfunction
Impaired renal excretion of H^+ ions
Load of administered titratable acid
Load of administered cationic amino acids
Arginine
Lysine
Histidine
Hypertonicity of infusates
Impaired renal excretion of solute

Hypophosphataemia, particularly in patients who are already severely malnourished at the time of instituting treatment, is becoming a well recognized complication of intravenous feeding[33–37]. Haemolytic anaemia, phagocytic dysfunction, platelet dysfunction, and neurological symptoms (e.g. paraesthesia, weakness, seizures and coma) may accompany the hypophosphataemia, and can be reversed by phosphate repletion. Table 17.7

shows the minimum serum inorganic phosphorus and haemoglobin concentrations in three of our patients which occurred during intravenous feeding following a period of severe malnutrition. The serum phosphorus and haemoglobin concentrations were corrected by phosphate supplementation. Hypophosphataemia may occur despite apparently adequate phosphate supplementation, and is probably related to compartmental 'shifts' of phosphate following the restoration of adequate quantities of intravenous nutrient substrates. If this is the case phosphate would be sequestered by

Table 17.7 Hypophosphataemia and anaemia during intravenous feeding in infants

Case	*Minimum serum inorganic phosphorus** (mg/100 ml)	*Minimum haemoglobin* (g/100 ml)
1	0.2	6.8
2	1.3	8.7
3	0.7	7.4

* Normal range 4.0–5.5 mg/100 ml

tissues undergoing rapid cellular turnover following their release from the mitotic arrest accompanying malnutrition, the phosphate substrate being required for synthesis of molecules such as DNA and proteins. In these circumstances non-dividing circulating cells would be at a competitive disadvantage and become phosphate depleted. Phosphate is an obligatory substrate for these circulating non-dividing cells with respect to the biosynthesis of adenosine triphosphatase and 2,3-diphosphoglycerate. Defective synthesis of these two molecules could account for all the clinical manifestations of hypophosphataemia.

Hyperglycaemia and glucosuria are not uncommon during the first few days of intravenous feeding regimes which utilize infusates containing high concentrations of glucose, and usually resolve spontaneously. Hypoglycaemia may follow abrupt termination of intravenous feeding. The mechanism is not clear, but it is possible that infused glucose and/or amino acids may stimulate insulin release, and that high levels of circulating insulin will persist after intravenous feeding has been discontinued. For this reason it is important to avoid abrupt termination of intravenous feeding (see later).

Trace metal deficiencies may accompany the anabolic phase which follows intravenous feeding[38–43], and the definition of the requirements of trace metals during intravenous feeding merits urgent investigation. Zinc deficiency, with manifestations similar to those seen in patients with acrodermatitis enteropathica, has been well documented[40,41,43]. Copper deficiency, with anaemia, leukopenia, neutropenia and skeletal abnormalities, has also been reported[38,39].

Hyper- and hypocalcaemia[6], essential fatty acid deficiency[44], and hepatic dysfunction[6] have all been documented in patients receiving intravenous feeding. Hyperuricaemia may be associated with the infusion of fructose-containing solutions[28], and high circulating levels of ammonia have been reported in infants receiving intravenous feeding[23].

It has been speculated that the metabolic events which accompany the correction of malnutrition may predispose the individual to infection[45], and it is our impression that malnourished children are most susceptible to infection during the initial period of intravenous feeding.

ORAL FEEDING DURING, AND AT TERMINATION OF, INTRAVENOUS FEEDING

Intravenous feeding can be used to complement oral feeding, or to exclusively provide nutrients by the intravenous route (i.e. 'total' intravenous feeding). The principles which we adopt during 'total' intravenous feeding and during its termination are illustrated in Figure 17.2. If possible, limited oral feeding is continued during 'total' intravenous feeding even in the face of severe

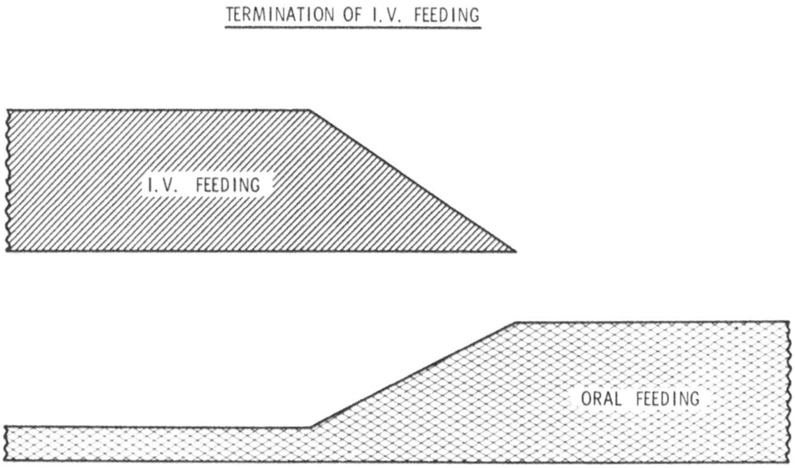

Figure 17.2 Principles of oral feeding during and at termination of 'total' intravenous feeding

diarrhoea, particularly when the duration of intravenous feeding is anticipated to be prolonged; the rationale is to maintain a continuous 'trophic' stimulus to the small intestinal mucosa. This approach is based on recent evidence that intraluminal substrates exert a trophic effect on the small intestinal mucosa, this effect being mediated by certain gastrointestinal hormones such as gastrin[46,47].

Termination of intravenous feeding should be anticipated, and oral feeding increased concurrently with the reduction of intravenous feeding.

This avoids the hypoglycaemia which may complicate abrupt termination of intravenous feeding, and allows for a 'rested' gastrointestinal tract to adapt to the re-exposure to increasing amounts of nutrients.

ETHICAL CONSIDERATIONS

The life-saving potential of intravenous feeding and the application of this form of treatment to certain patients is posing major ethical considerations. In our experience this applies particularly to protracted infantile diarrhoea of undetermined cause dating from birth[25], and in newborns following extensive small intestinal resections[48]. The following two case reports illustrate the ethical problems which may arise in such instances.

Case 1 (protracted infantile diarrhoea of undetermined cause dating from birth—see Figure 17.3)

L.P. was born at 36 weeks' gestation to healthy unrelated parents weighing 2.74 kg. The only previous sibling, a female, was born prematurely and birth was complicated by asphyxia. She developed severe watery diarrhoea from birth which persisted until the age of 4 months when she died of a combination of septicaemia, pulmonary embolus and congestive cardiac failure; extensive investigations had failed to reveal a cause for the diarrhoea, and autopsy was non-contributory. Intravenous feeding was necessary throughout her short life.

L.P. also developed severe watery diarrhoea of undetermined cause from

♀ L.P. PROTRACTED DIARRHOEA OF UNDETERMINED CAUSE FROM BIRTH

* ONSET OF SEVERE WATERY DIARRHOEA FROM BIRTH
* R. DYSPLASTIC KIDNEY
  - Urinary tract infections
* SIMILAR HISTORY IN ♀ SIBLING → † AGED 4 MONTHS

EXTENSIVE INVESTIGATIONS
DIETARY MANIPULATIONS
VARIOUS DRUGS
I.V. FEEDING

* CURRENT STATUS
  Alive and intelligent
  Age 15 months
  Weight 4.5 kg.
  Stool volume 1000-2000 ml/24 hr

Figure 17.3 Protracted diarrhoea of undetermined cause dating from birth

birth. This was associated with a right dysplastic kidney and urinary tract infections. Despite a variety of dietary manipulations (e.g. exclusion of sugars, cow's milk protein and gluten from the diet), and the administration of various drugs (e.g. cholestyramine, corticosteroids, indomethacin, propranolol) the diarrhoea progressed in severity. Intravenous feeding has been necessary for the vast majority of her life. At the time of writing she is aged 15 months and weighs only 4.5 kg, but is astonishingly bright and responsive. Remarkably her stool volume varies from 1000 to 2000 ml/24 h. Table 17.8 lists the complications which have been encountered, many of which are similar to those which occurred in Case 2.

Table 17.8 Complications in a child with protracted diarrhoea of undetermined cause dating from birth and 15 months of intravenous feeding

Electrolyte disturbances
Metabolic acidosis
Hypophosphataemia
Anaemia
Thrombocytopenia
Leukopenia
Zinc and copper deficiency
Hepatic dysfunction
Septicaemia
Hypoalbuminaemia
Hypocalcaemia → Tetany and laryngospasm
Pneumonia
Extravasation of infusates → R. neck → Horner's syndrome
Extravasation of infusates → Retroperitoneum → Ileus

During the hospitalization of these two siblings, the mother lived in the same cubicle as her daughters, and with amazing fortitude. During L.P's hospitalization there have been a number of recent occasions when complications have not been treated 'aggressively' but despite such compromised medical care, she continues to survive. The strain on the parents, nursing and medical staff has been intolerable, and the parents' marriage very nearly disintegrated.

We presume that these two infants represent a genetically determined disorder of fluid and electrolyte transport by the gut, the precise nature of which has not been defined. The parents sought genetic advice and, despite being informed of at least a 1 in 4 risk of further children being similarly affected, decided to have another child. Happily a normal male infant was recently born and is thriving at the age of 2 months.

Case 2 (extensive small intestinal resection—see Figure 17.4)
Following an uneventful pregnancy, a healthy female infant (H.H.) was born at term weighing 3 kg and the neonatal period was uneventful. She remained well until the age of 8 months when she began to have recurrent episodes of bile-stained vomiting. The parents consulted a number of physicians, no

investigations were instituted and her symptoms were labelled as 'functional' in origin. At 2 years she was admitted to hospital with acute intestinal obstruction and an immediate laparotomy was performed. There was mid-gut malrotation and volvulus, with extensive gangrene of the small intestine. All but 13 cm of the small intestine was resected, and an end-to-end anastomosis of the duodenum to the ileum was performed. Her immediate post-operative course was uneventful and she was referred to us 2 days after the operation for further management. On clinical examination she was a well-nourished intelligent girl with no abnormalities outside the gastrointestinal tract.

♀ H. H. MASSIVE SMALL BOWEL RESECTION

- 8 MONTHS
  ONSET OF RECURRING BILE STAINED VOMITING

- 2 YEARS
  ACUTE INTESTINAL OBSTRUCTION
  MALROTATION → VOLVULUS → EXTENSIVE GANGRENE
  MASSIVE RESECTION
  13 cm VIABLE SMALL GUT

I.V. FEEDING

DIED $3\frac{1}{2}$ YEARS

Figure 17.4 Massive small bowel resection for malrotation and volvulus

Intravenous feeding was instituted, and continued for most of the remaining 18 months of her life, in the hope that the remaining short segment of small intestine would 'adapt' to a degree sufficient to maintain life. This, however, was not the case. Table 17.9 lists the many complications which occurred. It is of interest that two episodes of zinc deficiency coincided with *Candida* septicaemia, in view of the relationship between zinc and cell-mediated immunity[49–51].

During this 18-month period the patient, her parents and siblings became progressively more depressed and emotionally disturbed. The two siblings developed gastrointestinal symptoms which were established as being non-organic following investigation. The parents were informed that the chances of survival were poor, and after a few months were given an almost hopeless prognosis. They were a deeply religious couple and could not accept the almost inevitable fate of their child, and were clearly aware of her dependence on intravenous feeding. As time passed complications were treated in a progressively less 'aggressive' fashion and she died at the age of 3½ years. Permission for autopsy was not obtained.

Table 17.9 Complications in a child following extensive small bowel resection and 18 months of intravenous feeding

Electrolyte disturbances
Metabolic acidosis
Hypophosphataemia
Anaemia
Thrombocytopenia
Leukopenia
Zinc and copper deficiency
Hepatic dysfunction
Septicaemia
Thrombosis of major vessels
Pneumonia

Survival following small intestinal resection is related to the length of remaining bowel, the presence of the ileocaecal valve, normal birth weight, successful surgery and a lack of associated anomalies[48]. Less than 15 cm of remaining small bowel, even in the absence of any of the above disadvantageous factors, is almost certainly incompatible with long-term survival. The surgeon has an intolerable responsibility at operation when faced with a situation such as described above. Untwisting of the volvulus, in the hope that some of the apparently unviable bowel will recover, and a second laparotomy 24 h later would seem a reasonable compromise to an ethical dilemma.

CONCLUSIONS

Intravenous feeding represents a major therapeutic advance and, in carefully selected patients, has revolutionized management, particularly in young infants. The optimal intravenous requirements of all types of nutrients, however, have not been defined clearly. The risk of infection, the metabolic complications and the techniques of delivering intravenous nutrients, continue to present major problems. Complications are particularly likely to occur during the anabolic phase following mitotic arrest in malnourished patients, often during the early period of intravenous feeding. Intravenous feeding has generated serious ethical problems in patients who have conditions which are unlikely to be compatible with long-term survival.

ACKNOWLEDGEMENTS

I am grateful to the surgeons and physicians of The Hospital for Sick Children for allowing me to continue my interests in their patients who are receiving intravenous feeding, and for helpful and stimulating discussions with many colleagues.

References

1. Dudrick, S. J. (1966). Total intravenous feeding and growth in puppies. *Fed. Proc.*, **25**, 481
2. Peaston, M. J. T. (1968). Parenteral nutrition in serious illness. *Hosp. Med.*, **2**, 708
3. Filler, R. M., Eraklis, A. J., Robin, V. G. and Das, J. B. (1969). Long-term total parenteral nutrition in infants. *N. Engl. J. Med.*, **281**, 589
4. Johnson, D. G. (1970). Total intravenous nutrition in newborn surgical patients: A three-year perspective. *J. Paed. Surg.*, **5**, 601
5. Harries, J. T. (1971). Intravenous feeding in infants. *Arch. Dis. Childh.*, **46**, 855
6. Heird, W. C., Driscoll, J. M., Schullinger, J. N., Grebin, B. and Winters, R. W. (1972). Intravenous alimentation in pediatric patients. *J. Pediat.*, **80**, 351
7. Bryan, M. H., Wei, P., Hamilton, J. R., Chance, G. W. and Swyer, P. R. (1973). Supplemental intravenous alimentation in low-birth-weight infants. *J. Pediat.*, **82**, 940
8. Pildes, R. S., Ramamurthy, R. S., Cordero, G. V. and Wong, P. W. K. (1973). Intravenous supplementation of L-amino acids and dextrose in low-birth-weight infants. *J. Pediat.*, **82**, 945
9. Lee, H. A. (1974). Intravenous nutrition. *Br. J. Hosp. Med.*, May, 719
10. Sinclair, J. C., Driscoll, J. M., Heird, W. C. and Winters, R. W. (1970). Supportive management of the sick neonate. *Ped. Clin. N. Amer.*, **17**, 863
11. Friss-Hansen, B. (1971). Body composition during growth: In vivo measurements and biochemical data correlated to differential anatomical growth. *Pediatrics*, **47**, 264
12. Widdowson, E. M. (1968). Growth and composition of the fetus and newborn. In N. S. Assali (ed.). *Biology of Gestation*, Vol. II, p. 1. (New York: Academic Press)
13. Rose, W. C. (1949). Amino acid requirements of man. *Fed. Proc.*, **8**, 546
14. Holt, L. E., Jr. (1967). Amino acid requirements of infants. *Curr. Ther. Approach*, **9**, 149
15. Harries, J. T., Piesowicz, A. T., Seakins, J. W. T., Francis, D. E. M. and Wolff, O. H. (1971). Low proline diet in Type I hyperprolinaemia. *Arch. Dis. Childh.*, **46**, 72
16. Jurgens, P. and Dolip, D. (1968). Die beteutung nichtessesentieller aminosäuren für den stickstoffhaushalt des menschen unter parenteralerar ernähbrung. *Klinische Wochenschrift*, **46**, 131
17. Sturman, J. A., Gaull, G. and Raiha, N. C. R. (1970). Absence of cystathionase in human fetal liver: is cystine essential? *Science*, **169**, 74
18. Stegink, L. D. and Baker, G. L. (1971). Infusion of protein hydrolysates in the newborn infant: plasma amino acid concentrations. *J. Pediat.*, **78**, 595
19. Wigglesworth, J. S. (1969). Malnutrition and brain development. *Development. Med. Child Neurol.*. **11**, 792
20. Stoch, M. B. and Smythe, P. M. (1976). 15-year developmental study on effects of severe undernutrition during infancy on subsequent physical growth and intellectual functioning. *Arch. Dis. Childh.*, **51**, 327
21. Ghadimi, H., Abaci, F., Kumar, S. and Rathi, M. (1971). Biochemical aspects of intravenous alimentation. *Pediatrics*, **48**, 955
22. Logan, R. W., Young, D. G., Ross, D. A., Stewart, B. R., Kubo, M. and Tryfonas, G. (1974). Comparison of an oral and an intravenous feeding regimen in the newborn. *Arch. Dis. Childh.*, **49**, 200
23. Johnson, J., Albritton, W. L. and Sunshine, P. (1971). Hyperammonemia complicating parenteral nutrition in infants, In *Combined Programme and Abstracts, Meeting of the American Pediatric Society, Inc. and the Society for Pediatric Research*, April, p. 102 (Atlantic City, New Jersey).
24. Harries, J. T. (1972). Metabolic acidosis during intravenous feeding of infants. In A. W. Wilkinson (ed.). *Parenteral Nutrition*, p. 266. (Edinburgh and London: Churchill Livingstone)
25. Larcher, V. F., Shepherd, R., Francis, D. E. M. and Harries, J. T. (1977). Protracted diarrhoea in infancy: an analysis of 82 cases with particular reference to diagnosis and management. *Arch. Dis. Childh.*, (In press).
26. Harries, J. T. (1974). Parenteral feeding—complications. *Arch. Dis. Childh.*, **49**, 824
27. Sahebjami, H. and Scalettar, R. (1971). Effects of fructose infusion on lactate and uric acid metabolism. *Lancet*, **i**, 366

28. Woods, H. F. and Alberti, K. G. M. M. (1972). Dangers of intravenous fructose. *Lancet*, **ii**, 1354
29. Aynsley-Green, A., Baum, J. D., Alberti, K. G. M. M. and Woods, H. F. (1974). Hyperlactataemia during intravenous feeding in childhood. *Arch. Dis. Childh.*, **49**, 647
30. Chan, J. C. M. (1972). The influence of synthetic amino acid and casein hydrolysate on the endogenous production and urinary excretion of acid in total intravenous alimentation. *Pediat. Res.*, **6**, 789
31. Chan, J. C. M., Malekzadeh, M. and Hurley, J. (1972). pH and titratable acidity of amino acid mixtures used in hyperalimentation. *J. Am. Med. Assoc.*, **220**, 1119
32. Kaplan, M. S., Mares, A., Quintana, P., Strauss, J., Huxtable, R. F., Brennan, P. and Hays, D. M. (1969). High calorie-nitrogen infusions. *Arch. Surg. Chicago*, **99**, 567
33. Jacob, H. S. and Amsden, T. (1971). Acute hemolytic anemia with rigid red cells in hypophosphatemia. *N. Engl. J. Med.*, **285**, 1446
34. Silvis, S. E. and Paragas, P. D. (1972). Paresthesias, weakness, seizures, and hypophosphatemia in patients receiving hyperalimentation. *Gastroenterology*, **62**, 513
35. Craddock, P. R., Yawata, T., VanSanten, L., Gilberstadt, S., Silvis, S. and Jacob, H. S. (1974). Acquired phagocyte dysfunction: A complication of the hypophosphatemia of parenteral hyperalimentation. *N. Engl. J. Med.*, **290**, 1403
36. Yawata, Y., Hebbel, R. P., Silvis, S., Howe, R. and Jacob, H. (1974). Blood cell abnormalities complicating the hypophosphatemia of hyperalimentation: erythrocyte and platelet ATP deficiency associated with hemolytic anemia and bleeding in hyperalimented dogs. *J. Lab. Clin. Med.*, **84**, 643
37. Ricour, C., Millot, M. and Balsan, S. (1975). Phosphorus depletion in children on long-term total parental nutrition. *Acta Paediatr. Scand.*, **64**, 385
38. Karpel, J. T. and Peden, V. H. (1972). Copper deficiency in long-term parenteral nutrition. *J. Pediat.*, **80**, 32
39. Vilter, R. W., Bozian, R. C., Hess, E. V., Zellner, C. D. and Petering, H. G. (1974). Manifestations of copper deficiency in a patient with systemic sclerosis on intravenous hyperalimentation. *N. Engl. J. Med.*, **291**, 188
40. Kay, R. G. and Tasman-Jones, C. (1975). Zinc deficiency and intravenous feeding. *Lancet*, **ii**, 605
41. Arakawa, T., Tamura, T., Igarashi, Y., Suzuki, H. and Sandstead, H. H. (1976). Zinc deficiency in two infants during total parenteral alimentation for diarrhea. *Am. J. Clin. Nutr.*, **29**, 197
42. Bozian, R. C. and Shearer, C. (1976). Copper, zinc, and manganese content of four amino acid and protein hydrolysate preparations. *Am. J. Clin. Nutr.*, **29**, 1331
43. Tucker, S. B., Schroeter, A. L., Brown, P. W., Jr., and McCall, J. T. (1976). Acquired zinc deficiency. Cutaneous manifestations typical of acrodermatitis enteropathica. *J. Am. Med. Assoc.*, **235**, 2399
44. Fleming, C. R., Smith, L. M. and Hodges, R. E. (1976). Essential fatty acid deficiency in adults receiving total parenteral nutrition. *Am. J. Clin. Nutr.*, **29**, 976
45. Murray, M. J. and Murray, A. B. (1977). Starvation suppression and refeeding activation of infection. An ecological necessity? *Lancet*, **i**, 123
46. Feldman, E. J., Dowling, R. H., McNaughton, J. and Peters, T. J. (1976). Effects of oral versus intravenous nutrition on intestinal adaptation after small bowel resection in the dog. *Gastroenterology*, **70**, 712
47. Johnson, L. R. (1976). The trophic action of gastrointestinal hormones. *Gastroenterology*, **70**, 278
48. Wilmore, D. W. (1972). Factors correlating with a successful outcome following extensive intestinal resection in newborn infants. *J. Pediat.*, **80**, 88
49. Endre, L., Katona, Z. and Gyurkovits, K. (1975). Zinc deficiency and cellular immune deficiency in acrodermatitis enteropathica. *Lancet*, **i**, 1196
50. Moynahan, E. J. (1975). Zinc deficiency and cellular immune deficiency in acrodermatitis enteropathica in man and zinc deficiency with thymic hypoplasia in Friesian calves: a possible genetic link. *Lancet*, **ii**, 710
51. Endre, L. and Katona, Z. (1976). Aetiology of cellular immune deficiency in acrodermatitis enteropathica. *Lancet*, **i**, 91

18
Study of the use of total parenteral nutrition in neonates suffering from necrotizing enterocolitis

A. B. JONES

Parenteral feeding of infants is not new. Protein hydrolysates became commercially available some forty years ago, and what might be termed hypoalimentation occurred on a rather smaller scale. However Heird and Winters[1] drew attention recently to an infant reported by Helfrick and Abelson in 1944 who was fed intravenously with a mixture of 50 % glucose and 10 % casein hydrolysate plus a lipid emulsion for 5 days with apparent weight gain[2]. A boost was given to parenteral feeding in the 1950s by the development of lipid infusates; however this initial boost turned out to be a false result in North America because of their apparent toxicity. During the 1960s parenteral feeding was again practised, more with the infusion of blood products as a last resort, than as a scientific exercise in nutrition.

The technical advance of central vein infusion of hypertonic solutions (described by Dudrick in the mid 1960s) has indeed produced a great leap forward by encouraging the development of more appropriate nitrogen-containing solutions, and encouraging a scientific appraisal of the metabolic consequences of parenteral feeding, both with carbohydrate and later with lipid, as energy sources.

Parallel with these most recent advances in intravenous nutrition have been advances in knowledge and technology of neonatal care, associated with a proliferation of neonatal intensive care units. More infants are surviving extreme prematurity or respiratory distress syndrome, but succumb to malnutrition as evidenced for instance by pneumonia, sepsis or poor wound-healing after surgery. There has also been an increase in the incidence of previously uncommon disorders such as necrotizing enterocolitis, a disease with devastating effects on the gut as well as the nutritional state of the infant.

INDICATIONS

During the past $6\frac{1}{2}$ years the use of parenteral nutrition in our intensive care nursery has advanced from approximately six cases per year to the present sixty-six cases during the past 16 months, the period of time that we have been using Travasol amino acid mixture.

Indications for parenteral nutrition in the nursery have fallen into two general categories: (a) surgical problems, and (b) non-surgical gut insufficiency. The surgical problems include congenital anomalies of the gastrointestinal tract such as atresia, stenosis, obstruction from other causes, gastroschisis/omphalocele, and gut perforation. The non-surgical gut insufficiencies include the hypomotility disorder of prematurity, recurrent apneic spells, severe respiratory distress, extreme prematurity, and necrotizing enterocolitis (NEC).

It is recognized that the medical indications other than NEC at present remain controversial. Studies by Bryan[3], Brans[4] and others have suggested that while premature and low birth-weight infants may lose less weight during the first days of life, and may initially gain weight more rapidly if parenterally supplemented, nevertheless the final discharge weight, length of stay in hospital and overall mortality rate is not affected by intravenous nutritional supplementation. Despite this, many neonatologists[5] prefer to use intravenous supplementation in small infants who appear unable to tolerate adequate oral, nasogastric or nasointestinal feeding.

In studying these patients, we find that growth initially has been poor. Two causes come to mind. The first is that most of these infants have some degree of hypoxaemia and respiratory acidaemia, usually with the addition of a metabolic acidaemia. The second problem is initial inadequate nutritional intake due to procrastination or caution in feeding. Intralipid, a valuable caloric source, must be used with extreme caution at this time because of the increased danger of kernicterus due to low bilirubin albumin binding capacity, and the deleterious effect of Intralipid on this[6]. Intralipid infusion, if used at all, should be guided by serial bilirubin and albumin binding capacity determinations.

Necrotizing enterocolitis (either suspected or proved) has been the largest single contributor to the increase in the use of TPN in our nursery, and accounts for about 60% of the infants being fed. This report presents data on twenty of these infants, plus a further eight referred to below who were studied in regard to amino acid patterns.

METHOD AND MATERIALS

Infants are usually managed by our resident house staff in the nursery; this results in some variation in nutritional intake and concentration of components of the infusate. The majority of the infants receive TPN via a peripheral vein. Umbilical vessels are not used. Complications have been minor. There has been no sepsis attributable to the infusions. Occasional small areas of skin necrosis have occurred on the scalp, rarely greater than 0.5 cm in diameter. There is the occasional difficulty in maintenance of the peripheral infusion, resulting in caloric shortfall and slowing of weight gain. At our sister unit in the Royal Alexandra Hospital, central venous catheters are used with greater frequency. Usually used is a $3\frac{1}{2}$ Fr Argylle Umbilical Artery Catheter, placed into the external or internal jugular vein, or into a more peripheral vein such as antecubital or saphenous, and advanced centrally.

The amino acid/dextrose/electrolyte solution includes the following components. Glucose concentration is normally maintained at about 10%. Build-up to this level is rarely necessary since the infants usually already have a glucose infusion running. This concentration of glucose supplies 9–16 g/24 h/kg or about 375–670 mg/kg/h, depending on the infusion rate.

Electrolyte concentrations are modified potentially on a daily basis, but generally supply 2.5–3.5 mEq of sodium and 1.5–2.0 mEq of potassium/kg/day. Calcium has varied widely. In our nursery, infants are given 0.5–1.0 mEq/kg/day of calcium as calcium gluconate; however our sister unit has been giving around 3.0 mEq/kg/day. The effect of this difference has so far not been studied, but serum calcium levels in our nursery remain within normal limits. Magnesium is provided in abundance, usually 1–1.5 mEq/kg/day, but effects have not been specifically assessed. No extra phosphate is added, as there is sufficient in the solution. Trace minerals have not ordinarily been used; however the infants receive frequent blood transfusions to maintain haemoglobin levels. A multiple vitamin infusion is added on a daily basis.

The amino acid component is usually started at 0.5–1.0% and increased so as to provide 2 g/kg/day of protein equivalent. Actual amino acid intake however tends to vary widely, between 0.9 and 3.5 g/kg/day, with an average of 1.76 g/kg/day. This provided between 6 and 12% of caloric intake, a figure approximating breast milk and commercial infant formulae.

Amino acid chromatograms in plasma were studied in eight infants receiving TPN and five control infants receiving breast milk only. One parenterally-fed and one milk-fed infant were between 900 and 950 g and approximately 30 weeks post-conception. The other eleven infants were larger, one at 1800 g and 33 weeks' gestation, the rest between 2 and 3 kg and 36–42 weeks post-conception.

An infant receiving a steady infusion of nutrients over several days or even weeks cannot be considered to be in a fasting state. Therefore stopping the infusion would not reflect the 'normal' state for that infant; therefore infusions were not stopped prior to blood being drawn for amino acids or other determinations. Blood was withdrawn from a radial artery. These conditions will produce results which are as close as possible to the steady state in the infant, and most representative of the anomalies produced by the infusion itself.

The control infants were being fed at 2–3-h intervals, and blood was taken 60–120 min after the previous feed. There is a circadian rhythm in plasma amino acids, with the peak around noon and the trough in the very early morning[7]. Blood was taken in the late morning or afternoon in all infants. The blood for amino acids was taken into heparinized tubes, the plasma deproteinized with 5′sulphosalacylic acid 30 mg/ml, and after separation was analysed on a Technicon dual column ion exchange amino acid analyser, using standard techniques.

RESULTS

The NEC infants were on TPN alone for a mean of 7.5 days (range 2–19 days). Supplemental breast milk was then started gradually over 2–3 days and the infusion weaned off. The mean total time of parenteral nutrition in this particular group was 12.6 days with a range of 4–26 days. Intralipid 10% was usually continued for a further 2–3 days and provided 20–25% of calories during this time.

There were no complications ascribed to the amino acid infusate. Clinically apparent hyperammonaemia (which had been seen in one infant as lethargy and twitchiness several years ago while we were using a casein hydrolysate) was not seen. Blood ammonia levels monitored over the last year while using Travasol have shown a mean of 135μ mole, range 76–230, with mean weight of the infants 1.42 kg.

Serum glutamic oxaloacetic transaminase, 5′nucleotidase and serum creatinine, measured prospectively in seven of the eight infants, were uniformly normal.

Retrospective analysis of blood urea nitrogen levels showed only two infants with levels greater than 18 mg/dl. One infant was thought to have some renal tubular damage secondary to severe cold stress, shock and acidaemia, the indications for admission to the unit; and the second infant had congestive heart failure due to a patent ductus and was on diuretics.

Blood glucose levels were almost uniformly normal. Two infants had single determinations between 200 and 250 mg/dl, one on the second day of infusion while receiving 720 mg glucose/kg/h, a level subsequently tolerated. The second infant's high glucose was unexplained and was normal on recheck.

Hyperchloraemic acidosis has been discussed extensively in the literature[8]. We note occasional serum chloride values above 107 mEq/l in almost every infant; maximum 115 mEq/l. It was interesting to note however that 32% of the infants had a level of greater than 107 mEq/l before TPN, maximum 116 mEq l and nearly 80% of infants who had serum chloride values measured after all parenteral nutrition had been finished had levels above 107 mEq/l. Further studies are necessary to assess chloride homeostasis in these small infants.

A mild fall in total plasma CO_2 to a range of 16–20 mEq/l occurred in the majority of the infants. This is in keeping with the data of Heird, Winter and others[8,9].

Weight gain on TPN alone occurred in all infants on parenteral nutrition for more than 3 days (Figure 18.1). There was a significant correlation

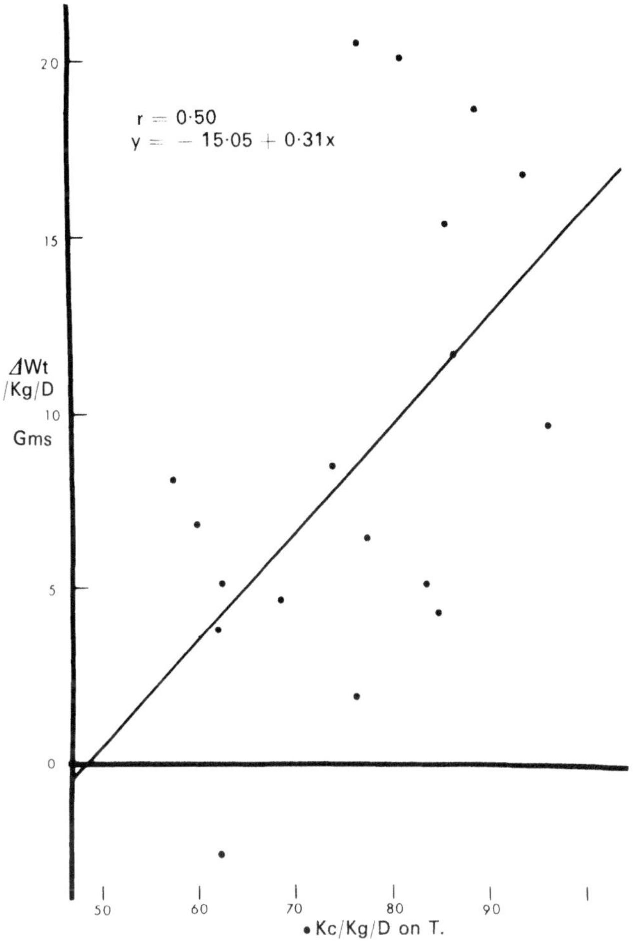

Figure 18.1 Weight gain (loss) versus caloric intake in infants with necrotizing enterocolitis on TPN

between caloric intake and weight gain as expected, although due to the variability in illness, and to duration of pure TPN feeding, there was a wide scatter. The relatively isothermal environment of the incubator or servo-controlled infant warmer is probably a great advantage in allowing weight gain at a lower caloric intake than might otherwise be necessary. The smallest infants tended to gain more weight relative to size than the larger infants

(Figure 18.2). It must be accepted that some of the initial weight gain is an expanded extracellular water mass, as shown by Brans and co-workers[10]. The explanation for the expanded water mass remains obscure, but might be related to increased free amino acid levels consequent upon the infusion None of our infants developed clinical oedema; however there was generally a slight weight loss of 10–20 g or a plateau in weight gain for 2–3 days after the amino acid/dextrose infusion was stopped.

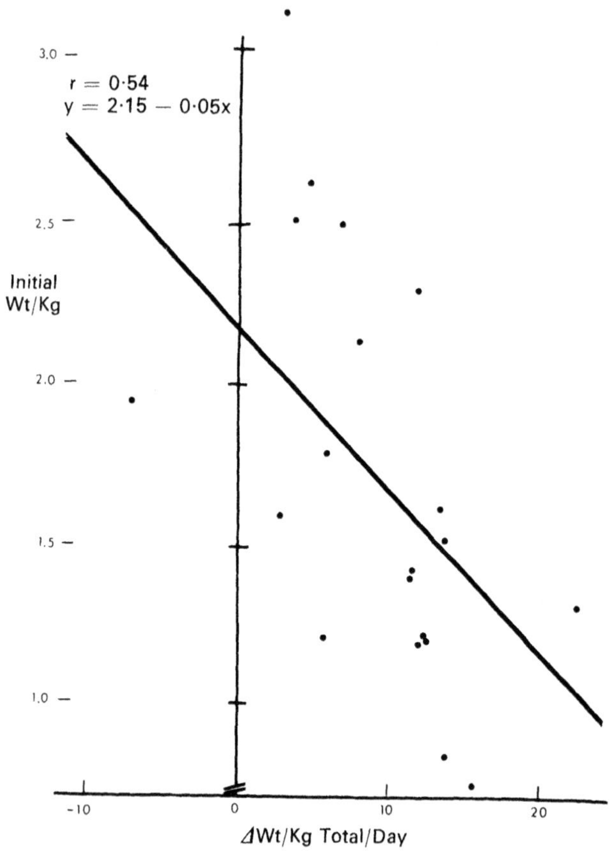

Figure 18.2 Birth weight related to weight gain (loss) on TPN

As mentioned, there was a correlation between weight gain and caloric intake, but not between weight gain and amino acid intake. Indeed there was a slight negative correlation between weight gain and the proportion of calories provided as amino acid (Figure 18.3). This was actually due to lower calorie intake when Intralipid 10% was either not being used, or could only be used in small amounts due to raised bilirubin levels. These observations suggest that as long as adequate nitrogen was being infused, the limiting factor in weight gain was total calorie intake, consistent with current concepts of protein–energy relationships.

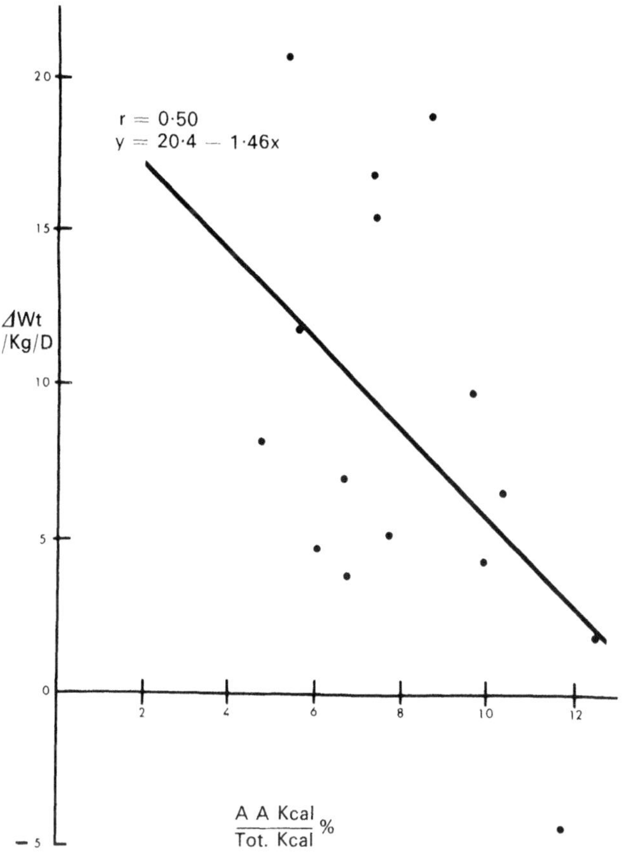

Figure 18.3 Weight gain (loss) related to percentage of caloric intake from nitrogen source

PLASMA AMINO ACID VALUES

Dickinson and co-workers[11,12] and Stegink[13] have studied plasma amino acid levels in newborns and found certain characteristic differences compared to older children and adults. In particular raised glycine, serine, asparagine, glutamine, taurine and methionine have been noted. In the following figures, the open points refer to the control breast milk-fed infants, and the closed points to the infants on TPN. Our results in the milk-fed infants are striking; the smallest infant (950 g) had markedly raised levels of glycine, arginine and methionine and to a lesser extent of alanine, threonine, serine, histidine, phenylalanine and citrulline. The blood was taken a few minutes before a feed and about 90 min after the previous feed, suggesting that this may be an expected pattern for a very small premature breast milk-fed infant. When compared to the infant of similar size on the Travasol amino acid infusion, the milk-fed infant was further from 'normal' on every measurement except aspartic acid and asparagine. In particular, the methionine level was more than twice as high as the level in the Travasol-fed infant, and about eight times the mean for normal fasting term infants.

The amino acid data for the parenterally fed group have been divided into three portions: three infants with a mean amino acid intake of 1.13 g/kg/day (range 0.63–1.71); four infants with a mean intake of 2.43 g/kg/day (range 2.0–2.75); and a single of 900 g. The infants on the low dose had amino acid levels mostly falling within 'normal' fasting levels, except for raised glycine, aspartic acid and tyrosine. The four infants on a mean intake of 2.43 g/kg/day

A

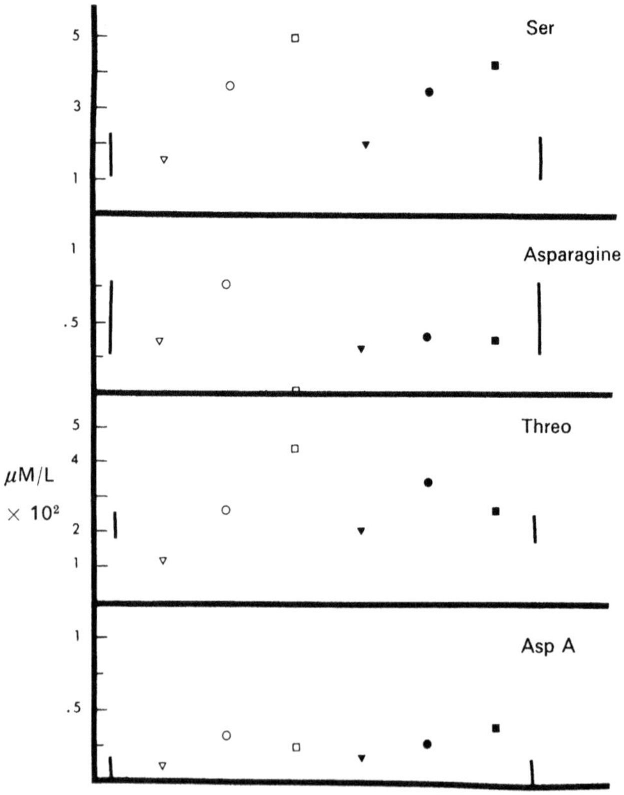

Figure 18.4 Plasma amino acid levels in infants on TPN with Travasol amino acid mixture and in infants on oral feeding with breast milk. ▽: Breast-fed 2 h p.c. full term; ○: breast-fed 60–90 min p.c. full term; □: breast-fed 90 min p.c. 900 g; ▼: TPN mean amino acid intake 1.13 g/kg/day; ●: TPN mean amino acid intake 2.43 g/kg/day; ■: TPN 900 g

B

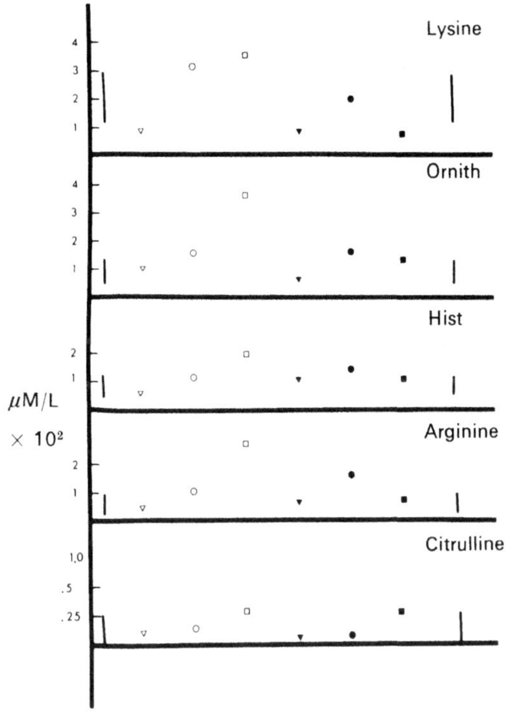
Lysine
Ornith
Hist
Arginine
Citrulline
μM/L
× 10²
1,0
.5
.25

C

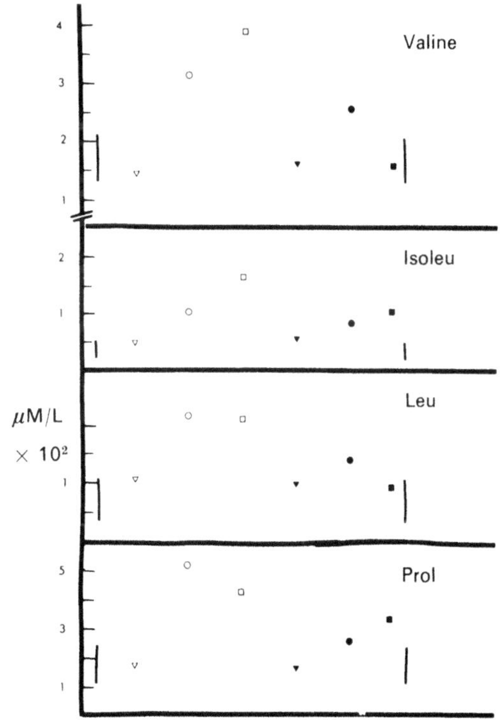
Valine
Isoleu
Leu
Prol
μM/L
× 10²

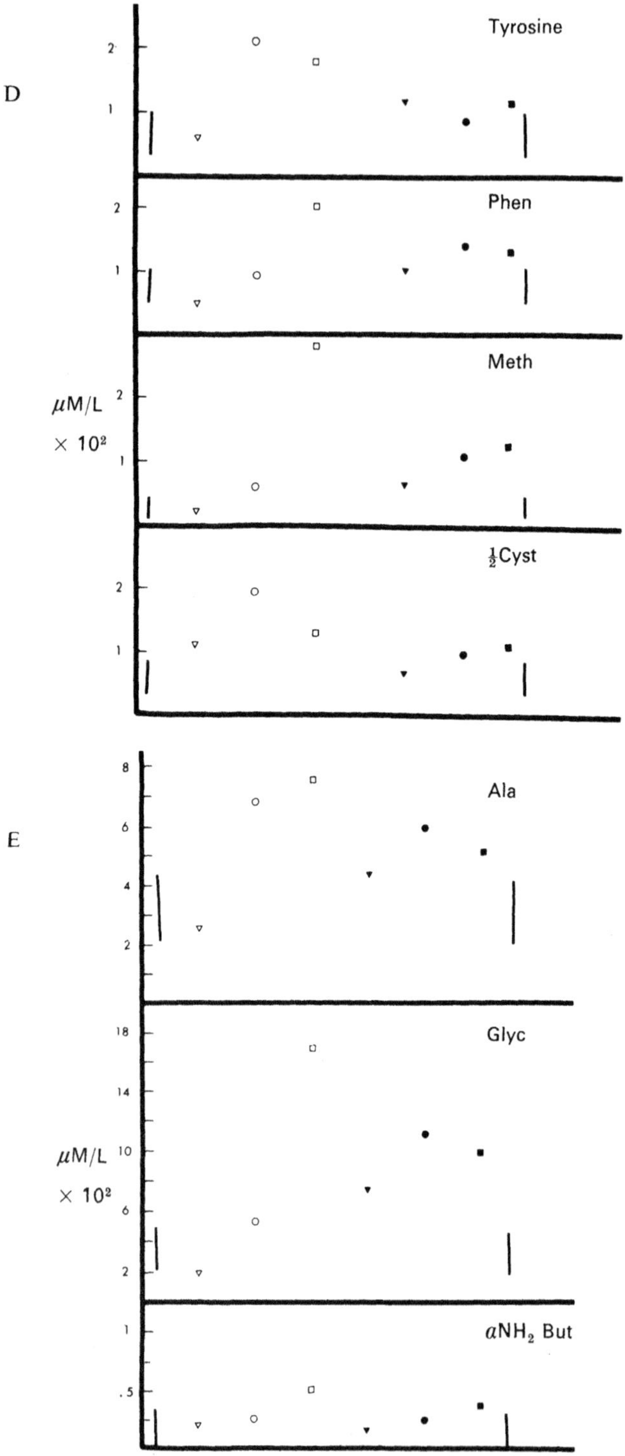
D
Tyrosine
Phen
Meth
½Cyst
μM/L
× 10²
2
1
E
Ala
Glyc
αNH₂ But
8
6
4
18
14
10
.5

had levels comparable to the 60–90 min post-feeding infants, except for glycine and methionine, both raised to levels of about twice the upper limit of 'normal'.

The high glycine levels are presumably related in part to the glycine load in the infusate and in part to whatever the mechanism of the normally seen high glycine levels in premature and normal-weight newborns. There would not at the present time appear to be any cause for concern regarding the raised glycine levels. The group of disorders termed 'hyperglycinaemia' do not appear to have their symptom complex completely related to the raised glycine levels, but to the underlying metabolic disorder causing these high levels. In particular, lethargy, seizures and ketosis were not evident in any of our infants.

The raised serine and threonine levels may be related to the raised glycine levels, since threonine is partly catabolized via glycine and this route may be impeded by high glycine. Glycine is converted to serine, and thus may contribute to the raised serine levels.

An important observation is the normal cystine levels. Because of the recognized cystathionase deficiency in the normal newborn, resulting in raised methionine levels, concern has been expressed that cystine levels might be below normal due to inadequate production and no intake from the infusion. This concern has not been borne out by our studies.

SUMMARY

In summary, Travasol* amino acid mixture in association with adequate calories provided by glucose and Intralipid 10% has proved a safe and effective nitrogen source to allow healing of damaged bowel in neonates with necrotizing enterocolitis, and to provide for appropriate weight gain. Plasma amino acid levels have generally been in the range of post-prandial breast milk-fed infants.

There is a definite dose response, indicating that too much *may* produce toxic effects, while too little *may* provide inadequate nitrogen for normal growth. At present, 2.0–2.5 g amino acid/kg body weight/day appears to be the most appropriate dose.

* Synthamin.

References

1. Heird, W. C. and Winters, R. W. (1975). Total parenteral nutrition. State of the art. *J. Pediat.*, **86,** 2
2. Helfrick, F. W. and Abelson, N. M. (1944). Intravenous feeding of a complete diet in a child: report of a case. *J. Pediat.*, **25,** 400
3. Bryan, M. H., Wei, P., Hamilton, J. R., Chance, G. W. and Swyer, P. R. (1973). Supplemental intravenous alimentation in low birth weight infants. *J. Pediat.*, **82,** 940
4. Brans, Y. W., Sumners, J. E., Dweck, H. S. and Cassady, G. (1974). Feeding the low

birth weight infant: orally or parenterally? Preliminary results of a comparative study. *Pediatrics*, **54,** 15

5. Schiff, D. Personal communication
6. Andrew, G., Chan, G. and Schiff, D. (1976). Lipid metabolism in the neonate. II. The effect of Intralipid on bilirubin binding in vitro and in vivo. *J. Pediat.*, **88,** 279
7. Feigen, R. D. and Haymond, M. W. (1970). Circadian periodicity of blood amino acids in the neonate. *Pediatrics*, **45,** 782
8. Heird, W. C., Dell, R. B., Driscoll, J. M., Jr., Grebin, B. and Winters, R. W (1972). Metabolic acidosis resulting from intravenous alimentation mixtures containing synthetic amino acids. *N. Engl. J. Med.*, **287,** 943
9. Heird, W. C. (1975). Disorders of acid base metabolism. In R. W. Winters and E. G. Hasselmeyer (eds.). *Intravenous Nutrition in the High Risk Infant* (New York: John Wiley)
10. Brons, Y. W., Sumners, J. E., Dweck, H. S., Bailey, P. E. and Cassady, G. (1976). Feeding the low birth weight infant: orally or parenterally? Corrected bromide space in parenterally supplemented infants. *Pediatrics*, **58,** 809
11. Dickinson, J. C., Rosenblum, H. and Hamilton, P. B. (1965). Ion exchange chromatography of the free amino acids in the plasma of the newborn infant. *Pediatrics*, **36,** 213
12. Dickinson, J. C., Rosenblum, H. and Hamilton, P. B. (1970). Ion exchange chromatography of the free amino acids in the plasma of infants under 2500 gms at birth. *Pediatrics*, **45,** 606
13. Stegink, L. D. and Baker, G. L. (1971). Infusion of protein hydrolysates in the newborn infant. Plasma amino acid concentrations. *J. Pediat.*, **78,** 595

19
Use of Travasol* in paediatric patients

M. T. STE-MARIE

INTRODUCTION

Total parenteral nutrition is being used widely in paediatric patients with a variety of disease states in order to prevent malnutrition and meet the requirements for normal growth and development when oral intake is insufficient or impossible to achieve. Indications for total parenteral nutrition in patients of this age group include infants with surgical disease of the gastrointestinal tract, chronic diarrhoea of infancy, and certain severe malabsorption states. Several groups have extended the use of total parenteral nutrition or intravenous supplementation of oral feedings to pre-term very low birth-weight neonates. Positive nitrogen balance, weight gain and growth have been achieved by continuous infusion of an amino acid mixture or protein hydrolysate with a concentrated glucose solution through an indwelling central-vein catheter[1,2] or by peripheral vein infusion using a fat emulsion as the calorie source[3].

Premature and immature infants whose birth-weight is below 1500 g are at a greater risk of developing calorie insufficiency because of the low energy reserve in their body fat and the high metabolic rate per unit of body mass. Total metabolic expenditure in these neonates can exceed 100 kcal/kg/day if one takes into account the added stress of pulmonary, cardiovascular, renal or metabolic complications which are frequent in this group of patients. Finally, an inadequate calorie intake in this group could also adversely influence brain development[4].

We have recently started a study of total parenteral nutrition in low-birth-weight premature neonates using a peripheral infusion of glucose, a crystalline amino acid mixture (Travasol*) and a soya bean oil fat emulsion (Intralipid, Vitrum Co. A.B. Stockholm, Sweden). Weight gain and positive nitrogen balance were achieved in all patients.

* Synthamin.

Table 19.1

	Birth weight (g)	Gestational age (weeks)	Sex	Days on total parenteral nutrition	Outcome	Diagnosis
PATIENTS WITH BIRTH WEIGHT LESS THAN 1000 g						
1. B.A.	750	29	M	30	Alive	Prematurity, intra-uterine malnutrition, periodic apnea, hyperbilirubinaemia, patent ductus arteriosus
2. L.E.	1000	27½	F	21	Alive	Prematurity, neonatal asphyxia with respiratory insufficiency, patent ductus arteriosus, hyperbilirubinaemia
3. D.U.	936	26	M	6	Dead	Immaturity, severe neonatal asphyxia, periodic apnea, respiratory insufficiency, patent ductus arteriosus, esophageal atresia, trisomy 21, hyperbilirubinaemia
4. M.O.	785	26	F	6	Dead	Immaturity, neonatal asphyxia, hyperbilirubinaemia, renal insufficiency
PATIENTS WITH BIRTH WEIGHT LESS THAN 1600 g						
1. J.A.	1070	27	M	12	Alive	Prematurity, neonatal asphyxia, periodic apnea, hyperbilirubinaemia, patent ductus arteriosus with cardiac insufficiency
2. B.E.	1550	32	M	34	Alive	Prematurity, respiratory insufficiency, periodic apnea, hyperbilirubinaemia, patent ductus arteriosus, intracerebral haemorrhage
3. B.R.	1300	34	M	8	Alive	Prematurity, neonatal asphyxia, intra-uterine malnutrition
4. B.E.R.	1060	27	M	39	Alive	Prematurity, periodic apnea, hyperbilirubinaemia
5. L.A.	1550	31	F	20	Alive	Prematurity, hyaline membrane disease, hyperbilirubinaemia, renal insufficiency

SUBJECTS AND METHODS

Patients

Nine patients whose birth weight was lower than 1600 g were studied. Four patients (two males, two females) had a birth-weight below 1000 g (mean, 867.8 g; range, 750–1000 g) and five patients (four males, one female) had a birth-weight of less than 1600 g (mean, 1306 g; range, 1060–1550 g). Total parenteral nutrition was given for an average period of 19.5 days (range, 6–39 days). The mean gestational age was 27.1 weeks in the first group and 30.2 weeks in the second group. Table 19.1 lists the clinical conditions of these patients.

Composition of infusate

Requirements for a suitable parenteral fluid mixture are shown in Table 19.2. The sources used in the preparation of our infusate are italicized. The composition of the final infusate is indicated in Table 19.3. The total caloric

Table 19.2 Requirements for total parenteral nutrition

Requirement	*Source**
Amino acids	Hydrolysates *crystalline amino acid mixtures*
Calories	*Glucose*, fructose, lipid, alcohol, *fat*
Electrolytes (Na, K, Cl)	*Additives*
Minerals (Ca, Mg, P)	Additives, *plasma*
Fat- and water-soluble vitamins	*Additives*
Essential fatty acids	*Intravenous lipid* *Plasma*
Trace minerals (Zn, Cu, etc.)	*Plasma*

* The sources used in our infusate are italicized

Table 19.3 Composition of the final infusate

Constituent	*Amount*
Amino acids (Nitrogen)	3.25 g/kg/day
Glucose	12.5–15 g/kg/day
Fat	2 g/kg/day
NaCl	2–4 mEq/kg/day
KH_2PO_4 or KCl	2–4 mEq/kg/day
Ca gluconate	0.5 mEq/kg/day
$MgSO_4$	0.5 mEq/kg/day
MVI	2 ml/day
Vitamin K	2 mg/week
Vitamin B_{12}	500 μg/month
Plasma	10 ml/kg/week
Total volume	125 ml/kg/day

Table 19.4 Amino acid concentrations in final infusate (mg/kg/day)

ESSENTIAL AMINO ACIDS		
Isoleucine	157	
Leucine	199	
Lysine	186	
Phenylalanine	199	
Methionine	186	
Cystine–cysteine	—	
Threonine	139	
Tryptophan	58	
Valine	147	
Histidine	141	
Tyrosine	13	
Total		1425 mg
NON-ESSENTIAL AMINO ACIDS		
Alanine	676	
Glycine	676	
Arginine	338	
Proline	135	
Total		1825 mg

Table 19.5 Monitoring parameters

	First week	*Thereafter*
1. METABOLIC PARAMETERS		
Blood		
Electrolytes (Na^+, K^+, Cl^-)	Daily	3 × weekly
Acid–base status	Daily	3 × weekly
Glucose	Daily	3 × weekly
Total calcium and inorganic phosphorus	3 × weekly	2 × weekly
Total proteins	3 × weekly	2 × weekly
Blood urea nitrogen	3 × weekly	2 × weekly
Haemoglobin	2 × weekly	weekly
Transaminases	weekly	weekly
Ammonia	weekly	weekly
Magnesium	weekly	weekly
Urine		
Glucose	3 × daily	3 × daily
2. GENERAL MEASUREMENTS		
Volume of infusate	daily	daily
Urinary output	daily	daily
3. GROWTH PARAMETERS		
Weight	daily	daily
Length	weekly	weekly
Head circumference	weekly	weekly

intake of 91 cal/kg/day was distributed as follows: 66% from carbohydrates, 20% from fat and 14% from protein. The maximum nitrogen to calorie ratio was 1 g to 150 calories. The infusate was started at half-strength with respect to the amino acid, glucose and fat concentrations at a rate of 85 ml/kg/day and gradually increased to the 125 ml/kg/day full-strength solution over a period of 2–4 days. The composition of Travasol at an amino acid concentration of 3.25 g/kg/day is given in Table 19.4. The essential to total amino acid ratio is 43.8%. Osmolarity of the total infusate is 820 mOsm/kg of water. Trace minerals and essential fatty acids were provided by weekly infusions of human plasma at a dose of 10 ml/kg of body weight.

The nitrogen balance was calculated as the difference between the total intake and the urinary loss. Growth and metabolic variables were measured in each infant according to the schedule shown in Table 19.5. Daily volume of infusate and urinary output were recorded and bacterial studies of the infusate material and intravenous solutions were carried out twice weekly.

RESULTS

Two deaths occurred in the group of patients whose birth weight was lower than 1000 g. The cause of death was not related to parenteral nutrition; one infant died from an intra-cerebral haemorrhage and another from severe respiratory failure and cardiac arrest. No sepsis or bacteraemia was documented in any of our patients. As shown in Figure 19.1, during total parenteral nutrition with a full-strength formula, weight gain averaged 8.4 g/kg/day and the mean positive nitrogen balance was 0.44 g/kg/day. Metabolic complications were encountered in infants whose weight was below 1000 g at the start of the intravenous feeding regime (6 patients). These infants had a greater difficulty in metabolizing nutrients and therefore required a longer period of time to achieve an intake of 125 ml/kg/day of the full-strength formula. Metabolic disturbances in this group occurred mostly in the first week to 10 days of total parenteral nutrition but responded rapidly to appropriate adjustments. Hypernatraemia developed in three patients (serum sodium higher than 150 mEq/l); the serum levels returned to normal in 24–48 h when the sodium intake was reduced. Hyponatraemia was not documented. No significant glucosuria was detected and serum glucose concentrations higher than 150 mg/100 ml were rarely present; none of the patients required insulin to help utilize carbohydrate.

Hyperlipaemia as judged by moderate or severe serum turbidity was not present in patients receiving 2 g/kg/day of fat emulsion. Azotaemia defined as a blood urea nitrogen (BUN) higher than 25 mg/100 ml was present in all of the six smaller patients. In three of them a high BUN was associated with an increase in serum creatinine. However, renal insufficiency was a transient phenomenon and responded to higher fluid intake in most patients. Protein intake was not reduced and serum BUN returned to normal levels in all patients after 48–72 h. Patients with severe periodic apnea or patent ductus arteriosus with cardiac insufficiency were more likely to develop complications and in one of them (J.A.) emergency closure of the ductus had to be performed because of clinical deterioration. Thereafter increased tolerance to nutrients developed and appropriate weight gain was noted for the first time since birth. Except for this patient, fluid intake was well tolerated.

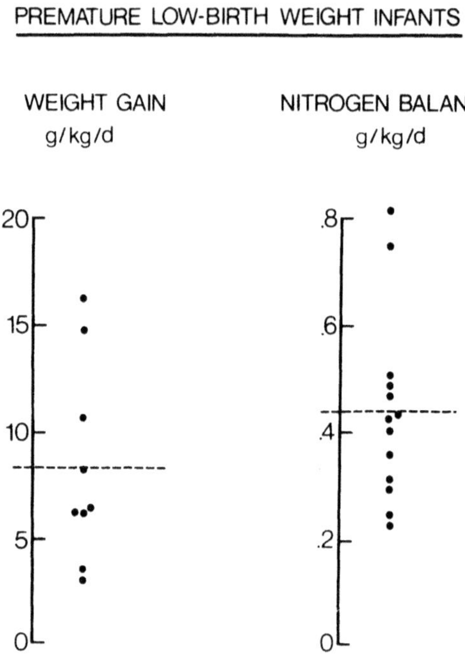

Figure 19.1 Average weight gain (g/kg/day) and nitrogen balance (g/kg/day) in low-birth-weight infants on total parenteral nutrition

Acidosis (blood pH lower than 7.30) was usually mixed respiratory and metabolic; base excess in these patients however was never less than −7 mEq/l and responded well to intravenous bicarbonate infusion. In most infants, alkalis were needed only for a short period of time to maintain normal blood pH and bicarbonate levels; thereafter metabolic acidosis was not encountered after the first week of intravenous nutrition. Chloride levels remained normal throughout the study period. Hyperammonaemia was not present in any of the infants on total parenteral nutrition. Hepatotoxicity defined as elevated serum transaminases and alkaline phosphatase and/or conjugated hyperbilirubinaemia was not present in any of the infants. Hepatomegaly was found in two patients and was attributed to cardiac insufficiency associated with patent ductus arteriosus; the liver size regressed after appropriate treatment. Indirect hyperbilirubinaemia was documented in almost all patients; no infant required exchange transfusion and they all responded to a short course of phototherapy. Finally, coagulation studies and platelet counts were normal.

DISCUSSION

In accord with previous publications[3,5], this study confirms that adequate weight gain and positive nitrogen balance can be achieved by total parenteral nutrition via peripheral vein infusion, thus eliminating the need of central venous catheterization and its potentially serious complications.

Protein intake level of 3.25 g/kg/day was chosen in this study in order to compare our results with those of O'Neill *et al.*[6] who also used Travasol at this concentration as a nitrogen source. 27 of their 62 neonates studied had a birth-weight below 1500 g. Average nitrogen retention in these patients was 0.31 g/kg/day which is similar to our own results. Transient azotaemia developed in eleven low-birth-weight infants and was corrected by diminishing the rate of infusion. As in this study, the elevation of BUN was attributed partly to renal immaturity, although serum creatinine levels were not determined. Incomplete utilization of amino acids can also explain this metabolic disturbance; a lower protein intake of 2.5 g/kg/day, as recently advocated by several groups[1,5,7], maintains a positive nitrogen balance, provides satisfactory weight gain and is not associated with azotaemia. Studies are currently in progress in our unit in order to confirm these observations using Travasol at this lower concentration.

The average daily intake of individual amino acids by neonates in this study compares well with average requirements recommended by others[8]. As in other synthetic formulae, the amino acid mixture is deficient in cystine–cysteine and low in tyrosine with high concentrations of methionine and phenylalanine. Premature infants have lower or non-existent levels of some enzyme systems required in the metabolism of various amino acids including methionine[9] and phenylalanine[10], so that a decrease in the concentration of these amino acids is desirable for prolonged use in neonates. If further studies confirm recent evidence showing that taurine may be an essential amino acid in premature neonates[11], addition of this amino acid to the mixture will have to be considered. Finally, the adequate amount of arginine received by the infants on full-strength formula (338 mg/kg/day) might explain the absence of biochemical and clinical evidence of hyperammonaemia.

Intolerance to fat emulsion concentrations higher than 2 g/kg/day developed consistently in our patients as manifested by an increased serum turbidity. Neonates in another study[3] however could tolerate amounts up to 3.5 g/kg/day. The concentration of fat infusion should be monitored individually especially in very low-birth-weight neonates. Relative inactivity of the gastrointestinal tract with decreased bile flow and sepsis have been implicated in the pathogenesis of hepatic cholestasis. Hepatic toxicity was not found using usual liver function tests in our study; patients were not receiving any oral feedings and had no evidence of sepsis or bacteraemia. Thus, the role of sepsis and parenteral nutrition in the aetiology of neonatal cholestasis may be of major importance[12].

In summary, weight gain and positive nitrogen balance can be achieved in very low-birth-weight premature infants by using a peripheral infusion of glucose, fat emulsion and crystalline amino acid (Travasol*) mixture. Metabolic complications are transient and respond well to individual adjustments. High blood urea nitrogen values can be avoided by infusing the amino acid mixture at a rate not exceeding 2.5 g/kg/day.

ACKNOWLEDGEMENTS

We wish to thank Dr Charles Carrier, Head of the Neonatal Intensive Care Unit, and the nursing staff for their collaboration in this study; also Jacinthe Larochelle, Research Technician, for the nitrogen balance determinations.

* Synthamin.

References

1. Winters, R. W. (1975). Total parenteral nutrition. The state of the art. *J. Pediat.*, **86**, 2
2. Peden, V. H. and Karpel, J. T. (1972). Total parenteral nutrition in premature infants. *J. Pediat.*, **81**, 137
3. Cashore, W. J., Sedaghatian, M. R. and Usher, R. H. (1975). Nutritional supplements with intravenously administered lipid, protein hydrolysate and glucose in small premature infants. *J. Pediat.*, **56**, 8
4. Winick, M. and Rosso, P. (1969). Effects of severe, early malnutrition on cellular growth of brain. *Pediat. Res.*, **3**, 181
5. Fox, H. A. and Krasna, I. H. (1973). Total intravenous nutrition by peripheral vein in neonatal surgical patients. *Pediatrics*, **52**, 14
6. O'Neill, J. A., Jr, Meng, H. C., Caldwell, M. D. and Stahlman, M. T. (1976). Metabolic evaluation of a synthetic amino acid mixture for parenteral nutrition in infants and children. *J. Paed. Surg.*, **11**, 979
7. Seashore, J. A. and Seashore, M. R. (1976). Protein requirements of infants receiving total parenteral nutrition. *J. Paed. Surg.*, **11**, 645
8. Winters, R. W. (1975). Summary of conference: average of amino acid requirements proposed by S. E. Snyderman, A. E. Harper and L. Stegink. In R. W. Winters and E. T. Hasselmeyer (eds.). *Intravenous Nutrition in the High Risk Infant*, p. 468. (New York: John Wiley and Sons)
9. Sturman, J. A., Gaull, G. E. and Raiha, N. C. R. (1970). Absence of cystathionase in human fetal liver: is cystone essential? *Science*, **169**, 74
10. Nicholson, J. F. (1973). Inborn disorders of intermediary metabolism. In R. E. Behrman (ed.). *Neonatalogy: Diseases of the Fetus and Infant*, p. 408. (St. Louis: C. V. Mosby Co.)
11. Sturman, J. A., Rassin, D. K., Hayer, K. C. and Gaull, G. E. (1977). Taurine in the developing kitten: nutritional importance. Presented at the *American Pediatric Society* and the *Society for Pediatric Research* meeting, April 27–29, San Francisco.
12. Manginello, F. P., Kok, E. and Javitt, N. B. (1977). Neonatal cholestasis: role of sepsis and intravenous alimentation. Submitted at the *American Pediatric Society* and the *Society for Pediatric Research* meeting, April 27–29, San Francisco.

20
Abnormalities of amino acid metabolism in the newborn

H. N. TUCKER

INTRODUCTION

Great advances in the understanding of protein, amino acid and carbohydrate utilization have led the physician to rely heavily on the clinical biochemistry laboratory for monitoring pertinent concentrations which might be altered by a disease state[1]. One or more biochemical processes may be defective from birth or become defective either temporarily or permanently due to disease later in life. Under these conditions the concentration of normal metabolites may change and in some cases new, abnormal metabolites may appear[2,3]. Early and accurate recognition of an altered metabolic process is important in any of the inborn errors of metabolism. In many instances a disorder is associated with mental or developmental retardation that may be prevented by early diagnosis and treatment[4].

Observed disturbances of amino acid concentrations are of particular interest during the newborn period. The concentration of amino acids is elevated in the urine of the newborn infant. The aminoaciduria of the premature infant is even more pronounced and may persist for several months. In addition to the large amounts of certain amino acids usually excreted in older children, asparagine, methionine, leucine, valine, tyrosine, proline, and hydroxyproline are elevated during this period. Monitoring urinary and plasma amino acids is mandatory for metabolic assessment.

An abnormality of urinary amino acid excretion may be seen as the elevation of a single amino acid, a group of amino acids, or all of the amino acids. A generalized aminoaciduria, with rare exceptions (Fanconi's or Lowe's syndrome) is usually due to a defect in renal tubular function or to the administration of excessive amino acids. The metabolic disturbances that result in a generalized aminoaciduria are those in which there is a destruction of tissue. Acute febrile states and acute liver failure may also show generalized elevations.

In high-risk paediatric populations, there is a special need to assess the individual metabolic ability to handle the nutritional amino acid profile whether administered parenterally or enterally. Techniques useful for diagnosis of metabolic faults are easily applicable for monitoring parenteral therapy and should be more frequently utilized for the evaluation of amino acid utilization.

GAS CHROMATOGRAPHY AS A DIAGNOSTIC TOOL IN METABOLIC FAULTS

The complexity of physiological fluids presents a unique analytical problem testing the versatility of the instrumentation and the ingenuity of the investigator. Classical ion-exchange or liquid column chromatography procedures that rely heavily on visualization of separated ninhydrin-positive components have failed to meet the challenge of easy adaptability and versatility in biomedical applications. The prohibitive expense, encumbrance of large buffer systems, and lengthy separation times have led to new applications of analytical instrumentation not routinely found in the clinical laboratory. The existing techniques for quantitation of amino acids are applicable to protein hydrolysates, prepared amino acid mixtures, and large quantities of physiological fluids. The semi-micro technique for free plasma amino acids[5] requires 5 ml of plasma. Routine studies of the neonatal patient are not feasible if such large quantities of sample have to be obtained. Recently modifications of the Gehrke procedure have been devised to insure that adequate quantities of blood for the complete determination of plasma amino acids are easily obtained from a finger or heel stick.

Gas chromatography has several advantages over the currently employed analytical techniques. The initial expense of a complete gas chromatographic system is quite low and the investment is greatly enhanced by the extreme versatility of a system that can be used for the separation of any compound that is volatile or can be made volatile by the preparation of a derivative. Gas chromatography (GC) was first successful in analytical chemistry applications for extreme accuracy at very low concentrations. Modern temperature-programmed ovens lend great speed to the system. Naturally occurring plasma amino acids may be separated and quantitated by a 32 min program from as little as 50 μl of sample[6]. In instances of unidentifiable components, the sample prepared for GC is ready to be introduced directly for mass-spectral analysis without further delay. Combination GC/MS investigations allow even smaller sample sizes (1 μl) with sensitivity to the femtomole level[7].

NORMAL PAEDIATRIC RANGES

The establishment of ranges for amino acid concentrations found in biological fluids of paediatric patients was imperative for adequate interpretation of gas chromatographic data. GC paediatric studies had not been reported on which to base an interpretation. Clinically normal paediatric patients, whose ages ranged from birth to 4 years, were used for the establishment of baseline data.

Plasma amino acid concentrations

Mean plasma concentrations based on thirty-one clinically normal paediatric patients are listed in Table 20.1. The concentrations of glutamic acid and aspartic acid include glutamine and asparagine respectively. Glutamic acid, alanine, and valine always dominated the plasma profile and were the most variable. A comparison of the mean paediatric ranges by ion-exchange chromatography (Table 20.1) showed very close agreement in the five different populations. Population D gave lower values (with the exception of proline and isoleucine) than the other three populations quantitated by ion-exchange chromatography. Column B gave a relatively low mean for isoleucine.

Table 20.1 Comparison of mean plasma amino acid concentrations determined by ion-exchange and gas chromatography

Amino acid	*Ion-exchange* (μmol/ml)				*GC* (μmol/ml)
	A	*B*	*C*	*D*	*E*
Alanine	0.348	0.292	0.271	0.214	0.267
Valine	0.220	0.161	0.181	0.127	0.181
Glycine	0.240	0.213	0.219	0.170	0.238
Isoleucine	0.067	0.039	0.044	0.044	0.067
Leucine	0.120	0.077	0.090	0.075	0.138
Proline	0.189	0.193	0.176	0.115	0.116
Threonine	0.135	0.177	0.145	0.060	0.143
Serine	0.129	0.131	0.121	0.092	0.194
Methionine	0.025	0.018	0.016	0.021	0.023
Hydroxyproline	0.011	—	—	0.049	0.028
Phenylalanine	0.057	0.055	0.047	0.040	0.049
Aspartic acid	0.013	0.019	0.016	0.002	0.161[F]
Glutamic acid	0.051	—	—	—	0.441[F]
Tyrosine	0.055	0.054	0.045	0.045	0.059
Ornithine	0.058	0.050	0.046	0.040	0.039
Lysine	0.165	0.135	0.130	0.087	0.132
Tryptophan	0.055				0.016

A. Helen K. Berry, Chromatography Report Sheet
B. Twenty-five infants, studied before first feeding (Scriver, 1973)
C. Twelve infants, 16 days to 4 months (Scriver, 1973)
D. Twenty children, 9 months to 2 years (Scriver, 1973)
E. Thirty-one children, 0 to 4 years by GC
F. Asparagine and glutamine are measured with aspartic acid and glutamic acid

Aspartic acid and glutamic acid cannot be compared, since ion-exchange does not separate asparagine and glutamine. With the exception of aspartic acid, glutamic acid, and tryptophan (for which only one value was given), the average of the four ion-exchange determinations was never greater than one standard deviation from the mean calculated from the gas chromatographic quantitation.

Urinary amino acid concentrations

Urinary concentrations of amino acids based on thirty-one clinically normal paediatric patients are listed in Table 20.2. The urinary concentration range is very wide. Careful consideration of the total amino acid concentration proved to be helpful in determining abnormalities. A mean value for each

Table 20.2 Urinary amino acid concentrations

	Range	*Mean*	*Standard deviation*	*Average percentage of total*
Alanine	0.051–1.250	0.414	0.363	10.5%
Valine	0.120–0.137	0.061	0.035	2.1%
Glycine	0.255–2.022	0.704	1.125	32.0%
Isoleucine	0.007–0.098	0.041	0.028	1.1%
Leucine	0.014–0.177	0.063	0.045	1.2%
Proline	0.010–0.208	0.098	0.055	3.5%
Threonine	0.030–0.268	0.123	0.082	3.1%
Serine	0.040–0.499	0.240	0.144	6.8%
Methionine	0.010–0.086	0.033	0.020	1.6%
Hydroxyproline	0.010–0.149	0.070	0.042	3.1%
Phenylalanine	0.010–0.150	0.052	0.039	2.1%
Asparagine and aspartic acid	0.084–0.563	0.259	0.148	7.3%
Glutamine and glutamic acid	0.089–0.695	0.347	0.201	13.0%
Tyrosine	0.010–0.222	0.081	0.062	2.3%
Ornithine	0.014–0.070	0.035	0.016	1.7%
Lysine	0.030–0.308	0.157	0.073	7.2%
Tryptophan	0.018–0.098	0.043	0.030	1.9%

amino acid was calculated relative to the total amino acid excretion. The percentage of the total amino acid excretion for each amino acid was narrower in range than was the value for absolute concentration in μmole/ml. Additional calculation compensated for the net effect of urinary dilution or concentration.

DIAGNOSTIC PATIENT STUDIES

The metabolic disease laboratory of the University of Tennessee Child Development Center received referrals of patients suspected of having metabolic faults from two separate sources. Primarily, urine or plasma samples are sent directly from regional hospitals for metabolic screening and/or quantitative amino acid determinations. Secondly, patients are automatically referred after receiving a positive result on the State of Tennessee's mandatory bacterial inhibition assay for elevations of plasma phenylalanine concentration.

Diagnostic gas chromatography

Diagnostic follow-up of an abnormal metabolic screen indicating an abnormality of aminö acid metabolism was done by gas chromatography.

Figure 20.1 is a composite of several GC recordings made during the investigation of one patient that exhibited the clinical manifestations of an inborn error of metabolism. Figure 20.1A is a recording of a standard run of known amino acids of equimolar concentrations (2.5 μmol/ml). Figure 20.1B is the strip-chart recording of the amino acid profile of a clinically normal patient. The profile is dominated by the glutamine–glutamic acid peak (Figure 20.1B, 2) appearing before the internal standard.

Figure 20.1C is the plasma profile of a patient (A.M.H.), showing a marked elevation of the valine peak (Figure 20.1C, 1). Leucine and proline also appeared to be slightly elevated, but were within normal limits. The urinary profile (Figure 20.1D) of a casual specimen, collected at the time of the first examination, shows a marked increase in valine (Figure 20.1D, 1) concentration. The identity of the peaks in the patient was confirmed by mass-spectral analysis by Finnigan Laboratories, Sunnyvale, California 94086. The profile for cerebrospinal fluid (Figure 20.1E) from the same patient was not remarkable, only glutamine–glutamic acid being found in measurable amounts (Figure 20.1E, 2).

Further evidence of an inborn error of metabolism was sought by evaluating the branched-chain amino acid pathways. Loading tests requiring serial sampling could be accomplished easily using 50 μl for each sample. Separate oral loading tests were done on consecutive days, in which L-isomers of valine, leucine, isoleucine, and a phenylalanine control were used. All plasma amino acid concentrations were unaffected except for the four involved in the study (Figure 20.2). Phenylalanine concentrations (for phenylalanine loading only) were measured by the modified fluorescence technique of McCaman and Robins[8]. In the fasting patient, phenylalanine concentrations as measured by the spectrofluorometric and GC methods agreed closely (Figure 20.2). The plateau in valine concentration was delayed, occurring at 2 h with a decreased rate of plasma clearance. Close agreement between all amino acid concentrations other than the elevation of the exogenous amino acid provides additional evidence of the GC quantitative method. Valine was inexplicably decreased during the isoleucine load. The purity of each of the administered amino acids was checked and no contaminating compounds were found.

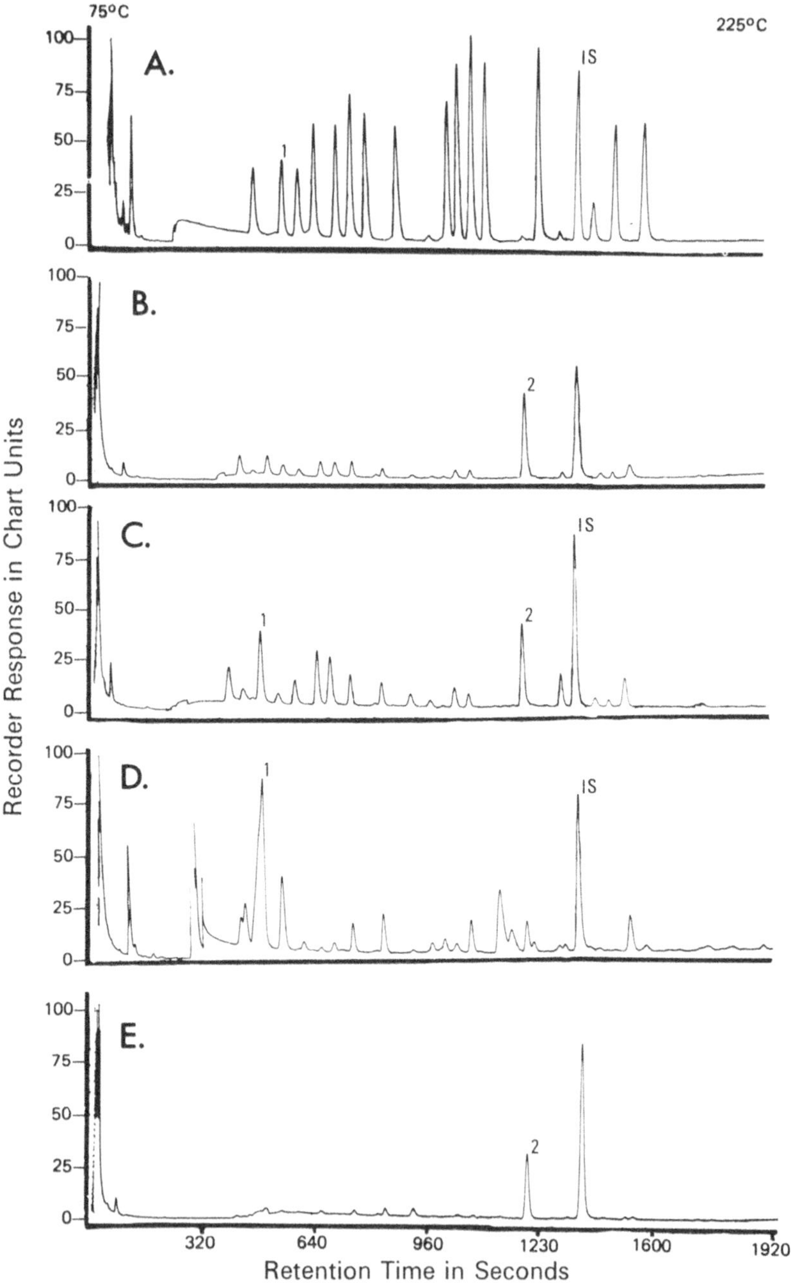

Figure 20.1 Strip-chart recordings of GC analysis of biological samples. A: Standard solution of known amino acids (each 2.5 mol/ml). B: Amino acid profile of normal plasma. C: Amino acids found in plasma of patient A.M.H. D: Urinary amino acids seen at admission of patient A.M.H. E: Amino acid profile of cerebrospinal fluid. IS: Internal standard. 1: valine. 2: glutamine–glutamic acid

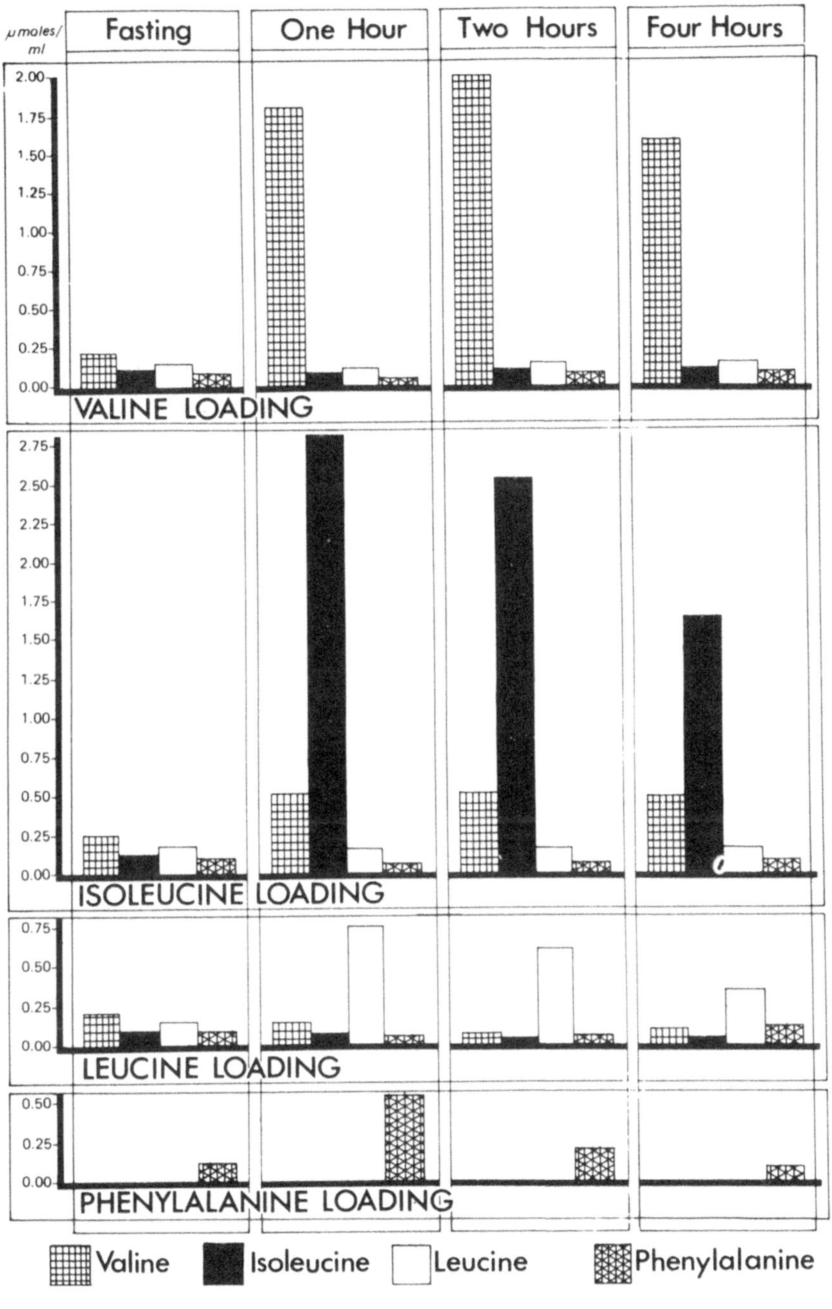

Figure 20.2 Results of oral loading tests with amino acids

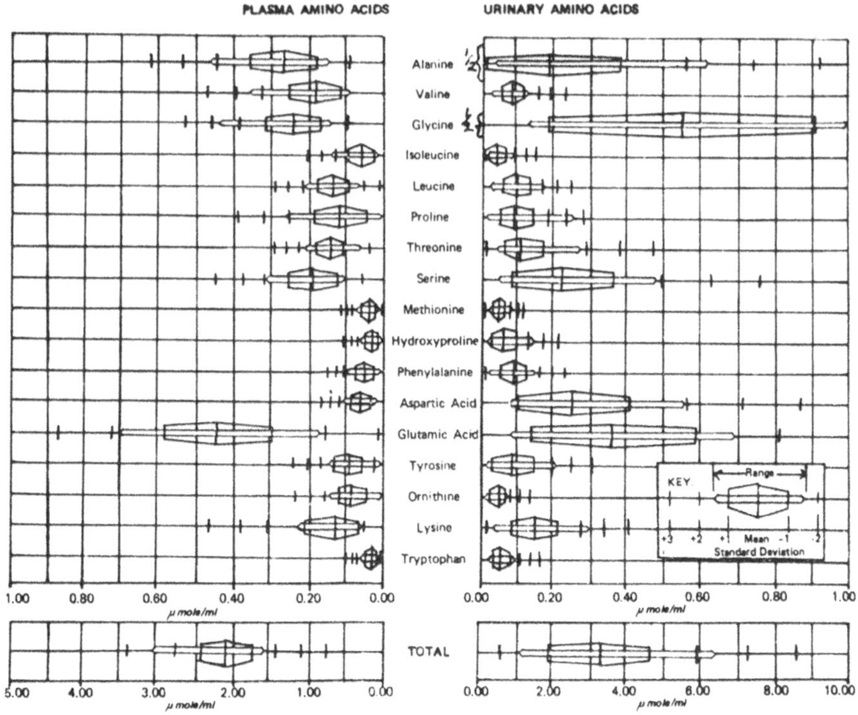

Figure 20.3 A graphic display of normal values to be used as a report form on which to indicate determined patients' amino acid profiles

Diagnostic evidence of abnormal valine metabolism supported dietary therapy with a valine restricted formulation. Careful monitoring of plasma amino acids was continued to judge the appropriate dietary inclusion of valine, isoleucine, and leucine.

In order to simplify the presentation of the complex biochemical data from both plasma and urinary quantitative amino acids, a graphic display of normal values (Figure 20.3) is used. The patient information is plotted in μmol/ml over the appropriate amino acid. The figures indicate mean, range, and standard deviations. Easy correlation of plasma and urinary profiles can be accomplished even if the user is unfamiliar with numerical values.

Differential diagnosis of the hyperphenylalaninaemias

The most common and best understood metabolic disease involves the conversion of phenylalanine to tyrosine. Because of the success of early dietary intervention in the treatment of phenylalanine elevations, screening is required by law in forty-three states in the United States.

Metabolic screening programmes, regardless of their scope, are useless

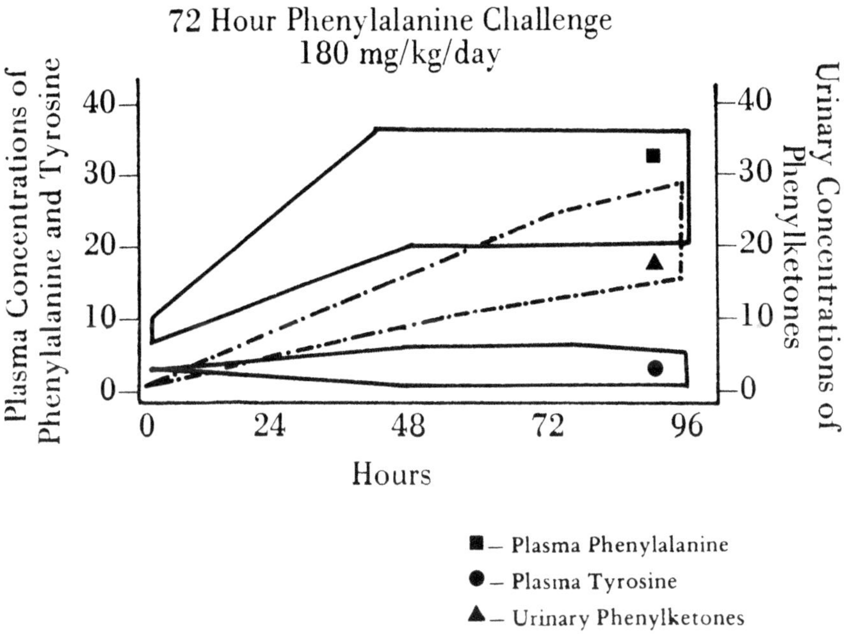

Figure 20.4 Ranges of typical responses of type I or II hyperphenylalaninaemic patients to the phenylalanine challenge

without proper diagnosis, evaluation, and subsequent follow-up. Patients with positive laboratory findings in the Tennessee's Guthrie Screening programme for phenylketonuria are now referred to the University of Tennessee Child Development Center, Clinical Biochemistry Department, for spectrofluorometric quantitation of phenylalanine, tyrosine, and histidine with provisions for complete evaluation, dietary management, and medical care at the Child Development Center for those who are not false positives.

Approximately 95% of the patients had transient elevations and were within established normal ranges when the test was repeated.

Classical phenylketonuria (PKU) is associated with very high levels of plasma phenylalanine (greater than 25 mg/dl). In recent years, an increasing number of patients have been found to have elevated plasma levels of phenylalanine (5–27 mg/dl) without mental retardation. It is extremely important to establish a differential diagnostic procedure to determine the need for dietary intervention.

The neonates with persistent plasma elevations of phenylalanine above 12 mg/dl were considered at risk and were given a phenylalanine restricted dietary intake with very close monitoring of the plasma amino acid levels. After age 3–6 months, the enzyme systems of the liver have matured, and a reproducible differential diagnosis is possible. Recommended follow-up is shown in Table 20.3.

Table 20.3 Recommendations based on laboratory results

Phenylalanine concentrations	*Recommendations*
1–4 mg/dl (0.6–0.25 mM)	Normal, no repeat
4–8 mg/dl (0.25–0.5 mM)	Repeat in 2–3 weeks with continued follow-up as necessary
8–12 mg/dl (0.5 mM–0.75 mM)	72 h phenylalanine challenge at 3–6 months with frequent continued follow-up
12.0 mg/dl or above (0.75 mM or above)	Immediate repeat. Consider institution of dietary intervention if above 16 mg/dl or 1 mM. Monitor all biochemical and clinical parameters. Mandatory phenylalanine challenge at 3–6 months

A standardized 72 h challenge diet consisting of 180 mg/kg/day of phenylalanine from natural protein has been recommended by the National Collaborative Study of Children Treated for Phenylketonuria to establish a definitive diagnosis. The response of a patient during challenge must meet specific requirements for diagnosis of classical phenylketonuria.

Plasma phenylalanine concentration must be above 20 mg/dl on two consecutive days during the 72 h challenge, abnormal phenylalanine metabolites (phenylketones) must appear in the urine and the tyrosine levels should remain within the normal paediatric ranges.

A classification scheme has been recommended[9] which recognizes several forms of hyperphenylalaninaemia based on the response to the challenge diet. A typical range of responses for a type I or II hyperphenylalaninaemic (classical PKU) is shown in Figure 20.4. A complete spectrum of responses can be seen during challenges, from normal to grossly abnormal. Appropriate and frequent monitoring must be used to determine the necessity of dietary intervention.

CONCLUSION

The summary of metabolic faults given in Table 20.4 indicates that a population referred because of previous screening and/or clinical indications of metabolic disease has, as would be expected, an increased frequency of positive results. Fast, accurate, and inexpensive microtechniques of amino acid profile estimation by high voltage paper electrophoresis and quantitation by fluorometric, ion-exchange or gas chromatography are of indisputable value both for diagnosis and clinical monitoring of treatment.

An obvious parallel exists during the intravenous administration of amino acids. Monitoring techniques can and should be applied more frequently to intravenous feeding. The estimation of appropriate amino acid profiles necessary to meet different clinical situations must continue until the practitioners of TPN are convinced that the perfect solution is being administered.

Table 20.4 Major metabolic faults detected

Metabolic fault	*Detected per* 3000	*Reported incidence per* 100,000
Phenylketonuria	10	8
Hyperphenylalaninaemia	3	3
Cystinuria	3	7
Cystathioninuria	1	(9 total)
Galactosaemia	3	1.4
Argininosuccinicaciduria	4	0.4
Maple syrup urine disease	1	0.4
Fanconi syndrome	1	0.4
Hypervalinaemia	1	(1 total)

ACKNOWLEDGEMENTS

Appreciation is expressed to the Inborn Errors of Metabolism Clinic and to Dr Samuel V. Molinary, Ms Dianne Brooks and Ms Ava Schaffer.

The training service and research of the University of Tennessee Child Development Center is funded by Special Project Grant No. 900, Division of Health Services Material and Child Health Service HSMHA, United States Department of Health, Education, and Welfare and National Institute of Health Grant No. RR-00211.

References

1. Stanbury, J. B., Wyngaarden, J. B. and Frederickson, D. S. (1972). *The Metabolic Basis of Inherited Disease*. 3rd Ed. (New York, N.Y.: McGraw Hill)
2. Jellum, E., Stokke, O. and Eldjarn, L. (1973). Application of gas chromatography, mass spectrometry, and computer methods in clinical biochemistry. *Anal. Chem.*, **54**, 1099
3. Jellum, E., Stokke, O. and Eldjarn, L. (1972). Combined use of gas chromatography, mass spectrometry and computer in diagnosis and studies of metabolic disorders. *Clin. Chem.*, **18**, 800
4. Berry, H. K., Leonard, C., Peters, H., Granger, M. and Chunecamai, N. (1968). Detection of metabolic disorders. *Clin. Chem.*, **14**, 1033
5. Gehrke, C. W., Roach, D., Zumwalt, R. W., Stalling, D. L. and Wall, L. (1968). Quantitative gas–liquid chromatography of amino acids in proteins and biological substances. Analytical Biochemistry Laboratories, Inc. Columbia, MO.
6. Tucker, H. N. and Molinary, S. V. (1973). Gas chromatography in diagnostic biochemistry of abnormal valine metabolism. *Clin. Chem.*, **19**, 1040
7. Petty, F., Tucker, H. N., Molinary, S. V. Flynn, N. W., and Wander, J. D. (1976). Quantitation of glycine in plasma and urine by chemical ionization mass fragmentography. *Clin. Chem. Acta.*, **66**, 111
8. McCaman, M., and Robins, E. (1962). Fluorometric method for the determination of phenylalanine in serum. *J. Lab. Clin. Med.*, **59**, 885
9. Blaskovics, M. E., Schaeffler, G. E. and Hack, S. (1974). Phenylalaninemia: differential diagnosis. *Arch. Dis. Childh.*, **49**, 835

Discussion

W. P. T. James: (UK) If I calculate the data correctly an increase in body protein amounting to 30% of weight-gain can be achieved. That would normally be considered to be entirely appropriate for the increasing protein mass which a premature baby would be expected to have if that baby had not been born. Can we establish the basis of the nitrogen balance. Is it urinary excretion? Is there any figure for skin loss, or gut loss?

M. Ste Marie: (Canada) We calculated the nitrogen balance as the difference between the intake (which is well regulated in the neonates, because it is by constant pump infusion) and the urinary protein nitrogen as a loss.

James: I am sure that Dr Ste Marie is familiar with the problem as set out by Widdowson, Dauncey, and Shaw in Cambridge and London[1], whereby they based the requirements on body compositional data of premature babies. As I understand it they are suggesting that there is, in addition to the very high protein requirements of the premature baby, the very important elemental requirements which are very difficult to achieve by the administration of any fluid intravenously. There is also a lot of data specifically relating to trace elements, suggesting that there is a very high requirement—and perhaps the word 'trace' is a misnomer. For example would 10 ml of plasma provide a sufficient quantity of trace elements to these children.

Ste Marie: I am not aware of data that specifically state the exact amounts of trace elements that a premature baby should receive per day. The plasma infusion that we give is in order to counteract the fact that up until now major hyperalimentation regimens have not provided these trace elements.

A. B. Jones: (Canada) Our babies were given blood quite frequently, not intentionally to give trace elements. It presumably gave some, but in micro-amounts.

Luckily the majority of babies are being supplemented only, not totally parenterally fed. Most of them are on breast milk at the same time, particularly the type of infants which Dr Ste Marie may be discussing who are apnoeic, and are on a respirator, etc., who cannot take total oral feeding. The babies that I was describing, with enterocolitis, are usually on intravenous feeding for 10 days at the most, and therefore not likely to run out of trace elements. However, babies with complicated surgical problems are likely to be on TPN for much longer than that. One of the first babies that we ever treated was fed intravenously for several months, and this was before we had a trace element solution in the hospital. He grew at a normal rate; at a 90 percentile for age and he was not fed at all via his intestines for the first 8 weeks, and we gave him no trace elements. Indeed the volume of blood needed to measure zinc, copper, etc., was more than we could have taken from him anyway, which is another problem.

We need more knowledge about what these babies require if they are being totally fed parenterally, for a long time. I am sure that the requirements are much greater than average.

Ste Marie: There is a need for caution in TPN in very-low-birthweight premature neonates. I agree with Dr Jones that this is not a procedure to be carried out automatically in these babies.

The patients we studied were acutely ill infants with a variety of clinical conditions, mostly severe hyaline membrane disease, respiratory insufficiency, cardiac insufficiency, etc. They needed intravenous feeding because we could not give them anything by mouth. This should not be a regular procedure for the very-low-birthweight prematures where I would prefer oral nutrition.

James: The difficulty with balance studies in infants is that if balance is achieved one does not know whether it is appropriate without the fundamental data on the increases to be expected under normal circumstances. There is a distinct difference between applying balance data in an adult and applying that concept to the premature baby who normally has to undergo such an enormous accretion of different elements.

J. T. Harries: (UK) I think perhaps in respect to zinc there is some evidence[2, 3] that both the experimental animal and man may be on the brink of zinc deficiency. The provision of zinc in some form would seem to be of great importance in intravenous feeding schemes in children and adults.

Jones: Clinically zinc deficiency will present in infants as acrodermatitis enteropathica, and none of our babies have had that. Obviously that is gross zinc deficiency, and it has been produced in adults who are on parenteral feeding without adequate zinc replacement, but at least as yet we have not seen that syndrome in infants on TPN.

Harries: Using PHA stimulation of lymphocytes in children with acrodermatitis enteropathica who have been successfully treated with zinc, and after zinc supplementation, their PHA response returns to normal; this can be reversed to an abnormal response within a few days of stopping their zinc supplementation, when they are very well, and their nutritional status is excellent.

Fell: One practical point. One does not know how much zinc one is giving in all the other fluids. There is a substantial amount of contamination in certain of the amino acid preparations and other fluids, so that one is giving far more than one thinks. This may be why gross deficiency rarely occurs; although I would support the view that the avoidance of acrodermatitis is rather a poor index as to whether an optimal amount is being given.

S. J. Karran: (UK) I got the impression that Dr Ste Marie was not totally happy with some of the constituents and proportions of the amino acid mixture used, and that there is no ideal mix available at the moment. Has she formed any firm conclusions as to what she would like for these neonates and come up with an ideal solution?

Ste Marie: No. Not even in theory. I do not think that enough work has been done in this particular area. One of the best examples is the recent work on taurine in New York[4]. Nobody had heard about taurine until a year ago, and then suddenly it became an essential amino acid for premature babies.

Jones: All our babies had what our laboratory considered to be normal taurine levels. Obviously more work needs to be done on amino acid formulations. It would be nice to have a little methionine. It probably would be advantageous to have cystine, but that needs further work, particularly in relation to the fact that our babies had normal cystine levels. Glycine could quite reasonably be less, as long as one could find a reasonably economic alternative to provide the non-essential nitrogen.

H. A. Krebs: (UK) I should like to comment on the question of special solutions for neonates, with special reference to Dr Ste Marie's comment that cystine and taurine may be essential. It is well established that, for the adult, methionine can supply all the cysteine, cystine and taurine. However, I gather from what Dr Jones has said that the enzymes handling the conversion from methionine to cysteine—those involving cystothionine—are not fully developed in the neonate. That would imply that the derivatives of methionine are not readily made in the neonate or premature infant. There would then be a case for making additions to the amino acid solutions.

Cystine or cysteine are not manageable, cystine because it is so insoluble, and cysteine because it is readily oxidized to cystine, but the addition of taurine would be warranted on the basis of general considerations. The very special situation of the neonate, quite different from that of the adult, warrants modification of the Travasol formula.

D. B. Allardyce: (Canada) Might I ask the three paediatricians about the technique of administration of parenteral solutions to infants. They all alluded to using scalp-vein and centrally-placed catheters. Dr Harries had septicaemia listed in the complications in both instances. Were these septicaemias traceable to the central catheter in these children? If Dr Jones or Dr Ste Marie used central catheters, was there any appreciable incidence of fungal or bacterial septicaemias in any of the infants that were fed for extended periods?

Harries: We are able to maintain infants on total intravenous feeding entirely by peripheral veins for periods of up to about 3 weeks. In the two patients that I illustrated, central venous catheters were necessary. Central venous catheterization of these children was probably directly related to the septicaemic episodes that they had. For example, we did grow the same organism from the tip of the catheter as we did from the blood.

On the other hand, there were a wide number of other variables in these very sick children, on intravenous feeding for periods of up to 18 months. In 4 kg infants after that period of time the veins begin to run out. Septicaemia certainly occurred during periods of central venous catheterization, and in our experience was extremely rare during peripheral vein catheterization.

Ste Marie: I have no evidence of septicaemia in my cases, probably because we always use peripheral veins. We have been able to maintain some of these neonates, particularly those after surgery of the gastrointestinal tract and short gut—for periods of up to 6 or 7 months with peripheral infusion only.

Jones: In relation to plasticizers and enterocolitis as suggested in a recent *Lancet* editorial[5], some of these infants were having intravenous feeds running when they developed necrotizing enterocolitis. Others were not. I suspect that necrotizing enterocolitis is a multi-factorial disease involving a number of different aetiologies. One is absolutely certainly infectious, and there have been outbreaks of necrotizing enterocolitis associated with infectious agents.

R. K. Ausman: (USA) In what is obviously a very short period of time there have been immense changes in therapy and we are now faced with the problems cited by Dr Harries. He mentioned that the zinc deficiency has been related to immune deficiency. I wonder if he could expand so that we could identify it further, because it is the first explanation that I have heard which gives support to the changes that occurred in terms of the causes of septicaemia or the types of septicaemia.

From 1965 to 1970, the literature rarely speaks of *Candida* septicaemia. From 1970 on there was a radical change and *Candida* septicaemia becomes almost a dominant feature, not because it is discussed so much, but because it has such a high incidence. We know that from

1970 on parenteral nutrition was an important part of care. We understand now to some extent that zinc deficiency occurs more frequently and earlier than we had ever expected, so a correlation might exist.

Harries: There is some information from Dr Colin Mills at the Rowett Institute, on experimental animal work[2], that zinc may be important in terms of immune function as judged by PHA stimulation of lymphocytes.

In our patient zinc deficiency was diagnosed by plasma levels of zinc, which I agree are not a very good index of total body zinc. Nevertheless, there was a triad of *Candida* septicaemia, zinc deficiency as judged by very low circulating levels of zinc, and an impairment in PHA stimulation of lymphocytes.

H. N. Tucker: (USA) I have a question for Dr Jones concerning reported elevations of methionine in his patients. We know that even in severely compromised enzyme systems, if we wish these to progress even marginally, we increase the precursor to stress that enzyme system. Do you consider that to be the case in achieving normal cystine levels in your patients?

Jones: We use only 0.5 cc deproteinized plasma for the amino acid analysis, so we have used only 2 cc blood for the total analysis. We are setting up the amino acid system on a GLC as well.

I do not know the answer to Dr Tucker's question in relation to the methionine and the cystine. I do not know how long it takes to induce the cystathionase or whatever enzyme system is necessary to produce cystine. We take the blood on the fifth day of TPN because by that time they are usually getting fairly close to taking breast milk. Whether 5 days would have been enough to induce enzyme activity I am not sure.

H. F. Woods: (UK) I was interested when Dr Tucker said that there is a potential danger in infusing amino acid solutions in the neonate because one might happen to come across a child who has a congenital defect in amino acid metabolism. I myself know of no case which has been well documented but one need not actually limit oneself to that group of patients. Particularly where we are discussing phenylketonuria, it really depends on what sort of mechanisms one is interested in, in terms of the biochemical pathogenesis of the central nervous system damage in phenylketonuria. It is relevant in the very young patient, the neonate, and the premature infant, Mayor and his group[6] working in Spain have described recently that many of the alternative products of phenylalanine metabolism are inhibitors of those enzymes which are involved in the utilization of ketone bodies in the brain. Therefore it does not matter whether the child has phenylketonuria, but if sufficient phenylalanine were to be infused and spill over from the hydroxylation pathway into transamination, deamination and decarboxylation pathways, and it was to be spilled out with sufficient concentrations of these alternative phenylalanine and tyrosine products, then one could postulate that this may be disadvantageous in terms of possible use of ketone bodies as an energy substrate by the brain.

Tucker: I do agree with Professor Woods' comment. I did not mean to imply that a metabolic fault was the only indication for monitoring amino acid concentrations. The point I made was that I think it is important to monitor this at all times during amino acid administration.

I feel, however, that it would be very difficult to raise the phenylalanine level in the normal infant to the 16 mg/dl that might cause spillage of abnormal metabolic products. It is very difficult, even in heterozygotes, to get any response whatsoever to increased infusion of amino acids.

References

1. Widdowson, E. M., Dauncey, J. and Shaw, J. C. L. (1974). *Proc. Nutr. Soc.*, **33,** 275
2. Mills, C. F., Quaterman, J., Chesters, J. K., Williams, R. B. and Dalgarno, A. C. (1969). *Am. J. Clin Nutr.*, **30,** 612
3. Halstead, J. A., Smith, J. C. and Irwin, M. S. (1974). *J. Nutr.*, **104,** 347
4. Sturman, J. A., Rassin, D. K., Hayes, K. C. and Gaul, G. F. (1977). *Paed. Res.*, **11,** 4, 450
5. Editorial (1977). *Lancet*, **i,** 459
6. Mayor, F., Benavides, J., Guninez, C. and Valdivieso, F. (1975). *Proc. Int. Soc. Neurochem.*, **194,** 267

Section VII
Control of Infection in Parenteral Nutrition

21
Microbial hazards in the assembly of intravenous infusions

R. B. KUNDSIN

INTRODUCTION

Factors that influence the rate of contamination of infusions can be described as a result of cultures of 1737 infusions in plastic containers with an overall contamination rate of 0.69 %. Preparation of the infusions in various hospital wards of a teaching hospital was tested by requesting duplicates of actual infusions designated for patient use. While statistical significance could not be calculated because of the low rate of contaminants, certain trends were found to be consistent. Attachment of the administration set to the container resulted in 0.40 % contamination of infusions. With one additive, the incidence was almost doubled (0.78 %); with two additives, incidence was again doubled (1.51 %). Each additive was therefore a calculated microbial risk as manipulation sequentially doubled the contamination.

Environmental micro-organisms have been incriminated in infections of patients undergoing cardiac and urinary tract catheterization as well as in infections of patients undergoing surgery, inhalation therapy, and haemodialysis. This study has extended this relationship to include the area of preparation of infusions to the rate of contamination. Areas with a higher number of environmental micro-organisms resulting from multiple activities were associated with a higher rate of contamination.

CULTURING PROCEDURE

Formulations to be tested were made up in duplicate on the nursing units. Identical additives, syringes, and infusion tubing were used. Customary personnel performed the task with the usual technique at the usual location.

One of the two systems that had been prepared for infusion was chosen for sterility testing.

The duplicate specimen was cultured in the laboratory using the following technique. The needle adaptor on the infusion set was connected to the inflow portal of a Millipore field monitor fitted with a 0.45 micrometer filter. The plastic plugs of the field monitor were removed and stored in 70% ethyl alcohol during the procedure. Sterile sampling tubing leading to a sterile flask was attached to the discharge portal of the field monitor, as shown in Figure 21.1, and the entire quantity of solution was filtered by gravity at the same rate as intended for the patient. The effluent sampling tubing was directed into a sterile flask as retrograde contamination can occur. A sterilized assembly of a Swinnex 13 filter (Millipore) and 20 gauge needle was used to perforate the disinfected medication site of the bag. As the bag was designed to prevent the solution from draining the set, complete emptying of the assembled apparatus was accomplished by admitting filtered air.

After the solution drained completely through the monitor, the appropriate medium was added with a syringe and needle through a disinfected site on the infusion set as shown in Figure 21.1. The most versatile culture medium for the growth of bacteria was found to be Bacto-tryptose phosphate broth (Difco) of one and one-half times normal strength.

The medium was added as follows: (1) The distal end of the infusion tube was isolated by clamping. (2) The injection site was wiped with 70% ethyl alcohol. (3) 3 ml of 1.5 times normal strength sterile Bacto-tryptose phosphate broth was added with a sterile syringe from individual test tubes containing 3 ml. (4) The tubing was held vertically above the monitor to ensure media flow into the monitor and not back into the line. The medium usually drained through the monitor without suction. If necessary, a 5 ml syringe attached to the lower portal was sufficient to pull the medium through the filter. The suction was stopped as soon as the medium disappeared from the tip of the filter. (5) The plastic plug (stored in the interval in 70% ethyl alcohol) used to occlude the lower portal of the monitor was replaced. The infusion tubing was dielectrically sealed or mechanically clipped above the flashball site and cut, leaving the monitor isolated.

The monitor was incubated at 37 °C for five days, and inspected daily for growth without opening. On the fifth day, the monitor was opened and searched for colonies. If there was growth, the number of colonies was counted, smears were Gram-stained, and a subculture made for identification. The filter was then stained with 1% malachite green and immersed in a preserving solution.* If no colonies were visible, the filter was simply stained with 1% malachite green. All stained filters were retained as a permanent record.

The procedures listed in Steps 1 to 5 were carried out under an ultraviolet

* Preserving solution: 8 ml of glycerol; 17 ml of distilled water; 15 ml of 40% formaldehyde.

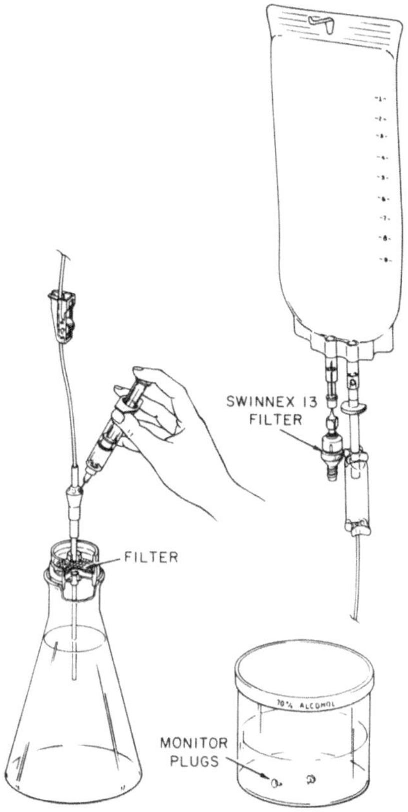

Figure 21.1 Technique for in-use testing of infusions in plastic containers

lamp (2,537 A) to minimize chance contamination with environmental micro-organisms at the time the infusion line was attached to the field monitor and when the medium was injected through the flashball site, the only two occasions when laboratory contamination could occur[1]. It is conceivable that some contamination can be attributed to the testing laboratory although a control test of 100 bags with no prior manipulations did not result in any isolations.

THE RESULTS OF CULTURES

The results of culturing the liquid from 1737 bags, duplicates of those prepared for administration to patients, are shown in Table 21.1. The number of additives for each bag is indicated. Twelve out of a total 1737 bags were found with contaminants, an incidence of 0.69% (Table 21.1). Five bags had fungi (*Pullularia pullulans*, *Mycelia sterila*, *Aspergillus* spp., *Aspergillus glaucus*, and *Paecilomyces* spp.). Four bags had colonies of *Bacillus* species, one bag had micrococci, one a diphtheroid, and one bag had *Bacillus* species

Table 21.1 Contamination as related to number of additives, December 1971–March 1977

No. additives	*(Viaflex) No. Cultured*	*Number contaminated*	*Percentage contaminated*
0	756	3	0.40
1	767	6	0.78
2	199	3	1.51
3	15	0	0
	1737	12	0.69

and *Corynebacterium xerosis*. The *Bacillus* species and fungi are both microorganisms suggesting environmental sources. The microccoci, diphtheroid and *Corynebacterium xerosis* suggested human sources. The contamination when found, was low, usually one colony, indicating casual contamination not originating in the solution. Each manipulation doubled the rate of contamination. The percentage of isolates increased with the number of additives, 0.40% with none, 0.78% with one, and 1.51% with two additives—an apparent association between contaminants and the number of manipulations on the ward. A bag with no additives still had one manipulation involving attachment of the administration set, thus accounting for the one organism recovered from a no-additive bag.

ENVIRONMENTAL FACTORS RELATING TO CONTAMINATION

Table 21.2 shows the percentage of contamination found in different hospital areas where infusions were prepared. It became apparent that certain areas were more prone to have contaminated bags than others. Investigation

Table 21.2 Contamination as related to area of preparation, December 1971–March 1977

Pavilion	*Viaflex (No. of solutions)*	*Number contaminated*	*Percentage contaminated*
A Main	57	0	0
A Second	53	1	1.89
A Third	54	0	0
Dialysis Unit	325	1	0.33
B Ward	25	0	0
C Main	307	2	0.65
C Second	160	1	0.63
D Main	119	2	1.68
D Second	204	1	0.49
Bartlett Unit	76	0	0
E Second	135	3	2.22
F Main	137	0	0
F Second	72	1	1.39
The Clinical Center	1	0	0
Pharmacy	12	0	0
	1737	12	0.69

revealed that all the second floor medication rooms had facilities for cooking, eating and congregating, while the first floor medication rooms did not condone such diverse activities. Because of the low overall rate of contamination no statistical significance could be calculated for this relationship.* There did, however, appear to be a trend towards a higher rate of contamination in areas where higher numbers of environmental micro-organisms were found, as shown in Table 21.3.

Table 21.3 Environmental microbiology of medication rooms used for preparation of infusions

Description	*Proportion of solutions contaminated*	*Air*		*Surfaces (Percentage with 25 VP/25 cm²)*
		Wells VP/ft³ (average)*	*Fallout VP/ft²/min (average)*	
Medication/Storage (5 rooms)	0.32% (1/311)	5	5	40
Medication/Storage with kitchen (7 rooms)	1.19% (5/420)	11	6	55

* VP = viable particles

Three types of environmental cultures were done: volumetric air samples indicative of small particles wafted on air currents expressed as viable particles per cubic foot; fallout or viable particles settling out per square foot per minute; accumulations on surfaces as determined by a 25 cm² impression plate (Rodac). All three culture parameters were higher in medication rooms with a wider range of activity.

EDUCATIONAL IMPACT OF RANDOM MONITORING

Monitoring of the microbiology of the Viaflex bags was accomplished with the cooperation of the staff on each ward. Culture results were reported back to the personnel involved in the study on a regular basis. Such communication resulted in a consistent reduction in the rate of contamination over the years of the study. From 1971 to 1976 the rate of contamination was decreased by over 50% as shown in Table 21.4.

Table 21.4 Contamination as related to period of monitoring

Years	*Viaflex (no. of solutions)*	*Number contaminated*	*Percentage contaminated*
1971–1972	667	6	0.90
1973–1976	482	3	0.62
1975–1976	485	2	0.41

* Consultation with Marjorie Drolette, Ph.D., Associate Professor of Biostatistics, Harvard School of Public Health.

GENERAL CONCLUSIONS

Intrinsic contamination of infusions in glass containers due to faulty sterilization procedures has been reported[2,3]. Extrinsic contamination can also occur during formulation of the solutions for administration on a ward. This second type of contamination is sporadic and depends on the technique and bacteriologic understanding of the individual adding constituents to the infusion. The results of this study indicate that extrinsic contamination can occur during manipulation of plastic containers. The number of additives and the area of preparation appeared to influence the rate of contamination.

The overall rate of contamination was found to be low (0.69%) and each contamination was usually due to very few organisms. Nevertheless, microbial growth is unpredictable and organisms with a proclivity for growth under most adverse conditions of incubation are known to exist. One appropriate organism with luck can proliferate at a wide range of pH values, temperatures, and even nutrients. *Pseudomonas* species are known to grow rapidly in distilled water. Thus, maintenance of an intact system for infusions is paramount.

Recommendations for the preparation of infusions are:

(1) The surface where manipulations are made should be disinfected daily. Protection by ultraviolet irradiation is recommended. A laminar air flow hood is an expensive luxury.

(2) Infusions should be prepared immediately prior to administration.

(3) Delayed infusions or refrigeration should be avoided. Waste of outdated mixtures is eliminated.

(4) Random monitoring of infusions should be done. The educational impact of monitoring is substantial.

References

1. Kundsin, R. B., Walter, C. W. and Scott, J. A. (1973). In-use testing of sterility of intravenous solutions in plastic containers. *Surgery*, **73** (5), 778

2. Duma, R. J., Warner, J. F. and Dalton, H. P. (1971). Septicemia from intravenous infusions. *N. Engl. J. Med.*, **284**, 257

3. (1971). Epidemiologic notes and reports: Follow-up on septicemias associated with contaminated Abbott intravenous fluid. *Mortality and Morbidity*, **20**, 91

22
Bacterial contamination of intravenous infusions due to faulty technique

C. W. WALTER

A review of the literature and a survey of hospital practices was carried out to gain the perspective for the design of a protocol for the investigation of the bacterial contamination of parenteral fluids in general hospital practice. Breaks in technique were discovered that indicate the need for a fingerproof design of the infusion apparatus and reform in the behaviour of personnel administering parenteral fluid. Either disinfected hands or sterile gloves must be used for the manipulation of the infusion apparatus. An aseptic conscience must dominate such manipulations.

Reports in the literature showed widely scattered rates of septicaemia associated with parenteral therapy. There was insufficient detail to permit comparison of techniques used. Confusion and contradiction were common.

A survey of hospital practices revealed little standardization of technique or coordination of practices throughout the complex of a general hospital. Practices prevalent during the day bear little relation to those pursued during the evening, at night, over the weekend or on a holiday. The protocol developed by a specialized team to manage total parenteral nutrition is ignored elsewhere in the same hospital. Expediency and carelessness prevail as a backdrop for the excellence of the few who are dedicated to perfection in the infection-prone field of parenteral therapy. The patient falls victim to the behaviour of chance individuals involved in the technical aspects of his infusion. Errors and carelessness are compounded with change in the location of patient care, the increase in duration of the infusion from hours to days, and the complexity in the composition of the parenteral fluid. The diversity in technique can be appreciated by following a patient through a common sequence: the induction room, operating room, recovery room, intensive

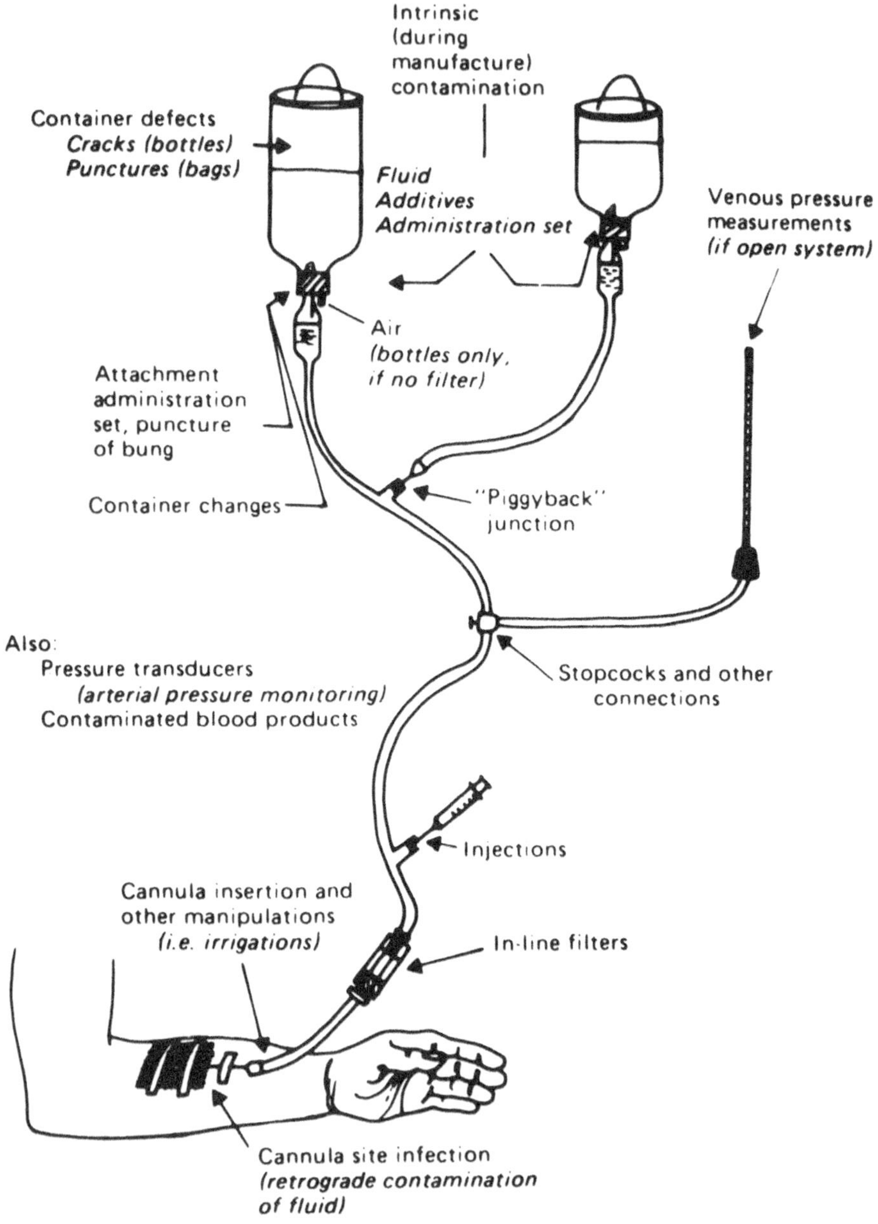

Figure 22.1 Potential sources for contamination of infusion fluid

care unit, and the nursing unit. Lack of continuity in responsibility for good practice is the glaring fault.

Figure 22.1 graphically itemizes the many portals of entry for bacteria[1]. The majority are created by the concepts and habits of persons starting or maintaining the infusion. A common error is depicted. That 'dry sterile' gauze dressing applied to protect the wound of entry frequently becomes wet with blood, tissue fluid, or solution from a leaking connection. The skin macerates, bacteria grow and penetrate the interface between the cannula—either a needle or catheter—and the skin. A strip of Micropore* tape applied over the puncture site effectively immobilizes the cannula, permits moisture to evaporate, and excludes fingers and insects.

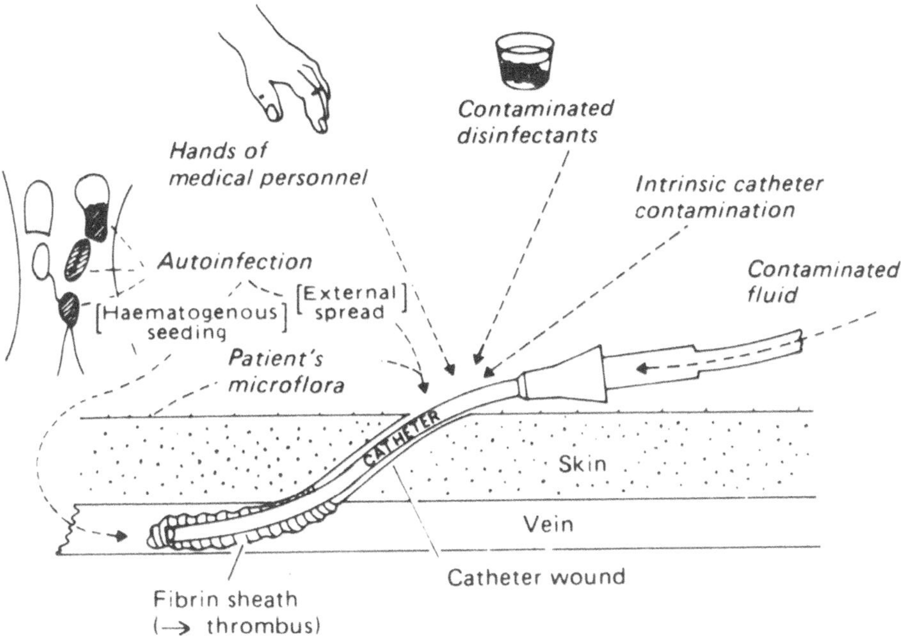

Figure 22.2 Sources of intravenous cannula-related infection

Figure 22.2 further details the sites for entry of bacteria[1]. Several elaborations are pertinent. The term 'contaminated disinfectants' is a misnomer. It is a synonym for ignorance on the part of the physician, nurse, pharmacist, or administrator. It is indicative of the neglect that dominates 'that trivial procedure', phleboclysis. A suitable disinfectant correctly formulated, properly dispensed, and intelligently used is self-disinfecting.

* Micropore Brand Surgical Tape, 3-M Company, St. Paul, Minnesota, U.S.A. 55101.

Disinfection of the skin merits examination. Figure 22.3[2] depicts the problem. It is a photomicrograph of a plug of skin that was incubated in broth. Growth of bacteria visualized their location in the complex structure of the skin. The black layer on the surface represents colonies of transient bacteria. These reflect the bacterial exposure of recent contacts. The black mass beneath the desquamating layers consists of colonies of transients that have taken up domicile in the cuticle. Both sites of bacterial accumulation are removed by scrubbing. The black masses in the ducts of the skin glands are bacteria resident in the structures of the dermis. These are not subject to removal by scrubbing and lie beyond the reach of most antiseptics other than chlorine[3]. Their growth can be suppressed by bacteriostatic agents applied to the skin daily for 4 or 5 days. Eventually desquamation rids the skin of the dormant bacteria. Resident bacteria also yield to systemic antibiotics; this was demonstrated when plugs of cadaver skin were taken to measure disinfection. The untreated control plugs were sterile. Systemic antibiotics are an evident factor in the success of parenteral therapy in certain patients despite flaws in technique.

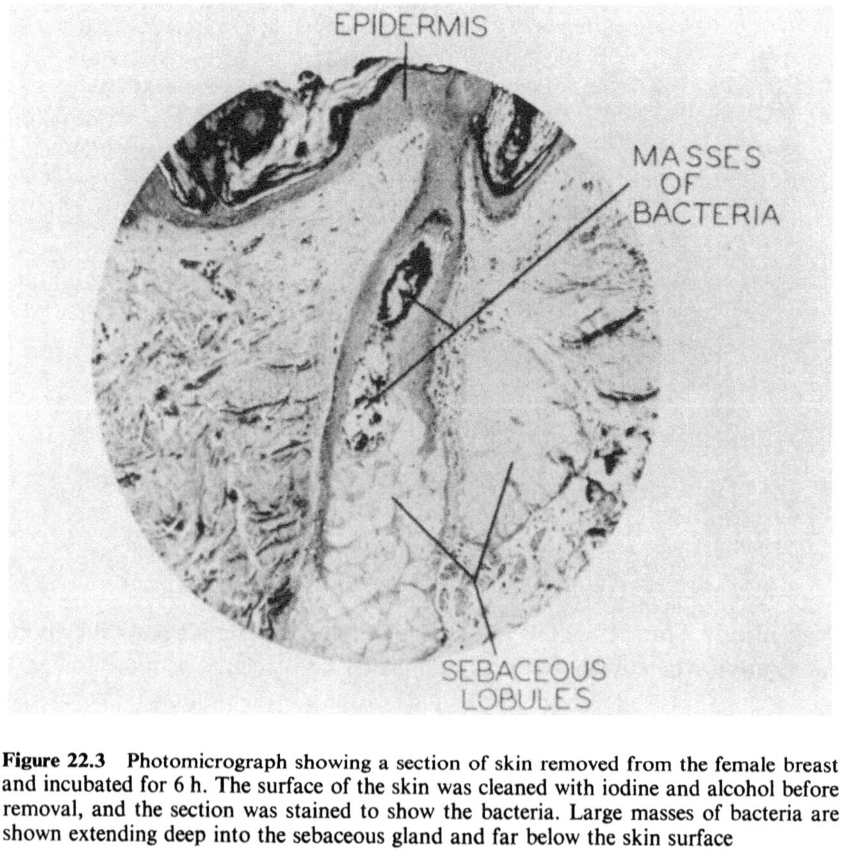

Figure 22.3 Photomicrograph showing a section of skin removed from the female breast and incubated for 6 h. The surface of the skin was cleaned with iodine and alcohol before removal, and the section was stained to show the bacteria. Large masses of bacteria are shown extending deep into the sebaceous gland and far below the skin surface

Figure 22.4 pictures a series of five sponges, alternately wetted with contrasting antiseptic detergents, that were used to scrub the antecubital skin of a blood donor. Despite her appearance of impeccable cleanliness, the fingerprints of the first sponge show the soil scrubbed off with 1:750 aqueous Zephiran*. The second sponge shows the cuticle subsequently removed by 60% isopropanol. Note the diminishing shadows with sequential scrubbing. The fifth sponge was grossly clean. The underlying epidermis was eventually exposed to the antiseptic effects of Zephiran and isopropanol. The scrubbing

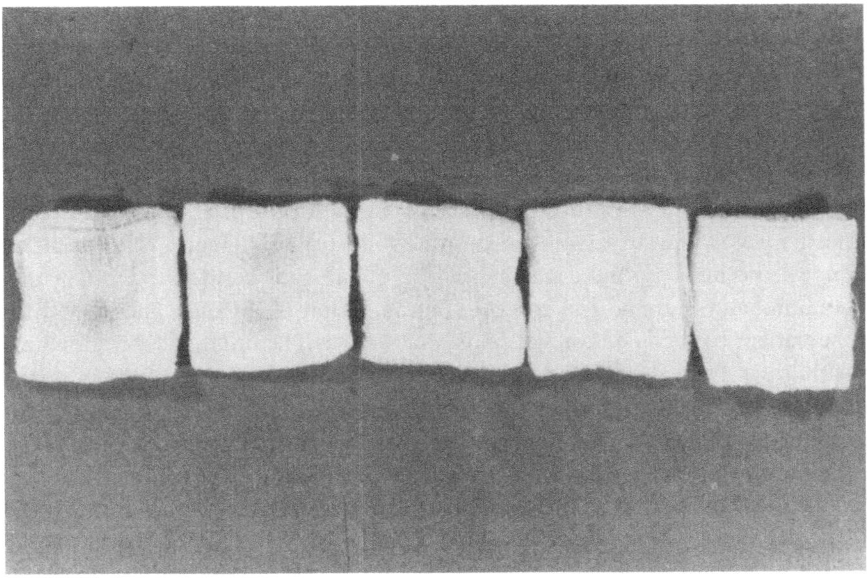

Figure 22.4 Soil scrubbed from apparently clean antecubital skin

provided time for antiseptic action—a critical requisite omitted by the quick swipe. An antiseptic, simply painted or sprayed on skin, forms a film over the surface of the cuticle. Some underlying bacteria may remain to contaminate the needle.

Growth of resident bacteria in the skin is provoked by the cannula. Until 1950 needles punched a hole through the skin. The core was displaced, plugged the lumen of the needle or embolized. Needles are now designed to lance the skin to initiate penetration. Further insertion stretches the puncture to accommodate the cannula. The adjacent taut skin becomes ischaemic.

* Zephiran chloride. Unadulterated benzalkonium chloride is designated because it does not support growth of Gram-negative bacteria as does the generic 1:750 aqueous benzalkonium chloride U.S.P. which contains up to 40% ammonium acetate as a buffer that supports growth of certain *Pseudomonas cepacia* strains. Winthrop Laboratories, 90 Park Avenue, New York, New York 10016, U.S.A.

Resident bacteria multiply in the ring of necrosing dermis and it becomes an intracutaneous source of bacteraemia.

The fibrin film about the cannula illustrated in Figure 22.2 initially deposits as a monomolecular layer[4,5]. It also forms on the wall of the lumen when blood is 'flashed back' to demonstrate a patent venepuncture. The Luer connector provides a cavity (Figure 22.5) where a blood clot as well as fibrin are deposited. When flow is established, a fluid path forms through the cavity leaving the peripheral deposit stagnant. This accumulation of clotted fibrin and blood can serve as a nidus of bacteraemia.

A more glaring fault of the Luer slip connector is its liability to contamination during manipulations inherent in its use. Figure 22.6 is a view of the connection as it is grasped to withdraw the needle from its protective sheath. A firm grasp is required to prevent the connector from being pulled from the hub of the needle. The skin of the index finger and thumb imprints the exposed hub of the needle and the taper of the connector. Figure 22.7 illustrates the bacterial contamination that occurs. The pad of the thumb was painted with a 4 h broth culture of *Escherichia coli* and air-dried. The needle was withdrawn from its sheath as illustrated in Figure 22.6 and the end of the hub imprinted on the surface of the agar beside the print of the contaminated thumb. The contact contamination is obvious. The import to the patient of such contamination is also shown. The original connector was withdrawn from the hub of the needle to permit replacement of the administration set. The first 10 ml of fluid from the newly connected set was caught in a pour-plate as it spurted from the needle. The entrainment of *E. coli* from the hub contaminated by contact with the thumbprint is obvious.

Residual clotted fibrin or blood inside the hub are thus readily contaminated. Bacteria grow in the clot suspended in the eddy currents in the throat of the needle and embolize. During manipulation of the joint, doses of bacteria are injected causing a sudden chill and peak of fever.

Figure 22.8 demonstrates that the Luer joint can be penetrated by bacteria. The administration set was plugged into the needle and the assembly withdrawn from the needle sheath by a contaminated thumb. The needle was flushed with 5% dextrose and saline prior to occluding it aseptically. The assembly was then incubated for 48 h at 37 °C. The *E. coli* had spread throughout the liquid in the set and could be cultured from the tip of the piercing coupler. The retrograde growth of bacteria probably explains why contamination has been found in administration sets so often that many advocate daily replacement. The source of bacteria, the needle, is left indwelling.

It is obvious that intravenous apparatus must be manipulated by sterile gloves until bacteria-proof connections become available. Contact contamination of the Luer hub is the likely cause of the confusing and contradictory results described in the literature.

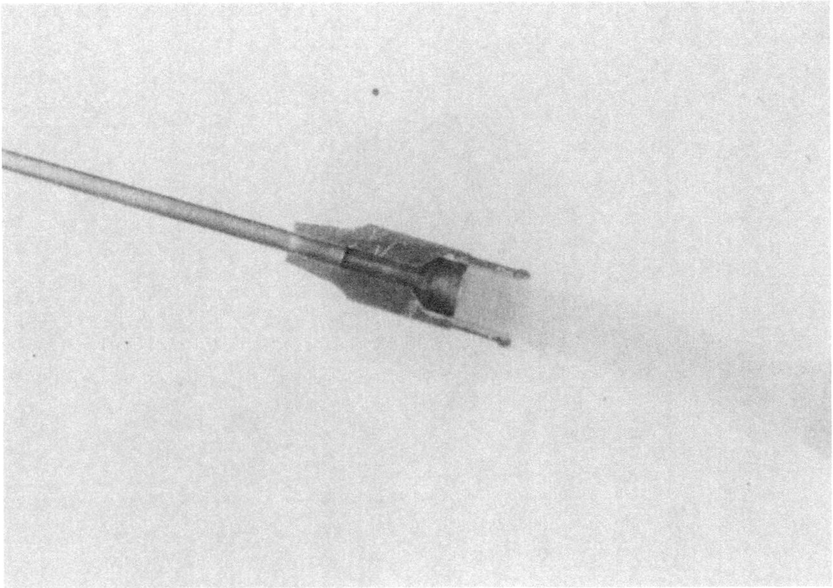

Figure 22.5 Longitudinal section of Luer hub and connector shows cavity that harbours blood and fibrin

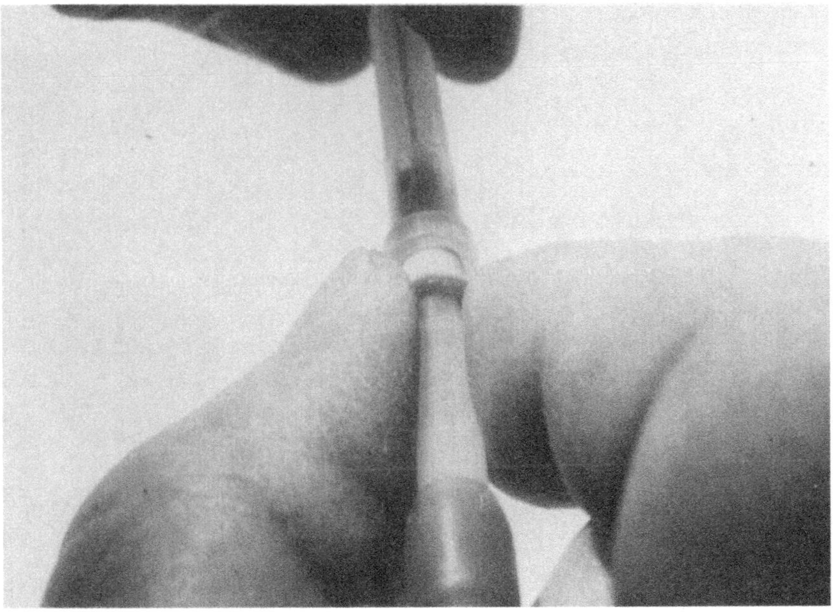

Figure 22.6 Skin of thumb and index finger imprints Luer hub and slip

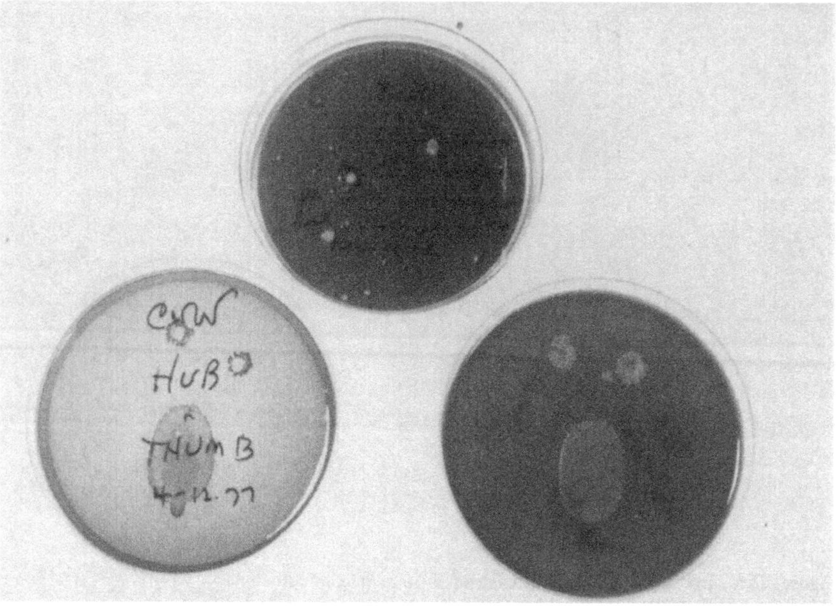

Figure 22.7 Culture plates demonstrating contamination from skin

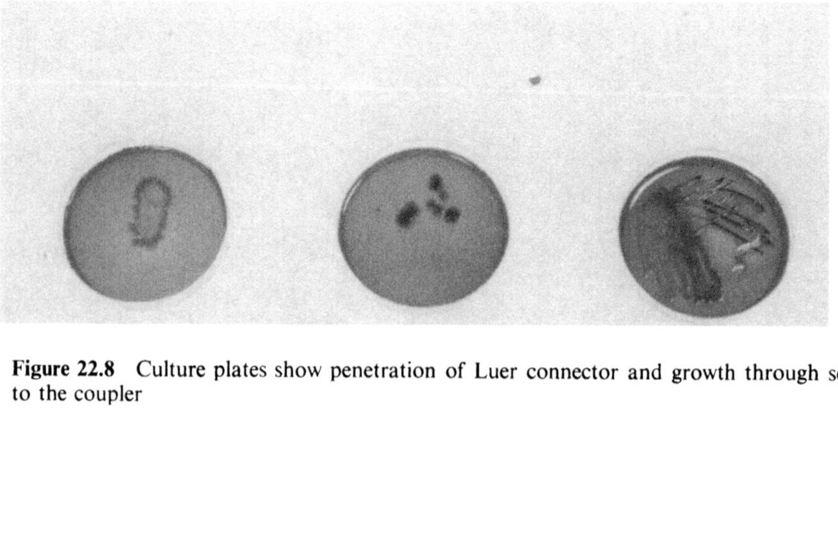

Figure 22.8 Culture plates show penetration of Luer connector and growth through set to the coupler

Exogenous contamination of the Luer hub is given a negligent dimension by the habit of grasping the needle sheath between the teeth when freeing the needle (Figure 22.9). Oral bacteria also are inoculated on the tubing of the administration set when the tubing is folded on itself and inserted between the teeth to maintain occlusion while the operator fishes for the vein. After each thrust of the needle the tubing is released to demonstrate flow. Each miss results in folding the tubing and reinserting it between the teeth, effectively contaminating the fingers. Facial hair or dangling tresses compound the bacterial hazard.

Several other breaches in technique merit discussion. The bacterial hazard of phlebotomy and phleboclysis differ. The phlebotomist places a tourniquet to effect distension of the peripheral vein. The needle is then inserted directly into the vein through the skin overlying the prominent vein (Figure 22.10). The puncture in the skin is apposed to that in the vein. The bacterial hazard is minimal when the needle is withdrawn promptly. When the needle is left for phleboclysis, bacteria invade the contiguous vein from the intracutaneous inflammatory reaction around the foreign body.

A needle intended for phleboclysis should be inserted through the skin at either side of the vein distal to the chosen site of venepuncture. It is then pushed through the subcutaneous tissue a centimetre or more before puncturing the vein (Figure 22.11). The fibroblasts lining the subcutaneous tunnel quickly form a barrier against invasion by bacteria. The cannula is stabilized in the tunnel by this technique.

Palpation of the distended vein is a frequent breach in asepsis. It results in insertion of the needle through skin imprinted with whatever contaminates the fingertip. When that finger has just been used to groom hair from the path of vision, or to stuff tubing between the teeth, the bacterial hazard is intensified. It is exceeded only by long hair dangling on the site of venepuncture. Long hair is an extension of the septic hand described by Semmelweis, and is a hazardous component of patient care.

Another breach was revealed at the Boston Blood Donor Center during World War II. Sterile cultures were reported on 60 658 consecutive bottles of blood sampled when the plasma was aspirated. Suddenly 5% of the cultures were positive[6]. These were traced to a single phlebotomist who had the reputation of being THE painless phlebotomist. The painless phlebotomy was done with needles she dragged across a thumbnail to cull the painful hooked needles! (Figure 22.12) The fact that the nail was wet with alcohol did little to enhance the sterility of the needle.

These examples of errant behaviour carry us back to a significant human experiment that occurred in 1847. You will recall that in May of that year, Ignatz Semmelweis demonstrated that hands could be freed of the septic matter that was acquired in the dissecting room[7]. He required everyone to scrub his hands with chlorinated lime on entering the obstetric clinic. Thereafter hands were washed with soap and water after each patient contact. Puerperal

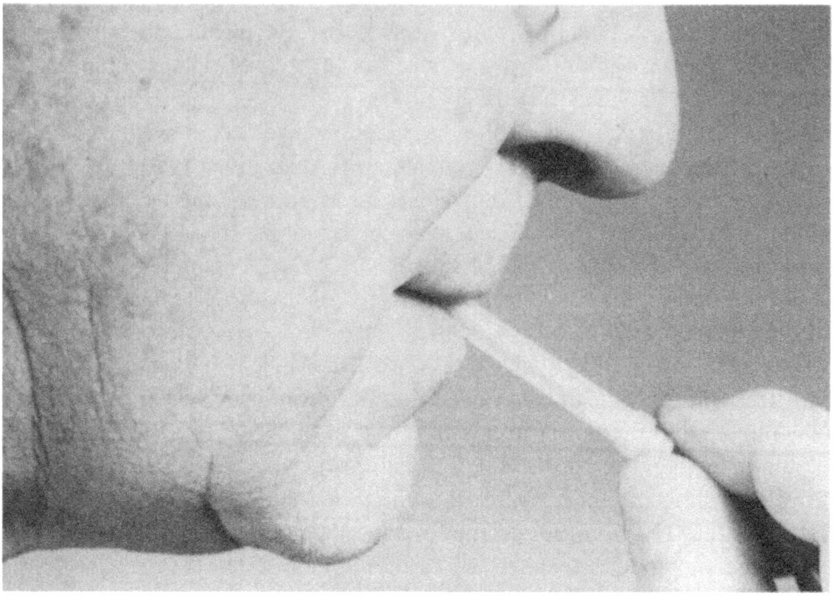

Figure 22.9 Negligent practice that enhances contamination

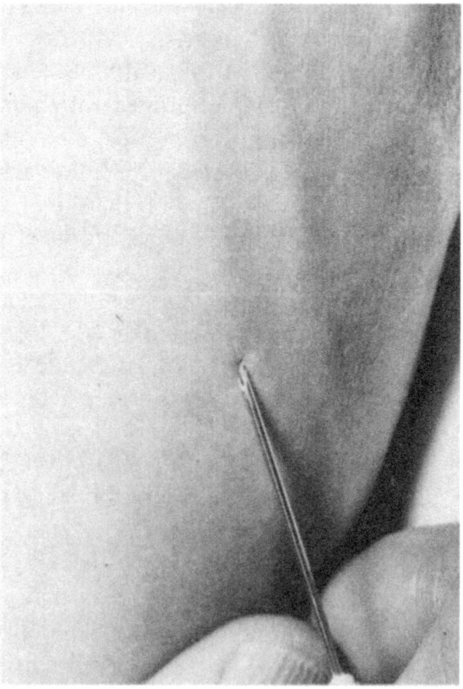

Figure 22.10 Venepuncture for phlebotomy

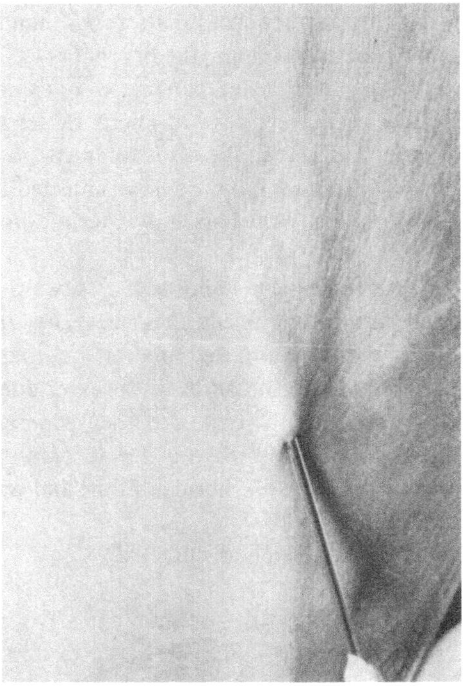

Figure 22.11 Venepuncture for phleboclysis

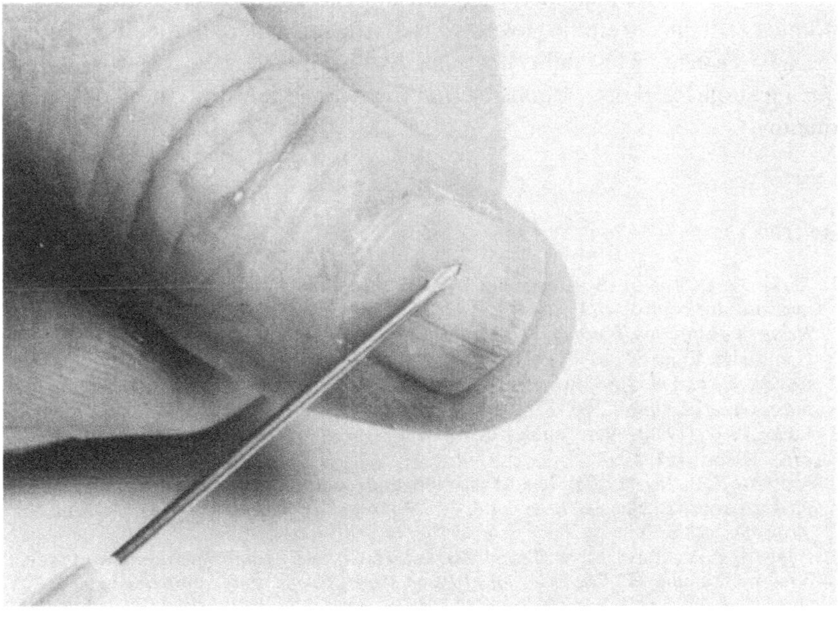

Figure 22.12 Culling hooked needle

sepsis was controlled. In October he entered the clinic with a group of students. Thirteen patients awaited examination. All hands were disinfected with chlorinated lime prior to examining the first patient. She had a sloughing cancer of the cervix. The other twelve patients were examined in sequence. Two days later eleven of them were dead of puerperal sepsis. Goaded by this horror, Semmelweis realized that sepsis also stemmed from sloughing tissue of the living patient and that hands must be disinfected after every patient contact. Simple hand-washing with soap and water did not suffice.

> 'The necessity for disinfecting the hand will . . . always be present, and in order to completely attain this object, it is necessary to oil the hand well before any contact with decomposed matter, so that the decomposed matter may not penetrate into the pores of the skin; after such occupation the hand must be washed with soap, and then exposed to the action of a chemical agent, capable of destroying the decomposed matter not yet removed; we use for this purpose chloride of lime and wash until the hands are slippery.
>
> A hand so treated is completely disinfected[7].

Yet, more than a century later the Communicable Disease Center admonishes hospital personnel to follow Semmelweis's example and wash their hands with soap and water[8].

Unsterile fingers are the cause of much of the sepsis that makes the literature in intravenous therapy confusing and contradictory. Either use of disinfected hands or sterile gloves is a requisite for manipulation of parenteral therapy systems. The ability to think like an invading microbe is a basic qualification for those responsible for the safe administration of parenteral therapy.

References

1. Maki, D. G. (1976). Sepsis arising from extrinsic contamination of the infusion and measures for control. In I. Phillips, P. D. Meers and P. F. D'Arcy (eds.). *Microbiological Hazards of Infusion Therapy*, Proceedings of an International Symposium, pp. 106, 120. (Lancaster, England: MTP Press Ltd.)
2. Lovell, D. L. (1945). Skin bacteria: their location with reference to skin sterilization, *Surg. Gynecol. Obstet.*, **80**, 174
3. Price, P. B. (1938). New studies in surgical bacteriology and surgical technic, *J. Am. Med. Assoc.*, **111**, 1993
4. Morrissey, B. W. (1977). The absorption and conformation of plasma proteins: A physical approach. In *The Behavior of Blood and Its Components at Interfaces. Ann. N. Y. Acad. Sci.*, **283**, 50
5. Cuypers, P. A., Hermens, W. T. and Hemker, H. C. (1977). Ellipsometric study of protein film on chromium. In *The Behavior of Blood and its Components at Interfaces. Ann. N. Y. Acad. Sci.*, **283**, 77
6. Walter, C. W. (1948). *Aseptic Treatment of Wounds.* 84. (New York: The Macmillan Company

7. Semmelweis, I. P. (1940–41). The etiology, the concepts and prophylaxis of childbed fever, C. A. Hartleben's Verlags—Expedition, Pest, Wien and Leipzig, 1861. Translated by Frank P. Murphy. Medical Classics, **5**, 350 (see p. 393)
8. Steer, A. C. and Mallison, G. F. (1975). Handwashing practices for the prevention of nosocomial infections. *Ann. Int. Med.*, **83**, 683

23
The incidence of nosocomial infection in patients receiving total parenteral nutrition

J. R. ALLEN

INTRODUCTION

Although attempts at intravenous alimentation with protein hydrolysates were reported as early as 1939[1], and intravenous catheters in the superior vena cava were being used for alimentation by 1948[2], little attention was paid to the potential infection hazards of this therapy during the three decades in which it was being developed. Following the initial reports by Dudrick, Wilmore and their colleagues in 1968 that total parenteral nutrition (TPN) could be employed safely for long-term nutrition with apparently normal growth, development and positive nitrogen balance[3,4], this technique was used widely. A review of published reports of TPN from the years 1969 and 1970 indicates that many centres were experiencing septicaemia rates of 14–23%[5–8], and one study reported a septicaemia rate of 93%[9]. It was not until 1972 when Curry and Quie published their experience reporting a combined bacterial and fungal septicaemia rate of 27% in patients receiving TPN[10] that the full significance of the infectious complications of this therapy was appreciated. The gravity of the situation was emphasized a year later when Heird and his colleagues[11] summarized the published experience with TPN in paediatric patients and reported a 37% septicaemia rate. By 1972, therefore, it was widely recognized that bacterial and fungal septicaemia was the major complication of TPN[12]. Only 5 years after this technique was introduced and heralded as the most significant advance in caring for patients who could not tolerate enteral nutrition, TPN received heavy criticism for not having been adequately evaluated for a risk : benefit ratio[13].

This paper reviews the progress which has been made in controlling the infection hazards of TPN therapy during the second 5 years of its use, briefly

Table 23.1 Incidence of septicaemia complicating total parenteral nutrition through central venous catheters

First author*	Year	Number of patients	Patient-days of TPN†	Rate of septicaemia (%)			Septicaemia rate/1000 Patient-days TPN	Comments
				Bacterial	Fungal	Total		
Wilmore[16]	1969	25	700	0	0	0	0.0	
Dudrick[5]	1969	22	NA	5	9	14	NA	
Filler[22]	1969	14	434	0	0	0	0.0	
Groff[6]	1969	18	396	—	—	17	7.6	
Filler[7]	1970	53	NA	6	11	17	NA	
Boeckman[9]	1970	15	885	53	40	93	18.1	
Ashcraft[8]	1970	22	NA	0	23	23	NA	
Curry[10]	1971	49	1274	10	16	27	10.2	
Owings[23]	1972	66	957	0	0	0	0.0	
Helmuth[24]	1972	4	8	0	25	25	125.0	
Peden[25]	1972	13	202	23	0	23	14.9	
Driscoll[26]	1972	9	167	0	11	11	6.0	
Johnson[27]	1972	23	NA	13	0	13	NA	
Parsa[28]	1972	307	NA	7	2	9	NA	Polyvinyl chloride catheter
		150	NA	—	—	1	NA	Silastic catheter
McGovern[29]	1972	25	NA	8	4	12	NA	
Asch[30]	1972	51	1275	8	4	12	4.7	
Freeman[20]	1972	33	660	(12)	21	21	10.6	Before starting TPN team
		78	1170	0	1	1	0.9	After TPN protocol, nurse
CDC Survey[31]	1972	2078	NA	3	4	7	NA	Survey of 31 hospitals

Miller[32]	1973	20	NA	10	10	20	NA	
Sanderson[33]	1973	100	2200	1	0	1	0.5	
Dillon[17]	1973	122	1952	2	2	4	2.6	
O'Neill[34]	1974	19	608	0	0	0	0.0	
Freeman[18]	1974	105	1414	11	3	14	10.6	Breaks in protocol observed
Copeland[35]	1974	35	770	0	0	0	0.0	Catheter sepsis suspected in 11%
Copeland[36]	1974	93	2325	0	2	2	0.9	
Ryan[19]	1974	200	4492	7	4	11	4.7	Breaks in protocol observed
Abel[37]	1974	64	847	0	0	0	0.0	
Myers[38]	1974	212	4749	0	2	2	1.1	
Popp[39]	1974	26	640	31	23	54	21.9	14 episodes sepsis in 7 burn patients
		(15)	—	—	—	(7)	—	Catheter through unburned skin
		(11)	—	—	—	(118)	—	Catheter through burned skin
Skoutakis[40]	1975	160	3280	0	1	1	0.3	
Hoshal[41]	1975	35	700	0	0	0	0.0	
Heird[42]	1975	35	1025	—	—	9	2.9	
Sanders[21]	1976	21	336	—	—	29	17.9	1970–72: Pre TPN team
		297	4346	—	—	8	5.3	1972–75: With TPN team
Filler[43]	1976	264	NA	9	7	16	NA	
Riella[44]	1976	43	15 930	16	2	19	0.5	Home TPN protocol

* Cited sources conform to text references
† Estimated from data provided
NA—data not available

reviews specific aspects of infection control practices for TPN therapy and comments on areas where further information is still necessary.

TPN ADMINISTRATION PRACTICES AND RISK OF SEPSIS

Comparison of septicaemia rates between different studies reported in the literature to evaluate the risk of infection with certain TPN administration or patient care practices is difficult because of the differences in protocols between institutions and the accepted fact that procedures as stated in a protocol frequently are not completely or properly carried out. Also, most investigators simply report anecdotal experiences with a series of patients and do not attempt to carry out controlled trials of patient-care practices to evaluate the relative risk of different patient-care procedures. Recommendations for the care of patients therefore are based almost entirely on evaluating experiences in different and non-comparable series of patients.

TPN via central venous catheters

Use of a catheter inserted percutaneously into the subclavian vein, or use of a central venous catheter inserted by cutdown with subcutaneous tunnelling of the catheter to a distant skin exit site, when carried out as originally described with strict aseptic technique[5,7,14,15], is compatible with a low frequency of sepsis and prolonged safe maintenance of the catheter (Table 23.1). In one of the original series by Wilmore and his colleagues[16] the catheters were changed only as necessary and were left in place for a mean of 24 days; in 700 patient-days of TPN therapy no patient experienced bacterial or fungal septicaemia. Most other investigators have described similar techniques of catheter insertion and maintenance, although in many series there was no guarantee that actual practices followed protocol requirements[17–19]. The results of a disorganized approach to TPN therapy are emphasized by Curry and Quie, who reported that: 'no uniform protocol was followed regarding technique of solution preparation or administration. Addition of dextrose, vitamins, etc., was usually done by personnel on the nursing stations. Albumin and blood were frequently administered through the same catheter as the protein hydrolysate solutions, and this intravenous line was often used to monitor central venous pressure as well[10].'

Other investigators, noting the high rate of septicaemia associated with an inadequately executed TPN protocol, significantly strengthened the stringent requirements for their protocols or began to employ some sort of team approach to the insertion and maintenance of TPN catheters. In a sequential study, Freeman and his colleagues[20] reported a septicaemia rate of 21% when there was no coordinated approach to TPN therapy by the pharmacy, medical or nursing staff. Following improvement of the pharmacy admixture services, the employment of a nurse to provide routine TPN catheter care, and the absolute refusal to allow the TPN catheter to be used for other purposes, the septicaemia rate fell to 1.3%. Freeman and Litton[18] subsequently reported a second series of TPN patients followed at another medical centre in which a compromise system allowed only partial supervision of TPN therapy; a TPN consultation team was available if requested although each physician maintained complete control over the care of his patients. In contrast to the low rate of septicaemia achieved with the team approach to care, 14% of the patients in this series developed septicaemia. The rate of 10.6 episodes of septicaemia per 1000 patient-days of TPN therapy is comparable to that reported by Curry and Quie[10] and Freeman *et al.*[20] prior to the institution of a team approach to TPN therapy. In eight of the eleven patients with infections caused by Gram-positive organisms the investigators documented a break in the TPN protocol or patient care practices, including catheter dressings soaked with TPN fluids and left unattended for more than 12 h; the use of piggy-back infusions or stopcocks in the TPN line; the administration of TPN fluid through a peripheral venous catheter; and irrigation of the TPN line by unauthorized personnel[18].

Dillon and his co-workers[17] observed that, although the TPN protocol did not permit the central venous catheter to be used for other purposes, it was used for central venous pressure measurements, infusion of non-TPN solutions, and administration of blood in 60% of their patients; however, the abuse of the TPN line in this series apparently was not associated with an increased risk of septicaemia. Ryan and his colleagues[19] found that 22.5% of the TPN catheters inserted in their patients were not managed according to the TPN protocol. Twenty per cent of the patients with these catheters developed septicaemia compared with only 3% of the patients in whom the catheters had been correctly maintained ($P<0.01$).

Sanders and Sheldon[21] have published recently the results of sequential studies in which they accomplished a 73% reduction in the rate of septicaemia, from 29% to 8% by instituting a TPN service for the hospital rather than leaving the total care of the patient and his TPN catheter in the hands of the Junior medical staff. During the last 12 months of the study, after an initial 2-year period with the TPN service, the rate of septicaemia decreased to only 4.7%.

These recent reports of TPN therapy in acutely ill patients emphasize that bacterial or fungal septicaemia is not an inevitable complication. A maximum rate of septicaemia of 1% to 2% of patients, or fewer than two episodes per 1000 patient-days of TPN therapy, can be achieved.

Team approach for TPN therapy

Each report of a series of patients receiving TPN through a central venous catheter was assigned to one of four categories of TPN patient care practices. The first category was one in which it was clear that no central authority or team approach was used to care for TPN patients. The second category included reports in which a central TPN authority or a partial team approach was used but in which there was not strict control of all aspects of TPN patient care. The third category included reports in which a full team approach to TPN therapy was used, with strict control of all aspects of fluid preparation and patient care. The fourth category included reports which could not be assigned definitely to one of the three preceding categories but in which it appeared from the description of the study that the investigator was the person primarily responsible for the care of the patient. Many of the reports

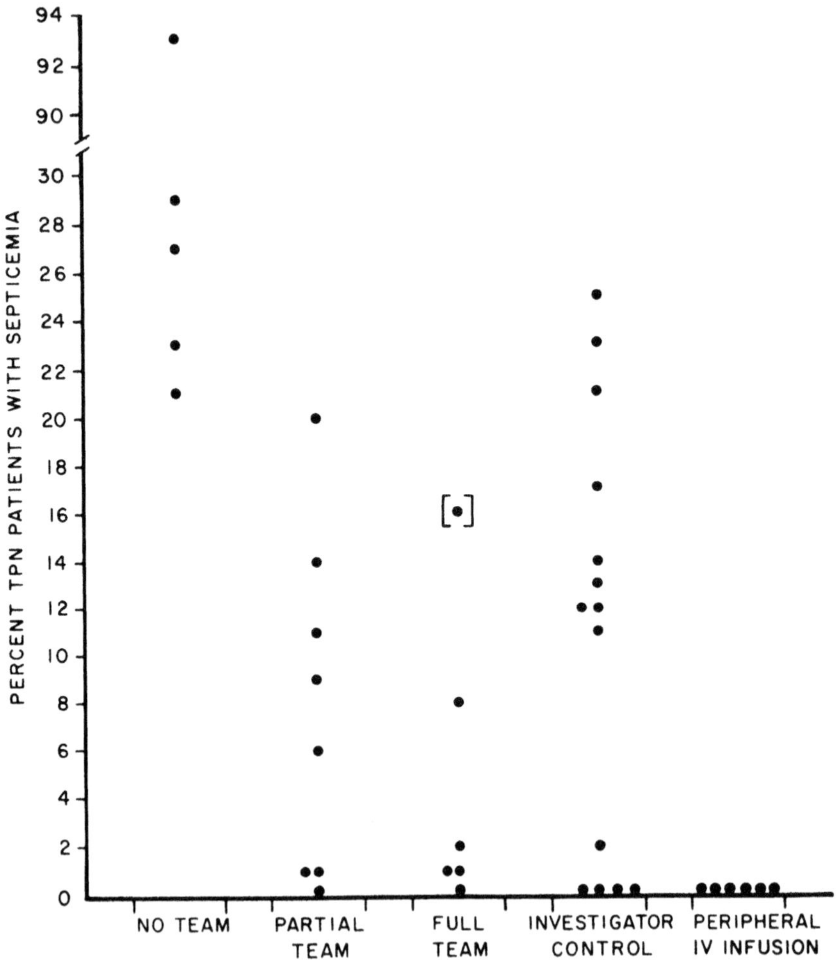

Figure 23.1 Percentage of patients receiving TPN who developed cannula-related sepsis, analysed by presence or absence of team approach to TPN therapy. Point in brackets is hospital allowing TPN team to administer or withdraw blood through TPN cannula. Peripheral intravenous infusion is with lipid emulsion TPN

falling in this category were investigational studies of TPN therapy published during the early years of its acceptance as a useful therapy. With the exception of the investigator-controlled series which ranged widely in reported rates of infection, the presence or absence of a team correlates quite strongly with high or low rates of septicaemia in the patient (Figure 23.1). The single report in the full-team category with an infection rate of 16% was one in which the investigators allowed the TPN team nurse to withdraw blood through the subclavian catheter[43]. It is unclear whether this practice alone could account for the difference in rates between this report and others in the same category. The same association of septicaemia rates with the team approach to providing care for TPN patients is apparent when the reports are analysed by septicaemia rate per 1000 patient-days of TPN therapy (Figure 23.2).

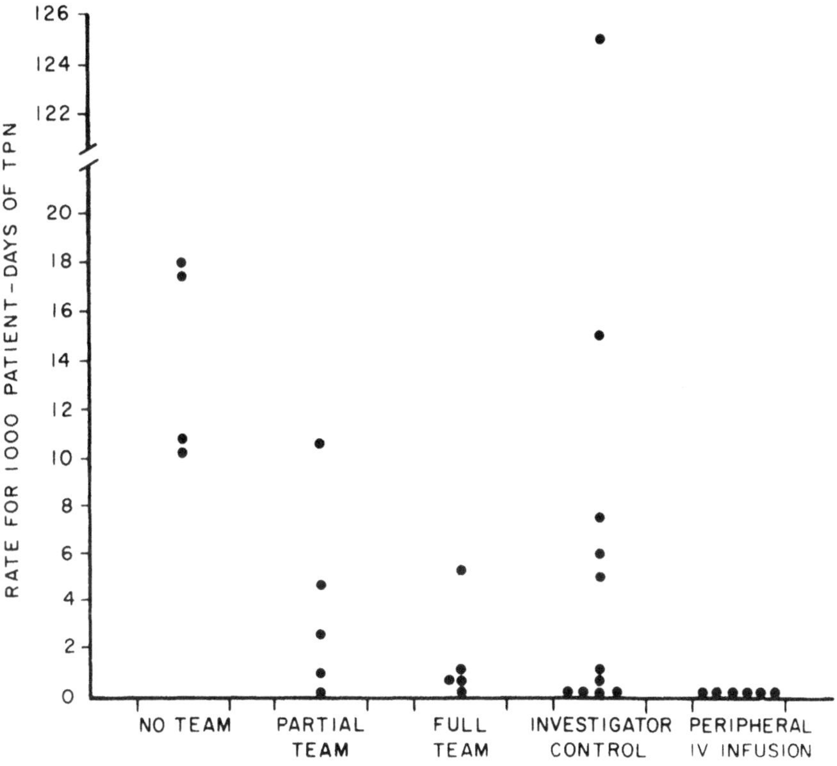

Figure 23.2 Rate of cannula-related sepsis in patients receiving TPN, analysed by presence or absence of team approach to TPN therapy. Peripheral intravenous infusion is with lipid emulsion TPN

Ambulatory patients receiving TPN

Riella and his colleagues[44] have recently reported maintaining forty-three

Table 23.2 Incidence of septicaemia complicating total parenteral nutrition through central venous catheters

*First author**	*Year*	*Number of patients*	*Patient-days of TPN†*	*Rate of septicaemia (%)*			*Septicaemia rate/1000 patient-days TPN*
				Bacterial	*Fungal*	*Total*	
O'Neill[34]	1974	4	98	0	0	0	0.0
Cashore[47]	1975	23	NA	0	0	0	—
Puri[48]	1975	15	282	0	0	0	0.0
Filler[43]	1976	80	NA	0	0	0	—
Hansen[49]	1976	292	6013	0	0	0	0.0
Allardyce[50]	1977	12	397	0	0	0	0.0

* Cited sources conform to text references
† Estimated from data provided
NA—data not available

patients on a home TPN programme for a total of over 44 patient-years of experience. The silicone rubber catheter is inserted by cutdown into the cephalic vein with the tip lying high in the right atrium, and the distal end of the catheter is tunnelled subcutaneously to emerge from the anterior chest wall midway between the nipple and the sternum. The patients in the study have a mean duration of catheter patency of over 9 months with the longest one remaining patent for 30 months. Each patient has been taught to maintain his own catheter at home, changing dressings, preparing and starting the intermittent TPN infusions, and preserving catheter patency with a heparin lock[45,57]. Eight episodes of sepsis have occurred in this series of patients – only one episode of septicaemia for every 5.5 patient-years of experience. While the patient risk factors in this group of ambulatory patients receiving TPN cannot be compared to a series of acutely ill hospitalized patients, it is apparent that if meticulous care is provided for the TPN catheter it can be maintained safely for a prolonged period of time. Other investigators have also successfully used this approach to long-term TPN therapy in ambulatory patients[46].

Lipid emulsions and peripheral intravenous TPN

TPN therapy with lipid emulsion delivered through peripheral intravenous needles is being studied widely (Table 23.2)[34,43,47–50]. These six series represent a minimum of 18½ patient-years of experience without one case of bacterial or fungal septicaemia related to the procedure being reported. All of the investigators meticulously prepared and handled the fluids and changed the needle routinely at least every 2–3 days or at the first signs of infiltration or phlebitis in order to prevent problems with thrombophlebitis. This complication is minimized with the combination of hypertonic solution (amino acids and glucose) and fat emulsion being infused simultaneously through the same needle since the presence of fat emulsion significantly reduces the frequency of thrombophlebitis seen with hypertonic TPN solution alone[50].

MICROBIAL PATHOGENS CAUSING TPN-ASSOCIATED SEPSIS

Generally, organisms causing TPN-associated septicaemia (Table 23.3) differ significantly in relative frequency from those causing nosocomial bacteraemia which are non-TPN associated[52,53]. Gram-positive cocci accounted for over 50% of isolates from reports in which actual numbers of all pathogens could be tabulated, with *Staphylococcus epidermidis* and *S. aureus* being isolated most often. Gram-negative bacteria were isolated relatively infrequently, especially in comparison to the frequency with which they caused septicaemia in TPN patients associated with primary infection at a site other than the TPN catheter[17,36].

Fungi caused approximately 46% of the cases of TPN-associated septicaemia reported (Table 23.1), although only 29% in those series in which all pathogens isolated were reported by species (Table 23.3). Conversely, reported series of patients with fungal sepsis of all causes have noted that a significant proportion of the patients developed their fungal disease in association with receiving TPN[54–56]. *Candida albicans* accounted for 59% of the fungal isolates causing sepsis in patients receiving TPN[9,10,19,51], with

Table 23.3 Microbial pathogens causing TPN-associated septicaemia*

Pathogen	*Frequency of isolation*		*Percentage*	
FUNGI	17		29	
Candida spp.		13		22
Torulopsis spp.		4		7
GRAM-POSITIVE COCCI	31		53	
Staphylococcus aureus		9		15
Staphylococcus epidermidis		18		31
Streptococcal species, alpha or non-haemolytic		3		5
Enterococcus		1		2
GRAM-NEGATIVE BACTERIA	10		17	
Klebsiella spp.		3		5
Pseudomonas spp.		3		5
Escherichia coli		2		3
Enterobacter spp.		1		2
Proteus rettgeri		1		2
ANAEROBIC BACTERIA	1		2	
Bacteroides spp.		1		2
TOTAL	59			

* Summary of six reports[17–19,21,32,33]

Table 23.4 Relative frequency of fungal species causing septicaemia in patients receiving total parenteral nutrition*

Fungal species	*Frequency of isolation*	*Percentage*
Candida albicans	33	59
Candida tropicalis	1	2
Candida parapsilosis	4	7
Candida parakrusei	2	4
Candida spp.	7	13
Torulopsis glabrata	9	16
TOTAL	56	

* Summary of nine reports[9,10,17–19,21,32,33,51]

other species of *Candida* being isolated less frequently (Table 23.4). *Torulopsis glabrata* sepsis also occurred fairly frequently[10,18,51].

GROWTH STUDIES OF BACTERIAL AND FUNG PATHOGENS IN TPN SOLUTIONS

Amino acid–dextrose solutions

The growth of certain bacteria and fungi in TPN solutions has been demonstrated by numerous investigators. Initial studies by Boeckman and Krill[9] and Brennan and his co-workers[58] demonstrated that *Candida albicans* could multiply in amino acid and amino acid–dextrose solutions at 30 °C or 37 °C, but not at 4 °C. In amino acid solutions without dextrose *Candida* had a highly selective advantage over other fungal species and Gram-negative bacteria which proliferated in 5% dextrose solutions.

Goldmann and his colleagues[59] extended these studies by inoculating small numbers of washed organisms into casein hydrolysate–dextrose and synthetic amino acid–dextrose TPN solutions. Both *C. albicans* and *T. glabrata*, as well as most of the selected bacterial organisms, showed rapid proliferation in the casein hydrolysate–dextrose solution within 24–48 h when

Table 23.5 Growth of fungi and bacteria in casein hydrolysate–dextrose total parenteral nutrition solution*

	Organisms per millilitre				
	0 time	*12 h*	*24 h*	*48 h*	*7 days*
Candida albicans	1	24.0	2.4×10^3	T‡	T
Torulopsis glabrata	1	15.0	1.7×10^3	T	T
Serratia marcescens	1	28.0	4.5×10^3	T	T
Klebsiella pneumoniae	1	12.0	2.2×10^3	T	T
Staphylococcus aureus§	1	5.0	1.4×10^3	T	T
Escherichia coli	1	3.0	1.1×10^3	$1\ 7 \times 10^6$	T
Enterobacter cloacae	1	4.7	96.0	1.0×10^6	T
Proteus mirabilis	1	1.9	27.0	7.2×10^4	T
Pseudomonas aeruginosa	1	2.7	1.6	1.1	0.13

* From Goldmann *et al.*[59], courtesy of *Am. J. Surg.*
† Mean concentration for five test strains of each organism, normalized to an inoculum of one organism per millilitre.
‡ Turbid.
§ Two strains failed to proliferate.

incubated at room temperature (Table 23.5). In synthetic amino acid–dextrose solutions, however, only the two fungal species demonstrated an ability to proliferate, although considerably more slowly than in the casein hydrolysate solution (Figure 23.3). None of the bacterial strains proliferated and many appeared to die out (Table 23.6).

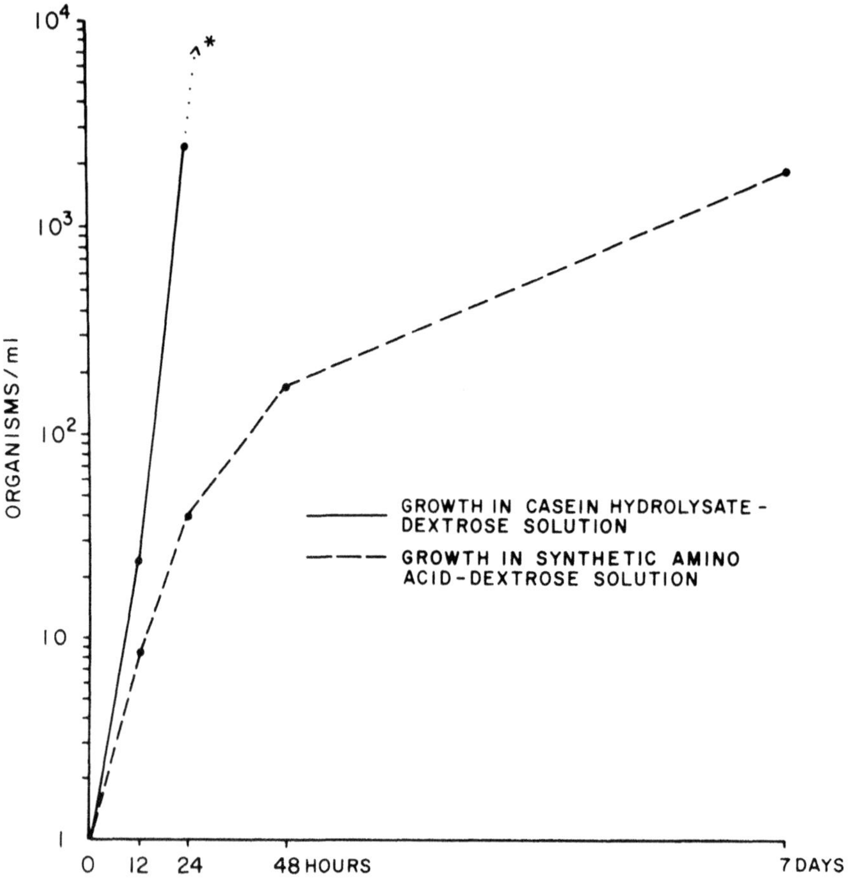

*REACHED TURBIDITY WITHIN 48 HOURS

Figure 23.3 Growth of *Candida albicans* in TPN solutions. Mean concentration for five test strains. (From Goldmann *et al.*[59], courtesy of *Am. J. Surg.*)

Table 23.6 Growth of fungi and bacteria in synthetic amino acid–dextrose total parenteral nutrition solution*

	Organisms per millilitre†				
	0 time	*12 h*	*24 h*	*48 h*	*7 days*
Candida albicans	1	8.5	49.0	1.7×10^2	1.7×10^3
Torulopsis glabrata	1	4.5	16.0	33.0	6.5×10^3
Serratia marcescens	1	2.5	3.0	0.77	1.5
Klebsiella pneumoniae	1	0.63	0.15	0.06	0.05
Staphylococcus aureus	1	0.66	0.24	0.01	0.09
Escherichia coli	1	0.89	0.67	0.46	0.18
Enterobacter cloacae	1	0.62	0.16	0.06	0.06
Proteus mirabilis	1	0.30	0.52	0.23	0.12
Pseudomonas aeruginosa	1	0.30	0.12	0.02	0.06

* From Goldmann *et al.*[59], courtesy of *Am. J. Surg.*
† Mean concentration for five test strains of each organism, normalized to an inoculum of one organism per millilitre.

Similar findings have been reported by other investigators, although differences between results and in the clinical applicability of the studies may be attributed to significant differences in technique between investigators[60]. Species of *T. glabrata* studied by Sanderson and Deitel[33] did not grow in the TPN solutions studied, although seven different species of *Candida* proliferated in the solutions. Gelbart *et al.*[61] compared the growth of *C. albicans* and nine strains of bacteria in multiple solutions, including TPN solutions with casein hydrolysate, fibrin hydrolysate, or one of two crystalline amino acid mixtures. After inoculating approximately 10^4 organisms/ml into the solutions and incubating them at 37 °C, they found that the two protein hydrolysate solutions selectively supported the growth of *Candida* species over that of the bacterial solutions, while the crystalline amino acid solutions did not support rapid growth of any of the species of organisms (Figures 23.4–23.6).

Several studies assessed the growth of bacteria and fungi in TPN solutions incubated at 4 °C[33,58,59]. No growth occurred with any of the organisms even when stored for as long as 1 month. When the contaminated solutions were again brought to room temperature rapid proliferation of the organisms occurred.

The *in vitro* growth studies in summary show that between 25 °C and 37 °C casein hydrolysate–dextrose solutions usually support the rapid growth of fungal species such as *Candida* spp. and *T. glabrata*, as well as the growth of bacterial species such as *S. aureus*, *E. coli*, *Proteus* spp., *Klebsiella*, *Enterobacter* spp., and *Serratia* spp. *Pseudomonas aeruginosa* does not grow well in this solution, although *P. cepacia* does. Synthetic amino acid–dextrose solutions support the growth of fungal species at a much slower rate than do the casein hydrolysate solutions, and generally do not support the growth of bacterial species.

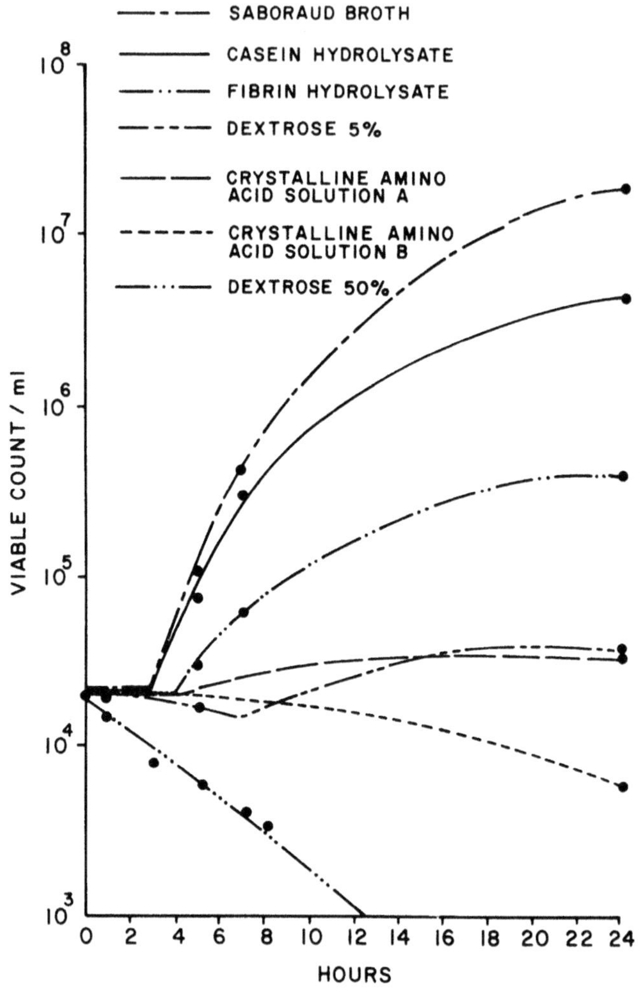

Figure 23.4 Growth of *Candida albicans* in various solutions at 37 °C. Protein hydrolysate and amino acid solutions are TPN solutions with dextrose. (From Gelbart *et al.*[61], courtesy of *Appl. Microbiol.*)

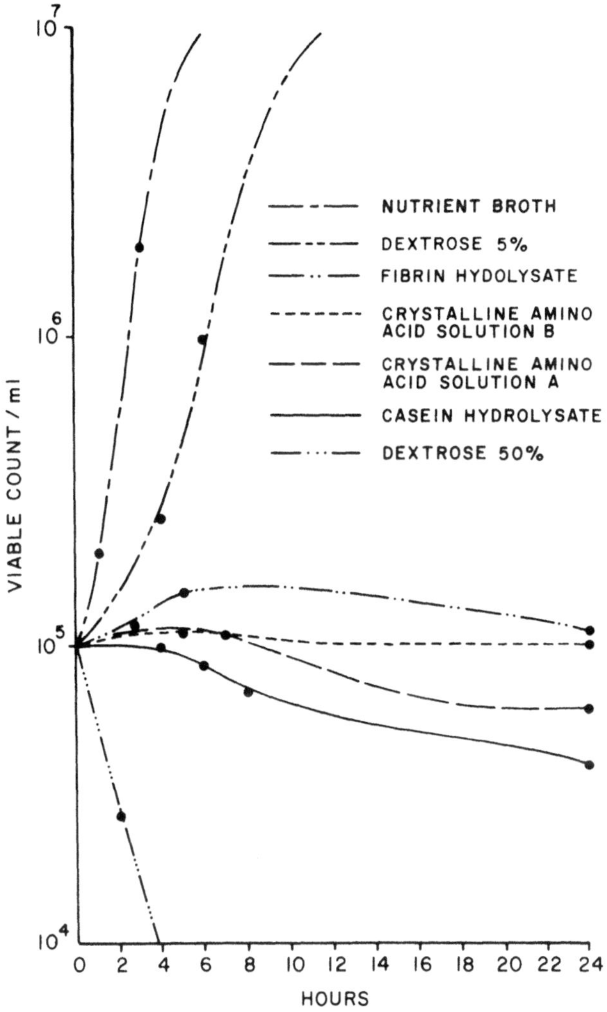

Figure 23.5 Growth of *Pseudomonas cepacia* in various solutions at 37 °C. Protein hydrolysate and amino acid solutions are TPN solutions with dextrose. (From Gelbart *et al.*[61], courtesy of *Appl. Microbiol.*)

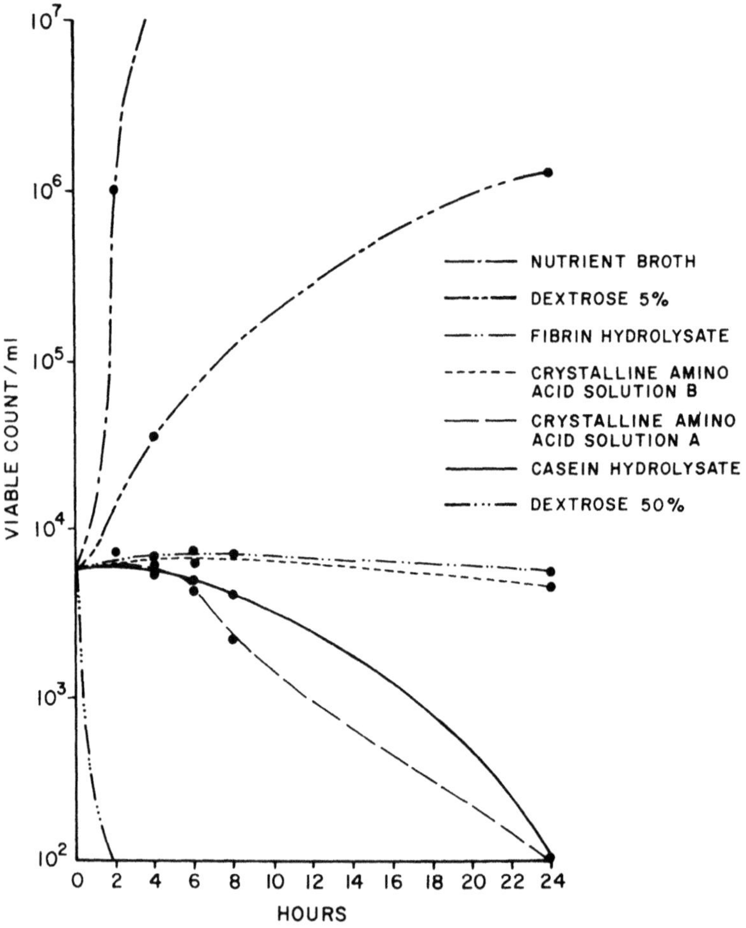

Figure 23.6 Growth of *Enterobacter cloacae* in various solutions at 37 °C. Protein hydrolysate and amino acid solutions are TPN solutions with dextrose. (From Gelbart *et al.*[61], courtesy of *Appl. Microbiol.*)

Failla and his co-workers[62] have demonstrated recently that the high concentrations of glycine in some crystalline amino acid preparations is inhibitory to bacterial growth although not to fungal growth. They suggested that since the amino acid balance of TPN solutions appears to significantly influence growth of bacterial organisms, the antibacterial activity of these solutions might be increased by decreasing the concentration of alanine and increasing that of glycine, if this is compatible with safe administration to patients.

Lipid emulsions

Lipid emulsions, which are being used increasingly frequently for TPN, also support bacterial and fungal growth. *Klebsiella*, *Pseudomonas* spp., *E. coli*. *S. aureus*, and *C. albicans* all proliferate to high levels in the emulsion within 24 h at room temperature[60,63,64] (Figure 23.7). Although current studies of TPN with lipid emulsion have not demonstrated a significant problem with associated septicaemias, especially if the TPN is delivered

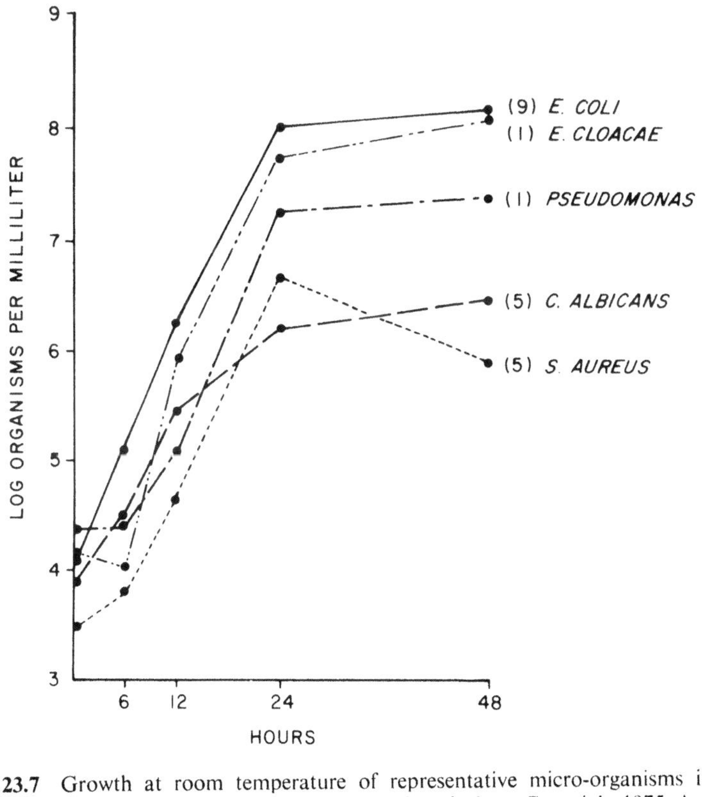

Figure 23.7 Growth at room temperature of representative micro-organisms in lipid emulsion for TPN. (From Melly *et al.*[64], courtesy of *Arch. Surg.* Copyright 1975, American Medical Association.)

through peripheral veins with steel needles, the potential for clinically significant contamination of this solution to occur is obvious.

CONTAMINATION OF TPN SOLUTIONS

Intrinsic contaminations

Although intrinsic contamination of intravenous colloid solutions has been well described[65–70], intrinsic contamination of components of TPN solutions as a source of clinical sepsis has not been documented. The potential for distributing intrinsically contaminated TPN component solutions must be as great as for intravenous colloid solutions, however, making it incumbent on the manufacturers of the solutions to maintain extremely high quality control standards over manufacture of the products and to employ appropriate sampling and microbiological techniques for end-product sterility testing[12,71,72].

Extrinsic contamination

Multiple opportunities for extrinsic contamination of TPN solution occur during admixture and administration. Only a few studies have cultured TPN fluids following admixture but prior to administration. All of these have shown low rates of contamination ranging from 0%[19,73] to 3%[35]. Most contaminants have been bacteria, with only one study reporting a pre-use contamination rate of 0.1% with fungi[74].

Studies of in-use contamination of TPN fluids have yielded far less consistent results[75]. Several studies which cultured the residual fluid from a combined total of over 1000 units of TPN solution found contamination, almost exclusively bacterial, in only 2–2.8% of the units[33,39,76]. Other studies, however, have found contamination rates as high as 39%[30,76]. Deeb and Natsios[73] were the only investigators to find a significant percentage of their units contaminated with fungi: 27% of the units sampled, or 72% of the contaminated units, grew a *Candida* sp., primarily *C. albicans*.

Miller and Gorgan[32,77] cultured 6750 TPN fluid samples or in-line millipore filter membranes from 1041 TPN administration systems and reported an overall rate of 7.6% of cultures positive or 33.2% of the systems contaminated on at least one culture. Most organisms isolated were normal skin flora, including diphtheroids (26%) and *S. epidermidis* (21%). *Candida* spp. (8%) and *S. aureus* (5%) were isolated much less frequently than their relative frequency as a cause of TPN-associated sepsis. Quantitative cultures to assess the degree of contamination of the fluid were not done in any of the studies.

In none of these studies on the extrinsic contamination of TPN solution did the finding of contaminated in-use TPN fluid correlate with bacterial or fungal septicaemia in the patient, suggesting that as with intravenous colloid solutions in-use contamination of the solution fortunately is usually not the source of significant clinical disease, although the potential for this is always present[78].

Pharmacy compounding of TPN solutions

The potential for extrinsic contamination of TPN fluids during compounding has resulted in stringent recommendations for admixture and storage of nutrient solutions, including having all TPN solutions compounded by a pharmacist using aseptic technique in a well-maintained laminar flow hood[31,79]. Following compounding, the fluid should be used immediately if possible or stored at 4 °C until use. TPN fluid must be administered within 24 h of compounding.

Meticulous pharmacy logs, both of the lot numbers of fluids and other pharmaceuticals used in compounding the TPN solution and of the administration records, should be maintained to facilitate epidemiologic investigation of complications of the therapy, including suspected contamination of the solution.

SUSCEPTIBILITY OF TPN PATIENTS TO INFECTION

Patients receiving TPN in a hospital are usually extremely ill. The debilitated, cachectic or malnourished patient who is in a catabolic state with negative nitrogen balance is also likely to have multiple deficiencies in his immunologic capabilities. Recent experimental evidence demonstrated the range of deficiencies in malnourished dogs to include serum immunoglobulins and C3, primary immune response to sheep red blood cells, lymphocyte count, lymphocyte response to phytohaemagglutinin, and neutrophil chemotaxis; most of these deficiencies were restored with TPN therapy of the animals[80].

In addition to the immunological deficits imposed by malnutrition, the serious underlying medical and surgical problems of the patients can increase their susceptibility to infections, particularly disseminated fungal disease. Included are conditions such as prematurity with its attendant complications[11,42,81]; immunosuppression, either from a primary disease such as lymphoma or leukaemia or because of cytotoxic drugs and irradiation; corticosteroid therapy; and therapy with broad spectrum and multiple antibiotic agents[10,16,51,54,55,82]. Burn patients receiving TPN are extremely susceptible to disseminated infection and suppurative central venous thrombosis, particularly if the catheter must be placed through burned skin[39,83,84]. Many patients receiving TPN are already infected at other sites, with a potential risk either of direct contamination of the catheter insertion site or septicaemic spread of infection to involve the catheter[17,36,85].

The TPN therapy itself may also contribute to increased risk of infection.

Cachectic patients receiving TPN may develop hypophosphataemia which can significantly reduce leucocyte ATP supplies with concomitant depression of chemotactic, phagocytic and bactericidal activity of granulocytes[86]. Other investigators have suggested that TPN infusion may cause a change in serum or systemic factors which predisposes the patient to infection, especially with *Candida*[9,29]. This concept is not uniformly believed, however[36]. Experimental evidence in animals indicated that acute alloxan-induced diabetes increased susceptibility to fungal infections, although this was not true for chronically diabetic animals or those with non-diabetic hyperglycaemia[87]. Because of the generally accepted susceptibility of diabetic patients to *Candida* infections[82], however, many investigators recommend carefully titrating the serum glucose level of patients receiving TPN to keep it within the normal range[36,84].

ORGANIZATION OF A TPN THERAPY TEAM

The impact which a TPN therapy team following a strict protocol can have on the incidence of septic complications has already been discussed. The team approach to TPN therapy has also been urged by others[31,75,88]. Several approaches to organization of a TPN team are possible[40,89,90], including the following:

1. Institution of a centralized, highly controlled system with all patients receiving TPN situated on a single nursing unit and total medical and nursing care being provided by team members.
2. Institution of a centralized but less highly controlled system in which patients remain on the original ward and receive TPN therapy as a consultant service with non-team members forbidden from inserting the catheter, providing routine catheter care, changing TPN solutions or orders, or manipulating the administration set. Management of the patient is handled jointly by the patient's regular physician and the TPN team.
3. Establishment of a central TPN consultation service which oversees administration of TPN therapy, provides instruction and assistance, and maintains quality control, but leaves all patient care to the medical and nursing personnel of the patient's ward. A small number of personnel on each ward are trained in TPN therapy techniques, certified as qualified for this, and are the only ward personnel allowed to provide care for the TPN catheter and administration set.

Each of these systems has certain advantages and disadvantages which must be carefully weighed in context with the entire hospital setting before which approach is best for any given hospital. If one of the less centralized approaches is selected, it is important that the chief of the TPN therapy team be given the authority to discontinue TPN therapy on any patient in whom the protocol is not being followed.

Two TPN therapy teams should provide a detailed and comprehensive protocol for all phases of TPN therapy, from compounding of the fluid in the pharmacy and insertion of the catheter to instructions for changing administration lines[91]. The team should be broad-based within the hospital, including representatives from pharmacy, nursing, administration, dietary and perhaps other departments, as well as physicians from all interested services and specialties and at multiple levels of training; team members should participate in regular meetings to establish or review policy and discuss problems. Formal and informal education programmes, including periodic staff conferences, must be established for hospital personnel involved in the care of patients receiving TPN; this is especially important for the less centralized programme. Education of patients in TPN therapy before they begin receiving it can help patient understanding and cooperation. Probably the most important function of the TPN therapy team is to facilitate each aspect of the programme, making it so convenient to follow the protocol that it is difficult not to do so[89,90].

INSERTION AND MAINTENANCE OF THE TPN CATHETER

Catheter composition

The relationship between composition of the catheter used for TPN therapy and the incidence of infections has not been studied in a controlled fashion, although Parsa *et al.*[28] reported anecdotally that the incidence of sepsis in their patients declined markedly coincident with a shift from plastic to silicone rubber catheters. Other clinical investigators have also commented on the frequency of tissue reaction and thrombus formation seen with polyvinyl and polyethylene catheters[43,92], and recommend the use of silicone rubber catheters which cause less tissue reaction and are less thrombogenic[43]. A theoretical reason for using the less thrombogenic catheters is that the thrombus surrounding the catheter is thought to 'cover' or 'hide' bacteria, allowing them to proliferate and cause subsequent sepsis or suppurative thrombophlebitis[93].

A controlled study in dogs comparing polyethylene and silastic catheters noted significantly less inflammatory reaction and thrombus formation with the silastic catheters[94]. An autopsy study on patients with indwelling subclavian central venous catheters at the time of death, however, demonstrated marked circumferential fibrin sleeve formation, occasionally adherent to the vein wall, on patients with all types of catheters: polyethylene, teflon, nylon and silicone rubber[95]. Significant thrombosis of the subclavian vein, innominate vein and superior vena cava was present in many patients even though this had not been suspected clinically. The significance of heparin bonding of catheters to reduce fibrin sheath formation and thrombosis is unresolved[95,96].

Recent clinical studies using newly designed silicone elastomer catheters, with stylets to simplify insertion, strongly suggest that these catheters are not only easy to use but are associated with significantly less tissue reaction and other complications than is seen with plastic venous catheters; catheter-related infections did not develop in any of the seventy-five patients with silicone elastomer catheters[41,97].

Skin preparations and disinfection

Aseptic insertion of a TPN catheter begins with meticulous preparation and disinfection of the skin at the site of insertion. Shaving the skin over the site of catheter insertion is frequently recommended although no studies have demonstrated the necessity of shaving areas of skin sparsely covered with hair[88]. Two reports in the surgical literature strongly suggest that using a depilatory agent rather than a razor to remove unwanted hair results in a significant decrease in the wound infection rate[98,99]. Whether the same relationship would be true for preparation of TPN catheter sites should be investigated.

Disinfection of the skin is a multi-stage process. The skin site should first be carefully scrubbed with soap or a detergent compound and water to remove dirt and organic debris which can inactivate antiseptics or protect bacteria from the antiseptics. Many investigators follow this by defatting the skin with ether or acetone[5,14], although the necessity of this is questionable. Substances in the skin surface lipid, including the free fatty acids, possess antimicrobial activity and significantly reduce the concentration of inoculated organisms including *S. aureus* and *C. albicans*[100,101]. Wiping the skin with acetone or ether removes the antimicrobial substances, although they appear to be replaced within 5 h[100].

The next phase of skin disinfection is scrubbing with an antiseptic. A 1% or 2% tincture of iodine allowed to remain on the skin for a minimum of 30 s is a safe, inexpensive and highly effective skin disinfectant[31,88,102]; this should be followed by a scrub with 70% alcohol to reduce the risk of iodine burns. An alternative skin disinfectant is an iodophor surgical scrub, although this must remain on the skin rather than being removed with alcohol since its antimicrobial activity depends on the sustained release of free iodine. A less desirable although acceptable disinfection procedure is the vigorous application of 70% alcohol. British investigators have successfully used other antiseptic compounds such as 0.5% chlorhexidine in 70% alcohol for skin disinfection[102,103].

Insertion of a TPN catheter

Institution of TPN therapy is always elective, allowing time for careful placement of the catheter under strict aseptic conditions as emphasized in the earliest reports of successful therapy[5,14]. The insertion of the catheter should be considered a surgical procedure, and should preferably be performed either in an operating room or treatment room[31]. Personnel participating in the procedure should scrub, and wear caps, masks, sterile gowns, and sterile gloves as would be required for other surgical procedures. Sterile drapes must be used to isolate the area of catheter insertion during the procedure.

Following insertion, the catheter must be anchored securely to reduce the risk of accidental dislodgement and to minimize slight motion of the catheter at the skin site which could be irritating and facilitate entry of organisms into the cannula wound site. Silicone rubber catheters are notoriously difficult to anchor securely, resulting in novel approaches to the problem[43,44]. Recent improvements in commercially available silicone elastomer catheters should eliminate problems of inserting and anchoring these soft flexible catheters[41,97].

Topical antimicrobial ointments

Because of the need to maintain TPN catheters aseptically for long periods of time, one question of major significance is whether a topical antibiotic ointment, such as one containing bacitracin, neomycin and polymyxin, or an antimicrobial ointment, such as an iodophor, reduces the frequency of intravenous or TPN cannula-related infection and sepsis. Although debated for over a decade, this question has not been satisfactorily answered. A few controlled studies of the use of topical antibiotic ointments were conducted years ago[104–107] and the results have been reviewed frequently[31,75,88]. No adequate trials have been conducted on the use of iodophor ointments applied to cannula sites, and none have been conducted on use of topical ointments for patients receiving TPN.

Most of the studies[104–107] demonstrated that use of the antibiotic ointment reduced the numbers of skin bacteria isolated from the cannula site as well as the frequency of contamination of the intravenous cannula tip. Although the cumulative results of the studies suggest that use of the ointments reduces the rate of cannula-associated infection, the number of patients in the studies was too small to establish the point conclusively. Major disadvantages of an antibiotic ointment are that the frequency of colonization of the catheter site with *Candida* is increased[104,106,107], particularly if the catheter remains in place for prolonged periods of time, and the selective proliferation of bacteria which are resistant to the antibiotics in the ointment is facilitated[104,107]. Use of ointment containing an iodophor, which has broad antibacterial and antifungal action, theoretically might overcome these disadvantages, but this has not been tested in a controlled study.

Of the TPN studies reviewed for this paper,[5–10,16–44] most investigators used a triple antibiotic ointment for routine application at the cannula insertion site. Four investigators, however, used iodophor ointments[19,26,29,44] and one used a combination of antibiotic ointment and nystatin ointment[20]; the rate of fungal septicaemia in these series was not different from that of studies using antibiotic ointment alone or not stating which, if any, agent was used. Although iodophor ointment has not been demonstrated to be superior to triple antibiotic ointment or none at all, use of it on the cannula insertion site is increasing[83,93].

Catheter site dressing and dressing changes

Virtually all the investigators in the studies reviewed[5–10,16–44] described using an occlusive dressing to cover the cannula insertion site. The purpose of this type of dressing is to reduce contamination by organisms from adjacent skin areas, the hands of attending hospital personnel, and the air. There was no standardization between studies on the definition of an occlusive dressing, however, and those described ranged from little more than a sterile gauze pad taped securely in place to a carefully applied waterproof dressing.

Although it is important to keep the dressing dry, and especially to prevent its becoming soaked with TPN fluid that would support the rapid proliferation of both bacteria and fungi, little consideration has apparently been given to the fact that a truly occlusive dressing alters the underlying skin flora. Moisture is essential for the growth of many types of bacteria, and the bacterial count under an occlusive dressing more than doubles from normal values within a few days[101]. The ability of *Candida* to survive and cause clinical infections on the skin of normal humans is also significantly increased under occlusive dressings; partially occlusive dressings, however, such as gauze held in place with tape, do not provide nearly as hospitable an environment for fungal growth[108]. The contribution of the altered cutaneous environment under occlusive dressings at the catheter insertion site to the increased incidence of *Candida* sepsis in patients receiving TPN has not been investigated.

The catheter site dressings in the vast majority of the studies reviewed[5–10,16–44] were changed routinely every 2–4 days. Although it is reasonable to assume that the same care given to preparing a skin site prior to insertion of the catheter is also used for maintenance care of that site, no studies have evaluated the frequency with which routine catheter site care should be given. Myers and his co-workers[38] recommend changing the dressing and providing catheter site care only once a week to minimize movement of the catheter at the site of insertion. They state that more frequent catheter care and dressing changes do not prevent local infection or septicaemia and may actually increase the risk of these complications. In contrast, Wilmore recommends daily catheter site care and dressing changes for burn patients[84], and Dillon *et al.*[17] provided daily catheter site care for their series of patients.

Definitive recommendations on catheter site dressings must await further studies. Reasonable recommendations based on evidence from the literature would be to provide a sterile, partially occlusive, gauze dressing; this should be changed immediately if it becomes wet, especially with TPN fluid. Special care probably should be given to placing an occlusive waterproof dressing over the catheter insertion site in patients with tracheostomies, burns or open wounds adjacent to the site[14]. Routine catheter site care and dressing changes probably should be made two or three times each week. Aseptic technique should be used, including gloves and mask; the catheter insertion site should be scrubbed either with tincture of iodine followed by 70% alcohol or an iodophor compound, the antimicrobial agent, if used, applied, and a sterile dressing taped securely in place.

Duration of catheterization for TPN

The demonstrated risk of infection with intravenous catheters for conventional fluid therapy has led to strong recommendations that the catheters be left in place for no longer than 48 h[88,109,110]. This recommendation is impractical for patients receiving TPN therapy, since these patients receive therapy for a median of 22 days[5–10,16–43] with some receiving therapy continuously for months. Although individual investigators differ significantly in their views on the maximum time which TPN catheters may be safely left in place, and whether the duration of catheterization correlates with the frequency of septicaemia, for most patients receiving TPN therapy the duration of catheterization does not correlate highly with the risk of developing catheter-associated septicaemia.

Dillon *et al.*[17] demonstrated an increasing risk of catheter-associated septicaemia during the first 3 weeks in which their patients were catheterized, but none of the twenty-four patients with a TPN catheter in place for over 21 days developed septicaemia. Sanders and Sheldon[21] found that the average duration the catheter was left in place in patients who developed septicaemia was the same as for patients who did not, although patients who developed septicaemia received a considerably longer total course of TPN therapy. Ryan *et al.*[19] found no increased risk of septicaemia in TPN patients in whom a single catheter was used for over 30 days, although Dudrick and his colleagues[5] found that several infants developed septicaemia after the catheter had been in place for over 35 days. Because of this experience they recommended that the catheter be changed routinely every 30 days. McGovern[29] took this one step further and recommended that the catheters be changed routinely every 2 weeks. Because of the heavy density of surface microorganisms on burn patients, Wilmore[83] has recommended that the catheter be left in place no longer than 3 days and that the insertion site be rotated routinely between the subclavian and external jugular veins if they are not involved with the burn. Usually the site of catheterization is changed when a new catheter is inserted, although Myers *et al.*[38] replaced the subclavian catheters in their TPN patients routinely every 2–3 weeks by inserting a new catheter into the same site over a guide wire.

Many investigators currently recommend that a TPN catheter which is inserted using aseptic technique and which is maintained carefully may be left *in situ* for weeks to months without increasing the risk of septicaemia[15,22,36,44,111]. The catheter should be discontinued or changed only for specific reasons, such as clinical septicaemia or fever without an identifiable origin. It has been suggested that patients with sepsis who are continued on TPN therapy may need to have the catheter replaced routinely every 1–3 days for the duration of the infection[35,109], although others continue to use the same catheter for therapy if a non-catheter source of the sepsis is identified[33,36].

ADMINISTRATION OF TPN SOLUTION

Management of the administration set

Because of the potential for growth of many microbial pathogens in TPN fluid and the significantly increased risk of contamination of the TPN administration set or catheter with manipulation of the system, it is imperative that the TPN administration system be maintained as a closed system. It should be kept as simple as possible with as few tubing connections as is practical and with no extraneous equipment such as stopcocks. Manipulation of the system, or correction of problems with the system, should be performed only by designated TPN team personnel who are aware of the hazards of contamination of the system and the precautions to take[91,93]. One protocol requires that two persons assist with any changes or manipulation of the system to ensure that sufficient hands are present to perform the task without compromising techniques[93]. Use of the TPN administration system for 'unauthorized' procedures such as measurement of the central venous pressure (CVP) or administration or withdrawal of blood has been linked by some investigators with an increased risk of TPN-associated infection[10,18,19].

Although many investigators in the past have changed TPN administration sets only every second day[9,32] or third day[16,18,23] or less often[33], currently accepted practice for TPN therapy is to change all components of the administration set down to the catheter at least every 24 h[17,19,31,34,38]. Guidelines promulgated by the National Coordinating Committee on Large Volume Parenterals state that new administration tubing should be attached to every container of TPN fluid in the pharmacy so that the only procedure in the patient care area is to connect the new set to the extension tubing from the catheter[79].

No studies have been conducted which suggest that disinfection of the administration set tubing routinely, or of the tubing junctions immediately before manipulation of the system is necessary or effective in reducing contamination of the internal portion of the system and the TPN fluid or in preventing septicaemia. Several investigators, however, recommend wiping the administration set lines at least daily, and immediately before any manipulation of the system with tincture of iodine or iodophor solutions[43,45], and using iodophor ointment held in place with a sterile gauze sponge at all tubing and catheter–tubing joints[93]. If a metal connector is used on the end of the catheter, it has been suggested that this can be disinfected more reliably by flaming it briefly in an alcohol flame at the time the administration set is changed than by using chemical disinfectants[112].

In-line millipore filters

In-line millipore filters have been suggested for years for intravenous and TPN fluid therapy[76]. Although the usefulness of the filters in reducing the incidence of phlebitis in conventional fluid therapy is accepted by many[113,114], others have demonstrated in a controlled study that the frequency of neither infusion thrombophlebitis nor positive bacterial cultures of cannula tips was reduced with the use of millipore filters[114a]. Additional controlled studies have been urged[75,88] and are still needed, however, to determine the efficacy of in-line filters at reducing the incidence of infusion-related septicaemia.

Filters with 0.45 μm pore size trap fungi and most bacteria for at least 6 h, while those with 0.22 μm pore size trap all bacteria but reduce the rate of fluid flow to the point that infusion pumps may be required[115]. Although they are useful for trapping micro-organisms which are present in the fluid above the filter, they are of no use in preventing contamination of the fluid or system at any point between the filter and the patient. Particulate matter from the fluid, and air bubbles from the infusion line are also trapped by the filters. A major difficulty however is their tendency to become blocked[114a] or develop an air-lock, a problem which is resolved only by manipulating the device or by replacing the filter; both solutions require breaking the closed administration system and result in increased risk of contaminating the system[18]. Filters incorporated as an integral part of the infusion system prevent manipulation of the system, but might require changing the entire administration set if the filter became blocked. New designs for filters which incorporate large filtration areas and air vents have eliminated some of the problems of blockage and air-locks[116].

In-line millipore filters inserted terminally between the administration set and the catheter were used in the majority of studies of TPN therapy reviewed[5–10,16–44], although in none of the studies was the efficacy of filter use in reducing the incidence of phlebitis or septicaemia evaluated.

Miller and Grogan[77] studied the effect of placing a single, double or triple 0.22 μm filter in the administration lines of patients receiving TPN therapy. They concluded there was little correlation between clinical infection and positive cultures from the filters or fluid. They also found that adding the second and third filters resulted in an increased risk of contamination of the system, and postulated that this occurred because of the more numerous junctions in the system and the opportunity or need for manipulation of the system which this entailed.

Freeman and Litton[18] found retrospectively that the small number of TPN patients for whom an in-line filter had been used had a 32% rate of TPN-associated sepsis, while only 8% of those patients in whom no filter was used had similar infections. The authors observed that administration sets with filters required many more manipulations than did systems without filters, and postulated that this might have been the source of the infections. Although this was not a controlled study, the findings emphasize the need to investigate this question thoroughly.

With the information currently available it is difficult to recommend that final filtration of TPN fluid with filters which will remove bacteria and fungi is essential. If the TPN fluid is prepared carefully and handled prior to administration there is little risk of significant microbial contamination of the fluid reaching the patient, and perhaps a greater risk arises from particulate contamination of the fluid. Filters of 1–5 μm are adequate for removing particulate matter from fluids[21,114] and do not have the disadvantage of clogging, or of reducing fluid flow to the point that a pump is required. The theoretical advantage of the fine-pore filters in perhaps reducing the risk of septicaemia in patients receiving TPN needs to be confirmed. Continuing evaluation of the potential benefits of these devices also needs to be conducted as new products which attempt to eliminate the defects of older devices are introduced into the market.

SEPSIS IN TPN THERAPY PATIENTS

Sources of sepsis in patients

The sources of sepsis in patients receiving conventional intravenous fluid therapy have been reviewed recently[75,88]. Most of the potential sources and types of transmission are equally applicable to TPN therapy, including external catheter-associated infections, intrinsic or extrinsic contamination of the TPN fluid or delivery system, and transient bacteraemia from other sites which seed the fibrin sleeve surrounding the catheter.

Catheter-associated sepsis

As with plastic intravenous catheters for conventional fluid therapy, the TPN catheter must always be considered a primary source of sepsis in a patient who develops signs or symptoms of septicaemia. TPN catheter sepsis is defined as an episode of systemic infection for which no distant locus can be identified and which resolves with removal of the catheter. Positive blood cultures confirm the infection; positive catheter tip cultures assist in confirming the source. Primary contamination of the TPN fluid should be excluded.

Migration of micro-organisms from the catheter insertion site on the skin along the catheter tract to the fibrin sheath which surrounds the intravascular portion of the catheter, or growth of micro-organisms along the inside of the catheter following contamination of the delivery system, probably account for a majority of TPN-associated infections. Prevention of these sources of contamination of the catheter depend on strict adherence to techniques for inserting[117] and maintaining the catheter and caring for the administration set. Of importance in preventing migration of micro-organisms along the catheter insertion tract is the distance between the skin insertion and the venous insertion sites. Angling the catheter to increase this distance in subclavian vein insertions or tunnelling the catheter subcutaneously in external jugular vein cutdowns[5,22] is thought to reduce the frequency of infection by this route. This procedure has also been used successfully in ambulatory TPN patients[44,46].

Contamination of the skin of patients in hospital is inevitable[118], including organisms derived from the patient's own microflora or that transported by medical personnel. Several studies have demonstrated the presence of organisms found on the skin to be the same as those contaminating catheters at the time of removal or causing septicaemia[21,36,119]. Patients with tracheostomies, enterostomies, fistulae, burn or infected wounds, and infected urinary tract catheters are sources of heavy contamination of their own skin, which may result in catheter-related sepsis. In burn patients, catheter-associated infections frequently occur following colonization of the burn wound or other sites with *Candida* or other opportunist organisms[84]. Special care must be taken to protect the catheter insertion site in these patients[14,15]. Medical personnel carrying bacteria on their hands or at other sites are often the means of transmission of organisms to patients[120] which may result in TPN catheter-associated infection.

Routine culturing of TPN catheters at the time of removal may yield useful information to the TPN therapy team about the success of aseptic practices used by the team. A semi-quantitative method of culturing the catheters as described by Maki[75,120a] correlates reasonably well with simple contamination of the catheter tip or heavy contamination of the catheter likely to be associated with septicaemia.

Infection of other sites

Experience in patients with central venous catheters not used for TPN suggests that the presence of clinical infection at a site distant to the catheter predisposes to haematogenous seeding of the catheter with the same organism[109,119]. In many series of patients receiving TPN, the majority of patients had active infections preceding or during therapy[17,19,35,36,85]. Despite this, haematogenous spread was not a major complication of the infections[19], especially if a specific source of infection was known and being treated, or if blood cultures were negative[35,36]. Dillon *et al.*[17] studied patients receiving TPN who developed suspected sepsis and concluded that although it was not possible to define non-catheter versus catheter-associated sepsis at the time of the acute episode, non-catheter sepsis occurred almost three times as frequently as did catheter-associated sepsis. Rea[85] reported the use of TPN in extremely ill patients with complicated oesophageal perforation or with septic pulmonary complications (abscess, empyema, mediastinitis, fistula); the mortality in patients receiving TPN was less than 20% that of the non-TPN control group although the TPN patients were generally more ill than the controls. Complications with secondary seeding of the catheter did not occur.

Although infection at a site distant from the TPN catheter may result in bacteraemia with haematogenous seeding of the fibrin sheath surrounding the catheter, this complication does not occur nearly as frequently as might be expected from the incidence of bacteraemia[15,17]. Bacteraemia secondary to infection at another site usually can be managed with recognition of the primary site of infection and appropriate treatment of the infection[15,17], replacing the TPN catheter only if necessary.

Prophylactic antibiotics for TPN therapy patients

Observations on the use of antibiotics in patients with intravenous cannulae suggest that they are not useful in decreasing the incidence of contamination of the catheter tip[117], although one study did demonstrate a significant reduction in the rate of contamination of the catheter in patients who had received antibiotics[107]. Another study noted that all patients developing Gram-negative rod bacteraemia or fungaemia had received prior systemic antibiotics[121]. Overuse of antibiotics has been recognized as one contributing cause of serious infections with multiple antibiotic-resistant organisms and with fungal and other opportunist pathogens. Prophylactic antibiotics, by altering the normal flora of the host, may interfere further with the already compromised host defences of patients receiving TPN, and may contribute to overgrowth of organisms, particularly *Candida*, which can cause TPN-related sepsis[9,10,15,36,84]. Curry and Quie[10] noted that eighteen of twenty-two of their TPN therapy patients who developed *Candida* sepsis had received multiple broad-spectrum systemic antibiotics prior to onset of the infection, and Boeckman and Krill[9] stated that all six of their patients had received antibiotics prior to developing *Candida* sepsis.

Antibiotics must be used judiciously in patients receiving TPN to treat documented infections[36]; they should not be used prophylactically in an attempt to prevent TPN-associated sepsis[15,29,43].

Brennan *et al.*[122] studied the usefulness of flushing TPN catheters several times a week with amphotericin B solution to prevent *Candida* infection.

Although they concluded this probably was effective, it has only received anecdotal support[51] and has never been studied in a prospective controlled trial. Other authors specifically state that this is not a necessary procedure to prevent *Candida* infections[35,36,19] and that it may create more hazards than it prevents[15] because the procedure requires an additional break and manipulation of the closed administration system. Flushing the administration set with amphotericin B is not recommended as prophylactic care against *Candida* infection. Meticulous attention to all aspects of catheter insertion and care and maintenance of the infusion system is usually adequate to prevent this complication.

TPN-associated sepsis

Diagnosis of sepsis

Patients receiving TPN frequently have infections at other sites[17,19,21,36,85], making evaluation of the patients difficult if they develop fever, chills, leucocytosis, deteriorating clinical or mental status, failure to gain weight, or unexplained glycosuria. Clinical evidence of sepsis demands expert clinical acumen and laboratory support to confirm the presence of infection and locate the source as accurately and rapidly as possible. An essential aspect of the evaluation is obtaining blood cultures from a vein not involved with the TPN therapy, as well as through the TPN catheter. If a non-catheter site of infection is found, appropriate therapy should be initiated.

Initial evaluation of the TPN system as a possible source of sepsis includes inspection of the catheter insertion site for erythema[21] and culturing the TPN solution and administration set according to standard recommendations[31]; the TPN fluid and administration set down to the catheter should be replaced immediately. Although one group of investigators recommend aseptically removing and culturing the TPN catheter as part of the initial evaluation of a septic patient[17], others recommend waiting 12–24 h to evaluate the patient's response to the measures taken; if the patient remains febrile without a known site of infection, the catheter should be removed and cultured[19–21,35,36], preferably using semiquantitative culture methods[75]. Patients in shock should be presumed to have catheter-associated sepsis and should have the catheter removed immediately. Catheter-associated sepsis may occur concurrently with infection at another site[21]. In one study over 75% of the TPN catheters removed were not the source of sepsis in the patients and in retrospect did not need to be discontinued[19]. Ryan has emphasized, therefore, that even though excellent clinical judgment is essential to recognize catheter-associated sepsis and remove the catheter, even better judgment is required to decide which catheters are not causing sepsis and can be safely continued[15].

Although septicaemia is not necessarily a contraindication to instituting or continuing TPN therapy[35], many investigators recommend waiting at least

24–48 h after removing a TPN catheter from a septic patient before inserting a new catheter[19,21,35]. Although this recommendation is reasonable, it is empirical, and the necessity for delaying catheter insertion has not been established. It is possible that the delay will prevent haematogenous seeding of organisms to the catheter[19].

Establishing a diagnosis of fungal sepsis is more difficult than diagnosing bacterial sepsis. Venous blood cultures from patients even with systemic *Candida* infections frequently remain negative[123,124], and clinical manifestations frequently are non-specific. Arterial blood cultures may be helpful in establishing the diagnosis[123,125]. Heavy colonization of the patient with *Candida* may call attention to potential problems[86]; persistent isolation of *Candida* from the urine[125] or finding lesions of fungal endophthalmitis[126,133] may assist in diagnosis. Intraleucocytic fungal forms on blood smear confirm a diagnosis of fungal septicaemia[127]. *Candida* has been found growing in the fibrin sheath and thrombus surrounding TPN catheters, and it has been suggested that blood culture or smear obtained directly through the catheter may enhance the ability to demonstrate candidiasis[128]. Although serologic diagnosis of serious *Candida* infection is still experimental and only marginally reliable[123,129], recent studies of *Candida* precipitins by double immunodiffusion[130], crossed immunoelectrophoresis[131], and other techniques[132] may result in a readily available and reliable test in the future.

Management of sepsis

The majority of patients with either bacterial or fungal catheter-related sepsis can be treated simply with prompt removal of the catheter[8,19,21,31,33,93,123], although some investigators suggest treating bacterial septicaemia with antibiotics initially[36,93]. If tissue invasion with fungus has occurred[123,128] or if other septic bacterial foci are identified, treatment with catheter removal alone is not adequate, and appropriate antibiotics or antifungal agents in adequate dosages for systemic therapy should be given.

Careful observation of the patient is essential following removal of a catheter causing sepsis. If the clinical picture is compatible with persistent or serious infection or if blood cultures remain positive, appropriate antibiotic or antifungal therapy should be instituted. Latent foci of infection following septicaemia may become clinically apparent only at a later time[19,20,82].

CONCLUSIONS

In reviewing the first decade of widespread use of TPN therapy, the first 5 years were ones in which the technique was used frequently without sufficient appreciation of infections and other complications. As more information became available, however, and the complications became better understood, methods of care were developed that could prevent them. For infection, this clearly has meant meticulous attention to aseptic technique at every point throughout therapy.

The only practical method of managing all aspects of this multi-faceted system is to establish a TPN therapy team with representatives from all departments or services involved to coordinate and oversee the care provided. Key members of the team include nurses or technicians who provide daily patient care such as changing solutions and administration sets and maintaining the catheter and insertion site. It is important to remember that this care must be available 24 hours a day 7 days a week; programmes that have provided less than this have found that major problems occur when the team is not available. Another important function of the team is to educate nurses and physicians who are not on the team about the intricacies and techniques of TPN therapy, and to work with these other hospital personnel in providing complete and coordinate care.

Many aspects of care currently provided for TPN therapy patients are based on uncontrolled clinical experience. Carefully designed, prospective, controlled clinical trials are needed urgently to provide solid information about the best techniques and procedures so that the risks of TPN therapy can be minimized and the patients provided with the best possible care.

A brief list of questions or areas which need to be evaluated in careful clinical trials includes:

1. The use of antibiotic or antiseptic ointments at the catheter insertion site.
2. The use of an occlusive dressing versus a sterile but not occlusive one.
3. The efficacy of a fine-mesh, in-line filter in preventing septicaemia or infection.
4. The relative importance of TPN catheters versus TPN fluid as sources of bacterial and fungal sepsis.
5. The best way to manage intermittent heparin-locks on TPN catheters if cyclic therapy is employed[45,134].
6. Careful evaluation of new products and techniques which are developed and offered for general use without adequate testing.

Acknowledgements

I acknowledge and greatly appreciate the assistance of Richard E. Dixon, M.D., Chief, Hospital Infections Branch, and John V. Bennett, M.D., Director, Bacterial Diseases Division, Bureau of Epidemiology, Center for Disease Control, for their influence in formulating many of the concepts in this chapter and for their helpful criticism and review of the manuscript.

References

1. Elman, R. and Weiner, D. O. (1939). Intravenous alimentation with special reference to protein (amino acid) metabolism. *J. Am. Med. Assoc.*, **112**, 796

2. Dennis, C., Eddy, F. D., Frykman, H. M., McCarthy, A. M. and Westover, D. (1948). The response to vagotomy in idiopathic ulcerative colitis and regional enteritis. *Ann. Surg.*, **128**, 479
3. Dudrick, S. J., Wilmore, D. W., Vars, H. M. and Rhoads, J. E. (1968). Long-term total parenteral nutrition and growth, development, and positive nitrogen balance. *Surgery*, **64**, 134
4. Wilmore, D. W. and Dudrick, S. J. (1968). Growth and development of an infant receiving all nutrients exclusively by vein. *J. Am. Med. Assoc.*, **203**, 860
5. Dudrick, S. J., Groff, D. B., and Wilmore, D. W. (1969). Long term venous catheterization in infants. *Surg. Gynecol. Obstet.*, **129**, 805
6. Groff, D. B. (1969). Complications of intravenous hyperalimentation in newborns and infants. *J. Ped. Surg.*, **4**, 460
7. Filler, R. M. and Eraklis, A. J. (1970). Care of the critically ill child: Intravenous alimentation. *Pediatrics*, **46**, 456
8. Ashcraft, K. W. and Leape, L. L. (1970). *Candida* sepsis complicating parenteral feeding. *J. Am. Med. Assoc.*, **212**, 454
9. Boeckman, C. R. and Krill, C. E. (1970). Bacterial and fungal infections complicating parenteral alimentation in infants and children. *J. Ped. Surg.*, **5**, 117
10. Curry, C. R. and Quie, P. G. (1971). Fungal septicaemia in patients receiving parentera hyperalimentation. *N. Engl. J. Med.*, **285**, 1221
11. Heird, W. C., Driscoll, J. M., Schullinger, J. N., Grebin, B. and Winters, R. W. (1972). Intravenous alimentation in pediatric patients. *J. Pediat.*, **80**, 351
12. Schaffner, W. (1972). Microbiological safety of solutions and delivery to the patient: problems in preparation and handling. In *Symposium on Total Parenteral Nutrition*, sponsored by Food Science Committee, Council on Foods and Nutrition, A.M.A., January 17–19, Nashville, Tenn., p. 125.
13. Duma, R. J. (1971). First of all do no harm. *N. Engl. J. Med.*, **285**, 1258
14. Wilmore, D. W. and Dudrick, S. J. (1969). Safe long-term venous catheterization. *Arch. Surg.*, **98**, 256
15. Ryan, J. A., Jr. (1976). Complications of total parenteral nutrition. In J. E. Fischer (ed.). *Total Parenteral Nutrition*, pp. 55–100. (Boston: Little, Brown and Company)
16. Wilmore, D. W., Groff, D. B., Bishop, H. C. and Dudrick, S. J. (1969). Total parenteral nutrition in infants with catastrophic gastrointestinal anomalies. *J. Ped. Surg.*, **4**, 181
17. Dillon, J. D., Jr., Schaffner, W., Van Way, C. W., III and Meng, H. C. (1973). Septicaemia and total parenteral nutrition. *J. Am. Med. Assoc.*, **223**, 1341
18. Freeman, J. B. and Litton, A. A. (1974). Preponderance of gram-positive infections during parenteral alimentation. *Surg. Gynecol. Obstet.*, **139**, 905
19. Ryan, J. A., Abel, R. M., Abbott, W. M., Hopkins, C. C., Chesney, T. McC., Colley, R., Phillips, K. and Fischer, J. F. (1974). Catheter complications in total parenteral nutrition. A prospective study of 200 consecutive patients. *N. Engl. J. Med.*, **290**, 757
20. Freeman, J. B., Lemire, A. and MacLean, L. D. (1972). Intravenous alimentation and septicemia. *Surg. Gynecol. Obstet.*, **135**, 708
21. Sanders, R. A. and Sheldon, G. F. (1976). Septic complications of total parenteral nutrition. *Am. J. Surg.*, **132**, 214
22. Filler, R. M., Eraklis, A. J., Rubin, V. G. and Das, J. B. (1969). Long-term total nutrition in infants. *N. Engl. J. Med.*, **281**, 589
23. Owings, J. M., Bomar, W. E., Jr. and Ramage, R. C. (1972). Parenteral hyperalimentation and its practical applications. *Ann. Surg.*, **175**, 712
24. Helmuth, W. V., Adam, P. A. J. and Sweet, A. Y. (1972). The effects of protein hydrolysate–monosaccharide infusion on low-birth-weight infants. *J. Pediat.*, **81**, 129
25. Peden, V. H. and Karpel, J. T. (1972). Total parenteral nutrition in premature infants. *J. Pediat.*, **81**, 137
26. Driscoll, J. D., Heird, W. C., Schullinger, J. N., Gongaware, R. D. and Winters, R. W. (1972). Total intravenous alimentation in low-birth-weight infants: A preliminary report. *J. Pediat.*, **81**, 145
27. Johnson, J. D., Albritton, W. L. and Sunshine, P. (1972). Hyperammonemia accompanying parenteral nutrition in newborn infants. *J. Pediat.*, **81**, 154
28. Parsa, M. H., Habif, D. V., Ferrer, J. M., Lipton, R. and Yoshimura, N. N. (1972).

Intravenous hyperalimentation: Indications, technique, and complications. *Bull. N.Y. Acad. Med.*, **48**, 920

29. McGovern, B. (1972). Septic complications of hyperalimentation. In G. S. M. Cowan, Jr., and W. L. Scheetz (eds.). *Intravenous Hyperalimentation*, pp. 165–174. (Philadelphia: Lea and Febiger)
30. Asch, M. J., Huxtable, R. F. and Hays, D. M. (1972). High calorie parenteral therapy in infants and children. *Arch. Surg.*, **104**, 434
31. Goldmann, D. A. and Maki, D. G. (1973). Infection control in total parenteral nutrition. *J. Am. Med. Assoc.*, **223**, 1360
32. Miller, R. C and Grogan, J. B. (1973). Incidence and source of contamination of intravenous nutritional infusion systems. *J. Ped. Surg.*, **8**, 185
33. Sanderson, I. and Deitel, M. (1973). Intravenous hyperalimentation without sepsis. *Surg. Gynecol. Obstet.*, **136**, 577
34. O'Neill, J. A., Meng, H. C., Caldwell, M. and Otten, A. (1974). Variations in intravenous nutrition in the management of catabolic states in infants and children. *J. Pediat. Surg.*, **9**, 889
35. Copeland, E. M., MacFayden, B. V. and Dudrick, S. J. (1974). Prevention of microbial catheter contamination in patients receiving parenteral hyperalimentation. *South. Med. J.*, **67**, 303
36. Copeland, E. M., MacFayden, B. V., McGown, C. and Dudrick, S. J. (1974). The use of hyperalimentation in patients with potential sepsis. *Surg. Gynecol. Obstet.*, **137**, 377
37. Abel, R. M., Fischer, J. E., Buckley, M. J. and Austen, W. G. (1974). Hyperalimentation in cardiac surgery: A review of sixty-four patients. *J. Thorac. Cardiovasc. Surg.*, **67**, 294
38. Myers, R. N., Smink, R. D. and Goldstein, F. (1974). Parenteral hyperalimentation—five years' clinical experience. *Am. J. Gastroenterol.*, **62**, 313
39. Popp, M. B., Law, E. J. and MacMillan, B. G. (1974). Parenteral nutrition in the burned child. *Ann. Surg.*, **179**, 219
40. Skoutakis, V. A., Martinez, D. R., Miller, W. A. and Dobbie, R. P. (1975). Team approach to total parenteral nutrition. *Am. J. Hosp. Pharm.*, **32**, 693
41. Hoshal, V. L. (1975). Total intravenous nutrition with peripherally inserted silicone elastomer central venous catheters. *Arch. Surg.*, **110**, 644
42. Heird, W. C. and Winters, R. W. (1975). Total parenteral nutrition. The state of the art. *J. Pediat.*, **86**, 2
43. Filler, R. M. and Coran, A. G. (1976). Total parenteral nutrition in infants and children: Central and peripheral approaches. *Surg. Clin. North Am.*, **56**, 395
44. Riella, M. C. and Scribner, B. H. (1976). Five years' experience with a right atrial catheter for prolonged parenteral nutrition at home. *Surg. Gynecol. Obstet.*, **143**, 205
45. Broviac, J. W. and Scribner, B. H. (1974). Prolonged parenteral nutrition in the home. *Surg. Gynecol. Obstet.*, **139**, 24
46. Solassol, C. and Joyeaux, H. (1976). Ambulatory parenteral nutrition. In J. E. Fischer (ed.). *Total Parenteral Nutrition*, pp. 285–301. (Boston: Little, Brown and Company)
47. Cashore, W. J., Sedaghatian, M. R. and Usher, R. H. (1975). Nutritional supplements with intravenously administered lipid, protein hydrolysate, and glucose in small premature infants. *Pediatrics*, **56**, 8
48. Puri, P., Guiney, E. J. and O'Donnell, B. (1975). Total parenteral feeding in infants using peripheral veins. *Arch. Dis. Childh.*, **50**, 133
49. Hansen, L. M., Hardie, W. R. and Hidalgo, J. (1976). Fat emulsion for intravenous administration. *Ann. Surg.*, **184**, 80
50. Allardyce, D. B. and Williams, B. J. (1977). Parenteral solutions for nutritional support in surgical patients. *Am. J. Surg.*, **133**, 315
51. Rodrigues, R. J. and Wolff, W. I. (1974). Fungal septicemia in surgical patients. *Ann. Surg.*, **180**, 741
52. McGowan, J. E., Barnes, M. W. and Finland, M. (1975). Bacteremia at Boston City Hospital: Occurrence and mortality during 12 selected years (1935–1972), with special reference to hospital-acquired cases. *J. Infect. Dis.*, **132**, 316
53. Scheckler, W. E. (1977). Septicemia in a community hospital 1970 through 1973. *J. Am. Med. Assoc.*, **237**, 1938

54. Rose, H. D. and Varkey, B. (1975). Deep mycotic infection in the hospitalized adult: A study of 123 patients. *Medicine*, **54**, 499
55. Rubinstein, E., Noriega, E. R., Simberkoff, M. S., Holzman, R. and Rahal, J. J. (1975). Fungal endocarditis: Analysis of 24 cases and review of the literature. *Medicine*, **54**, 331
56. Gaines, J. D. and Remington, J. S. (1972). Disseminated candidiasis in the surgical patients. *Surgery*, **72**, 730
57. Ivey, M., Riella, M., Mueller, W. and Scribner, B. (1975). Long-term parenteral nutrition in the home. *Am. J. Hosp. Pharm.*, **32**, 1032
58. Brennan, M. F., O'Connell, R. C., Rosol, J. A. and Kundsin, R. (1971). The growth of *Candida albicans* in nutritive solutions given parenterally. *Arch. Surg.*, **103**, 705
59. Goldmann, D. A., Martin, W. T. and Worthington, J. W. (1973). Growth of bacteria and fungi in total parenteral nutrition solutions. *Am. J. Surg.*, **126**, 314
60. Maki, D. G. (1976). Growth properties of microorganisms in infusion fluid and methods of dectection. In I. Phillips, P. D. Meers and P. F. D'Arcy (eds.). *Microbiological Hazards of Infusion Therapy*, pp. 13–48. (Lancaster, England: MTP Press, Ltd.)
61. Gelbart, S. M., Reinhardt, G. F. and Greenlee, H. B. (1973). Multiplication of nosocomial pathogens in intravenous feeding solutions. *Appl. Microbiol.*, **26**, 874
62. Failla, M. L., Benedict, C. D. and Weinberg, E. D. (1975). Bacterial and fungal growth in total parenteral nutrition solutions. *Antonie van Leeuwenhoek*, **41**, 319
63. Crichton, E. P. (1973). Infusion fluids as culture media. *Am. J. Clin. Pathol.*, **59**, 199
64. Melly, M. A., Meng, H. C. and Schaffner, W. (1975). Microbial growth in lipid emulsions used in parenteral nutrition. *Arch. Surg.*, **110**, 1479
65. Phillips, I., Eykyn, S. and Laker, M. (1972). Outbreak of hospital infection caused by contaminated autoclaved fluids. *Lancet*, **i**, 1258
66. Felts, S. K., Schaffner, W., Melly, M. A. and Koenig, M. G. (1972). Sepsis caused by contaminated intravenous fluids: Epidemiologic, clinical, and laboratory investigation of an outbreak in one hospital. *Ann. Int. Med.*, **77**, 881
67. Mackel, D. C., Maki, D. G., Anderson, R. L., Rhame, F. S. and Bennett, J. V. (1975). Nationwide epidemic of septicemia caused by contaminated intravenous products: Mechanisms of intrinsic contamination. *J. Clin. Microbiol.*, **2**, 486
68. Maki, D. G., Rhame, F. S., Mackel, D. C. and Bennett, J. V. (1976). Nationwide epidemic of septicemia caused by contaminated intravenous products. I. Epidemiologic and clinical features. *Am. J. Med.*, **60**, 471
69. Center for Disease Control. (1973). Septicemias associated with contaminated intravenous fluids. *Morbid. Mortal. Weekly Rep.*, **22** (11), 99
70. Center for Disease Control. (1973). Follow-up on septicemias associated with contaminated intravenous fluids. *Morbid. Mortal. Weekly Rep.*, **22** (13), 115
71. DeMerre, L. J. (1972). Current regulatory practices regarding solutions and equipment in total parenteral nutrition. In *Symposium on Total Parenteral Nutrition*, sponsored by Food Science Committee Council on Foods and Nutrition, A.M.A., January 17–19, Nashville, Tenn., pp. 201–213
72. Dixon, R. E. (1976). Intrinsic contamination—the associated infective syndromes. In I. Phillips, P. D. Meers and P. F. D'Arcy (eds.). *Microbiological Hazards of Infusion Therapy*, pp. 145–160. (Lancaster, England: MTP Press, Ltd.)
73. Deeb, E. N. and Natsios, G. A. (1971). Contamination of intravenous fluids by bacteria and fungi during preparation and administration. *Am. J. Hosp. Pharm.*, **28**, 764
74. Hak, L. J., Long, J. M., Ruberg, R. L. *et al.* (1971). Contamination incidence in I.V. solutions with additives. Presented to the Annual Meeting of the American Society of Hospital Pharmacists, 31 March 1971
75. Maki, D. B. (1976). Sepsis arising from extrinsic contamination of the infusion and measures for control. In I. Phillips, P. D. Meers and P. F. D'Arcy (eds.). *Microbiological Hazards of Infusion Therapy*, pp. 99–143. (Lancaster, England: MTP Press, Ltd.)
76. Wilmore, D. W. and Dudrick, S. J. (1969). An in-line filter for intravenous solutions. *Arch. Surg.*, **99**, 462

77. Miller, R. C. and Grogan, J. B. (1975). Efficacy of inline bacterial filters in reducing contamination of intravenous nutritional solutions. *Am. J. Surg.*, **130**, 585
78. Maki, D. G., Anderson, R. L. and Shulman, J. A. (1974). In-use contamination of intravenous infusion fluid. *Appl. Microbiol.*, **28**, 778
79. National Coordinating Committee on Large Volume Parenterals (1975). Recommended methods for compounding intravenous admixtures in hospitals. *Am. J. Hosp. Pharm.*, **32**, 261
80. Dionigi, R., Zonta, A., Dominioni, L., Gnes, F. and Ballabio, A. (1977). The effects of total parenteral nutrition on immunodepression due to malnutrition. *Ann. Surg.*, **185**, 467
81. Winters, R. W. (1975). Total parenteral nutrition in pediatrics: The Borden Award address. *Pediatrics*, **56**, 17
82. Louria, D. B., Skiff, D. P. and Bennett, B. (1962). Disseminated moniliasis in the adult. *Medicine*, **41**, 307
83. Wilmore, D. W. and Pruitt, B. A., Jr. (1976). Parenteral nutrition in burn patients. In J. E. Fischer (ed.). *Total Parenteral Nutrition*, pp. 231–252. (Boston: Little, Brown and Company)
84. Wilmore, D. W. (1975). Parenteral nutrition in the thermally injured patient. In H. Ghadimi (ed.). *Total Parenteral Nutrition*, pp. 483–505. (New York: John Wiley and Sons)
85. Rea, W. J. (1975). The role of TPN in thoracic surgery. In H. Ghadimi (ed.). *Total Parenteral Nutrition*, pp. 507–514. (New York: John Wiley and Sons)
86. Craddock, P. R., Yawata, Y., VanSanten, L., Gilberstadt, S., Silvis, S. and Jacob, H. S. (1974). Acquired phagocyte dysfunction resulting from parenteral hyperalimentation. *N. Engl. J. Med.*, **290**, 1403
87. Sheldon, W. H. and Bauer, H. (1962). The role of predisposing factors in experimental fungus infections. *Lab. Invest.*, **11** (Part 2), 1184
88. Maki, D. G., Goldmann, D. A. and Rhame, F. S. (1973). Infection control in intravenous therapy. *Ann. Int. Med.*, **79**, 887
89. Fischer, J. E. (1976). The organization of a parenteral nutrition unit. In J. E. Fischer (ed.). *Total Parenteral Nutrition*, pp. 127–131. (Boston: Little, Brown and Company)
90. Colley, R. (1976). Education of the hospital staff. In J. E. Fischer (ed.). *Total Parenteral Nutrition*, pp. 111–125. (Boston: Little, Brown and Company)
91. Phillips, K. J. (1976). Nursing care in parenteral nutrition. In J. E. Fischer (ed.). *Total Parenteral Nutrition*, pp. 101–110. (Boston: Little, Brown and Company)
92. Jones, M. V. and Craig, D. B. (1972). Venous reaction to plastic intravenous cannulae: Influence of cannula composition. *Can. Anaesth. Soc. J.*, **19**, 491
93. Filler, R. M., Eraklis, A. J. and Das, J. B. (1975). Total parenteral nutrition in pediatrics, rationale and clinical experience. In H. Ghadimi (ed.). *Total Parenteral Nutrition*, pp. 445–482. (New York: John Wiley and Sons)
94. Welch, G. W., McKeel, D. W., Silverstein, P. and Walker, H. L. (1974). The role of catheter composition in the development of thrombophlebitis. *Surg. Gynecol. Obstet.*, **138**, 421
95. Hoshal, V. L., Ause, R. G. and Hoskins, P. A. (1971). Fibrin sleeve formation on indwelling subclavian central venous catheters. *Arch. Surg.*, **102**, 353
96. Peters, W. R., Bush, W. H., McIntyre, R. D. and Hill, L. D. (1973). The development of fibrin sheath on indwelling venous catheters. *Surg. Gynecol. Obstet.*, **137**, 43
97. MacDonald, A. S., Master, S. K. P. and Moffitt, E. A. (1977). A comparative study of peripherally inserted silicone catheters for parenteral nutrition. *Can. Anaesth. Soc. J.*, **24**, 263
98. Cruse, P. J. E. and Foord, R. (1973). A five-year prospective study of 23 649 surgical wounds. *Arch. Surg.*, **107**, 206
99. Seropian, R. and Reynolds, B. M. (1971). Wound infections after preoperative depilatory versus razor preparation. *Am. J. Surg.*, **121**, 251
100. Aly, R., Maibach, H. E., Shinefield, H. R. and Strauss, W. G. (1972). Survival of pathogenic microorganisms on human skin. *J. Invest. Dermatol.*, **58**, 205
101. Marples, R. R. (1975). *Bacterial Infections*, Section I. Fundamental cutaneous micro-

biology. In S. L. Moschella, D. M. Pillsbury, and H. J. Hurley, Jr. (ed.). *Dermatology*, pp. 482–491. (Philadelphia: W. B. Saunders Company)

102. Selwyn, S. and Ellis, H. (1972). Skin bacteria and skin disinfection reconsidered. *Br. Med. J.*, **1**, 136
103. Lowbury, E. J. L. and Lilly, H. A. (1973). Use of 4% chlorhexidine detergent solution (Hibiscrub) and other methods of skin disinfection. *Br. Med. J.*, **1**, 510
104. Levy, R. S., Goldstein, J. and Pressman, R. S. (1970). Value of a topical antibiotic ointment in reducing bacterial colonization of percutaneous venous catheters. *J. Albert Einstein Med. Ctr.*, **18**, 67
105. Moran, J. M., Atwood, R. P. and Rowe, M. I. (1965). A clinical and bacteriologic study of infections associated with venous cutdowns. *N. Engl. J. Med.*, **272**, 554
106. Norden, C. W. (1969). Application of antibiotic ointment to the site of venous catheterization—a controlled trial. *J. Infect. Dis.*, **120**, 611
107. Zinner, S. H., Denny-Brown, B. C., Braun, P., Burke, J. P., Toala, P. and Kass, E. H. (1969). Risk of infection with intravenous indwelling catheters: Effect of application of antibiotic ointment. *J. Infect. Dis.*, **120**, 616
108. Rebora, A., Marples, R. R. and Kligman, A. M. (1973). Experimental infection with *Candida albicans*. *Arch. Dermatol.*, **108**, 69
109. Henzel, J. H. and DeWeese, M. S. (1971). Morbid and mortal complications associated with prolonged central venous cannulation. *Am. J. Surg.*, **121**, 600
110. Smits, H. and Freedman, L. (1967). Prolonged venous catheterization as a cause of sepsis. *N. Engl. J. Med.*, **276**, 1229
111. Shils, M. E. (1972). Guidelines for total parenteral nutrition. *J. Am. Med. Assoc.*, **220**, 1721
112. Holm, I. and Wretlind, A. (1975). Prophylaxis against infection and septicemia in parenteral nutrition via central intravenous catheter. *Acta Chir. Scand.*, **141**, 173
113. DeLuca, P. P., Rapp, R. P., Bivins, B., McKean, H. E. and Griffen, W. O. (1975). Filtration and infusion phlebitis: A double-blind prospective clinical study. *Am. J. Hosp. Pharm.*, **32**, 1001
114. Evans, W. E., Barker, L. F. and Simone, J. V. (1976). Double-blind evaluation of 5-μm final filtration to reduce post-infusion phlebitis. *Am. J. Hosp. Pharm.*, **33**, 1160

114a. Collin, J., Tweedle, D. E. F., Venables, C. W., Constable, F. L. and Johnston, I. D. A. (1973). Effect of a millipore filter on complications of intravenous infusions: A prospective clinical trial. *Br. Med. J.*, **4**, 456

115. Rusmin, S., Althauser, M. B. and DeLuca, P. P. (1975). Consequences of microbial contamination during extended intravenous therapy using inline filters. *Am. J. Hosp. Pharm.*, **32**, 373
116. Rapp, R., Bivins, B., Schroeder, H. and DeLuca, P. P. (1975). Evaluation of a prototype air-venting inline intravenous filter set. *Am. J. Hosp. Pharm.*, **32**, 1253
117. Bernard, R. W., Stahl, W. M. and Chase, R. M. (1971). Subclavian vein catheterizations: A prospective study. II. Infectious complications. *Ann. Surg.*, **173**, 191
118. Pollack, M., Charache, P., Nieman, R. E., Jett, M. P., Reinhardt, J. A. and Hardy, P. H., Jr. (1971). Factors influencing colonization and antibiotic-resistant patterns of gram-negative bacteria in hospital patients. *Lancet*, **ii**, 668
119. Mogensen, J. V., Frederiksen, W. and Jensen, J. K. (1972). Subclavian vein catheterization and infection: A bacteriologic study of 130 catheter insertions. *Scand. J. Infect. Dis.*, **4**, 31
120. Knittle, M. A., Eitzman, D. V. and Baer, J. (1975). Role of hand contamination of personnel in epidemiology of gram-negative nosocomial infections. *J. Pediat.*, **86**, 433

120a. Maki, D. G., Weise, C. E. and Sarafin, H. W. (1977). A semiquantitative culture method for identifying intravenous-catheter-related infection. *N. Engl. J. Med.*, **296**, 1306

121. Bentley, D. W. and Lepper, M. H. (1968). Septicemia related to indwelling venous catheter. *J. Am. Med. Assoc.*, **206**, 1749
122. Brennan, M. F., Goldman, M. H., O'Connell, R. C., Kundsin, R. B. and Moore, F. D. (1972). Prolonged parenteral alimentation: *Candida* growth and the prevention of candidemia by amphotericin instillation. *Ann. Surg.*, **17**, 265

123. Goldstein, E. and Hoeprich, P. D. (1972). Problems in the diagnosis and treatment of systemic candidiasis. *J. Infect. Dis.*, **125**, 190
124. Gaines, J. D. and Remington, J. S. (1973). Diagnosis of deep infection with *Candida*. *Arch. Int. Med.*, **132**, 699
125. Stone, H. H., Kolb, L. D., Currie, C. A., Geheber, C. E. and Cuzell, J. Z. (1974). *Candida* sepsis: Pathogenesis and principles of treatment. *Ann. Surg.*, **179**, 697
126. Freeman, J. B., Davis, P. L. and MacLean, L. D. (1974). *Candida* endophthalmitis associated with intravenous hyperalimentation. *Arch. Surg.*, **108**, 237
127. Portnoy, J., Wolf, P. L., Webb, M. and Remington, J. S. (1971). *Candida* blastospores and pseudohyphae in blood smears. *N. Engl. J. Med.*, **285**, 1010
128. Anderson, A. O. and Yardley, J. H. (1972). Demonstration of *Candida* in blood smears. *N. Engl. J. Med.*, **286**, 108
129. Filice, G., Yu, B. and Armstrong, D. (1977). Immunodiffusion and agglutination tests for *Candida* in patients with neoplastic disease: Inconsistent correlation of results with invasive infections. *J. Infect. Dis.*, **135**, 349
130. Everett, E. D., LaForce, F. M. and Eickhoff, T. C. (1975). Serologic studies in suspected visceral candidiasis. *Arch. Int. Med.*, **135**, 1075
131. Glew, R. H., Buckley, H. R., Rosen, H. M., Moellering, R. C. and Fischer, J. E. (1975). Value of prospective *Candida* precipitins in fungemia in patients with hyperalimentation. *Surg. For.*, **26**, 113
132. Kozinn, P. J., Galen, R. S., Taschdjian, C. L., Goldberg, P. L., Protzman, W. and Kozinn, M. A. (1976). The precipitin test in systemic candidiasis. *J. Am. Med. Assoc.*, **235**, 628
133. Dellon, A. L., Stark, W. J. and Chretien, P. B. (1975). Spontaneous resolution of endogenous *Candida* endophthalmitis complicating intravenous hyperalimentation. *Am. J. Ophthalmol.*, **79**, 648
134. Blackburn, G. L. and Bistrian, B. R. (1976). Nutritional care of the injured and/or septic patient. *Surg. Clin. North Am.*, **56**, 1195

24
Tracing sources of infection associated with parenteral infusions

I. PHILLIPS AND S. EYKYN

INTRODUCTION

Since 1969, the Department of Clinical Microbiology, St Thomas' Hospital, London, has recorded the clinical progress of all patients with bacteraemia. Our experience has included most of the described variants of infusion-related sepsis, and it is our purpose now to give an account of infusion-related bacteraemia in one hospital.

St Thomas' is a busy general hospital with about 600 acute medical and surgical beds. There is no special interest in total parenteral nutrition, and we have not studied it specifically. Intravenous infusions are set up largely by the junior medical staff, and intravenous admixtures are usually made as required in the open wards. There is no team charged solely with the care of intravenous therapy.

The procedure for the diagnosis of bacteraemia (and we have used the term to include the clinical condition of septicaemia) follows a strict pattern. If a clinician believes that one of his patients is bacteraemic he speaks to a medical or senior technical member of the laboratory staff, and the two agree on the number and type of blood cultures required. Blood cultures are therefore performed only on patients who are ill, and never as a routine, and the laboratory doctors know about them at an early stage. Blood cultures are then made with few exceptions by members of the laboratory technical staff. Positive blood cultures are reported immediately to the clinician and a laboratory doctor visits the patient and starts a clinical record based on a temperature chart. Thus we now have records of almost 1000 cases of bacteraemia.

An additional means of gathering information is possible in regular internal laboratory meetings at which technical and medical staff discuss interesting bacteriological results, and also when reports are finally scrutinized by laboratory doctors. In this way, information on, for example, infected infusion sites is made known at the earliest opportunity, even if the clinician does not consult the laboratory himself and merely sends a sample.

A final important point is that we identify fully all clinically-important organisms, and hold many of them for typing should the need arise.

As we have never made a specific study of the incidence of catheter-related sepsis, we have no denominators in our results.

INFUSION-RELATED BACTERAEMIA

Among 930 cases of bacteraemia included in this study no less than seventy-two (8%) were associated with intravenous therapy. Table 24.1 lists the organisms that we isolated from the blood of these patients. Almost half the cases were caused by *Staphylococcus aureus* and infusion-related staphylococcal bacteraemia accounts for 25% of all cases of staphylococcal bacteraemia.

Table 24.1 Organisms isolated from the blood of seventy-two patients with intravenous infusion-related bacteraemia. St. Thomas' Hospital, 1969–76

Organisms	*Number of cases*
S. aureus	31
S. aureus and *Strep. pyogenes*	1
and *Strep. faecalis*	1
S. epidermidis	6
S. epidermidis and *Strep. sanguis*	1
Strep. agalactiae (Group B strep.)	1
Pseudomonas aeruginosa	2
Ps. acidovorans	1
Ps. cepacia	3
Ps. fluorescens	1
Ps. maltophilia	2
Ps. pseudoalkaligenes	1
Ps. thomasii	10
Ps. spp.	1
Klebsiella spp.	4
Enterobacter cloacae	2
Proteus mirabilis	1
irregular Enterobacteriaceae	2
Candida albicans	1

In fifty-five instances there was overt clinical infection at the infusion site, and this was true in all thirty-three cases with *S. aureus* infection. The ten patients with *Pseudomonas thomasii* infection were, with some of the other pseudomonads, associated with intrinsic contamination of our own pharmacy's intravenous fluids in an outbreak that we have already described in detail[1]. There was only one case of fungaemia in the whole series.

In the fifty-five cases not associated with intrinsic contamination of the infused fluid, our investigations included assessments of four factors that influence infusion-related sepsis. These are the site of catheterization, the area of the hospital in which the catheter was inserted, the interval between the insertion of the catheter and the onset of sepsis, and finally the influence of prior antimicrobial chemotherapy.

Among the fifty-five cases there were sixteen with catheters inserted in the antecubital fossa, four with femoral vein catheters, and no less than thirty-five in the jugular vein. These latter were often multipurpose lines used for pressure measurements, sampling and therapy, and we presume that continued manipulation is one of the more important factors associated with sepsis.

Twenty-four catheters were inserted in the wards, twenty-one in the intensive care unit (all neck lines with the exception of two femoral catheters) seven in operating theatres (six of them antecubital catheters) and one in the Special-care Baby Unit. Only two of the fifty-five patients had catheters inserted in other hospitals.

Table 24.2 shows the relationship between sepsis and duration of catheterization. Because we have no knowledge of the uninfected patients we can

Table 24.2 Interval between insertion of catheter and signs of local sepsis or bacteraemia in 49/55 cases for whom the information was available

Time interval (days)	*Site of insertion*			
	Arm	*Neck*	*Femoral*	*All*
2	3	3	1	7
3	6	6		12
4	2	8		10
5	2	1		3
6		2	1	3
7	7	2		3
8–10		3		3
>10		7	1	8
TOTAL	14	32	3	49

only point out that infection may become apparent, either locally or as bacteraemia at any time after about 48 h of catheterization, and that more of the sepsis associated with neck lines presents late, presumably due to the longer duration of neck-line catheterization.

Table 24.3 shows the relationship between prior chemotherapy and the organism causing bacteraemia in the fifty-five patients. None of the *S. aureus* bacteraemias arose in patients receiving chemotherapy: we do not know how many catheterized patients received antistaphylococcal antibiotics, and thus do not have any information on their prophylactic value. Other organisms were more often isolated in the face of chemotherapy, most often inappropriate for the organism. Infection with these other organisms might be the price to be paid if antistaphylococcal prophylaxis were attempted.

Table 24.3 The prior use of antibiotics in fifty-five patients with infusion-related bacteraemia and catheter site sepsis

	Systemic antimicrobial in use:			
Organism	*At the time of septicaemia*	*In the previous week*	*None in previous week*	*Total cases*
S. aureus	0	1 (R)	32	33
S. epidermidis	2 (R, S*)	0	5	7
Strep. agalactiae	0	1 (R)	0	1
Ps. aeruginosa	2 (R)	0	0	2
Pseudomonas spp.	1 (R)	0	3	4
Klebsiella spp.	0	2 (R, S)	2	4
Enterobacter cloacae	1 (R)	1 (R)	0	2
Proteus mirabilis	0	0	1	1
Candida albicans	1 (R)	0	0	1

* Resistant (R) or sensitive (S) to the antimicrobials used

Exogenous infection

In twenty-five cases we identified an exogenous source. In twenty-two of these the intravenous infusion fluid was contaminated either because of faults in the manufacture of our own intravenous products[1] (10 *Ps. thomasii*, 2 *Ps. maltophilia*, 1 *Ps. acidovorans*, 1 *Ps. pseudoalkaligenes*, 1 *Ps. flourescens*, 1 *Pseudomonas* sp.) or because the glass bottle was cracked (2 irregular Enterobacteriaceae, 1 *Klebsiella* sp.) or the infusion apparatus was contaminated (3 *Ps. cepacia* from contaminated pressure monitors[2]). We have seen no case of infection caused by contaminated infusion fluid since 1972.

In three cases the exogenous source was shown to be the medical attendants. Two patients were infected with *S. aureus* phage type 187, an unusual type known to be carried by the doctor who inserted the intravenous catheters under difficult circumstances. A third was infected with phage type 29/52A/80, also carried by the doctor who inserted the catheter. It seems likely that this is a route of infection for other patients, but we seldom knew the carrier status of the doctor who set up the infusion, so we cannot prove this.

Endogenous infection

We were able to suggest a highly probable endogenous source in fourteen cases on the evidence that the patient was either infected or colonized with the same organism before the infusion was set up. Ten patients were colonized without being clinically infected. Two were shown to carry, in their anterior nares, *S. aureus* of the phage type that later caused infection, and it seems likely that had we investigated carriage in all our patients we would have found more cases of autoinfection. Eight patients had abnormally colonized respiratory tracts, largely as a result of tracheostomy and mechanical ventilation. *S. aureus* was again implicated in three patients with the same phage type in blood and the carrier site in each case. The other patients had *Ps. aeruginosa* (2, same pyocine, serological and phage type), *Klebsiella aerogenes* 1, same serotype), *Enterobacter cloacae* (1) and *Strep. agalactiae* (1, same serotype).

Four patients had had previous clinical infection and presumably still carried the organism although we did not attempt to demonstrate it. There were three patients with wound infections, with *S. aureus* of the same phage type and one with a previous urinary tract infection with *Proteus mirabilis* of the same Diene's type.

Epidemiology in St Thomas' Hospital

As a result of our clinical, microbiological and epidemiological investigations, we were able to identify a convincing source of infection in thirty-nine of the seventy-two patients. We were least successful with staphylococci. In the case of *S. aureus* we were able to decide between autoinfection and cross-infection in only eleven of the thirty-three patients, and in eight of these autoinfection was responsible. It is impossible to know whether this represents the true proportion.

The source of *S. epidermidis* in the seven infected patients was not identified. We never knew the carrier status of the patients or attendants, and although it seems likely that the pattern of infection is similar to that for *S. aureus* we have no evidence for either. We were able to identify the source of the *Strep. agalactiae* but not the *Strep. sangius*. *In toto* we had good evidence for a source for only twelve out of the forty-one Gram-positive organisms.

For the Gram-negative organisms we were more successful and identified a highly probable source for twenty-seven out of the thirty, of which seventeen came from the infusion fluid at a time when the risk of such contamination was not fully appreciated.

We were unable to assign a source to the single episode of candidaemia.

Clinical effects

In most of our patients recovery from infusion-associated bacteraemia was uneventful upon removal of the catheter and the exhibition of correct chemotherapy.

In a few patients the course was catastrophic, and a brief case history will illustrate the problems. Following coronary artery surgery, a 58-year-old woman was given prophylactic flucloxacillin. Her management necessitated the constant use of jugular venous lines: the first set was inserted at operation and changed after 10 days, the second set changed after 10 days for femoral catheters, replaced after about 1 week. Her sputum and then the site of insertion of the jugular lines became colonized with *Ps. aeruginosa* about 1 week post-operatively and shortly afterwards she became bacteraemic. During the next month all of the blood cultures collected on eleven different days yielded *Ps. aeruginosa* despite treatment with gentamicin to which the organism appeared partially sensitive, and carbenicillin, and finally tobramycin and carbenicillin. We were unable to sterilize the blood while intravenous catheterization remained essential. She died, with sterile blood cultures, almost 2 months after her operation.

CONCLUSIONS

Careful liaison between clinicians and microbiologists, and full identification and typing of bacteria causing bacteraemia and associated sepsis in patients with intravenous catheters, has enabled us to identify most of the known infection hazards among patients in a single general hospital. In some instances, as for example in those due to contaminated infusion fluid, we have been able to take steps to prevent recurrence. In others we have been unable to persuade our clinical colleagues of the feasibility of possible preventive measures, as for examples, against *S. aureus*, which remains our major problem.

References

1. Phillips, I., Eykyn, S. and Laker, M. (1972). An outbreak of hospital infection caused by contaminated autoclaved fluids. *Lancet*, **i**, 1258
2. Phillips, I., Eykyn, S., Curtis, M. A. and Snell, J. J. S. (1971). *Pseudomonas cepacia* septicaemia in an intensive care unit. *Lancet*, **i**, 375

Discussion

A. B. Jones: (Canada) Would the authors care to comment on the value of having a millipore filter in the line. This seems to be the subject of controversy lately. Some feel that it increases the incidence of infection, while others think that it filters out any inadvertently introduced contamination.

R. B. Kundsin: (USA) As a result of our work we found that organisms can often go right through the filter. We have also seen fungi grow right through and form colonies on both sides of millipore filters. Our feeling is that a millipore filter does not add much.

Jones: Do the nurses mix the whole solution?

Kundsin: These are not total parenteral hyperalimentation solutions. Those are made up in the pharmacy. I am discussing regular infusions.

J. T. Harries: (UK) What is meant by additives and their relationship to contamination? Would the authors comment on how specifically this relates to contamination of the fluids.

Kundsin: There are various things that are added and they are tailored for individual patient's needs. The nurse simply takes the syringe and adds the prescribed solution to the bag. What was interesting was that, even without an additive, the simple process of inserting the administration set into the bag resulted in a very small level of contamination; and we can relate everything to that. The environment in which these procedures is carried out is extremely important. The contamination is predominantly *Bacillus* species and fungi. We had diphtheroids on two occasions and micrococci once, but predominantly they were environmental organisms and not organisms from people. That is why the place where this is done has to be bacteriologically clean.

P. Vinay: Was there any opportunity to culture Intralipid bottles? One of our hospitals reported strange organisms in Intralipid bottles, which are not usually found in hospitals or as skin contaminants.

Kundsin: We did not examine any Intralipid, but it does not surprise me. One can always find some organism that will grow in any solution. The idea is to keep them all out.

S. J. Karran: (UK) Is the philosophy of the preparation of all TPN solutions by the pharmacy completely acceptable to hospital practitioners in the US?

Kundsin: I have personal feelings about it. Most of those working in the pharmacy do not have adequate training in microbiology, and therefore I feel that a microbiologist should be involved in the environmental testing that has to be done to ensure that the work is carried out in a clean area. Pharmacists are becoming more concerned about the microbiology.

Jones: It was suggested that laminar airflow hoods may be an expensive luxury. Is it a waste of money to get laminar airflow hoods for mixing TPN solutions?

Kundsin: I think that it may be. Unless one is really actively aware of the mechanisms of contamination, a laminar airflow is no magic solution. If there is a laminar hood available, one should test it, check it out and see that there are no micro-organisms around. The hoods have to be tested and the filter changed regularly.

Ultraviolet light is extremely effective in destroying micro-organisms. If the working surfaces are kept clean, and irradiated with U-V, then solutions can be prepared under U-V light. U-V light is perfectly satisfactory to work under as it has no penetration and will not do any harm.

Jones: Our practice is to prepare all TPN solutions in a laminar airflow hood and there are special pharmacists' aides who have been trained to do it. All batches are monitored bacteriologically and our contamination rate is effectively zero. They are providing for 16 to 20 patients a day, and providing 60, 80 or 100 bags a day. It is a very satisfactory system. Obviously in smaller hospitals one will run into problems with people not being sufficiently well trained.

N. Zöllner: (Germany) Did the authors go back to the ward and find out what happened to the patients who got the contaminated infusions? Did any symptoms arise?

Kundsin: We had no reports of any symptoms. These contaminants were of a very low order (one or two colonies) and we got them immediately. Our rate of contamination *is* extraordinarily low. However, I do think that when something is given intravenously, it should be sterile and there should be no excuse. Let us not speculate whether it takes five *Candida* to make someone sick or ten. We do not know. One patient might get sick with one and another not get sick with fifty.

G. L. Blackburn: (USA) In our own hospital we have a protocol which involves changing the catheter dressing on Mondays, Wednesdays and Fridays, with the patients masked, using gloves, and following a most meticulous aseptic technique. Freeman and his colleagues[1] have tried to determine which of the various procedures besides aseptic technique diminishes the flora. They studied a mechanical scrub, and different antibiotic ointments. They found that with a daily mechanical scrub they were able to reduce the plate count. Their conclusion was that the mechanical preparation, rather than the ointment, was the key factor.

I. Phillips: (UK) I do not know the complete answer but all the attempts that I have seen at applying antibiotic ointments have led to resistance problems and the topical preparation not working. We have experience with Fucidin which is perhaps rather an unfortunate choice because it has built-in potential for resistance. However, in individual patients resistance occurs.

J. Allen: (USA) My own feeling would be for antibiotic ointments not to be used. I agree on meticulous preparation of the site and the maintenance of a very clean, dry dressing. I have some concern over the occlusive dressing. This has not really been looked at. But, as Dr Walter has pointed out, it is essential to keep that dressing clean and dry.

There is nothing to allow us to comment on the ideal frequency of cleaning and preparation with any surety. The one team that changed it only once a week was concerned that the manipulation of the catheter skin junction with the to-and-fro movement caused by the cleaning might serve to introduce further bacteria, even though their catheter-associated septicaemia rate was about 2%, which is a good low average.

C. W. Walter: (USA) My feeling is that mechanical cleansing of the catheter site every day or two, with some detergent germicide, is very effective. Most of my experience has been with access sites for dialysis. Patients may even learn how to scrub up the sites for themselves. It is important to use a germicide that does not cause smarting, and leaves some residual on the skin so that the skin is self-sterilizing. I have had success with 1–750 Zephiran. I admit that this is the quaternary that everybody curses, but they forget that Zephiran is chemically pure benzalkonium chloride and that it is very effective, whereas the USP benzalkonium chloride is loaded with ammonium acetate and it is not effective. The buffer neutralizes a great deal of its effectiveness and certain *Pseudomonas* grow in it easily.

As for disinfecting the original site, scrubbing is important. I have described the technique that we used but ordinary soap and water was also successful. Flood the soap and water with 2% aqueous iodine; leave it on for a minute and then wash it off with 60% isopropyl alcohol. That was the mainstay of disinfecting the donor sites, and we had good results with that.

G. Hardy: (UK) Could someone elaborate on the role of the pharmacist and the microbiologist in the TPN team. In the UK pharmacists are reasonably well trained in microbiology, but very few of them are involved in TPN. Where they are, the Medicines Inspectorate of the Department of Health recommend that they carry out the manipulations in laminar flow conditions rather than under ultraviolet light as does the CDC (Centre for Disease Control).

Allen: I do not think that the CDC has come out with any recommendation to the effect that ultraviolet light should not be used. It is perhaps an appropriate adjunct. It is extremely important—as Dr Kundsin has already stressed—to have a clean work area that is disinfected at least daily. I feel that a well-maintained laminar flow hood with the filter changed periodically with work surfaces disinfected and which is kept running 24 hours a day is an ideal area in which to prepare solutions. It is also important for the pharmacist to be trained in microbiology so that he knows what he is doing.

Walter: Would the pharmacist be recommended to wear sterile gloves? Is Dr Allen satisfied with the laminar flow hood? Having done the bacteriology for many years, I hold them in utter contempt.

Allen: I will bow to Dr Walter on that. Obviously I have not done that sort of work. Again it depends on how they are maintained. I have seen some that are poorly maintained, and have solutions spilled on the work-surfaces, that are encrusted with chemical precipitates on the roof. They are obviously an incredibly bad area in which to do this sort of careful preparation.

Walter: Laminar flow or unidirectional flow has the airstream coming towards the operator. He must keep his hands behind the container, he must wear a mask—because any trajectory will go against it. Any fall-out of bacteria from the manipulating fingers eddies right around the very area that one is trying to protect. Everything has to be handled very carefully from the point downstream from the insertion site. If one tries to teach this technology one finds that it is almost impossible for people to do it. Ultra violet light (25 microwatts per cm^2) coming straight down, is an enormously effective way of dealing with any contamination from the operator.

One has to wear goggles as otherwise one would get conjunctivitis. It costs very little and power need only be used when one is working, and it almost never wears out.

R. K. Ausman: (USA) Would anyone comment on the increased *Candida* septicaemia that has occurred, or appears from literature references to have occurred, since 1970, and which most of us associate with the advent of parenteral nutrition, particularly central vein parenteral nutrition?

Walter: I can only comment from my own hospital. The microbiologists did not appreciate the presence of *Candida* until they started looking for it vigorously. For a long time every Gram-negative organism was discarded, and then we started to study it and now we have a great increase in incidence. I believe that it is only an increased awareness on the part of the microbiologist as to what is going on.

Allen: Probably there is an increased association of fungal septicaemias, particularly *Candida* septicaemias, in patients receiving TPN therapy as opposed to patients receiving routine intravenous therapy. There are probably a number of reasons for that. Perhaps one of them is associated with the fact that the fungi do grow much better in TPN fluids while they virtually do not grow in routine intravenous fluids.

I shall temper that statement immediately by saying that I do not think that contamination of the fluid is the source of most of the septicaemias that occur; it is probably catheter-associated. On the other hand, the patient most likely to receive TPN therapy will be extremely ill or debilitated, frequently having had surgery. Many of the patients are also receiving steroids, other immuno-suppressive agents, or broad-spectrum antibiotics. These predisposing situations would lead to fungal septicaemia in the sort of patients that frequently receive TPN.

I do not think that there have been adequate studies to see how many of the patients who get fungal septicaemias might have these other predisposing factors.

Kundsin: I have some details from our hospital between January 1976 and April 1977; the blood culture data of patients on intravenous hyper-alimentation. We had two *Candida albicans* out of thirty-four positive bloods, and one *Candida tropicalis*—a total of three in something like a year and a quarter. However we had nine *Staph.* coagulase negative and four *Klebsiella ammoniae*. There is more of everything else and very little *Candida*—Now.

Allen: I suspect that as other studies are published they will show the same trend. I think the better care that is being given to patients receiving TPN will probably influence this trend.

I would also comment that the series that have been published differ one from another as to the organisms causing disease. Some hospitals will report that almost all their infected patients have fungal infections, while there are others that will have almost none. Part of these differences, as Dr Walter suggested, might be due to how good the microbiology laboratory is at isolating and identifying organisms.

Phillips: I wonder about the relevance of laboratory cultures of intravenous fluids. The results are dependent on inoculum, how many organisms are put in, what the organisms are taken from, the medium of suspension, and whether they are habituated to the particular solution used. We have had widely different results by varying these various parameters.

Allen: That is why I emphasized the study of Goldman[2] and his colleagues. They inoculated a concentration of 1 organism per ml in an attempt to simulate more of a real-life situation. Certainly other studies would indicate that organisms isolated from the patient are more viable than those that have been grown in the laboratory and then transferred.

Walter: A lot of organisms from the patient also have a nice inoculum in the foreign body in which the organism has been growing, e.g. dried pus, or squames. One of our anaesthetists had a mycosis under her finger-nails which was dangerous because the caseous material was a good inoculum and she could finger nothing without shedding organisms. The long hair that droops all over the phlebotomy is all the time raining dandruff and organisms onto the site.

References

1. Jarrard, M. M. and Freeman, J. B. (1977). *J. Surg. Res.*, **22,** 521
2. Goldmann, D. A., Martin, W. T. and Worthington, J. W. (1973). Growth of bacteria and fungi in total parenteral nutrition solutions. *Am. J. Surg.*, **126,** 314

Section VIII
Biochemical Aspects of Parenteral Nutrition

25
Acid–base balance during parenteral nutrition with Travasol*

D. BOURBEAU, P. VINAY, G. LEMIEUX, A. GOUGOUX AND A. DURANCEAU

INTRODUCTION

Parenteral nutrition (TPN) is mandatory in patients unable to feed themselves by the oral route or in which intestinal absorption is either reduced or absent. The daily nitrogen intake necessary to establish and maintain a positive nitrogen balance was initially met by administration of an hydrolysate of casein or fibrin[1]. No systemic acidosis usually occurred with this procedure[1]. However following the recent introduction of synthetic crystalline amino acid mixtures, a high incidence of hyperchloraemic metabolic acidosis was observed[2,3]. The present study describes the hydrogen ion load given during TPN and describes plasma and urinary acid–base parameters following the short-term administration of one of these crystalline amino acid mixtures, Travasol*, while caloric requirements were ensured by glucose and lipid administration.

METHODS

Patients

Seven patients with an inability to achieve adequate nutrition via the oral route and referred to the Surgery Service of the Hôtel-Dieu Hospital of Montreal were selected for this study (Table 25.1). Patients with chronic or acute renal failure, insulin-dependent diabetes or active infections were excluded. All patients were cared for by the same medical team, and a special nurse supervised the TPN administration, care of the catheters, and collection of the various specimens.

* Synthamin.

Table 25.1 Description of patients on TPN protocol

Patients	*Sex*	*Age*	*Weight*	*Height*	*Primary diagnosis*
Travasol ($n = 7$)			kg	m	
L.A.	M	60	61.5	1.67	Gastroduodenal stenosis
P.O.	M	72	72.0	1.76	Acute pancreatitis
R.C.	F	52	54.0	1.60	Ileitis; ileovaginal fistula
S.A.	M	49	56.6	1.83	Chronic pancreatitis
M.G.	F	72	54.0	1.62	Biliary fistula
P.J.	M	28	75.4	1.70	Ruptured Meckel's diverticulitis
L.R.	F	65	55.7	1.57	Carcinoma of pancreas
Mean ± SEM		56.9 ± 5.9		61.3 ± 3.4	

Solutions

All solutions were prepared in a sterile fashion by a clinical pharmacist who ensured the exact formulation of the infusions. No nutrients were given orally for 4 days prior to and during parenteral nutrition. Each patient received daily a fixed intake of 12.6 g of nitrogen as a 10% amino acid solution (0.75 of Travasol, Baxter Laboratories, Malton, Ontario, Canada), 750 g of glucose and 100 g of lipids (Intralipid, Pharmacia Canada Ltd, Montreal, Canada) giving a total of 3600 non-protein cal in a volume of 4.5 l. The daily electrolyte intake provided with this regimen is given in Table 25.2. Vitamins were added to the solutions but no trace metals were given.

Table 25.2 Daily electrolytes intake during TPN protocol

	mEq/day
Na^+	98
K^+	165
Mg^{2+}	15
Ca^{2+}	10
Cl^-	172
PO_4^{2-}	93
SO_4^{2-}	75
Acetate$^-$	112

Experimental design

The patients were studied for 4 days (referred to as −4 to −1) prior to TPN and for 10 days (referred to as +1 to +10) during TPN. Control blood values have been pooled in two groups, the first one representing the data for day −4 and −3 and the second for day −2, −1 plus the data collected on the morning of day + 1 before the installation of the intravenous nutrients. Blood data obtained during intravenous feeding have been grouped in three periods: day +1 to +3, day +4 to +6, and day +7 to +10. Urinary data are presented on a daily basis.

Analytical methods

Venous blood pH and pCO_2 were determined anaerobically at 37 °C with appropriate electrodes using an Instrumentation Laboratory ultramicro Duo-matic pH and blood gas analysing system, model 123–S1. Urine was collected under mineral oil, and urinary pH and pCO_2 were determined on the same apparatus. Bicarbonate concentration was calculated from the Henderson–Hasselbach equation using a pK' of 6.1 and a CO_2 solubility coefficient of 0.0301 for plasma and 0.0309 for urine. Urinary net acid excretion was taken as the sum of ammonia plus titratable acid minus bicarbonate. Urinary or plasma, sodium, potassium, chloride ammonia and titratable acid were determined by methods previously reported[4]. Phosphorus in plasma and urine were determined on the AutoAnalyzer[5]. Osmolarity of plasma or infusates was measured on an Advanced Instruments osmometer.

Blood for determination of pyruvate, lactate, β-hydroxybutyrate and acetoacetate was deproteinized immediately with an equal volume of chilled 10% (weight/vol) perchloric acid[6]. These organic acids were measured enzymatically by spectrophotometry[4]. Glomerular filtration rate was calculated from endogenous creatinine clearance. Results are presented as means ± SEM.

RESULTS

Characteristics of the infusates

Since the measured osmolarity of the Travasol–dextrose mixture is 1590 mOsm/l (Table 25.3), all solutions were infused through a central venous catheter. The measured sodium, potassium and chloride content of these solutions are in good agreement with the manufacturers' description of the product. pH, titratable acid, and electrolyte content of the solutions used in this study are shown in Table 25.3. One litre of 10% Travasol (pH 6.01) contains 50 mEq of titratable acid. There is no titratable acid in dextrose 33% (pH 2.85) indicating the complete absence of buffers in this solution. When Travasol and dextrose are mixed, the titratable acid is diluted to 14 mEq/l.

Table 25.3 Measured parameters on TPN solutions

	pH	*Titratable acid* (mEq/l)	*Na^+* (mEq/l)	*K^+* (mEq/l)	*Cl^-* (mEq/l)	*Osmolarity* (mOsm/l)
10% Travasol	6.01	50	76	62	69	1260
Dextrose 33%	2.85	0	0	0	0	1672
10% Travasol + dextrose 33%	5.83	14	19	15	17	1590
10% Intralipid	7.50	0	0	0	0	275

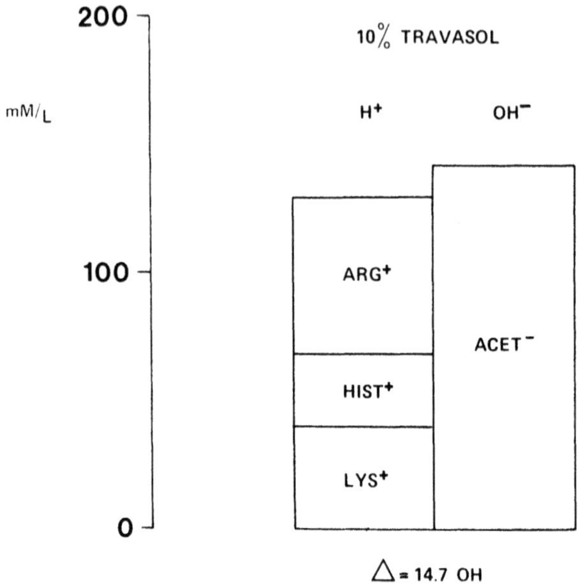

Figure 25.1 Distribution of cationic amino acids and organic anions in 1 l. of Travasol solution

Figure 25.1 presents the cationic amino acids in 1 l. of 10% Travasol. The incorporation of these amino acids into protein leads to a stoichiometric production of H^+. To compensate for this additional acid source, 150 mEq of acetate are provided in 1 l. of the crystalline amino acid mixture. Obviously, 95% of this acetate will be in the anionic form at pH 6.0.

Its metabolism will thus generate an equivalent amount of bicarbonate. The administration of the organic cations and anions contained in 1 l. of 10% Travasol thus generates 14.7 mEq of bicarbonate (Figure 25.1). The net acid–base effect of the administration of 1 l. of Travasol/dextrose mixture, will be the generation of 14 mEq of H^+ (Table 25.4). 1 l. of Intralipid containing 24 mM of phosphates as phospholipids will also liberate 27 mEq of

Table 25.4 Sources of H^+ during TPN with Travasol and Intralipid (mEq/l)

	10% Travasol	*33% Dextrose*	*10% Travasol 33% dextrose*	*10% Intralipid*
Free H^+ ion	0.0010	1.4	0.0015	0
H^+ from titratable acid	50	0	13.5	0
H^+ from $\frac{\text{cations}}{\text{anions}}$ balance	−14.7	0	−3.68	0
H^+ from phospholipids	0	0	0	+27
Net H^+*	+35.3	+1.4	+14.0	+27

* Approximate value.

H^{+} [7]. The net H^{+} intake induced by our protocol with Travasol and Intralipid can be calculated as 56.5 mEq/day (Table 25.5).

Table 25.5 Net H^{+} intake during TPN protocol (mEq/day)

Free H^{+}	+ 0.0045
H^{+} from titratable acid	+40.5
H^{+} from $\frac{\text{anions}}{\text{cations}}$ balance	−11.04
H^{+} from phospholipids	+27
Net H^{+} intake	+56.5

Effect of TPN on plasma and urinary acid–base parameters

Figure 25.2 presents the venous blood pH, $p\mathrm{CO_2}$ and bicarbonate before and during TPN. No significant changes in the blood acid–base parameters can

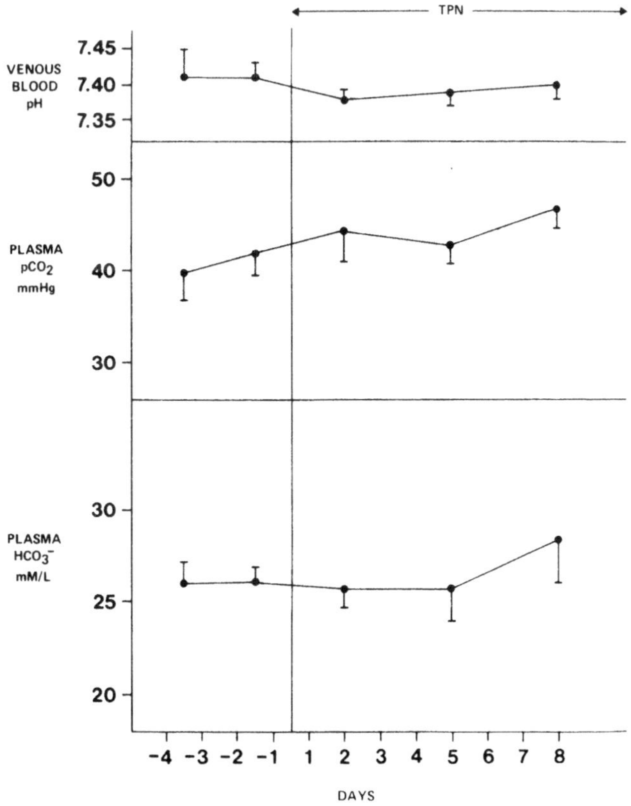

Figure 25.2 Venous blood acid–base parameters before and during TPN with Travasol

be detected. Table 25.4 presents the net changes in the various organic acids after 5 or 8 days of TPN. Following the carbohydrate load, a small increase in blood lactate and pyruvate was observed. The ketone bodies were only elevated slightly during the control period despite a negative nitrogen balance (Vinay *et al.*, chapter 4). The intravenous fluids including 5% dextrose given during the control period prevented the establishment of a more severe ketosis.

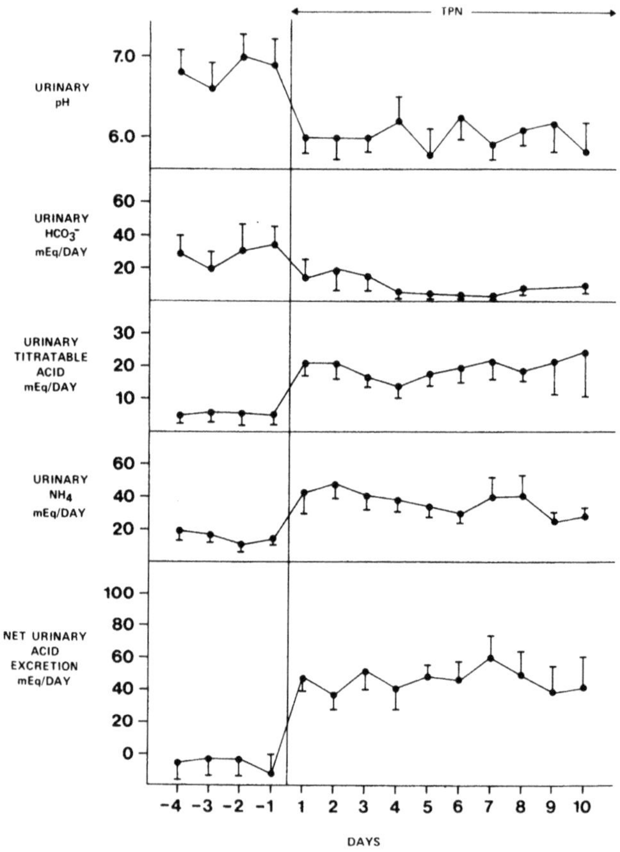

Figure 25.3 Urinary acid–base parameters before and during TPN with Travasol

Following TPN the blood concentration of ketones fell. The net effect of these organic acid changes was the accumulation of 42 mM/l of organic anions in the blood. The mean plasma sodium fell at the same time by 4 mEq/l after 8 days while the plasma chloride fell by 8 mEq/l. The fall in plasma chloride coincides with the fall in the sodium, the rise in bicarbonate and the gap.

Urinary acid–base parameters are presented (Figure 25.3), the mean urinary pH in the control period is around 6.8 and a significant loss of bicarbonate is observed as most of these patients had significant acid losses from gastric drainage and were correcting a small metabolic alkalosis. As the bicarbonate output nearly equals the sum of urinary titratable acid plus ammonia, the mean net acid excretion for these patients is around 0. Following administration of TPN, a rapid fall in urinary pH and urinary bicarbonate was observed while the titratable acid and ammonia excretion rose. The net acid excretion was about 45 mEq/day, a value significantly lower than the H^+ load administered to the patients during TPN. However, if allowance is made

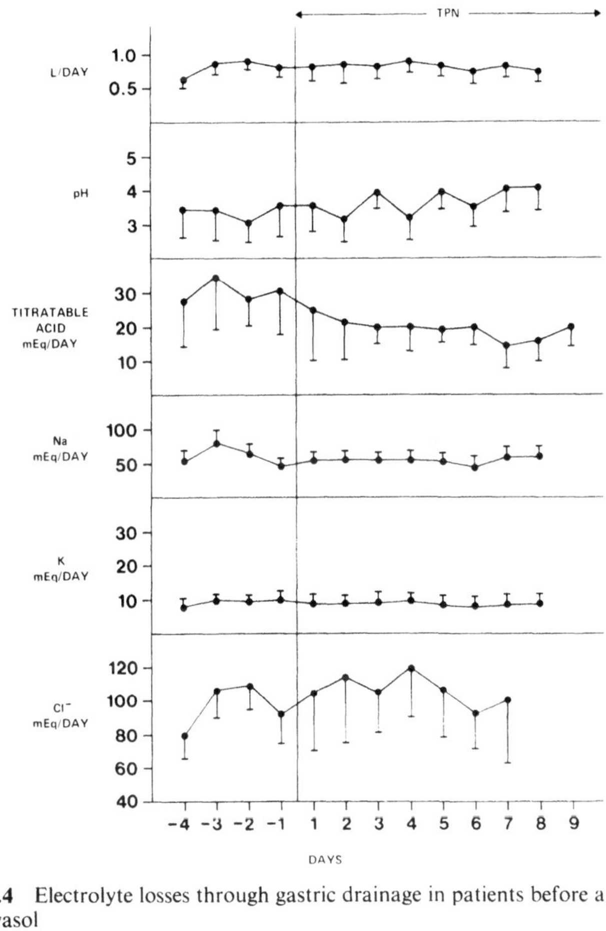

Figure 25.4 Electrolyte losses through gastric drainage in patients before and during TPN with Travasol

for the 20 mEq/day extrarenal losses of hydrogen ion presented in Figure 25.4, the hydrogen ion input agrees with the measured output.

Figure 25.5 presents the urinary electrolyte excretion before and during TPN. On a fixed intake of 98 mEq/day of sodium, the mean sodium loss decreased from 160 to 60 mEq/day. If the gastrointestinal daily losses of sodium are taken into account, a zero balance for sodium was observed (Figures 25.4 and 25.5). The renal and extrarenal losses of potassium rose to

110 mEq/day (Figure 25.5), combined so that with a fixed intake of 163 mEq/day, a positive balance of around 50 mEq/day was observed. If the positive nitrogen balance is taken into account (Chapter 4) the potassium balance can be corrected to +40[8]. However as no data on the potassium excretion in the stools were obtained, an accurate balance cannot be calculated. Nevertheless these data suggest that potassium administration has corrected in part

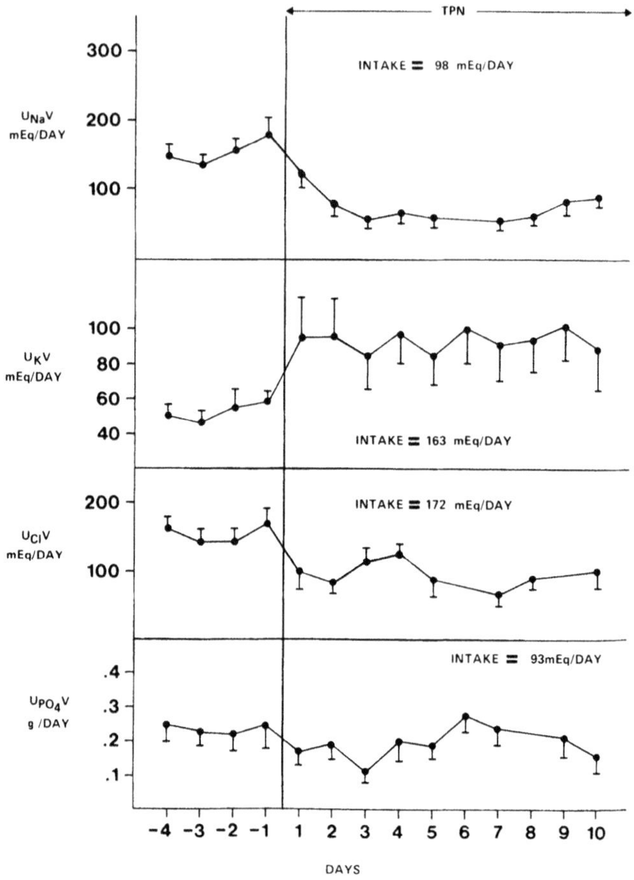

Figure 25.5 Urinary excretion of sodium, potassium, chloride and phosphate in patients before and during TPN with Travasol

a pre-existent potassium depletion in these malnourished patients. Furthermore a shift of potassium from extracellular to intracellular fluid secondary to carbohydrate administration was also present, as demonstrated by a significant hyperkalaemia observed in one patient in which TPN was interrupted abruptly. The chloride excretion in the urine (Figure 25.5) and the gastrointestinal losses (Figure 25.4) of around 180 mEq/day agrees closely with the fixed intake of 172 mEq/day.

Table 25.6 Blood organic acids and plasma anion gap before and during TPN with Travasol

	Control	△ *Day* 5	△ *Day* 8
Lactate (mM/l)	1.21	+1.97	+2.28
Pyruvate (mM/l)	0.08	+0.13	+0.13
β-OH-βutyrate (mM/l)	0.14	−0.11	−0.07
Acetoacetate (mM/l)	0.06	−0.04	0.04
Sum of △ org. acids		+1.95	+2.30
Plasma Na^+ (mEq/l)	137		133
Plasma Cl^- (mEq/l)	99		91
Plasma HCO_3 (mEq/l)	26		28
Anion gap (mEq/l)	12		14
△ Anion gap (mEq/l)			+2

DISCUSSION

Metabolic acidosis can occur during parenteral nutrition in three ways: an increment of the H^+ load, a diminution in the renal capacity for the excretion of hydrogen ion or extrarenal losses of bicarbonate. The H^+ load induced by TPN in part is due to the free hydrogen ions in the solutions. However, minute quantities of free hydrogen ions are present in these solutions (Table 25.4), there is only 1.4 mEq/l of hydrogen ion in 33% dextrose despite a pH of 2.85. However, significant amounts of hydrogen ions are present in acid solutions containing quantities of buffers. In Travasol at pH 6.0, 50 mEq/l of H^+ are present in the various buffers. Furthermore the incorporation into protein or the metabolic degradation of cationic amino acids will generate an equivalent amount of H^+ ions.

The frequent hyperchloraemic metabolic acidosis observed with the older preparations of synthetic amino acids was in fact due to the presence of excessive quantities of cationic amino acids in these solutions[1–3]. In 10% Travasol, the H^+ generated through this mechanism is compensated by the bicarbonate production through the metabolism of the accompanying anion acetate. The metabolism of sulphur-containing amino acids (absent in Travasol) and of phospholipids (contained in Intralipid), will generate sulphuric and phosphoric acid[9,10]. We have calculated that our protocol ensures a hydrogen ion load of around 57 mEq/day.

Kidney function should be able to respond to this moderate acid load by increasing its net hydrogen ion excretion. However, in the presence of a poor renal function (low glomerular filtration rate) or of a tubular defect in H^+ excretion, this adaptation could be deficient with secondary generation of a metabolic acidosis. Patients with malnutrition, like some patients in our study, are known to have a relative defect in their maximal capacity for hydrogen ion excretion[11]. This has been attributed to the poor availability of phosphate as buffers and to the low plasma level of amino acids used as precursors of the renal ammonia synthesis[11]. Finally extrarenal losses of bicarbonate through drainage of pancreatic juice for example could add its effect to the H^+ load produced by the intravenous feeding protocol and lead to the generation of a metabolic acidosis.

In the present study, it is clear that H^+ load produced by the intravenous feeding protocol did not change the systemic acid–base parameters as an adequate increase in H^+ excretion through the kidney occurred rapidly. It must be pointed out that, as the endogenous H^+ production and excretion is lower in malnourished patients than in normal subjects, the total H^+ excretion of 65 mEq/day observed in our study is close to the value of 1 mEq/kg/day observed in normal subjects on a normal diet[12]. Consequently we do not feel that bicarbonate should be added routinely to solutions used for total parenteral nutrition.

ACKNOWLEDGEMENTS

The authors are grateful to Y. Courchesne, S. Desjardins, D. Donaldson, L. Tessier, J. Sénécal for their kind assistance, as well as to all the physicians and nurses who were involved in this study. Travasol solution was kindly provided by Baxter Canada, Ltd.

References

1. Heird, W. C. and Winters, R. W. (1975). Total parenteral nutrition. The state of the art. *J. Pediat.*, **86**, 2
2. Heird, W. C., Dell, R. B., Driscoll, J. M., Jr., Grebin, B. and Winters, R. W. (1972). Metabolic acidosis resulting from intravenous alimentation mixtures containing synthetic amino acids. *N. Engl. J. Med.*, **287**, 943
3. Chan, J. C. M., Asch, M. J., Lin, S. and Hays, D. M. (1972). Hyperalimentation with amino acid and casein hydrolysate solutions: mechanism of acidosis. *J. Am. Med. Assoc.*, **220**, 1700
4. Vinay, P., Lemieux, G., Cartier, P., Ahmad, M. and Baverel, G. (1976). Effect of fatty acids on renal ammoniagenesis, in vivo and in vitro studies. *Am. J. Physiol.*, **231**, 880
5. Fiske, C. H. and Subbarow, Y. (1925). The colorimetric determination of phosphorus. *J. Biol. Chem.*, **66**, 375
6. Bergmayer, H. U. (1974). *Methods of Enzymatic Analysis*, p. 1446. (New York and London: Academic Press)
7. Wretlind, A. (1972). Complete intravenous nutrition. Theoretical and experimental background. *Nutr. Metab.*, **14** (Suppl. 1), 57
8. Reifenstein, E. C., Jr., Albright, F. and Wells, S. L. (1945). The accumulation, interpretation and presentation of data pertaining to metabolic balance, notably those of calcium, phosphorus, and nitrogen. *J. Clin. Endocrinol*, **5**, 367
9. Lemann, J., Jr. and Relman, A. S. (1959). The relation of sulphur metabolism to acid–base balance and electrolyte excretion: the effects of D, L-methionine in normal man. *J. Clin. Invest.*, **38**, 2215
10. Lennon, E. J., Lemann, J., Jr. and Relman, A. S. (1962). The effects of phosphoproteins on acid balance in normal subjects. *J. Clin. Invest.*, **41**, 637
11. Klahr, S., Tripathy, K. and Lotero, H. (1970). Renal regulation of acid–base balance in malnourished man. *Am. J. Med.*, **48**, 325
12. Relman, A. S., Lennon, E. J. and Lemann, J., Jr. (1961). Endogenous production of fixed acid and the measurement of the net balance of acid in normal subjects. *J. Clin. Invest.*, **40**, 1621

Discussion

J. T. Harries: (UK) Several people have reported a relationship between infusions of fructose-containing solutions and high circulating levels of lactic acid and metabolic acidosis. The risks of metabolic acidosis in young infants must be borne in mind because of the immaturity of their renal tubular transport systems to handle hydrogen ion. We have seen very severe metabolic acidosis in this age group when a fructose-containing solution has been used.

D. Bourbeau: (Canada) I agree completely. It is perfectly true that in small infants with immature or possible limited renal function, fructose might create significant lactic acidaemia. It might depend on the quantity of fructose infused.

H. F. Woods: (UK) Does Dr Bourbeau stand by his statement that a metabolic acidosis can only develop during the infusion of certain of these substrates if renal function is impaired? I am not sure that the renal route is in every case the controlling factor in the homeostasis of H^+ concentration in tissues and fluids.

P. Vinay: (Canada) It is clear that when an acid load which the kidney can cope with is given no systemic acidosis will develop as greater amounts of H^+ will be excreted. In some situations acid loads significantly greater than that which the kidney can cope with will cause acidosis.

We wished to emphasize that if Travasol solution is used as recommended, a very moderate load of H^+ will be given. A normal subject will excrete around 1.0 mEq of H^+ per kg per day, so for a normal 70 kg man that means about 70 mEq/day. A malnourished man would not put out this amount of H^+. He would put out around 30 mEq. When that 30 mEq is added to the 50 mEq load provided by Travasol, around 80 mEq requires to be excreted, and the difference between 80 mEq and the 70 mEq put out by a normal man is very slight. One would therefore not expect anybody with normal kidney function to develop metabolic acidosis with hyperalimentation. Other factors might come into the picture which may produce metabolic alkalosis: for example, if bicarbonate is lost, due to small bowel or pancreatic fistula, or for some other reason. The development of metabolic acidosis is completely independent of the chloride load. One could give twice or three times as much chloride and metabolic acidosis would still not occur.

* Synthamin.

26
Metabolic complications of parenteral nutrition

R. K. AUSMAN AND G. HARDY

INTRODUCTION

Nearly every therapy in medicine has a well-understood risk/benefit ratio after it has been in use for several years. Early experience, while a treatment or technique is being investigated, is designed to show that the benefits of therapy outweigh any disadvantages. During this period physicians learn to search for, recognize, evaluate, and manage adverse reactions and side effects. When this task is done well and the therapy has achieved its intended magnitude of efficacy, the risk/benefit ratio may be considered favourable. The treatment then becomes used more widely, providing secondary advantages: the appreciation of difficulties and their modulation or prevention.

It is clear now that great benefit can be obtained for suitable patients who receive amino acid solutions to support their nutritional needs or make up existing deficits. The fact that we have learned to deal with the complexities of this therapy is very encouraging; there are few clinical surprises mentioned in the literature any longer. The concensus of this symposium is that the risk/benefit ratio of parenteral nutrition is favourable and that the technique can be used effectively by the well-informed, attentive physician.

It is the purpose of this paper to describe some of the past encounters with clinical complications which are metabolic rather than mechanical or technical. Readers will understand that an exhaustive review is inappropriate. However, prominent, frequent, or spectacular difficulties are discussed and where possible, a description is provided, a cause identified, and corrective action (if one is needed) suggested.

METABOLIC ACIDOSIS

Two forms of metabolic acidosis related to parenteral nutrition have dominated the literature. Hyperchloraemic metabolic acidosis is the first, the cause for which is rather obvious in that it is associated invariably with the infusion of an amino acid solution with a high concentration of chloride. This type of acidosis is not different from any clinical condition associated with excess infusion or excess retention of chloride. The difficulty is overcome by diminishing the input of chloride as a definitive measure and by administering bicarbonate as a short-term expedient. Recently, acetic acid has been substituted by some manufacturers for hydrochloric acid as the acidifying medium during the preparation of crystalline amino acid solutions. Therefore, this form of acidosis should not occur in the future.

A second type of metabolic acidosis is more subtle in its manifestation and controversial as to its cause. Typically, the measurement of the cations (K and Na) and the anion (Cl) is normal in these patients. Likewise, the BUN is not elevated. The distorted parameter is CO_2 content which is low compared to normal values. Confirmation of acidosis comes from the determination of plasma pH and base excess, the former being below normal and the latter having a negative value.

Chan *et al.*[1] have stated that the genesis is an abnormally large intake of titratable acid (TA) in one particular crystalline amino acid mixture which has between 24 and 26 mEq/l of TA. He supports this contention by showing that reducing the infusion or giving a base such as bicarbonate corrects the base deficit.

An alternative cause has been suggested by Heird *et al.*[2,3] who say that the acidosis is induced by the delivery of solutions which have a cation gap, that is a dominance of amino acids which, when metabolized, produce excess H^+.

In previous work most investigators have not commented on the development of acidosis while administering a casein hydrolysate (Amigen). It is equally true that a 'gap analysis' of casein hydrolysates shows it to be weighted on the anion side. However, this evaluation presumes complete metabolism of the protein.

The formulation of the crystalline amino acid solution, Travasol*, results in a net anion gap. In addition, with one exception, the amino acids are buffered with acetate which, when metabolized, consumes H^+. Thus, no acid–base balance problems have been noted with the use of this solution.

Regardless of the correctness of the Chan or Heird hypothesis, it is clear that the clinical incidence of metabolic acidosis can be reduced with bicarbonate or its precursors.

Metabolic acidosis was not observed by Dale *et al.*[4] during post-operative feeding of newborn babies with a crystalline amino acid (Vamin), glucose, fat regime. Indeed, on four occasions a metabolic alkalosis was reported.

* Synthamin.

This clinical picture may be due to high concentrations of the bases glutamate and aspartate which are not balanced effectively by sufficiently high concentrations of arginine, to improve hydrogen ion homeostasis[4].

CHOLESTASIS AND JAUNDICE

Since the first report by Peden *et al.*[27] in 1971, several authors have described neonates in whom jaundice is observed shortly after parenteral nutrition is begun and it has recently been observed in adult patients (see Allardyce chapter 28). This finding persists throughout intravenous feeding and then abates rather rapidly. When long-term follow-up has been possible, there appears to be no permanent liver damage.

The cellular pathology associated with this problem is hepatocellular cholestasis with bile duct proliferation and eosinophilic periportal infiltration.

Several different theories have been advanced to explain the cause of this liver pathology. These include osmotic diuresis with dehydration, thrombosis of central and/or portal veins, nutritional imbalance with aminoacidaemia and fatty acid deficiency, copper deficiency, sepsis, an excessively burdened Krebs cycle due to hyperammonaemia[5,6] and failure to stimulate bile secretion because an oral intake of food is absent[8].

Some of these can be dismissed as not being the unique cause. For instance, absent oral intake was not part of the clinical picture in some of the reported patients[9]. Other authors have found no correlation[7] between the duration of parenteral nutrition or the peak elevation of ammonia with the highest bilirubin. No sepsis has been present in several patients[9]. Finally, autopsy studies frequently failed to demonstrate any vascular pathology of the type suggested by some.

Both hydrolysate[9,10] and crystalline[8] amino acid solutions have been used as a protein source in patients noted to have cholestasis. Intravenous fat has not been infused in all cases[8].

At this time no single cause has been established for the cholestasis of newborns receiving parenteral nutrition. Nearly all the patients seem to be premature or low-birth-weight infants, and all seem to demonstrate a relatively characteristic liver lesion. Until a specific aetiology is uncovered, the physician faced with this clinical side-effect of parenteral nutrition will have to balance the benefits of the therapy against the risk of the complication. The only way to overcome the problem is to discontinue the amino acid–glucose intravenous solution.

Two recently reported cases of jaundice have been related to acute folate deficiency[29]. Both patients were receiving broad-spectrum antibiotics along with the parenteral feeding regimen, thus preventing determination of serum folate levels. However, there was a rapid response to intravenous folate with a conversion to normal haemopoiesis and disappearance of the jaundice.

Poor oral intake of folate, increased folate demand by anabolic and catabolic processes, and interference with folate metabolism and erythropoiesis by sepsis are all factors which interfere with folate balance.

Ethanol is also known to impair folate balance and can act as a direct marrow toxin. In a prospective study of twenty-five surgical patients, Wardrop[11] and others found that intravenous nutrition with an amino acid/sorbitol/ethanol preparation correlated strongly with a fall in serum folate. Patients developed acute folate deficiency with pancytopenia and megaloblastic haemopoiesis after abdominal operations.

Folic acid treatment produced a response, and the authors drew attention to the risks of including ethanol in a feeding regimen for such patients.

AZOTAEMIA

Several reports by early users[12] of parenteral nutrition described a rapidly rising blood urea nitrogen. A retrospective analysis of clinical data by Ausman and Aust[13] has confirmed that this component in the blood is increased when insufficient non-protein calories are provided and the infused amino acid is used to meet immediate energy needs rather than stored for replenishing body protein. An animal study by Ausman and Meng[14] adds support to this concept.

It has been our experience that nearly every patient given parenteral nutrition has a disease which is accompanied by a hypercatabolic state. Non-protein calories at the level of at least 40 cal/kg body weight/day are enough in many instances to overcome the catabolism. In some patients the amounts required may be greater.

Monitoring the BUN indicates the adequacy of the caloric support being given to the patient. In this regard some advocate the advantages of glucose as the carbohydrate of choice (see Krebs, chapter 2; Woods, chapter 3). As the amount of glucose is increased, there is the possibility that exogenous insulin will be required to accomplish full utilization of the substrate. Urine glucose levels can be observed, as in the control of carbohydrate metabolism in diabetic patients. Insulin may be given subcutaneously or intravenously. If the latter method is chosen due to the certainty of absorption and availability, the insulin may be added to the parenteral fluid container. The anticipation of a large loss due to container surface absorption of insulin has been shown to be only a very minor issue by Nedich, chapter 27.

HYPOPHOSPHATAEMIA AND HYPOKALAEMIA

Several workers have observed and reported hypophosphataemia in association with parenteral nutrition. Many years ago Gröen[17] and associates provided a substantial insight into the likely cause by showing that marked redistribution of serum inorganic phosphate occurred during the metabolism of large quantities of glucose. Smaller amounts of glucose have a less marked, but similar effect[18].

An adequate understanding of the consequences of this derangement has been achieved recently with the elucidation of different clinical states. Travis *et al.*[19] described the depletion of red cell 2,3DPG with consequent increase in the affinity of haemoglobin for oxygen. An even more spectacular result follows severe hypophosphataemia when there is a depression of red cell ATP to 15% of normal levels[20]. The relation of red cell ATP to serum phosphate is quite good[21]. This condition results in red cell fragility and loss of biconcavity followed by acute haemolytic anaemia.

The continued administration of high level glucose without the addition of phosphate can have serious clinical consequences. Sheldon and Grzyb[22] have recommended a dose of 20 mEq of phosphate for each 1000 kcal infused. They recognized the specific relationship between glucose utilized and phosphate driven from the serum in defining the requirement. Others have employed greater quantities to be certain that any tendency to hypophosphataemia is covered completely.

The picture which emerges with this metabolic rearrangement is that specific attention must be given both to the utilization of phosphate and the exogenous supply required to prevent changes in the serum level.

More recently Guillou and Hill[23] in a study of post-surgical patients receiving simple dextrose–saline intravenous therapy have observed a degree of hypophosphataemia.

A dramatic lowering of the serum potassium level occurs during the infusion and metabolism of glucose usually with insulin. This treatment has been used to advantage for anuric or oliguric patients with life-threatening hyperkalaemia. Gröen *et al.*[17] have given insight into the dynamics of the changes in serum potassium accompanying the administration of glucose.

The treatment of this problem is the inclusion of sufficient potassium ion in the parenteral nutrition mixture to offset any loss into the cells. This flux may reach higher levels than would be considered safe under other circumstances. The physician should give potassium in relation to frequent serum measurements. The cardiac consequences of a failure to maintain the serum potassium within an acceptable range may be serious.

HYPERAMMONAEMIA

High levels of blood ammonia associated directly with the infusion of parenteral nutrition solution in infants were reported by Johnson and colleagues[24]. They observed this phenomenon when using either casein or fibrin hydrolysate and attributed the cause to the free ammonia content of these solutions. They recognized that the amount of NH_3 infused was quite small but wrote that along with other ammonia-producing reactions in the body the total might exceed the ability of an infant to produce urea. The same clinical condition was reported later in infants receiving a crystalline amino acid solution[25] having essentially no ammonia.

The cause of hyperammonaemia in association with parenteral nutrition remains uncertain.

Most authors have found, as reported initially by Fahey[26], that the use of therapeutic levels of arginine will suppress the further formation of ammonia and return the blood levels to within the normal range. However, success has not been uniform with this therapy.

If the level of blood ammonia continues to rise in spite of arginine therapy, the choice is to discontinue the amino acid infusion or risk the consequence of severe hyperammonaemia. The amino acid solution Travasol, which contains a substantial amount of arginine, has not been associated with hyperammonaemia in any clinical studies reported to date.

HYPEROSMOLALITY

Structural and functional neurological abnormalities develop during the rapid infusion of hypertonic glucose. An increase in serum osmolality precedes serious neurological problems and the possibility of hyperosmolar pre-coma must be remembered in a patient whose condition is deteriorating rapidly. Insulin is required in adequate doses when hyperosmolality has been demonstrated.

The first priority of the clinician is usually to reduce the hyperglycaemia to normal levels by administering insulin at whatever doses are necessary to accomplish the task quickly. The more correct treatment is to accomplish the same goal slowly.

During the increase of serum osmolality the cells of the central nervous system develop a protection against environmental hyperosmolality by producing sorbitol intracellularly in quantities sufficient to counteract the serum level. When a rapid reduction in serum osmolality follows insulin treatment, the intracellular osmolality is higher relative to the extracellular environments. Sorbitol moves slowly from the cell. Water is absorbed across the cell membrane, and clinical signs of brain edema become a real possibility. These signs may be misinterpreted as continuing evidence of high blood sugar levels, and even more insulin may be given.

The same sequence of events has been reported by Bischel and Barbour[28] during peritoneal dialysis. It is obviously better to avoid hyperosmolality during treatment, but if hyperglycaemia does develop, its management by insulin should continue over many hours to avoid swelling of cells in the central nervous system.

SUMMARY

In this paper several clinical conditions which deserve attention during parenteral nutrition are described. The complication can be prevented usually by appropriate attention to simple details including the selection of the solutions and additives used.

References

1. Chan, J. C. M., Asch, M. J., Lin, S. and Hays, D. M. (1972). Hyperalimentation with amino acid and casein hydrolysate solutions: mechanism of acidosis. *J. Am. Med. Assoc.*, **220**, 1700
2. Heird, W. C., Dell, R. B. and Grebin, B. (1971). Combined program and abstracts. Society for pediatric research, April, Atlantic City, N.J., 203
3. Heird, W. C., Dell, R. B. and Driscoll, J. M. (1972). Metabolic acidosis resulting from intravenous alimentation mixtures containing synthetic amino acids. *N. Engl. J. Med.*, **287**, 943
4. Dale, G. *et al.* (1976). Plasma amino acid changes in the post-surgical newborn during intravenous nutrition with a synthetic amino acid solution. *J. Paed. Surg.*, **11**, 17
5. Johnson, J. D., Albritton, W. L. and Sunshine, P. (1972). Hyperammonemia accompanying parenteral nutrition in new born infants. *J. Pediat.*, **81**, 154
6. Ghadimi, H., Abaci, F., Kumar, S. and Rathi, M. (1971). Biochemical aspects of intravenous alimentation. *Pediatrics.*, **48**, 955
7. Touloukian, R. J. and Seashore, J. H. (1975). Hepatic secretory obstruction with total parenteral nutrition in the infant. *J. Paed. Surg.*, **10**, 353
8. Rager, R. and Finegold, M. J. (1975). Cholestasis in immature newborn infants: Is parenteral alimentation responsible? *J. Pediat.*, **86**, 264
9. Rodgers, B. M., Hollenbeck, J. I., Donnelly, W. H. and Talbert, J. L. (1976). Intrahepatic cholestasis with parenteral alimentation. *Am. J. Surg.*, **131**, 149
10. Touloukian, R. J. and Downing, S. E. (1973). Cholestasis associated with long term parenteral hyperalimentation. *Arch. Surg.*, **106**, 58
11. Wardrop, C. A. J. *et al.* (1975). Acute folate deficiency in surgical patients on amino acid/ethanol intravenous nutrition., *Lancet*, **ii**, 640
12. Dudrick, S. J. *et al.* (1972). Parenteral hyperalimentation: metabolic problems and solutions. *Ann. Surg.*, 176, 259
13. Ausman, R. K., Aust, J. B. and Friend, J. E. (1976). Parenteral nutrition with a new amino acid solution. *Acta Surg. Scand.*, **466** (Suppl.), 32
14. Ausman, R. K. and Meng, H. C. (1976). The effect on nitrogen balance and other parameters of varying doses of intravenous protein and calories. *Acta Surg. Scand.*, **466** (Suppl.), 26
15. Hill, J. B. (1959). Adsorption of insulin to glass. *Proc. Soc. Exp. Biol. Med.*, **102**, 75
16. Weisenfeld, S. *et al.* (1968). Adsorption of insulin to infusion bottles and tubing. *Diabetes*, **17**, 766
17. Gröen, J., Willebrands, A. F., Kamminga, C. E., *et al.* (1952). Effects of glucose administration on the potassium and inorganic phosphate content of blood serum and the ECG in normal individuals and non-diabetic patients. *Acta Med. Scand.*, 141, 352
18. Hill, G. L., Gunn, E. J. and Dudrick, S. J. (1976). Phosphorus distribution in hyperalimentation induced hypophosphatemia. *J. Surg. Res.*, **20**, 527
19. Travis, S. F., Sugerman, H. J., Ruberg, R. L., *et al.* (1971). Alterations of red cell glycolytic intermediates and oxygen transport as a consequence of hypophosphatemia in patients receiving intravenous hyperalimentation. *N. Engl. J. Med.*, **285**, 763
20. Jacob, H. S. and Amsden, T. (1971). Acute hemolytic anemia with rigid red cells in hypophosphatemia. *N. Engl. J. Med.*, **285,** 1446
21. Lichtman, M. A., Miller, D. R. and Treeman, R. B. (1969). Erythrocyte ATP depletion during hypophosphatemia in a uremic subject. *N. Engl. J. Med.*, **280**, 240
22. Sheldon, G. F. and Grzyb, S. (1975). Phosphate depletion and repletion: relation to parenteral nutrition and oxygen transport. *Anal. Surg.*, **182,** 683
23. Guillou, P. J. *et al.* (1976). Hypophosphatemia: a complication of innocuous dextrose saline. *Lancet*, **ii**, 710
24. Johnson, J. D. *et al.* (1972). Hyperammonemia accompanying parenteral nutrition in newborn infants. *J. Pediat.*, **81**, 154

25. Heird, W. C. *et al.* (1972). Hyperammonemia resulting from intravenous alimentation using a mixture of synthetic L amino acids: a preliminary report. *J. Pediat.*, **81**, 162
26. Fahey, J. L. (1957). Toxicity and blood ammonia rise resulting from intravenous amino acid administration in man: The protective effect of L-arginine. *J. Clin. Invest.*, **36**, 1647
27. Peden, V. H., Witzleben, C. L. and Skelton, M. A. (1971). Total parenteral nutrition. *J. Pediat.*, **78**, 180
28. Bischel, M. D. and Barbour, B. H. (1973). Peritoneal dialysis with sorbitol versus dextrose dialysate. *Nephron*, **8**, 340
29. Green, P. J. (1977). Folate deficiency and intravenous nutrition. *Lancet*, **i**, 814

Discussion

A. W. Goode: (UK) We have developed a computer program to assist with intravenous feeding. Magnesium was one of the elements that we have looked at for serum levels, and it was surprising how often a patient, after two or three days on any regimen, developed hypomagnesaemia, with problems clinically similar to a potassium deficiency, such as muscular weakness. It was quickly corrected.

The other point to re-emphasize is that there is evidence that this particular syndrome is associated with the use of alcohol as a calorie source, as ethanol increases the renal loss of magnesium.

G. Hardy: (UK) When ethanol was used, was it necessary to add more magnesium?

Goode: In two or three patients, when we have specifically looked for it we have had to give magnesium supplements.

H. A. Krebs: (UK) It has been stated that Travasol* solution has not given rise to hyperammonaemia. This is because it contains arginine. The liver at all stages of life contain enough of the ammonia detoxicating enzymes of the urea cycle to deal with very large quantities of ammonia. Milk contains a fair amount of nitrogenous material. There are safeguards in milk, that prevent hyperammonaemia occurring. The safeguard depends on the presence of sufficient ornithine, which is supplied by the arginine in the Travasol formula.

There is a view, probably not very well-based, that arginine is not an essential amino acid. There can be no doubt that in the developing animal arginine cannot be synthesized from any other precursors. There may be enough synthesized in the adult under some conditions, but I doubt it, because the enzymes for the synthesis of arginine would probably be synthesized from glutamine by the reduction of the carboxyl group to the *semi-aldehyde* of glutamic acid, and then through transamination to ornithine, but these enzymes, if present at all, are very weak, so it would be essential to include arginine in parenteral nutrition, even though some may think that it is not an essential amino acid.

N. Zöllner: (Germany) Many do not recognize that when insulin is injected subcutaneously, that it takes from half an hour to an hour before the insulin reaches the circulation, because as a protein it has to travel quite a long way along the lymphatic pathway. That is the reason why insulin is taken before a meal, since the post-absorptive peak levels are only half an hour to an hour later. When one is in a hurry insulin will have to be given parenterally.

Secondly, it is very dangerous to give insulin subcutaneously in accidental hyperglycaemic states. One can never predict how long it will take for the bolus to disappear, whereas when an insulin infusion is turned off, insulin will disappear from the circulation within 5 minutes.

*Synthamin.

I have two further suggestions: many of the side effects that were described can be prevented by giving only half of the energy as carbohydrate, and the other half as fat; many of these complications are carbohydrate complications.

P. Vinay: (Canada) I would make a plea for the abandonment of the old nomenclature of base excess. In chronic respiratory disease, very acute acidosis can occur, with pH down below 7.0 with normal base excess as usually defined.

It is not the diminution of chloride in the Travasol solution that overcomes the acidosis problem, but the substitution of an inorganic anion chloride by an organic anion acetate that will generate bicarbonate.

The alkalosis problem occurs with solutions high in glutamate and aspartate. Metabolic alkalosis cannot be generated by giving bicarbonate, even where the bicarbonate is given in the form of an organic acid; it needs something else. The bicarbonate threshold level needs to be raised in some way. That can be achieved by contraction of extracellular fluid, or of chloride deficiency.

During the course of hyperalimentation with high quantities of glucose we have observed some hypokalaemia. It is easy to give potassium to correct the situation. However, when the hyperalimentation stops and the glucose drops, the shift of potassium from the extracellular fluid to the intracellular fluid will be reversed, and severe hyperkalaemia can occur after cessation of TPN.

Finally, a comment on ammonia levels. When a solution of Travasol is given into the systemic circulation, bypassing the liver, it provides an ammonia and an amino acid load, especially to the kidneys that are known to use some of these amino acids to produce ammonia. There have been no appropriate studies on the effect of the amino acid load on renal ammonia production. This might be of importance in metabolic alkalosis. In that situation the very important renal blood flow will drive more than 80% of the ammonia into the systemic circulation, and if for some reason the liver is not able to cope with the increase in ammonia production, hyperammonaemia might appear. This would be unlikely to be a problem in adults, but it could be a problem in infants.

G. L. Blackburn: (USA) I would hate the generation of urea to become a criterion of efficacy, because I hear about rising BUN as an indicator to cut down the protein intake. Often that only allows one to obtain nitrogen balance in people that were previously depleted, whereas really the efficacy of response would be one in which as much as 50 or 70 g of new protein would be generated beyond breakdown—in other words a positive 5–7 g nitrogen balance.

There are two ways to improve nitrogen balance: calories and nitrogen; but on a practical basis, and on a gram for gram basis, nitrogen intake in the form of amino acids is superior to raising the energy level. I am not aware of any toxicity until BUN levels get quite high. If a new high set point of BUN would allow the generation of plus-five or plus-seven g nitrogen/day, then I believe that would be the criterion of efficacy.

R. K. Ausman: (USA) That comment is entirely correct. Our paper referred to the adult incidence of azotaemia. In children, and in any patient with a heightened creatinine one needs to look for an organic cause rather than an iatrogenic cause.

I am sure that Dr Blackburn is aware of a paper that appeared in a Mayo Clinic Proceedings several years ago which could never be done again because of the manner of the experiment and the moral atmosphere in which we work today. On an artificial basis, the urea levels of patients undergoing dialysis were raised by including urea in the dialysate solution. Thereafter, on the following day, the study of the clotting mechanisms was performed and it was ascertained that platelet function and related parameters were abnormal in these patients. The blood urea levels that were achieved by these techniques were 100 mg%, and there would be a question in my mind, and I am sure in Dr Blackburn's, as to whether a level of 50 mg% is associated with a real but proportionately lower incidence of problems. All of us have worked with patients having BUNs of 100 mg%, and we have little reason for concern, particularly if the creatinine is near normal. It then becomes a choice of what one believes in terms of energy source. If one believes that carbohydrate is an important source of energy for the parenteral nutrition regimen that one is using, then we recommend, and believe, that the reduction of BUN should be accomplished because it is an indicator to the physician that he may be under-prescribing energy in the form of carbohydrate. If one prefers the non-carbohydrate approach, then the BUN can be expected to rise, and Dr Blackburn's explanation of its value and benefit is certainly meritorious and meets the needs of the patient.

Vinay: I agree with Dr Ausman. Urea *per se* is a non-toxic substance. It is not urea that makes one sick, even where there is renal insufficiency, so I do not see why a slightly higher BUN would be of any consequence.

27
The compatibility of extemporaneously added drug additives with Travasol* (amino acid) injection

R. L. NEDICH

COMPATIBILITY WITH DEXTROSE AS THE CARBOHYDRATE SOURCE

In North America one of the commonly used parenteral nutrition base solutions is the mixture of 500 ml of 5.5 or 8.5% Travasol* with 500 ml of 50% Dextrose Injection thus providing 1000 ml of a 2.75 or 4.25% amino acid solution in 25% dextrose. In general, pharmaceutical practices are such that storage prior to administration of the prepared base solution is controlled and limited. Accordingly, short-term stability of extemporaneously mixed parenteral nutrition solutions was considered to be a requirement. Data derived in these studies are shown in Tables 27.1 and 27.2 for a mixture composed of 2.75% Travasol and 25% Dextrose Injection stored in Viaflex parenteral containers. It is clear that within the analytical error associated with the gravimetric procedure utilized, dextrose concentration remains essentially constant, as do all electrolyte concentrations. These data suggest that the carbohydrate is stable and compatible in the prepared formulation over the time course evaluated. Similar data are available for a 4.25% amino acid solution in 25% dextrose.

Relative to the amino acid values derived in these studies, it should be mentioned that amino acid analysis by automated chromatographic equipment has a ±10% analytical variability. With this analytical constraint in mind, all the amino acid values remain within an acceptable range for the mixture stored up to 7 days at room temperature, or 30 days at 4–5 °C.

* Synthamin.

Table 27.1 2.75% Travasol and 25% dextrose injection, lot 2545-10, stability study No. 1470, laboratory scale study (room temperature storage)

Analysis	*Percentage of initial*	
	1 *Day*	7 *Days*
Sodium	102.8	102.8
Potassium phosphate, dibasic	100.0	104.0
Magnesium	100.0	100.0
Chloride	100.0	105.0
Alpha-amino nitrogen	97.3	100.0
Dextrose	101.2	100.8
pH	100.0	100.0
Lysine	98.0	92.7
Histidine	98.4	106.3
Arginine	100.4	101.0
Tryptophan	91.7	89.6
Threonine	103.7	100.0
Proline	101.8	102.6
Aminoacetic acid	100.7	98.2
Alanine	98.9	96.8
Valine	102.4	101.6
Methionine	102.7	98.6
Isoleucine	101.5	100.8
Leucine	100.0	101.7
Tyrosine	109.0	109.0
Phenylalanine	101.9	100.0

This study was performed to demonstrate short-term stability of the extemporaneously prepared amino acid and carbohydrate mixture stored in plastic parenteral containers stored at room temperature

Table 27.2 2.75% Travasol and 25% dextrose injection, lot 2545-10, stability study No. 1470, laboratory scale study (refrigerated storage)

Analysis	*Percentage of initial*		
	1 Day	*7 Days*	*30 Days*
Sodium	102.8	102.8	105.6
Potassium phosphate, dibasic	100.0	104.0	104.0
Magnesium	100.0	100.0	100.0
Chloride	105.0	105.0	100.0
Alpha-amino nitrogen	100.0	100.0	100.0
Dextrose	100.0	102.4	100.8
pH	100.0	100.0	101.7
Lysine	100.0	98.0	102.7
Histidine	100.0	110.3	103.2
Arginine	98.9	104.6	100.7
Tryptophan	97.9	89.6	106.2
Threonine	104.6	104.6	103.7
Proline	107.1	106.2	98.2
Aminoacetic acid	101.1	102.6	101.4
Alanine	99.1	103.5	101.4
Valine	106.4	105.6	104.0
Methionine	102.0	103.4	104.1
Isoleucine	101.5	103.8	102.2
Leucine	101.7	105.2	101.2
Tyrosine	109.1	109.1	109.1
Phenylalanine	101.9	105.6	104.4

This study was performed to demonstrate short-term stability of the extemporaneously prepared amino acid and carbohydrate mixture stored in plastic parenteral containers stored under refrigerated (5 °C) conditions

CONTAINER COMPATIBILITY

Flexible plastic containers, are used frequently for the administration of parenteral nutrition products. These containers provide a number of advantages such as reduced weight and bulk storage, and relative freedom from breakage as a result of careless handling or exposure to freezing. For parenteral nutrition mixtures the more positive advantage is related to the fact that the plastic container is a collapsible, non-air-dependent system.

In the presence of aqueous solutions the principal plasticizer di-(2-ethylhexyl) phthalate (DEHP), used in the plastic formulation has been shown to extract at a level of less than 0.05 ppm at room temperature throughout the product's expiration dating. Blood, however, being lipoidal in character has been shown to accumulate DEHP from PVC containers to the extent of approximately 0.25 mg/100 ml/day when stored at 4 °C[1]. In 1972 Rubin[2] reported that DEHP levels in aqueous protein hydrolysate injections stored for more than 1 year under a wide range of ambient temperatures contained DEHP levels not greater than his analytical blank.

DEHP concentrations were determined during the short-term storage evaluations previously described for Travasol–dextrose parenteral nutrition admixtures compounded in litre parenteral containers. DEHP values were obtained by organic solvent extraction and quantitated by vapour phase chromatography. All values obtained (Table 27.3) were found to be consistent with those normally obtained, i.e. less than 0.05 ppm, for simple aqueous solutions stored in these containers.

Table 27.3 DEHP concentration (ppm) in Travasol–dextrose parenteral nutrition mixtures store in plastic parenteral containers

A. 2.75% Travasol (amino acid) injection and 25% dextrose

Room temperature storage			*5 °C storage*			
Initial	*1 Day*	*7 Days*	*Initial*	*1 Day*	*7 Days*	*30 Days*
0.02	0.01	0.01	0.02	0.01	0.02	0.01

B. 4.25% Travasol (amino acid) injection and 25% dextrose

Room temperature storage			*5 °C storage*			
Initial	*1 Day*	*7 Days*	*Initial*	*1 Day*	*7 Days*	*30 Days*
0.01	0.02	0.01	0.01	0.03	0.02	0.02

COMPATIBILITY OF CALCIUM SALTS

In most marketing areas, Travasol is currently available as 5.5 and 8.5% amino acid solutions with and without electrolytes. Solutions with electrolytes present a fixed electrolyte profile found to be acceptable in a majority of clinical applications. No one single electrolyte formula, however, will provide adequate electrolyte supplementation for every patient. Formulations without electrolyte are now available so that the electrolyte profile may be tailored to the requirements of a particular patient. Calcium additives are extremely important, as dictated by a patient's metabolic requirements and electrolyte concentrations in blood.

While calcium phosphate precipitation in parenteral nutrition products have been reported[3,4], more information was required as a white precipitate had been reported on a number of occasions in extemporaneously prepared parenteral nutrition solutions and this required to be identified.

Travasol (amino acid) Injection with electrolytes provides a fairly complete electrolyte profile, thus reducing the manipulations required for preparation of the parenteral nutrition mixture. This is important since multiple-container entry provides an increased opportunity for microbiological contamination. Because of possible calcium phosphate formation during sterilization and storage, Travasol products do not contain calcium ions, so that a suitable calcium salt must be added when required. The onset and extent of any precipitation could be influenced both by concentration (ionic ratio as well as amount) and admixture pH.

In order to evaluate the effect of pH on calcium phosphate precipitation, parenteral nutrition solutions were prepared by mixing 5.5% Travasol with electrolytes (containing 60 mEq HPO_4^{2-}/l) and 50% dextrose in a 1:1 ratio. The resulting mixture provided a composition of 2.75% amino acids in 25% dextrose and contained 30 mEq/l (15 mmoles/l) phosphate as the divalent salt. Calcium salts chloride and gluconate were added and the mixtures were agitated. Admixture pHs were serially adjusted with sodium hydroxide and the samples were allowed to stand undisturbed at room temperature for 24 h. The samples were inspected visually and with the aid of a HACH turbidimeter for evidence of precipitate in order to determine the 24 h precipitation pH. The data from this study are in Figure 27.1. In the event of purposeful

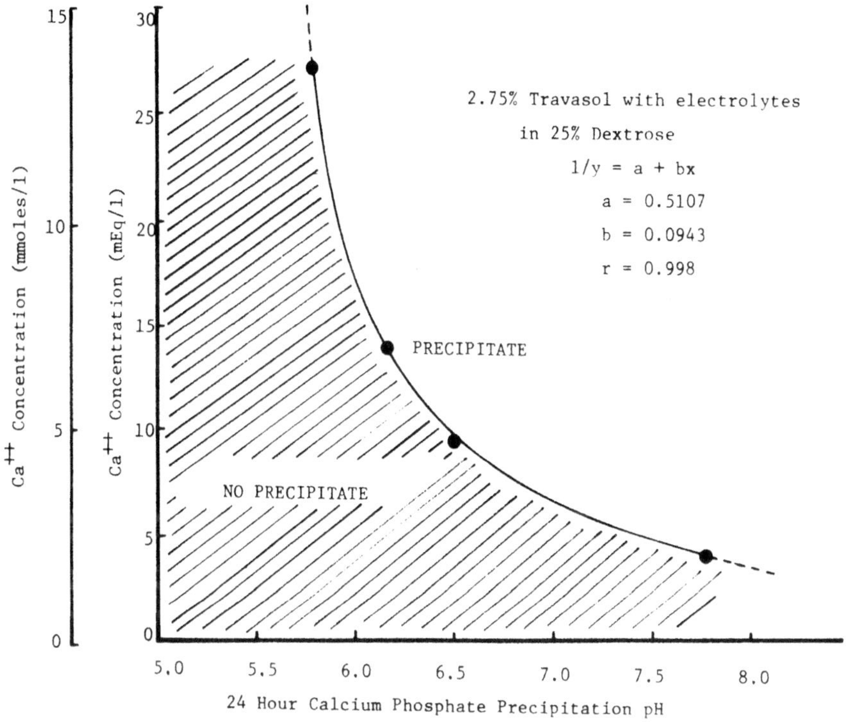

Figure 27.1 Calcium ion concentration in an extemporaneously prepared TPN solution as a function of admixture pH for calcium phosphate precipitation at 24 h. At any point below the curve no precipitate will be encountered for a mixture of the composition evaluated

pH adjustment or the addition of drug additives capable of overcoming the mixture's buffer capacity, calcium phosphate precipitation would not be expected to occur after 24 h if the extrapolated calcium-pH point lies below the curve (shaded area). Caution must be observed, however, since all intravenous products have allowable pH tolerances. Hence, pH adjustment to a borderline point on this curve may result in calcium phosphate precipitation.

It is difficult to modify the pH of the solution when the buffer capacity associated with amino acid–dextrose mixtures is considered. This being the case, it became important to evaluate concentration, i.e. ionic ratio, effects associated with phosphate and added calcium ions. Travasol solutions containing a fixed amount of phosphate (60 mEq or 30 mmoles/l calculated as the divalent species) were used in these evaluations. An assortment of admixtures was prepared using 5.5 and 8.5% Travasol without electrolytes with varying amounts of added calcium and phosphate. These admixtures

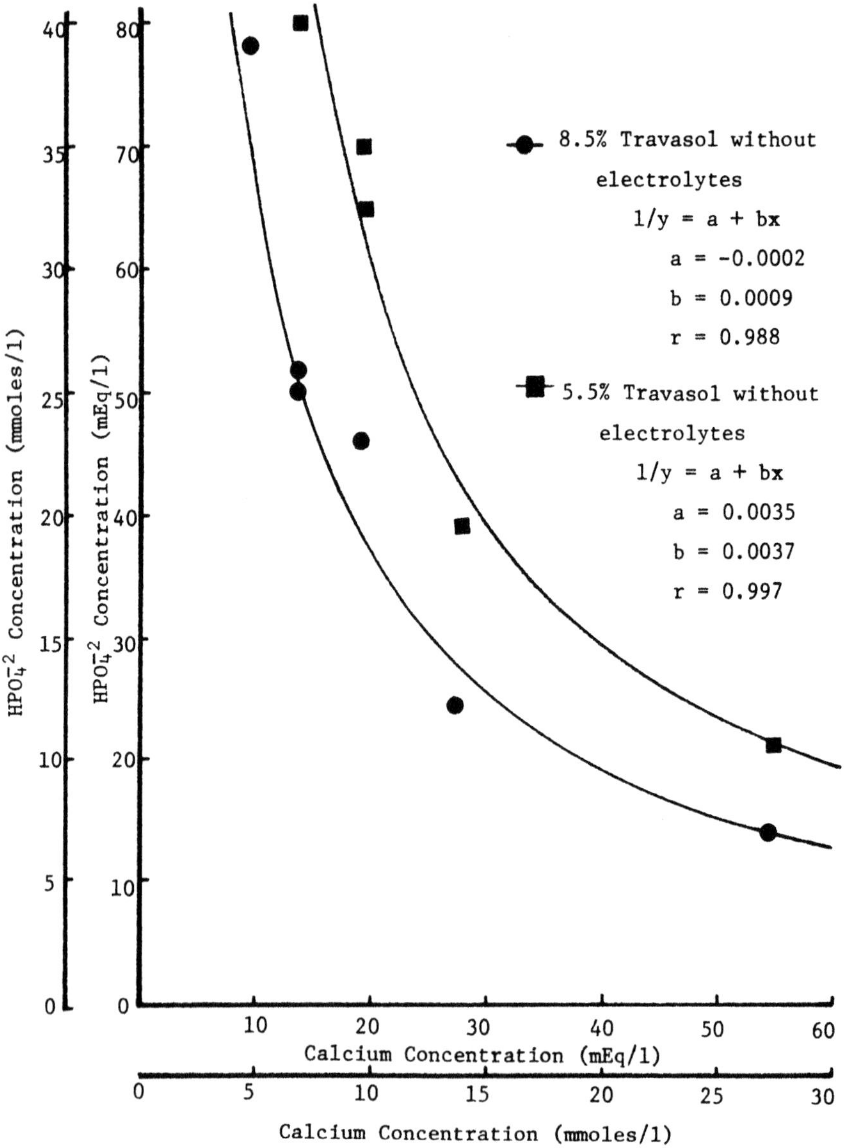

Figure 27.2 Phosphate ion concentration as a function of calcium ion concentration for calcium phosphate precipitation in undiluted Travasol for 24 h. At any point below the curves no precipitation will be encountered for products of the composition evaluated

were inspected visually before and after 24 h storage at room temperature in order to identify the calcium: phosphate ratio which caused gross precipitation. Once these concentrations and ratios were known, the technique was refined by the use of a HACH turbidimeter so that the exact concentrations could be determined. Data from these evaluations are detailed by the hyperbolic functions in Figures 27.2 and 27.3. Calcium phosphate precipitation would not be expected to occur during a 24 h storage-administration

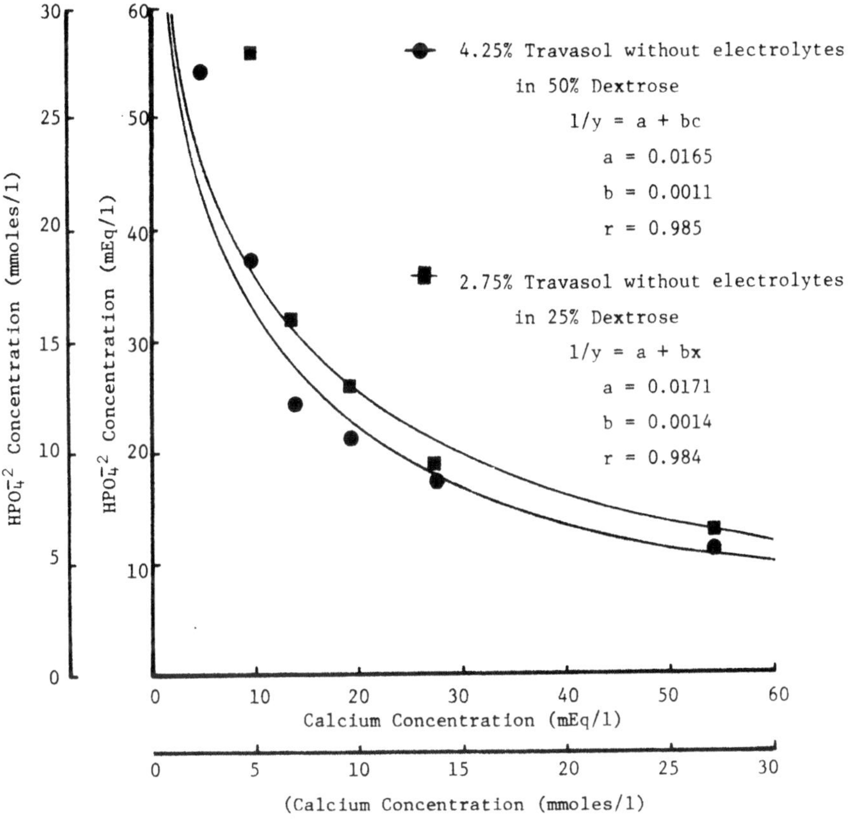

Figure 27.3 Phosphate concentration as a function of calcium concentration for calcium phosphate precipitation in parenteral nutrition mixtures at 24 h

period if the extrapolated calcium to phosphate concentration point lies below the curves. Admixtures with calcium:phosphate ratio at the borderline point on the curve may result in calcium phosphate precipitation. Such precipitation will be effected by admixture pH and particulate matter acting as nuclei for precipitation.

A summary of available calcium compatibility data is shown in Table 27.4. The calcium concentrations listed represent the maximum concentration evaluated and found to be both chemically and physically compatible.

Table 27.4 Maximum added calcium ion concentration evaluated and found to be chemically and physically compatible

Product of admixture	*pH*	*Conc.* HPO_4^{2-} (mEq/l)	*Conc.* Ca^{2+} (mEq/l)
3.5% Travasol M with electrolyte 45	5.8	15	80
5.5% Travasol with electrolytes	5.9	60	20
10% Travasol with electrolytes	6.0	60	29
2.75% Travasol with electrolytes and 25% dextrose	5.8	30	23
8.5% Travasol with electrolytes	5.9	60	26
4.25% Travasol with electrolytes and 25% dextrose	5.8	30	29
50% dextrose	4.0	0	80

INSULIN COMPATIBILITY

In order to fully use intravenous glucose it has become a common practice to add exogenous insulin directly to the parenteral nutrition solutions. This is thought to offer a high level of control of the insulin:carbohydrate ratio because the rate of insulin infusion is decreased or increased with changes in administration rate.

The potential for insulin adsorption to parenteral administration equipment has been described[5–7]. In a study at Eli Lilly and Company[8] insulin losses measured by radioimmunoassay were reported to be between 10 and 20% for 20–40 units of regular insulin added to plastic and glass containers with attached administration tubing. Insulin loss associated with adsorption was independent of container (glass or plastic) and parenteral solution (simple carbohydrates, electrolytes or their combinations). In 1974, Petty and Cunningham[9] reported a 55% adsorption of insulin by glass and plastic containers within 15 s of addition of the insulin. They reported that the PVC administration sets adsorbed an additional 50% of the insulin remaining in the intravenous fluid.

Peterson *et al.*[10] in 1976, reported that solutions containing 25 units of regular insulin in 500 ml of normal saline in plastic Viaflex containers provided delivery of 75% of the insulin for the first 50 ml of the infusion through the administration set and 100% thereafter if a 50 ml set 'washout' volume were utilized.

Because of the conflicting data on insulin adsorption reported in the literature, studies were designed to measure insulin loss to administration equipment in Travasol–dextrose mixtures. Preliminary data suggest that 80–90% of the added insulin is available for solutions stored at either 5 or 22 °C for 24 h.

Simulated infusion through administration sets using flow rates of 100 ml/h was included in the experimental design. These data are in accord with those accumulated for simple parenteral solutions by workers at Eli Lilly and Company.

In April 1977, Weber *et al.*[11] published a report entitled 'Availability of Insulin from Parenteral Nutrition Solutions'. These authors reported that amino acid solutions and protein hydrolysates combined with dextrose and 30 units of insulin 'failed to deliver approximately 44 to 47 percent of the added insulin'. They further state that 'the use of inline filters and PVC bags caused an even greater loss of insulin'.

The literature appears to provide a most confusing and contradictory situation. Unpublished data available through Eli Lilly and Company and the preliminary results generated at Baxter Travenol Laboratories appear to provide the only consistent data currently available. It would appear that in the clinical situation when insulin is added directly to nutrient solutions blood glucose levels appear to be controlled effectively.

SUMMARY AND RECOMMENDATIONS

Parenteral nutrition products presents a most complex situation, containing essential and non-essential amino acids, carbohydrates, electrolytes, oil- and water-soluble vitamins and insulin. Considering this complexity, the addition of drugs or electrolytes should be approached with caution. Where possible, additives should be instilled only to carbohydrate diluted amino acid solutions or to the carbohydrate itself. Thorough mixing between additions is recommended.

Specific recommendations include:

1. Phosphate salts should be added prior to the instillation of calcium salts. Thorough mixing should precede the addition of calcium.
2. Avoid purposeful pH adjustment to the physiological range when both calcium and phosphate ions are present.
3. Considering the labile nature of parenteral vitamin mixtures, parenteral nutrition solutions containing these products should not be stored prior to use.
4. Since a major cause of loss of insulin appears to be associated with administration tubing, the shortest length of tubing should be used.

References

1. Valeri, C. *et al.* (1973). Accumulation of di-2-ethylhexyl phthalate (DEHP) in whole blood, platelet concentrates and platelet poor plasma. 1. Effect of DEHP on platelet survival and function. *Environ. Health Persp.*, **3**, 103
2. Rubin, R. (1972). Storage of aqueous solutions for parenteral infusion. *Lancet*, **i**, 965
3. Hull, R. (1974). Physicochemical considerations in intravenous hyperalimentation. *Am. J. Hosp. Pharm.*, **31**, 236

4. Kaminski, M. *et al.* (1974). Electrolyte compatibility in a synthetic amino acid hyperalimentation solution. *Am. J. Hosp. Pharm.*, **31**, 244
5. Weisenfeld, D. *et al.* (1968). Adsorption of insulin to infusion bottles and tubing. *Diabetes*, **17**, 766
6. Hill, J. (1959). The adsorption of I^{131}-insulin to glass. *Endocrinology*, **65**, 515
7. Wiseman, R. and Baltz, B. (1961). Prevention of insulin-I^{131} adsorption to glass. *Endocrinology*, **68**, 354
8. Inman, G., Department Head, Insulin Testing, Eli Lilly and Company, Indianapolis, Indiana. (June 1972). Personal communication
9. Petty, C. and Cunningham, N. (1974). Insulin adsorption by glass infusion bottles, polyvinylchloride infusion containers and intravenous tubing. *Anaesthesiology*, **40**, 400
10. Peterson, L. (1976). Insulin adsorbance to polyvinylchloride surfaces with implications for constant-infusion therapy. *Diabetes*, **25**, 72
11. Weber, S. *et al.* (1977). Availability of insulin from parenteral nutrient solutions. *Am. J. Hosp. Pharm.*, **34**, 353

Discussion

N. Zöllner: (Germany) The best medical practice is surely not to add any additives to complex solutions such as mixtures of amino acids. I wonder whether some such warning should be issued. I cannot think of any metabolic situation where the patient should get calcium and amino acids at the same time.

I should like to draw attention to another point. Metals and highly oxidizable substances added to a large volume end up in very small concentrations and are liable to considerable oxidation. The wisest approach is not to add substances, but to give them when necessary, or when changing bottles.

R. L. Nedich: (USA) I have to agree totally. Trace elements are very subject to redox reactions. When one considers the complexity of these solutions, although we may be able to measure trace elements chemically, we really do not know what the biological availability of these trace metals is.

P. Vinay: (Canada) I was interested in the solubility problem with calcium phosphate. We have devised a protocol in which we match two different situations with the same electrolytes. We add calcium to one solution and phosphate to the other. This was done because of the possibility of precipitation. Nevertheless, it could happen that, in trying to devise special electrolyte intakes, calcium and phosphate could be added to the same bottle, and this is potentially dangerous.

I suggest that a danger notice be placed on the product so that both calcium and phosphate cannot be added to any of these bottles.

A. Goode: (UK) I should like to comment about the use of insulin as an additive. Wright, in Newcastle[1], has had patients where an insulin and glucose mixture has been given, cerebral edema developed and the patients became very ill. They were particularly malnourished patients where an anabolic substance seemed to be indicated. Wright suggests that perhaps these patients lose the intracellular ability to phosphorylate glucose as an energy source. He found the intracellular glucose content of the patients' red cells was enormous, and perhaps similar problems may be occurring in other cells as suggested by Frayn[2].

R. K. Ausman: (USA) We gave an explanation in the paper given by Dr Hardy[3] that seemed to explain the clinical phenomenon that Mr Goode has described. The same phenomenon has been reported in several instances in peritoneal dialysis centres.

Mixtures are certainly not without risk. As Dr Zöllner said, when they are put in complex solutions, the risks are incremental with the complexity of the solution. In addition each admixture carries with it its own risk of bacterial contamination, without any reassurance that whatever is put in will somehow stop any organisms multiplying.

References

1. Wright, P. D. Personal communication
2. Frayn, K. N. (1977). Endocrinology, **101,** 312
3. Ausman, R. K. and Hardy, G. (1978). *Advances in Parenteral Nutrition*, chapter 26 (Lancaster: MTP Press Limited)

Section IX
Clinical Aspects of Parenteral Nutrition

28
Clinical experience of total parenteral nutrition

D. B. ALLARDYCE

Intravenous feeding in the Vancouver General Hospital began in paediatric and adult Intensive Care Units, between 1967 and 1973, but evolved into a full programme by 1974. At present, from twenty to twenty-five patients daily require such special support. The programme has a paediatric, medical, and surgical component.

Table 28.1 100 cases intravenous feeding—VGH, 1975–1977

Enterocutaneous fistulae	
Small bowel fistulae	20
Oesophagocutaneous	2
Gastrocutaneous	4
Gastrojejunal anastomosis	1
Duodenal stump	5
Colocutaneous	2
Pancreatitis	
Acute oedematous pancreatitis	4
Pancreatic necrosis, abscess	9
Peritonitis, ileus or mechanical obstruction	16
Crohn's disease	9
Ulcerative colitis	3
Oesophageal carcinoma	1
Oesophageal stricture	1
Gastric retention after gastrectomy or vagotomy and drainage procedure	4
Intra-abdominal abscesses	10
Biliary fistula	3
Gastrocolic fistula (gastric ulcer)	1
Obstructed afferent loop after gastrectomy	1
Metastatic Zollinger–Ellison tumour	1

The 100 cases reported here were managed on the adult medical or surgical wards of the Vancouver General Hospital during the period 1975–77. The VGH has over 1200 acute beds. The TPN programme supports about ten adult and ten paediatric cases daily. Cases referred as possible candidates for TPN are screened carefully before instituting intravenous feeding.

Table 28.1 shows the primary illnesses or complication leading to the initiation of TPN in most of the 100 cases. Enterocutaneous fistulae were the commonest problem, followed by selected cases of pancreatitis and Crohn's disease.

ENTERAL NUTRITIONAL SUPPORT

Elemental diets and blended food preparations, taken orally by the patient, or administered continuously after intubation of the gastrointestinal tract (nasogastric or jejunal) have been a safe and very effective means of nutritional support. They have been used alone or in combination with intravenous feeding. If a significant portion of functional small bowel remains, and there is access to it, then enteral feeding should be the method of support. The use of the gastrointestinal tract is often dependent on the anticipation by the surgeon of the need for prolonged nutritional support, and the provision of access by the insertion of a jejunostomy feeding tube at the time of operation.

During the past two years, an extended period of enteral feeding with elemental diet was undertaken eight times. In these patients, this was the major form of nutritional support. This technique was used in combination with intravenous feeding in ten other patients. From the nutritional standpoint alone, an elemental diet (Table 28.2) administered slowly and continuously via the gastric or jejunal route was a highly successful means of

Table 28.2 Elemental diet composition

	g/1000 kcal		*Caloric contribution/1000 cal*	
Protein equivalent	24.07		96	
Protein hydrolysate powder		22.94		92
Added amino acids		1.13		4
Fat	34.29		304	
Soya bean oil (lightly hydrogenated)		26.63		240
MCT, 75% C_8 25% C_{10}		6.66		55
Lecithin		1.00		9
Carbohydrate	149.93		600	
Corn syrup solids		63.20		253
Sucrose		77.34		309
Tapioca starch		9.39		38
TOTAL	233		1000	

support[1]. In earlier studies this method was a much more effective means of support than intravenous feeding using a combination of a 5% protein hydrolysate, fructose, and Intralipid 10% (Table 28.3).

Table 28.3 Calorie and nitrogen intakes in ten patients receiving elemental diets

	Nasogastric feeding tube				*Jejunostomy*			
Patient	*Cal./day*	*g N/day*	*g N bal./day*	*Treatment period* (days)	*Cal./day*	*g N/day*	*g N bal. day*	*Treatment period* (days)
1	4066	12.4	+5.4	34	2660	9.8	+3.5	20
2	2680	9.7	+3.9	43	6500	20.0	+9.6	27
3	3962	16.7	+9.9	19	6000	21.0	+8.2	23
4	3800	16.0	+6.0	40	3320	10.8	+5.2	19
5					3255	11.6	+7.4	31
6					4371	18.8	+10.3	21
Av.	3627	13.7	+6.3	34	6351	15.3	+7.4	24
SD	±640		±2.5		±1578		±2.6	

SD, standard deviation

PERIPHERAL INTRAVENOUS FEEDING

The peripheral route was employed in 60 of the 100 cases reported. In 49, it was the sole means of nutritional support.

In our earlier experience, the peripheral route proved a safe and perhaps ideal means of sustaining a starving, but non-septic individual for periods up to 30 days. It was not possible, however, to show nitrogen gains; if the patient was septic the method did not provide for sufficient calorie and nitrogen intake, and the nutritional state deteriorated. (See data in Group 1, Table 28.5 compared with enteral support with an elemental diet in Table 28.3.)

The technique requires the simultaneous infusion of Intralipid, an amino acid solution and glucose via a butterfly needle into the peripheral veins of the upper extremity. Frequent (daily) changes in the infusion site are required. Nonetheless, this method was well tolerated by most patients. There were no instances of septicaemia, and no complications of catheter placement.

The failure to consistently induce positive nitrogen balance and weight gain in depleted patients using this system results from the limited amino acid intake provided by amino acid hydrolysates, and the separation of the calorie source (Intralipid) from the amino acid solution (doubling the volume for a given number of calories and grams of nitrogen given).

In 1975, the combination of a 10% amino acid solution (Travasol*) and 50% dextrose (Table 28.4), in combination with 10% Intralipid, was tried by the peripheral route[2]. In view of the considerable increase in the osmolality

* Synthamin.

Table 28.4 Composition of peripheral TPN solutions, using Travasol

	Protein/l	*cal./l*
Travasol 700 ml	70 g	350
50% dextrose 300 ml	—	600
	70 g	950
Intralipid (10%)		
Soya bean oil	—	900
Lecithin	—	200
TOTAL	70 g	2050 cal/2 l

of this preparation, an increase in problems with painful infusions, or very frequent changes of infusion sites, was anticipated.

The nitrogen balances of six patients receiving the mixture of 10% Travasol, 50% dextrose, and Intralipid were compared with data previously collected on patients receiving Amigen 800 and Intralipid (Table 28.5). Not only was

Table 28.5 Nitrogen and calorie intake with peripheral TPN

	GROUP 1 *Amigen* 800 *Intralipid* 10%				GROUP 2 *Travasol/dextrose* *Intralipid* 10%			
Patient	*Cal./ day*	N_2 *in per day*	$+N_2$ *bal./ day*	*Treatment period* (days)	*Cal./ day*	N_2 *in per day*	$+N_2$ *bal./ day*	*Treatment period* (days)
1	3210	10.2	+2.9	20	3128	19.7	+7.8	28
2	2244	7.2	−1.4	13	2563	17.2	+6.2	85
3	2677	9.5	+2.0	28	2761	19.2	+10.9	30
4	2754	8.4	−0.7	16	2476	16.1	−0.7	34
5	2510	7.3	+0.6	21	2489	16.9	+7.8	62
6	2336	8.0	+2.1	16	2870	17.2	+7.8	44
Av.	2622	8.5	+0.9	19	2714	17.7	+6.6	47
SD	±347		±1.7		±255		±3.9	

The difference in nitrogen balance/day between Group 1 and Group 2 is significant, $P < 0.005$

SD, standard deviation

the more concentrated mixture tolerated reasonably well, but modest nitrogen gains were demonstrated, even after moderate trauma or sepsis.

The peripheral technique remains our method of choice where the course of TPN is anticipated to be short (2–3 weeks) and metabolic requirements of the patients are not great.

CENTRAL VENOUS FEEDING

Placement of central catheters has been used when the gastrointestinal route was impossible or inadvisable, peripheral veins were unavailable, and when the period of intravenous support was anticipated to be prolonged. Access to the central veins was obtained by use of the Broviac catheter in thirty-nine patients and by subclavian and internal jugular percutaneous puncture with a Centrasil kit in eleven patients. The Broviac catheter was originally designed for home parenteral feeding and not for hospital use. The ease with which the line could be maintained for extended periods led to its use in patients in hospital where extended periods of support were anticipated. This line must be inserted in the operating room, usually under local anaesthesia. The catheter is fitted with a Dacron cuff which becomes anchored by fibrous tissue growth in the subcutaneous tunnel.

Using the central route, 3.5–4.0 l of TPN solution could be given daily. In thirty-two patients on prolonged TPN, on whom nitrogen balance studies were carried out, a mean of 2600 calories and 18.4 g of nitrogen was provided daily over an average period of 57 days.

The outstanding feature of the Broviac catheter was its long life and patient-acceptance. However, when used in a hospital environment for prolonged periods, an increased rate of catheter sepsis was encountered. For this reason, we now restrict its use to individuals in whom an extended period of TPN is required. When central venous feeding is necessary, and the predicted period of treatment is less than 30 days, we have employed recently a Centrasil Catheter via the internal jugular vein. One patient requiring TPN in hospital for 5 months received TPN through an arteriovenous shunt (PTFE graft) in the arm.

ENTEROCUTANEOUS FISTULAE

Fistulae from the gastrointestinal tract (usually post-operative complications) were the indication for instituting TPN in 35 individuals.

Tables 28.6–28.8 show that anastomotic leaks and peritonitis were the major factors leading to mortality and serious morbidity after resection and anastomosis at all levels of the gastrointestinal tract (1970–1973—VGH).

TPN played a major role in the support of these individuals. Operative

Table 28.6 1970–1973, *Gastrectomy for peptic ulcer*

136 Cases—no deaths
2 duodenal stump leaks
Revision gastrectomy
27 Cases
4 Deaths:
—2 Due to duodenal stump leak
—2 Due to gastrojejunal anastomosis leak
10 Major complications in 23 survivors:
—2 Leaks from stump
—2 From gastrojejunal anastomosis

Table 28.7 1970–1973, Oesophageal

resection for carcinoma—25
8 Deaths (32% mortality rate)
All 8 due to anastomatic leak
3 Major complications but survived
1/3 Leak
9 Anastomatic leaks, 8 died

Table 28.8 1970–1973, Small bowel surgery

Division of adhesions: (124 cases)
1 Small bowel fistula
Resection of small bowel (gangrene or operative damage to small bowel)—114 cases
9 Deaths (7.9%)
4 Anastomotic leaks
13 Major complications
4 Anastomotic leaks
(8 leaks, 4 deaths)

Table 28.9 Enterocutaneous fistulae

Source	*Total No.*	*Without operation*	*Required operation*
Oesophagocutaneous	2	2	0
Gastrocutaneous	4	3	1
Gastrojejunal Anastomosis	1	1	0
Duodenal stump	5	5	0
Colocutaneous	2	2	0
Small bowel	21	6	15
TOTAL	35	19	16

intervention was required ultimately to close fistulae in sixteen patients (Table 28.9).

Fistulae from the oesophagus, stomach and duodenum (including duodenal stump) were best managed, from the nutritional standpoint, by a jejunostomy feeding tube. This tube was placed at the time of the primary procedure (e.g. oesophagogastric resection) or during re-operation for a complication (e.g. duodenal stump leak and subhepatic abscess). Peripheral intravenous feeding is often employed initially, until small bowel function returned, and while jejunostomy feedings are being increased.

SMALL BOWEL FISTULAE

Enteral feeding is best avoided (and is usually unsatisfactory) in small bowel fistulae. This is particularly true in high output fistulae in the mid or upper small bowel. Our experience with twenty-one small bowel fistulae is summarized in Table 28.10, and reviewed in Table 28.11.

The appearance of a small bowel leak usually indicates that the patient will be without significant enteral intake for a period of weeks. TPN may be started via the peripheral route, while the site is being localized, early operation considered, and until the pattern of fistulous drainage is evident. If early operative intervention is not indicated, and the volume of drainage is moderate, TPN will probably be required for an extended period.

During this period of support, some fistulae will show a progressive fall in the volumes of drainage and will close. The fistulae which close spontaneously will be 'low output' fistulae and with long sinuses from the small bowel to skin. Provided there is no evidence of sepsis, forcing re-operation, these

Table 28.10 21 Cases—small bowel fistula

7 Immediate operative interventions:	
3 Successful	—2 exteriorized
	—1 repaired
4 Recurrent leak	—2 spontaneous closure
	—1 delayed operation successful
	—1 died
8 Delayed operative interventions:	
7 Successful closure small bowel fistula (2 died wound + abdominal sepsis)	
1 Persistent fistulae (died of septicaemia)	
6 Had no operation:	
5 Closed spontaneously—discharged (ileocolic anastomotic leaks)	
1 Died of unrelated cause (CVA)	
5 Deaths (25% hospital mortality)	
2 Deaths subsequent to discharge	

fistulae are best managed by prolonged TPN in anticipation of eventual closure. If, after an extended period of TPN, a fistula persists, re-operation will be less difficult, and the patient's nutritional status and tolerance of major surgery will be improved.

Although TPN is a vital component of the management of small bowel fistulae, excessive reliance must not be placed on it. TPN alone will not salvage a patient with a spreading faecal peritonitis from a disrupted anastomosis.

In seven of the patients in our series, immediate operation to exteriorize or repair the fistula was carried out, and TPN was utilized postoperatively to sustain the nutritional state and rest the gastrointestinal tract. In fourteen individuals, in whom there was no evidence of spreading peritoneal contamination, TPN was employed to rest the gastrointestinal tract and sustain or improve nutritional status, while spontaneous closure of the fistula was anticipated.

Table 28.11 Small bowel fistulas, 1975–1977

Patient	*Diagnosis*	*Route*	*Travasol*	*50% D*	*10% lipid*	*Total cal.*	*Duration feeding*	*Duration fistula*	*Outcome*
M.K.	Gangrene abdominal wall	Broviac	1100	400	1500	2300	45	10	Spontaneous closure
K.C.	Blunt trauma small bowel perforation	Broviac	1100	400	1500	2300	53	—	Immediate operation and repair
M.M.	Leak from ileocolic anastomosis	Peripheral	1100	400	1500	2300	35	28	Closed without operation
F.K.	Ileocolic anastomosis	Peripheral	1100	400	1500	2300	12	11	Closure without operation
A.J.	Mesenteric artery occlusion + resection	Broviac	1400	600	2000	3200	38	21	Closure after 2 attempted resections
R.M.	Crohn's disease leak ileocolic anastomosis	Broviac	1100	400	1500	2300	2 Years (Home)	28	Closed without operation but short gut
E.M.	Ileocolic anastomosis	Peripheral	1100	400	1500	2300	27	10	Closed without operation
B.B.	Ileocolic anastomosis	Peripheral	1100	400	1500	2300	11	32	Closed without operation
J.J.	Trauma to colon + small bowel	Broviac	1100	400	1500	2300	104	70	Resection + colostomy

W.I.	Dehiscence + small bowel fistula	Broviac	1100	400	1500	2300	33	20	Operation resection + anastomosis
S.L.	Total colectomy for ulcerative colitis	Broviac Flexical	1400	600	2000	3200	77	—	Closure without operation
L.J.	Appendiceal perforation of small bowel	Broviac	1100	400	1100	2300	64	—	Resection + Ileostomy delayed closure
E.J.	Leak from ileocolic anastomosis	Peripheral	1100	400	1500	2300	15	—	Anastomosis leak. Exteriorized
D.D.	Multiple small bowel fistulae	Broviac	1100	400	1500	2300	62	15	Died of over-whelming abdominal sepsis
V.H.	Small bowel fistula after Hartmann	Subclav	Amigen 800 1500	—	1500	2300	35	20	Small bowel fistula repaired. Died of abdominal sepsis
E.L.	Myonecrosis abdominal wall	Broviac	1100	400	1500	2300	150	150	Small fistulae remained. Patient died of septicaemia
R.L.	Small bowel fistula	Subclav	Amigen 800 1500	—	1500	2300	50	25	Fistula resected. Patient died from septicaemia
S.B.	Cystectomy ileal conduit	Peripheral	1100	—	1500	2300	32	10	Died CVA. Fistula still present
T.M.	Small bowel injury during oophorectomy	Broviac	1400	600	2000	3200	66	65	Delayed operation + resection
P.W.	Small bowel injury during colon anastomosis	Shunt	1400	600	2000	3200	150	90	3 small bowel resections

Six fistulae in this group did close without operation; in eight, operation was required. It is our observation that the longer that operation to resect or repair small bowel fistulae can be delayed, the easier the dissection and greater the chances of success. A 3-week delay is probably adequate, 6 weeks ideal, but little is gained by waiting more than 8 weeks.

If there is evidence of persisting sepsis, every effort should be made to detect and locate intra-abdominal abscesses and provide drainage by the most direct route possible.

CROHN'S DISEASE

Ten patients with Crohn's disease of the duodenum, small bowel and colon were given TPN via Broviac catheters during 1976–1977 (Table 28.12). The indications for starting intravenous feeding were:

1. An attempt in three patients to induce a remission of active disease, where there did not appear to be any clearly defined 'complication' of the disease deserving operative intervention. It was anticipated that the elimination of oral intake, and 'intestinal rest' would result in a remission of symptoms, perhaps permitting a reduction or elimination of other drug therapy (steroids, Imuran), and that these benefits would persist for a reasonable period after the resumption of oral intake. These patients were supported for 52, 43, and 40 days. They gained 8.2, 9.0, and 10.0 kg. Two of the three showed persistent tachycardia and leucocytosis at the conclusion of the course of TPN. Two of the three also developed cholestasis which reversed after TPN was stopped.

Surgery was required in two of the three patients, within 2 months of the TPN-induced 'remission'.

2. Complications had evolved in four patients which required major surgical intervention. The benefits of intestinal rest and nutritional support attained in these cases were considerable. The temperature and pulse rate fell, inflammatory masses resolved, diarrhea decreased with improvement in the appearance of the bowel mucosa. Abscess cavities contracted, and urinary symptoms in patients with enterovesical fistulae, were reduced. There were also dramatic improvements in nutritional status. Immediate or early surgery in complicated Crohn's disease is seldom indicated, but if it is, resection with no anastomosis should be carried out. Operation should be deferred ideally, pending a period of intestinal rest and TPN.

A wasted, febrile patient with an intra-abdominal inflammatory mass, incomplete small bowel obstruction and internal fistulae should not be subjected if possible to a major surgical procedure. In four patients, TPN was continued for 50, 43, 51, and 35 days. On each of these individuals operation was undertaken on the 25th, 35th, 46th, and 28th day respectively. The mean weight gain in the overall group was 10.2 kg, and in these four

Table 28.12 Crohn's disease in 10 patients 1975–1977, Travasol/dextrose/Intralipid

Patient	*Site involvement*	*Venous access*	*Initial weight*	*Weight at disease*	*Temp. fall*	*Pulse fall*	*WBC improve*	*Mass*	*Duration feeding*	*Day of operation*
L.R.	Colon and rectum	Broviac	41	51	✓	✓	✓	✓	43	35
R.K.	Duodenum + jejunum	Broviac	50	62	✓	✓	✓	—	50	25
J.C.	Ileum	Broviac	45	57	✓	✓	✓	✓	51	46
D.M.	Ileocolic	Broviac	42	51			0	—	35	28
J.C.	Ileum and caecum	Broviac	48	56	✓	0	0	—	52	Operation on next admission
R.M.	Ileum and jejunum	Broviac	44	65				—	Home programme	—
D.Mc.	Multiple ileal + jejunal	Broviac	43	58					Home programme	—
D.E.	Ileocolic	Broviac	48	53					40	—
B.B.	Ileocolic	Broviac	50	56	✓	0	0		48	Operation at another hospital
M.P.	Colon	Broviac	39	53					41	TPN after operation

patients the mean weight gain was 8.5 kg, prior to operation. Nitrogen gain in the four patients ranged from 3.2 to 6.0 g/day.

Two individuals treated earlier in the programme developed zinc deficiency with typical facial dermatitis—in both instances the manifestations resolved quickly after discontinuing the high protein intake (Travasol). Two patients also developed mild cholestasis which resolved when TPN was discontinued.

PANCREATITIS

Acute pancreatitis and its sequelae were frequent indications for TPN (Table 28.13). Pancreatitis is managed initially by nasogastric decompression and intravenous fluids. TPN is withheld initially, while problems related to blood flow, water and salt balance are managed. In instances where the process quickly subsides with a fall in serum amylase, pulse rate and temperature, and a prompt return of gastrointestinal function, a cautious resumption of oral intake is usually indicated.

In some patients, delayed gastric emptying, recurrence of pain and hyperamylasaemia demand a more prolonged period of intestinal rest. Five such individuals were managed by peripheral intravenous feeding for relatively short periods (10–35 days). This would appear to be an ideal method to meet requirements.

Patients with severe pancreatitis often developed secondary problems with pancreatic necrosis, pancreatic abscess, fistulae, pseudocysts, and duodenal and biliary obstruction. In these patients TPN was required for extended periods.

Surgical intervention was required in seven of eight in this latter group, usually to drain abscesses or evacuate necrotic tissue. A feeding jejunostomy tube was placed in four, and elemental diets via this route played a major role in their nutritional support. In three of eight patients, jejunal feeding of an elemental diet was the major component of nutritional support.

Four individuals were supported with Broviac catheters for periods of 22, 35, 42, and 61 days.

Only one patient in the group died. It is our opinion that this 'salvage' was the result of an aggressive approach to the detection and drainage of intra- and retroperitoneal abscesses, as well as early attention to the nutritional requirements.

CHOLESTASIS DURING TPN

Bilirubin and alkaline phosphatase levels rose in thirteen out of nineteen patients supported for extended periods (30–130 days) with mixtures of Travasol, Intralipid and 50% dextrose. The patients had complications of major surgery or inflammatory bowel disease (Table 28.14).

Thirteen developed cholestasis with bilirubin elevations ranging from

Table 28.13 Pancreatitis 1975–1977, 6 necrotizing pancreatitis

Patient		*Route*	*Travasol* (ml)	50% *dextrose* (cal.)	*Lipid*	*Elemental diet*	*Duration* (days)	*Outcome*
J.L.	Drainage of multiple pseudo cysts	Broviac jejunostomy	1100	400	1500	2500 ml 25% Flexical	39	Survived. Gained 7 kg
D.Mc.	Pancreatic necrosis + retroperitoneal abscess	Peripheral nasogastric	1100	400	1500	2500 ml 25% Vivonex	52	Survived. Gained 10.2 kg
L.P.	Subhepatic abscesses × 2	Broviac centrasil	1100	400	1500		20 25	Survived. Gained 3.0 kg
W.S.	L. subphrenic abscesses	Peripheral	1100	400	1500	1500 ml/day 25%	48	Survived. Gained 4.8 kg, drained twice
J.H.	Duodenal obstruction, gastrointestinal haemorrhage	Subclavian jejunostomy	1400	600	2000		40	Survived. Sustained initial weight
D.Y.	Recurring subhepatic abscesses	Centrasil jejunostomy	1400	600	2000	2000 ml/day 25% Vivonex	20 30	Died of CVA on 50th hospital day
D.H.	Retroperitoneal abscesses	Centrasil nasogastric	1400	600	2000	2500 ml/day 30% Vivonex	20 20	Survived after drainage abscess via 12th rib

Table 28.14 Cholestasis on TPN

Patient	*Diagnosis*	*Travasol* 10% (ml)	*Dextrose* (cal.)	*Lipid* 10% (ml)	*Initial*		*Peak Bilirubin*	*Peak Alkaline phosphatase*	*No. days until peak*	*Bilirubin after TPN stopped*
					Bilirubin	*Alkaline phosphatase*				
W.I.	Small bowel fistula	1100	800	1500	0.6	24	1.5	507	22	0.4
S.L.	Small bowel fistula	1100	800	1500	0.4	82	6.6	613	39	1.6
R.K.	Crohn's disease Duodenal obstruction	1400	1200	2000	0.2	116	4.1	279	49	0.4
L.J.	Small bowel fistula	1100	800	1500	0.5	216	3.0	767	50	0.6
J.C.	Crohn's disease with obstruction	1100	800	1500	0.9	65	1.5	284	50	0.4
D.W.	Ulcerative colitis	1100	800	1500	0.7	131	3.2	929	36	1.8
J.C.	Crohn's disease with obstruction	1100	800	1500	0.9	109	4.8	790	60	—
L.M.	Small bowel obstruction abscess	1600	400	2000	0.4	162	7.3	704	43	4.9*
D.E.	Crohn's colitis	1100	800	1500	0.4	68	8.7	237	32	2.5
J.S.	Duodenal stump leak	1100	800	1500	0.5	76	2.0	290	67	0.2
T.G.	Oesophageal perforation	1100	800	1500	0.5	738	4.0	1084	38	—

* Still in hospital

1.5 to 8.0 mg%. All of these patients showed coincidental elevation of alkaline phosphatase, and four other patients who did not develop bilirubin elevation had elevation of alkaline phosphatase.

Jaundice developed by 30 days of TPN in seven patients, and appeared by 60 days in the other six. Once jaundice was evident it progressed rapidly, usually requiring discontinuation or a major change in the TPN. Bilirubin levels dropped quickly once TPN was stopped. By sequentially eliminating the major components of TPN, it seemed evident that the amino acid solution (Travasol) was directly or indirectly responsible. Aside from the presence of cholestasis, no deterioration of liver function was evident. Serum albumin levels, and prothrombin levels were sustained. Mild SGOT elevation was present in most.

It is unclear at present whether cholestatic jaundice is a deficiency disease, or due to an excess of some component of TPN. In our experience, it has become almost a predictable, and relatively harmless side effect of TPN. In some individuals, however, it has forced discontinuation of TPN when this support was still required.

References

1. Allardyce, D. B. and Groves, A. C. (1974). A comparison of nutritional gains resulting from intravenous and enteral feeding. *Surg. Gynecol. Obstet.*, **139**, 179
2. Allardyce, D. B. and Williams, B. J. (1977). Parenteral solutions for nutritional support in surgical patients. A comparison of nitrogens employing 5% and 10% amino acid solutions. *Am. J. Surg.*, **133**, 315

Discussion

D. E. F. Tweedle: (UK) I gained the impression that the catheter was removed as soon as sepsis was suspected. It is fine if a patient who is being fed develops sepsis, and one suspects that there is a bacteraemia and removes the catheter. But if a patient who has a focus of sepsis, perhaps a pelvic abscess, shows an increase in temperature, that is not necessarily an indication for removing the catheter. For such patients I have frequently changed their antibiotic, and found that the temperature dropped and the catheter could be left *in situ*.

D. B. Allardyce: (Canada) I did not suggest that we would remove the catheter at the first flick of a temperature. We have tried to use some degree of common sense but we are a little concerned about our use of the Broviac catheter which takes considerable effort to insert and is not readily removed. We would be more inclined to take out a Centrasil catheter because this can be replaced more easily.

The reason why we remove catheters fairly soon if we think that there is a sepsis problem, is that we have had one or two cases of monilial septicaemia. We took Mr Tweedle's approach initially with antibiotics and trying to find the source of infection but very often we found very serious complications developed. In these situations we can stop parenteral nutrition and try to feed the patient enterally, even though that might not be the ideal route.

A. Goode: (UK) We looked at a very similar group of Crohn's disease patients given an elemental diet. Calculating roughly from the figures that Dr Allardyce presented, his group fed intravenously had a weight-gain of about 1.7 kg/week. Giving a similar group an elemental diet with 11 g nitrogen/day we produced a weight-gain of 1.9 kg/week. It would seem that in terms of effectiveness they are similar. The difference possibly was that the elemental diet group, who were fed for a thousand feeding days, were only in hospital for about 10% of that time.

J. M. Kinney: (USA) Could Dr Allardyce tell us how many patients he sees with excess fat in the liver? When they have it, does he find fat deposition in any other tissues?

Allardyce: I regret that we do not have liver tissue from patients parenterally fed for long periods of time, as I am afraid to do liver biopsies for that purpose alone. One thing we do see is the obvious increase in lipid in the subcutaneous fat. One of the basic problems that TPN has to conquer is the tendency to increase lymphocyte effectiveness and cause polymorphs to migrate faster, possibly raising the serum proteins, while it does nothing for the skeletal muscle mass while the septic patient is bed-ridden. If we give 5000 cal/day to a patient who is hypercatabolic, we end up with a truncally obese patient with about 4 inches of subcutaneous fat and withered limbs, which achieves nothing. Where the patient is ambulatory, as in Crohn's disease, there are considerable gains in skeletal muscle mass.

DISCUSSION

I. D. A. Johnston: (UK) Looking back on the patients who developed complications after surgery, was there any evidence that they might have been sub-nourished or undernourished as a group initially?

Allardyce: It is difficult to go into that in a general sense. In the bowel cases, most of them were emergency or elective operations for appendicitis, adhesive obstruction of the small bowel or elective operations for cancer of the right side of the colon, and they were basically fairly well-nourished people who had had a short period of deprivation, sometimes for a few days.

* Synthamin.

29
Protein sparing therapy during prolonged ileus

K. J. FOSTER, K. G. M. M. ALBERTI, N. ALLEN, J. JENKINS, R. M. KAMMERLING, S. J. KARRAN AND C. SMART

Some patients have an obvious need for parenteral nutrition. Such patients are unable to take an adequate oral diet and are already showing signs of malnutrition. Severe weight loss is said to be associated with a poor prognosis in surgical patients[1,2]. It is, however, not always easy to decide at what stage a well-nourished patient should start parenteral nutrition in order to prevent the development of overt malnutrition.

Patients may lose weight as a result of anorexia associated with their illness before operation. Recovery following operation may be protracted by the development of intestinal ileus or obstruction, or by fistula formation. This usually prolongs starvation, increasing the loss of weight, and particularly the loss of protein suffered by the patient. The stress associated with operation, especially in the event of infection, causes an acceleration of the rate of protein loss.

Such weight and protein loss are believed to impair recovery of patients from their operation. Recommendations for the use of total parenteral nutrition as early as 3 days after operation[3] are based on the premise that limiting protein loss might reduce the incidence of complications after surgery and might speed reparative processes.

Case history

The case of M.G. (Figure 29.1) illustrates the problem. M.G., a 60-year-old English woman, was admitted to hospital having had symptoms of intestinal obstruction for 4 days. She had been unable to tolerate oral fluids or food. Her health had been excellent and she had suffered no recent weight loss.

After rehydration, she improved enough to have a barium enema examination. This showed a carcinoma at the splenic flexure. Two days after admission she underwent left hemicolectomy with complete excision of the tumour.

Her post-operative course was prolonged. She restarted oral food 5 days after operation but developed pneumonia, and later an intra-abdominal abscess with a large wound infection. Her oral intake was inadequate, resulting in weight loss of 6 kg and the development of anaemia (Hb, 8.4 g/dl).

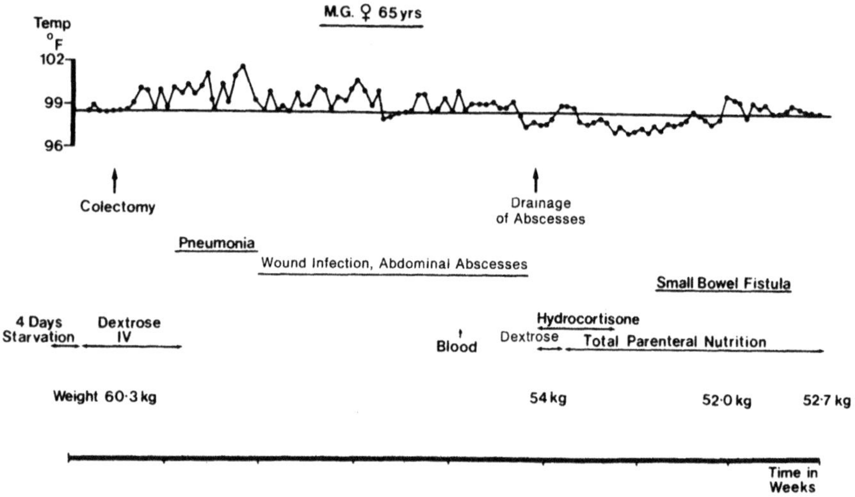

Figure 29.1 The temperature chart of M.G. (female, aged 65 years) admitted to hospital 4 days after developing symptoms of intestinal obstruction. A localized carcinoma of the colon at the splenic flexure was excised at the first operation. Time in hospital was 66 days after operation

Drainage of an intra-abdominal abscess was performed 1 month after her first operation, together with resection of a loop of small bowel. She was treated with antibiotics and hydrocortisone for septicaemia and started on intravenous feeding in anticipation of further delay in obtaining adequate oral nutrition. She then developed a high intestinal fistula which closed spontaneously after 3 weeks of parenteral nutrition.

M.G. spent 66 days in hospital after her first operation. She had already spent 6 days in a state of near-starvation when she underwent her first operation, and a further 5 days elapsed before she restarted oral food. Yet her eventual recovery, with the aid of parenteral nutrition, was complete. Furthermore, weight loss is only one feature of undernutrition[4].

Could M.G. have been helped by starting parenteral nutrition at the time of her first operation? Weight and nitrogen balance can be maintained in this way. Early use of parenteral nutrition can only be contemplated if the technique is shown to be safe.

The risks of parenteral nutrition have been assessed. These are either metabolic, e.g. hyperglycaemia, lactic acidosis and hypophosphataemia, or catheter-related. The need to provide a central venous catheter to administer the nutrient solutions has led to many complications. Overall one may expect complication rates in 5–10% of all cases receiving TPN in non-specialist units[5].

Septicaemia is the commonest complication, with rates reported of up to 27%[6]. By contrast septicaemia arising from peripheral venous cannulae is rare, probably less than 1%, though localized phlebitis is common. Peripheral infusion of isotonic amino acid solutions therefore might be a safer means of maintaining nitrogen balance in adequately nourished patients.

We have completed three studies to assess the extent of the problem and to test the effectiveness of isotonic amino acid infusions.

INCIDENCE OF PROTEIN DEPLETION BEFORE OPERATION

We surveyed the progress of 151 patients undergoing abdominal surgery. These comprised 45% of all patients undergoing abdominal surgery in a 101-bed surgical unit during a 6-month period. Patients having oesophageal surgery and trauma victims were excluded.

Using simple bedside tests we found that patients were generally well nourished, 95% were at or over 80% of average body weight[7] and 94% had 80% or more of average arm muscle circumference[8] before operation (Table 29.1). We found good agreement for the weight (as an index of average weight for height) with arm muscle circumference, which is possibly a more specific measure of protein reserve. In their own estimate only 12% had lost 10 kg body weight or more.

Weight loss was greatest in patients with carcinoma of the stomach and in patients with neoplasms generally. This latter group of patients was also older.

Intravenous 5% glucose and saline were used to maintain these patients in the immediate post-operative period. Two deaths occurred. Both these patients were less than 80% of average body weight and had had palliative procedures for disseminated carcinoma. Six patients developed complications requiring additional nutritional support with total parenteral nutrition (five for fistulae, one for intra-abdominal sepsis) and nine more had a prolonged convalescence with complications which did not preclude oral feeding. 90% of patients left hospital within 3 weeks of operation. Neither body weight, arm muscle circumference nor the patients' own estimate of weight loss served as good indications of the likelihood of serious complication or time to be spent in hospital. 90% of patients returned to oral feeding by the fifth post-operative day.

The outcome of surgery supported by 5% dextrose infusion is favourable in most cases. Whilst these figures are reassuring, we should not be complacent. There are still a number of patients who developed serious complications

Table 29.1 Weight loss and body weight of patients admitted to hospital for abdominal surgery. Average body weight (ABW) refers to values published from 'Build and Blood Pressure Study' of 1959 while Average arm muscle circumference (AMC) refers to the technique described by Jeliffe[8]

	Gastric surgery					*Colonic surgery*		*Others*	
	Inflam.	*Neoplastic*	*Cholecy-stectomy*	*Pancreatic surgery*	*Appendi-cectomy*	*Inflam.*	*Neoplastic*	*Inflam.*	*Neoplastic*
Total ops in 6 months	39		84	19	96	59		54	
No. studied	12	7	54	7	33	8	21	6	9
Mean weight loss (kg)	4	12	3	5	0	0	4	1	3
Wt % ABW	105	90	112	102	102	93	107	105	97
No. < 80%	1	2	0	1	1	1	0	0	2
No. > 120%	3	0	15	0	3	0	4	0	0
AMC % Av.	95	85	102	88	98	92	96	97	87
Mean age (yrs)	48	66	51	66	36	50	64	51	45

thus prolonging their stay in hospital, and a much larger number of patients suffered more minor complications. The role of isotonic amino acids in this situation remains speculative.

THE ROLE OF PARENTERAL NUTRITION AFTER TOTAL CYSTECTOMY AND URINARY DIVERSION USING AN ILEAL CONDUIT

The operation of total cystectomy and urinary diversion into an ileal conduit is formidable, with mortality rates of about 10% for a primary procedure and higher rates for operation after previous radiotherapy. Furthermore serious complication rates of 30–50% may be expected[9]; particularly when performed after previous radiotherapy, intestinal ileus is prolonged, usually lasting 5–10 days before oral feeding is possible. We have studied the effects of intravenous feeding during this early post-operative period.

Care of the patients and their intravenous feeding catheters was maintained by experienced urological surgeons who have used total parenteral nutrition post-operatively in these patients routinely since 1974. They have had a clinical impression of more rapid recovery during this period. The majority of these patients have had previous radiotherapy (usually 6000 rad. given externally from a linear accelerator).

Comparison of total parenteral nutrition and isotonic amino acid infusion methods

The effects of total parenteral nutrition and isotonic amino acids were studied on fifteen patients to assess the performance of the latter in maintaining nitrogen balance after total cystectomy. Table 29.2 shows pre-operative data on the patients and their feeding regimens. In general these patients lose little weight and every attempt is made to avoid the development of uraemia before operation. The operation was performed on five patients as an elective procedure for transitional cell carcinoma of the bladder, on seven for recurrent tumour after previous radiotherapy and on one patient for persistant haemorrhage due to radiation cystitis. One patient underwent partial cystectomy and caecocystoplasty for tuberculosis. He was receiving corticosteroid therapy.

Two intravenous feeding regimens (Table 29.3) were constructed from commercially available materials and adjusted to give isocaloric isonitrogenous amounts as a continuous infusion to facilitate comparisons. These are not necessarily the best of the currently available regimens. In fact the regimens were probably deficient in calories (providing 35 non-protein cals/kg body wt/day) this being fixed by our desire to limit the amount of sorbitol infused. Total parenteral nutrition regimen provided 0.21 g amino acid nitrogen per kg body weight and the Synthamin 3.5% amino acid solution provided 0.24 g amino acid per kg body weight. Aminoplex 5 was infused at a rate administering 0.22 g sorbitol/kg/h. Vamin glucose and Intralipid provides 32% of

Table 29.2 Details of patients receiving intravenous nutrition for prolonged ileus after total cystectomy and ileal conduit formation. Average body weight refers to values quoted in 'Build and Blood Pressure Study' 1959

	No.	*Mean age in years* (range)	*Mean Wt % of ABW* (range)	*Mean B. urea Pre-op. mmol/l* (range)
Aminoplex 5 (Geistlich)	5	65 (48–84)	96 (79–118)	7.5 (5.5–11.5)
Vamin glucose Intralipid (Vitrum)	4	58 (52–64)	90 (75–107)	6.7 (4.8–8.0)
Synthamin 3.5% (Travenol)	6	59 (35–83)	101 (73–130)	7.5 (5.5–9.4)

Table 29.3 Solutions used in parenteral nutrition for patients with ileus after total cystectomy and ileal conduit formation

	Nitrogen (g/l)	*Calorie source* (g/l)	*Electrolytes* (mmol/l)	*Daily infusion for 70 kg pt.* (l)
Aminoplex 5	5	Sorbitol 125 Ethanol 50	Na 35, K 15	2.90
Vamin glucose	9.4	Glucose 100	Na 50, K 20	1.54
Intralipid 10%		Soya bean oil emulsion 100 Glycerol 25	Mg 1.5, Ca 2.5, P 15	1.67
Synthamin 3.5%	5.6		Na 35, K 30, Mg 2.5, P 15	3.00

calories as glucose or glycerol (which enters the glycolytic pathway) and 68% as lipid.

Metabolic studies were carried out on the 3rd post-operative day and on the 7th day in those patients still unable to take any oral food. Methods used to estimate metabolites have been described previously[10]. Nitrogen excretion was derived from measurement of urea in urine and all aspiration and drainage specimens, as described by Lee, with correction for changes in blood urea.

Cutaneous losses of nitrogen are small and have been ignored. One patient receiving Aminoplex 5 died on the 4th day and three had returned to oral feeding by the 7th day. One each in the groups receiving Vamin glucose and Intralipid and the isotonic amino acid solution had returned to oral feeding by the 7th day. Therefore data for the 7th day are shown only for the isotonic amino acid group.

Nitrogen balance

Nitrogen loss was greater in the Synthamin group, but had improved by the 7th day. This was due no doubt to the increased time since operation as well as

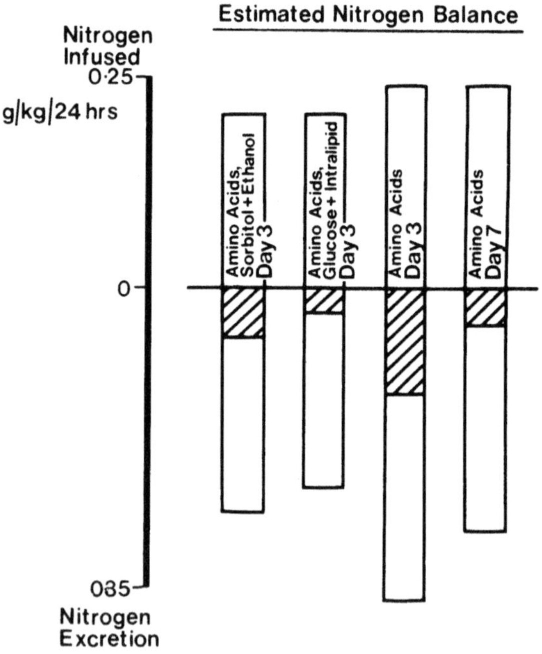

Figure 29.2 Nitrogen balance (estimated from urea excretion in urine and drainage specimens) for patients on the 3rd day after total cystectomy during infusion of various intravenous feeding regimes

physiological adaptation to altered caloric input. At this time the nitrogen loss was less than that seen during glucose infusion after less severe abdominal operations (Foster *et al.*, chapter 9, this volume).

Metabolites

Table 29.4 summarizes metabolic data on these patients. In neither intravenous feeding regime was hyperglycaemia a problem and although serum insulin levels were higher in patients receiving Vamin glucose and Intralipid, no additional insulin therapy was necessary to maintain blood glucose levels.

Table 29.4 Mean blood metabolite concentrations during various parenteral feeding programmes 3 days after total cystectomy (and 7 days for the group receiving Travasol)

	Mean blood glucose (mmol/l)	*Mean serum insulin* (mu/l)	*Mean blood lactate* (mmol/l)	*Mean blood ketone bodies* (mmol/l)
Aminoplex 5	7.6	16	1.79	0.05
Vamin glucose Intralipid	8.3	65	0.90	0.17
Synthamin 3.5% (Day 3)	5.8	16	0.81	0.59
Synthamin 3.5% (Day 7)	6.0	9	0.79	0.47

Sorbitol is a sugar alcohol which is metabolized to fructose, the infusion of which is associated with the risk of lacticacidosis in patients with hepatic or renal damage, and those who are also given ethanol are particularly prone to this complication. The highest lactate level recorded in this group was however only 2.1 mmol/l, in a patient with a serious infection. Nevertheless mean blood lactate was twice that found in the other groups and we believe that such solutions should be used with great care, especially products which contain ethanol.

Ketone bodies (acetoacetate and 3-hydroxybutyrate) were raised slightly during isotonic amino acid therapy. The mean level at 7 days however is not significantly different from the level on the 3rd day. These levels are much lower than those found during saline infusions after operation (Foster *et al.*, chapter 9). One patient, M.D., was receiving corticosteroid therapy throughout his Synthamin infusion. His metabolite and nitrogen excretion values were close to the means for the group as a whole and are included in those means. His insulin levels were markedly raised (50 and 48 mu/l respectively) and are excluded from the mean insulin levels. We have previously noted that metabolite levels are similar in the early post-operative period in normal patients and in those taking corticosteroids.

Compared with 5% dextrose, 3.5% Synthamin clearly limits nitrogen loss after operation and after a week of such therapy the loss is reduced to about

3–4 g daily. If parenteral nutrition does reduce complications after operation then isotonic amino acid infusions might also do so. We have therefore examined the effect of parenteral nutrition on recovery retrospectively from case records of patients undergoing total cystectomy since 1970.

Total cystectomy operations

This operation with formation of an ileal conduit was performed on seventy-one patients between January 1970 and December 1976. The series includes eleven of the patients referred to above including two who received Synthamin 3.5% amino acid solution. For purposes of analysis these two are regarded as having been fed intravenously.

Parenteral nutrition has been used from the first post-operative day since 1974 for prolonged ileus despite some complications arising from the central venous catheter. Feeding catheters were inserted by anaesthetic staff and maintained by the surgical team. One patient who received parenteral nutrition late after operation is regarded as not having been fed intravenously. Previous to 1974 5% dextrose and saline were used to maintain fluid and electrolyte balance.

Table 29.5 summarizes the pre-operative data on these patients. Age and blood urea were similar except for two patients with markedly raised blood urea secondary to bilateral ureteric obstruction, in the group with no prior radiotherapy which received parenteral nutrition in the post-operative period. Salvage for recurrent carcinoma after radiotherapy was the commonest indication for operation in both the fed group (46%) and in the group not fed intravenously (47%). Other indications included elective procedures (9% and 11% respectively), ureteric obstruction (9% and 11% respectively), haemorrhage (9% and 8% respectively) and small bladder syndrome (12% and 8% respectively). Thirty-three patients received early intravenous feeding; thirty-eight did not.

Table 29.5 Pre-operative characteristics of seventy-one patients undergoing total cystectomy and ileal conduit formation from 1970 to 1976 and receiving either full intravenous feeding or 5% dextrose and saline during the subsequent period of ileus

	Intravenous feeding		*Dextrose 5% intravenously*	
	Previous RT	*No RT*	*Previous RT*	*No RT*
No.	26	7	29	9
Mean age	65	64	62	64
(Range)	(48–84)	(53–74)	(33–75)	(46–72)
Mean pre-operative blood urea (mmol/l)	6.2	13.7	5.6	5.2
(Range)	(2.0–11.5)	(3.4–44.3)	(2.3–13.3)	(4.3–6.0)

RT = radiotherapy

RESULTS

The results are shown in Table 29.6. There was no difference in overall mortality in the groups fed or not fed intravenously from the first post-operative day. Time spent in hospital after operation was also similar for the survivors. Six deaths occurred early in the post-operative period, due to myocardial infarction (2), pulmonary embolus (1), tension pneumothorax (1), bowel infarction (1) and gangrene of the abdominal wall (1). Six later deaths occurred due to infection or failure of wound healing which one might have expected to have been influenced by parenteral nutrition. However, there were three such deaths in each group (this includes one death from *Staphylococcus aureus* septicaemia arising from the feeding catheter). Follow-up at 1 year, of survivors operated on up to April 1976, showed eight deaths from secondary spread in the thirty-two patients surviving operation and given dextrose infusions, and four deaths in the sixteen survivors treated with early parenteral nutrition.

Table 29.6 Influence of early intravenous feeding on recovery from total cystectomy compared with 5% dextrose intravenously (1970–76). (Radiotherapy (RT) denotes previous cystotomy and gold grain insertion or external irradiation)

	Intravenous feeding			*Dextrose 5% intravenously*		
	Previous RT	*No RT*	*Total*	*Previous RT*	*No RT*	*Total*
No. of patients	26	9	33	29	9	38
Deaths	5	1	6	3	3	6
Deaths in 1st week	2	1	3	1	2	3
Late deaths due to infection or wound breakdown	3	0	3	2	1	3
Time in hospital—days after operation	21.6	20.8	21.4	22.5	24.2	22.8
(Range)	(14–38)	(13–43)		(11–42)	(15–45)	

Complications

Complications arising from the need for a central venous catheter included one fatal pneumothorax, one fatal septicaemia due to *Staph. aureus* (in a patient with pre-existing severe intra-abdominal sepsis), a pleural effusion and one case of axillary vein thrombosis. No metabolic complications were recorded.

Phlebitis with 3.5% Synthamin

One clinical aspect of the use of 3.5% Synthamin has been the occurrence of severe phlebitis. It was necessary to change infusion sites a mean of 0.3 times in 72 h in each patient receiving dextrose–saline infusions, 0.5 times for 0.9% saline and 1.3 times during 3.5% Synthamin infusions. The phlebitis occurred sometimes within a few hours and was frequently so severe as to preclude further use of that arm for intravenous therapy. Though only Freeman *et al.*[12] using Freamine have reported this complication before, we also noted an increased rate of phlebitis during a pilot study with half-strength Vamin N (3.5% amino acid solution).

DISCUSSION

Recovery from an operation may be influenced by many factors including the nature and extent of the original lesion, the age of the patient, the presence or absence of associated diseases and the technique of the surgeon. Weight loss and protein depletion may be associated with more advanced lesions. However, there is widespread agreement that protein depletion impairs healing. In patients with upper gastrointestinal carcinoma, Williams and his colleagues were able to demonstrate some aspects of improved recovery after pre-operative parenteral nutrition[13].

Despite reports of a high incidence of malnutrition in surgical patients[14] it has been our experience that severe weight loss and protein depletion have been unusual at the time of operation. Protein depletion before operation has probably not been a major cause of severe complications although it may have been a contributory factor to the morbidity associated with abdominal operation. Steiger and his colleagues[15] found that total parenteral nutrition was beneficial in improving the health of experimental colonic anastomoses in malnourished rats (weight loss of 25% body weight before operation, but the same group was unable to show any improvement of the healing of anastomoses after infusions of isotonic amino acids into well-nourished rats[16].

After abdominal operation over 90% of our patients made a reasonable recovery and returned to oral feeding within 5 days. We were also unable to find any evidence of favourable influence by parenteral nutrition on the development of complications after total cystectomy, in our sequential retrospective series. Isotonic amino acid infusions are slightly less effective in maintaining nitrogen balance than conventional intravenous feeding regimen. There appears to be no evidence to support the routine use of isotonic amino acid therapy (or parenteral nutrition) in the immediate post-operative period in a prophylactic role, since most patients are not seriously malnourished, and recover quickly.

Malnourished patients and patients with more prolonged inability to tolerate oral food do benefit from parenteral nutrition. Fistula formation was the commonest indication in our patients and there can be no doubt of the value of parenteral nutrition in patients with high gastrointestinal fistulae[17]. Because of the seriousness of possible complications of intravenous feeding, the technique should only be employed for such specific indications. The 3.5% Synthamin electrolyte solution had an osmolality of 480 mOsm and was associated with severe phlebitis so that we have at times needed to use a central venous catheter to maintain infusions. For this reason we prefer to use total parenteral nutrition through a central catheter when required, and dextrose solutions at other times, through peripheral veins.

Acknowledgements

We would like to thank Mrs B. Lloyd, Miss P. Smythe, and Miss L. Hinks for expert technical assistance. We gratefully acknowledge financial support from Travenol Laboratories Ltd, and the British Diabetic Association.

References

1. Studley, H. O. (1936). Percentage weight loss. A basic indicator of surgical risk in patients with chronic peptic ulcer. *J. Am. Med. Assoc.*, **106**, 458
2. Lawson, L. J. (1965). Parenteral nutrition in surgery. *Br. J. Surg.*, **52**, 795
3. Lee, H. A. (1975). Intravenous nutrition. *Ann. R. Coll. Surg.*, **56**, 59
4. Law, D. K., Dudrick, S. T. and Abdon, N. I. (1973). Immuno competence in patients with protein calorie malnutrition. *Ann. Int. Med.*, **79**, 545
5. Ryan, J. A., Abel, R. M., Abbott, W. M., Hopkins, C. C., McChesney, T., Colley, R., Philips, K. and Fischer, J. (1974). Catheter complications in total parenteral nutrition. *N. Engl. J. Med.*, **290**, 757
6. Goldmann, D. A. and Maki, D. G. (1973). Infection control in total parenteral nutrition. *J. Am. Med. Assoc.*, **223**, 1360
7. Soc. of Actuaries, (1959). Build and Blood Pressure Study. Chicago.
8. Jeliffe, D. B. (1966). *The Assessment of the Nutritional Status of the Community*. (Geneva: W.H.O.)
9. Whitmore, W. F. (1975). Total cystectomy. In E. Cooper and R. Williams (eds.). *The Biology and Clinical Management of Bladder Cancer*. (Oxford: Blackwell Scientific Publications)
10. Batstone, G. F., Alberti, K. G. M. M., Hinks, L., Smythe, P., Laing, J., Ward, C., Ely, D. W. and Bloom, S. R. (1976). Metabolic studies in subjects following thermal injury. *Burns*, **2**, 207
11. Lee, H. A. (1974). *Parenteral Nutrition in Acute Metabolic Illness*. p. 315. (London: Academic Press)
12. Freeman, J., Stegink, L., Meyer, P., Thompson, R. and Den Beston, L. (1975). Metabolic effects of amino acid versus dextrose infusion in surgical patients. *Arch. Surg.*, **110**, 916
13. Williams, R. H. P., Heatley, R. V., Lewis, M. H. and Hughes, L. E. (1976). A randomised controlled trial of pre-operative intravenous nutrition in patients with stomach cancer. *Br. J. Surg.*, **63**, 667
14. Bistrian, B., Blackburn, G., Hallowell, E. and Heddle, R., (1974). Protein status of general surgical patients. *J. Am. Med. Assoc.*, **230**, 858
15. Steiger, E., Allen, T., Daly, J., Vars, H. and Dudrick, S. (1971). Beneficial effects of immediate post-operative total parenteral nutrition. *Surg. For.*, **22**, 89
16. Daly, J., Steiger, E., Vars, H. and Much, J. (1973). Post-operative intravenous use of 5% dextrose versus 5% amino acid solutions. Effects on body weight, colonic anastomotic strength and serum protein metabolism. *Surg. For.*, **24**, 84
17. Himal, H., Allard, J., Nadeau, J., Freeman, J. and Maclean, L. (1974). The importance of adequate nutrition in closure of small intestinal fistulas. *Br. J. Surg.*, 724

Discussion

N. J. Kartinos: (UK) Is there any evidence to support a conclusion that the egg phosphatide emulsifying agent in the fat emulsion is utilized?

Secondly, in comparing Travasol* with any other amino acid solutions, we should also compare the electrolyte concentrations, as the osmolarity will be influenced by the electrolyte profiles.

S. J. Karran: (UK) To take up the last point, we are aware that the osmolarity of this particular solution was somewhat higher than had been reported. Certainly it was higher than the Vamin solution that we used. We think that this is due to the electrolyte contents.

G. L. Blackburn: (USA) There was a report at the American Urological Association in May 1977[1] of a group of forty-four patients with bladder cancer from the MGH who had 4500 R before total cystectomy and ileal loop and also were randomized between dextrose with water and amino acid infusions. Nutritional assessment revealed 17 of 44 (39%) of the patients to be malnourished prior to operation. The postoperative complication rate was 33% in Group I(D_5W) versus 17% in Group II ($A_{3.5}W$). Cell-mediated immunity, determined by reactivity to a battery of recall antigens, revealed that 56% of the patients in Group I were able to maintain their skin test reactivity throughout their post-op. course while 94% of the patients in Group II maintained reactivity during the same period. Four nutritionally depleted patients in Group I required conversion to a forced feeding regimen (IVH) while none of the Group II patients required a change in their nutritional regimen.

There has also been an article by Hill *et al.*[2] confirming the Bistrian and Blackburn[3] study on the epidemiology of malnutrition, so the point is well taken that where there is no malnutrition, it is not likely that nutritional support will make any difference. The candidates for cholecystectomy are not likely to develop indices of malnutrition, and that would be a group where one would not need to worry about nutritional support; patients for major surgery with several days of starvation are those where the nutrition indices require to be measured and the effects of nutritional support studied.

Karran: It is important to know which patients will have to be brought in some time before operation for nutritional support, as this is quite expensive.

I. D. A. Johnston: (UK) Surely the point at issue is not whether intravenous feeding in certain patients will prevent complications, but whether under-nutrition at the time of admission to hospital is associated with a more protracted convalescence and a higher incidence of complications.

H. M. Shizgal: (Canada) There is some evidence that the patient who comes in depleted has a higher complication rate. At our centre a lot of data[4] have been collected showing that the patient who is anergic pre-operatively has a

* Synthamin.

high complication rate and mortality rate compared to the patient who reacts normally.

We have also collected some data[5] to demonstrate that if the nutritional status of the anergic patient is measured by means of body composition studies, and he can be repleted nutritionally, skin reactivity will return to normal.

Karran: Do they heal faster and get better quicker?

Shizgal: There is no question that the anergic patient who undergoes any form of surgery has a significantly higher mortality rate. The problem has been to quantitate nutritional status. Once that can be done one can show a difference.

Studies which look at crude complication rates or mortality rates will never give an answer, as one is dealing with a situation where the parameter being measured has a high variance and a high standard deviation; the demonstration of a significant difference will only be achieved by collecting large numbers—which is impractical.

H. F. Woods: (UK) It has always been assumed that the phosphate content as phospholipid in a fat solution is a way of administering phosphate during intravenous feeding. I know of no good evidence which shows that phosphate infused in the fat solution is available to the general phosphate pool. We have seen the severe hypophosphataemic syndrome in a neonate although he was being fed with enough Intralipid to provide more than his total daily phosphate requirement.

Goode: We have looked at cardiac surgical patients. Four of these had a significant loss of body cell mass of more than 10%, and they had four times the hospital stay in terms of days (59 days), as opposed to 16 for non-depleted patients. No other factor was operating in those patients apart from undernutrition which could have accounted for the increased stay.

Karran: I accept that entirely, but what we want to identify more readily in the District General Hospital patients with malnutrition without having to send them off for total body potassium measurements.

References

1. Hensle, T. W. (1978). *J. Urology*, **11,** (in press)
2. Hill, G. L., Main, W. S. T., Edwards, J. P. and Goligher, J. C. (1976). *Br. J. Surg*., **63,** 133
3. Bistrian, Blackburn, G. L., 1974, *J. Am. Med. Assoc*., **230,** 858
4. Pietsch, J. B. and Meakins, J. L. (1977). *Can. J. Surg*., **20,** 15
5. Spanier, A. H., Meakins, J. L., MacLean, L. D. and Shizgal, H. M., (1976). *Surg. Forum*, **27,** 332

30
Cholestatic jaundice during parenteral alimentation in adults

A. SITGES-CREUS, E. CANADAS AND L. VILAR

INTRODUCTION

Significant intrahepatic cholestasis has been reported during total parenteral alimentation in adults[1-5] and in premature infants[6]. The solutions used in these reports included dextrose synthetic L amino acids and protein hydrolysates.

Many clinicians have noted some alteration of liver function during intravenous feeding in ill patients. The patients reported in this study had marked elevation of serum transaminases, alkaline phosphatase and serum bilirubin. They also had evidence of intrahepatic cholestasis in liver biopsy specimens.

The three patients, in whom intrahepatic cholestasis was established, all received dextrose Intralipid 20% and casein hydrolysate or essential L amino acids. Their ages ranged from 31 to 80 years and they had lost between 10 and 20% of their body weight when total parenteral alimentation was started.

Two patients were fed intravenously for 22 and 32 days respectively. The third patient had four separate periods of parenteral nutrition ranging from 12 to 45 days on each occasion and averaging 29 days. This patient died from liver failure during the last period of treatment.

CASE HISTORIES

Case 1

An 80-year-old male patient with dysphagia for 2 months due to a carcinoma of the oesophagus was placed on parenteral alimentation. He had lost 12% of his body weight. Jaundice developed within 17 days and intravenous feeding was stopped after 24 days. A gastrostomy was performed for purposes of nutrition and a liver biopsy obtained on the 30th day. The jaundice persisted but cleared gradually during the next 20 days. The biochemical changes in this patient are shown in Figure 30.1. The serum bilirubin continued to rise after the parenteral nutrition was stopped. The transaminase levels fell slowly to normal but the alkaline phosphatase remained elevated.

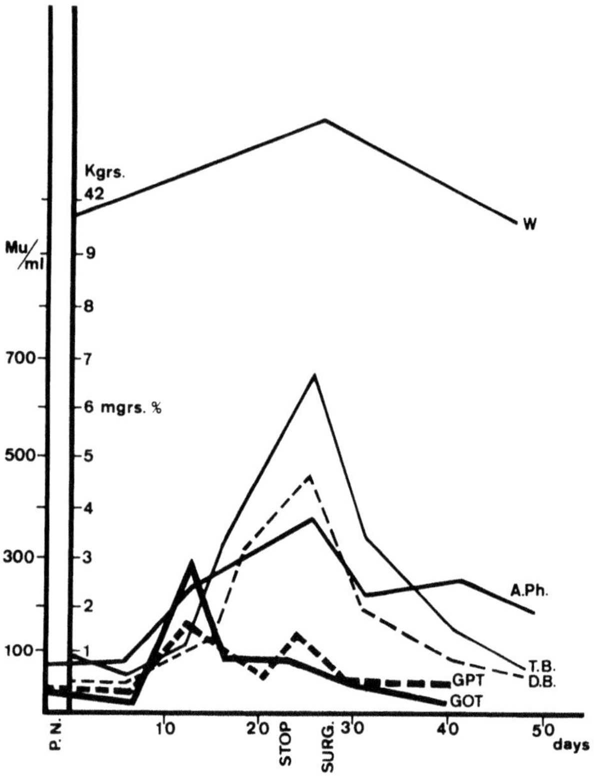

Figure 30.1 Changes in liver function tests during TPN in a patient with carcinoma of the oesophagus

Case II

A 31-year-old man had an injury to the cervical oesophagus during total thyroidectomy for papillary carcinoma. A fistula developed and gastrostomy was established 1 week later. The patient lost 11 kg. The fistula was closed at a subsequent operation and gastrostomy feeding was continued intermittently for 8 months, by which time he had regained his health-weight and returned to work.

A cervical wound abscess developed 5 months later and the fistula reopened. He rapidly lost 7 kg of body weight. A further gastrostomy was not possible and total parenteral alimentation was started.

Jaundice developed after 3 weeks of intravenous feeding which had to be discontinued after 1 month. A further fistula repair was attempted with only partial success, but oral feeding became possible. The relationship between altered liver function tests and parenteral nutrition is shown in Figure 30.2.

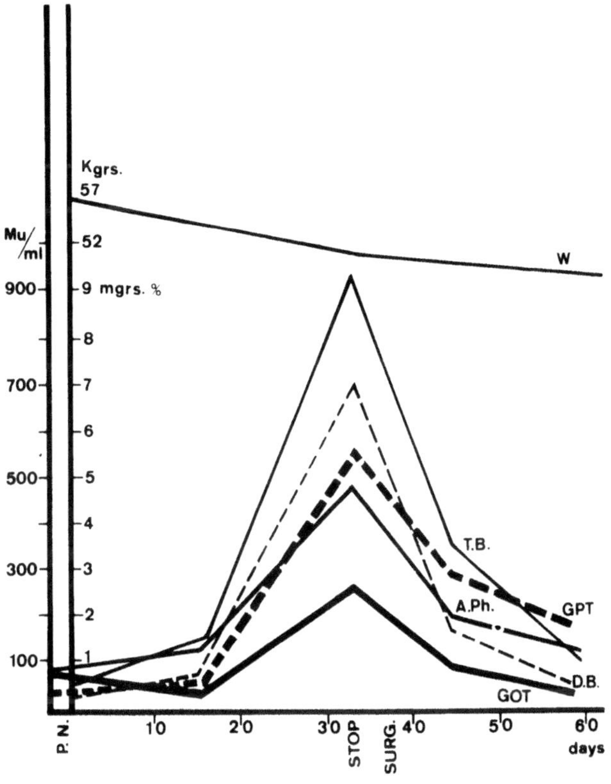

Figure 30.2 Changes in liver function during TPN in a patient with an oesophageal fistula

Case III

A 55-year-old man weighing 48 kg had a total oesophagectomy with oesophagostomy and gastrostomy as part of a staged procedure for carcinoma of the middle third of the oesophagus. He developed a post-operative wound infection and diarrhoea. He was given total parenteral alimentation and after 28 days jaundice developed. Intravenous feeding was continued for a further 22 days and stopped.

The patient developed an appendicular abscess a few days after stopping the intravenous feeding. A drainage operation was required and a liver biopsy was obtained. The abnormal liver function tests returned slowly to normal during the next 20 days (Figure 30.3).

This patient's nutritional state did not improve on gastrostomy feeding and further parenteral nutrition was indicated. The second period of parenteral alimentation followed a similar pattern to the first, except that jaundice and abnormal liver function developed earlier (Figure 30.4). A further liver biopsy was obtained during the second episode of jaundice. It became clear that further intravenous support was required. Amino acids were excluded

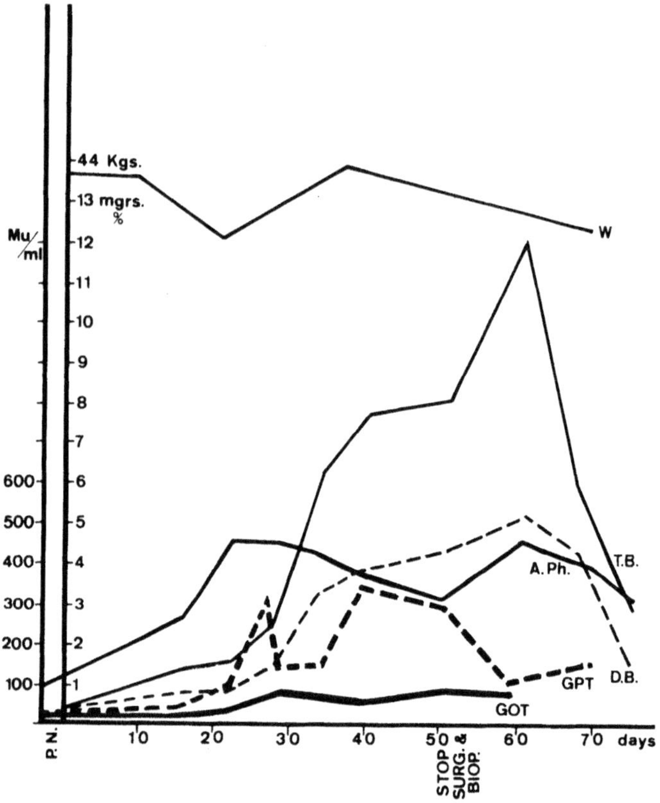

Figures 30.3–30.5 Changes in liver function tests during three separate periods of total parenteral alimentation in a single patient

initially and dextrose and Intralipid alone were given for several weeks. The hepatic enzyme levels and bilirubin levels did not alter during this time, but when amino acids were added the liver enzymes and bilirubin in the serum rose progressively and the intravenous feeding had to be stopped for a third time.

A decision was taken to proceed to further surgery to restore intestinal continuity and a further short course of 10–12 days' parenteral alimentation was planned (Figure 30.5). There was a sudden increase in serum bilirubin after 11 days of intravenous feeding. The patient went into hepatic coma and died 4 days later.

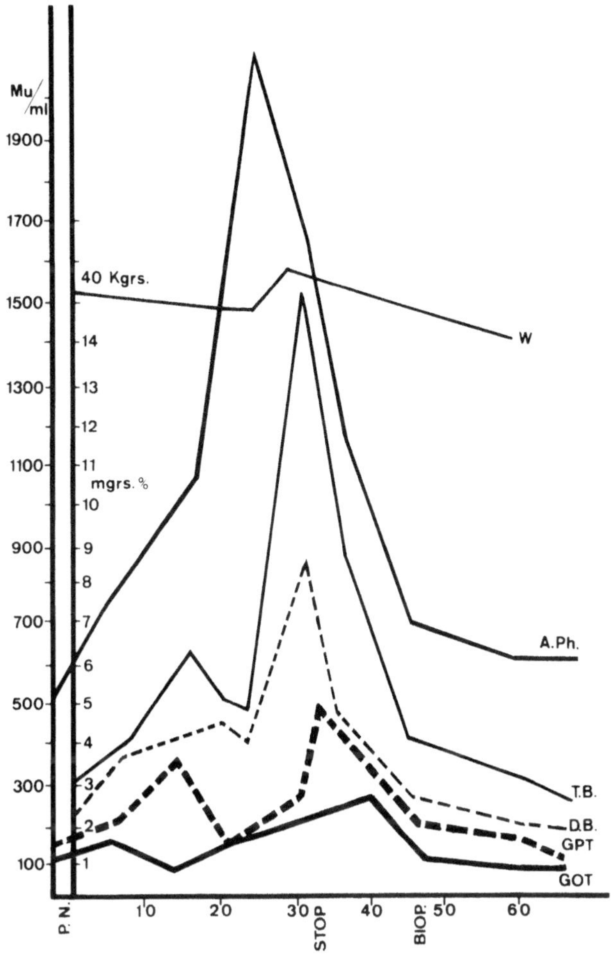

Figure 30.4

LIVER PATHOLOGY

The pathological findings in these patients consisted of changes of intrahepatic cholestasis similar to those described by other authors. The lobular pattern is preserved. Light microscopy shows minimal to moderate cholestasis, scattered areas of hepatocellular damage and variable activity of Küpffer cells. There is infiltration of the periportal space with round cells; some eosinophils and proliferation of bile ducts is also present.

Lesions were more marked in Case III, which received several courses of TPN. The liver cells have extensive ultrastructural changes (Figure 30.6). The bile canaliculi show severe dilatation with a decrease in the number of villi. There are occasional giant mitochondria showing a crystalloid pattern and increased number of mitochondrial granules (Figure 30.7).

The liver in Case III showed massive necrosis. Cholestasis was seen in some sections which were not totally destroyed and was centrilobular. There was marked proliferation of bile ducts and a massive round cell infiltration (Figure 30.8).

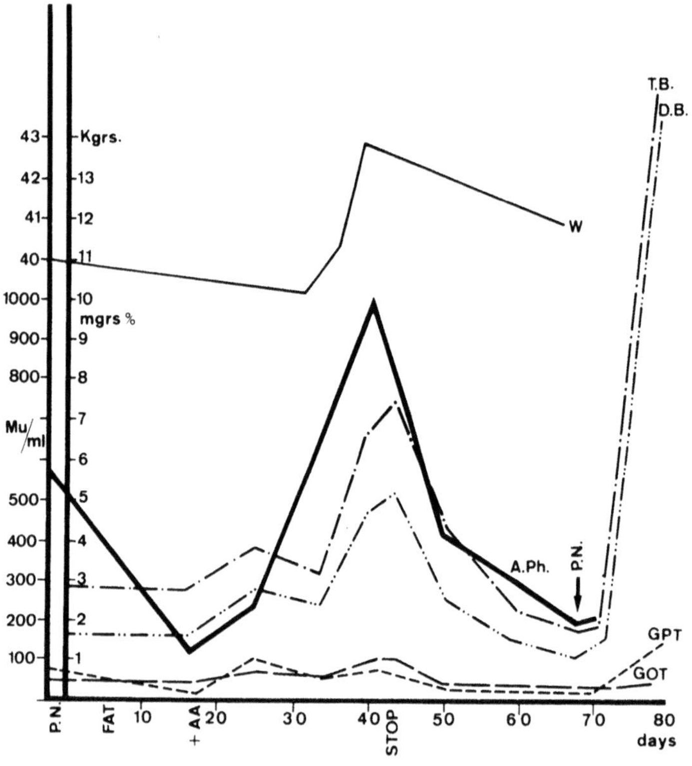

Figure 30.5

DISCUSSION

The aetiologic possibilities of the cholestasis in association with parenteral alimentation are multiple: failure of oral intake, malnutrition, sepsis, hypoxia, drugs, hyperammonaemia, amino acid imbalance, toxicity and hypersensitivity, have all been suggested.

All our patients have a common denominator: failure of oral intake and resultant malnutrition due to a lesion of the oesophagus. Both factors seem to predispose to the development of intrahepatic cholestasis in patients on TPN. It has not been determined whether the parenteral solutions are toxic. All the components of the mixtures used have been known to cause liver damage, and amino acids, either in crystalline form or as casein hydrolysate, have been associated, clinically and experimentally, with liver dysfunction.[8]

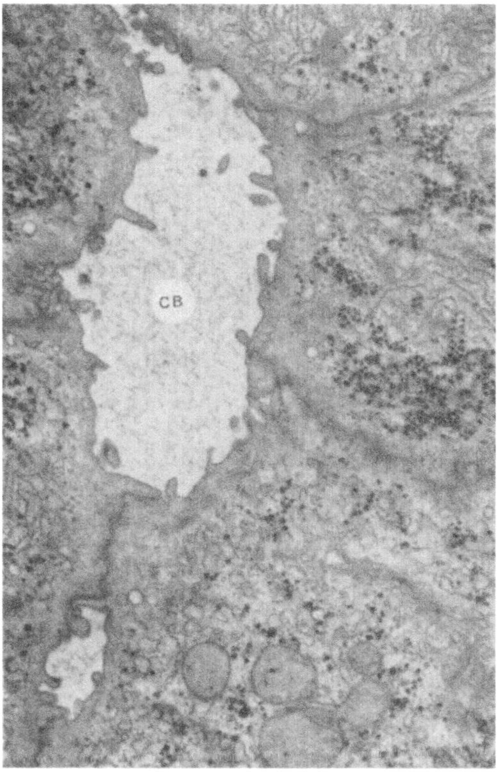

Figure 30.6 Ultrastructural changes in intrahepatic cholestasis. Case III. The bile canaliculi are enlarged.

In our experience discontinuing TPN was always followed by a decrease of plasma bilirubin, returning to normal within 1 month. Serum transaminases returned to normal at the same time, but alkaline phosphatase levels took longer to fall.

The exclusion of amino acids from one period of intravenous feeding in the third patient was not associated with any alteration in liver function, even though previous amino acid infusions had been followed by jaundice on two occasions.

Two patients had septicaemia during their intravenous nutrition, but changes in serum bilirubin and other liver function tests were not associated with periods of established septicaemia.

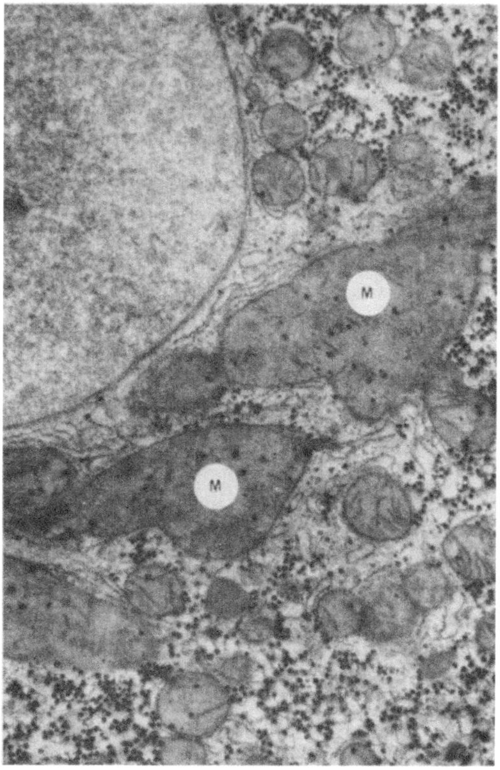

Figure 30.7 Electron microscopy section in intrahepatic cholestasis. The mitochondria are large and contain excess granules.

It has been postulated that a hypersensitivity reaction follows the infusion of amino acids. The jaundice, however, does not appear until 4 weeks of treatment have elapsed and although excess eosinophils in the blood were observed in the three patients studied there were only a few eosinophils in the portal triad in one patient.

Intrahepatic cholestasis associated with intravenous nutrition is a reversible condition and both the histological and biochemical changes disappeared within a few weeks of discontinuing treatment. Serious problems,

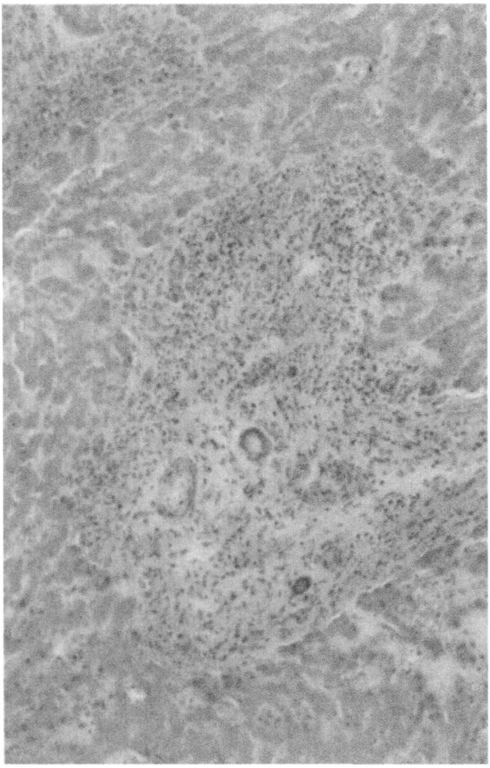

Figure 30.8 Proliferation of bile ducts and round cell infiltration in cholestasis. Case III

however, will arise in the future in patients with complete alimentary failure who require continuous intravenous nutrition to survive and who develop cholestasis.

Discussion

D. B. Allardyce: (Canada) I would like to report on a miscellaneous series of patients who were not septic. They were not receiving any drug which was common to them all. They were supported with a mixture of Travasol*, dextrose and Intralipid. All the patients started out with a normal bilirubin, and a normal serum alkaline phosphatase.

The shortest course before jaundice appeared was 22 days and the next shortest was 32. For the majority it was over 50 days of parenteral feeding. The bilirubin elevation appeared, usually after 20–30 days of alimentation and rose rapidly by 2 mg/day. The peaks ranged from 2 to 4 mg%. The highest bilirubin level was 8.7 mg%.

In every instance, as soon as the parenteral feeding was stopped, the bilirubin levels returned to normal, within a week to 10 days. There was a later, but delayed, fall towards normal in alkaline phosphatase.

We found that by changing the various components of the intravenous feeding, it was the omission of the Travasol (or in one case Freamine) that seemed to produce a fall in bilirubin. If we continued to support the patient on hypertonic dextrose, or Intralipid alone, or Intralipid combined with Amigen, we could usually get a remission of the jaundice.

There are two cases that did not develop jaundice. One of them has been on intravenous feeding for 150 days and the other for more than 360 days. These patients are at home on TPN on the same components exactly, but they are capable of eating moderate amounts of food.

M. T. Ste Marie: (Canada) Has Dr Allardyce studied the immunological status of his patients, either serum immunoglobulins or skin reactivity, to see if they were deficient in any way?

The two patients who are at home are feeding orally, and are stimulating the gut with food, and have not developed hyperbilirubinaemia. Instead of stopping the TPN in the other patients, has any attempt been made at giving them an elemental diet or food, without stopping the TPN, to see what happens to the hyperbilirubinaemia? The cholestasis might have something to do with gut stimulation with antigens, or the presence in the gut of immunological mechanisms which might be a defence against antigen uptake.

Neonates make a very good model because their gut is not stimulated. They are really like germ-free animals when they are started on TPN. If such is the case, and there are no normal gut defences with antigen stimulation, then there might be antigen uptake, and the first place where these antigens can go is to the liver. The liver either destroys these antigens and there is no cholestasis, or the liver cannot cope with them and there is cholestasis. If such is the case, then the serum bile acids are increased—as has been shown by Norman Javit and his group[1] at an APS Meeting in San Francisco (Spring 1977).

* Synthamin.

Allardyce: We did not do any immunological testing.

A. Sitges-Creus: (Spain) We did immunofluorescent studies in the liver and looked for an antigen–antibody reaction, but found nothing.

I. D. A. Johnston: (UK) Did any of the patients have intravenous fat?

Sitges-Creus: All of them.

U. Freund: (Israel) It is very difficult to make a 'clean' observation on cholestatic jaundice with these complex patients that have many other complications like sepsis. There seems to be a completely different phenomenon where there is Intralipid administration with amino acids and glucose, and when Intralipid is not used. The liver biopsies (of Sitges-Creus) were striking because of the fat infiltration. Where exactly was this fat? In the hepatocytes, or somewhere else in the liver? I would be inclined to link the Intralipid more than the amino acid administration to the cholestatic jaundice that Dr Sitges-Creus observed in his patients.

Sitges-Creus: We interrupted one of the periods of TPN, and after a rest period of more than a month we started parenteral alimentation with lipids and dextrose only for 17 days and we saw a real improvement. As soon as we gave amino acids, the problem recurred. In none of these cases have we seen hepatic steatosis.

D. W. Wilmore: (USA) The liver avidly loves endotoxin and endotoxin is taken up as if in a sponge by the liver. I would suggest that we are seeing only the tip of the iceberg by looking at the liver function studies that were presented to us. More sophisticated studies of liver function will show these people to have dysfunction long before 4 weeks. This may occur in many patients, and along with the thesis that there may be antigen–antibody reactions or bacteria crossing the intestinal mucosa, we must also keep in mind that endotoxins can damage the livers of these critically ill people.

N. Zöllner: (Germany) If I understood Dr Allardyce correctly, his pathologists considered the sample from the liver to be compatible with obstructive jaundice. However, I could not see much evidence of obstructive jaundice in the paper from Dr Sitges-Creus. Where does the bilirubin stop flowing if it is obstructive jaundice. Could it be hepatic obstruction, say in the gliosomes or the periportal spaces, or is it just cholestasis similar to what we see in drug jaundice and in antigen–antibody reactions?

Allardyce: I showed a slide where the liver architecture is quite well preserved, and the liver cells looked—by ordinary light microscope—to be fairly normal. The characteristic features are bile duct proliferation in the triads with a few inflammatory cells and in the more pronounced case–some fibrosis and bile duct proliferation. Bile plugs and lakes are very characteristic, and the pathologist considered that it had most of the features of extrahepatic biliary obstruction which disappeared subsequently when TPN was stopped.

I might add that, of the other liver function tests, prothrombin time is well sustained in these patients and their serum albumin levels are normal. This is uncharacteristic of a patient who is going into liver failure. It seems to be a cholestatic problem, but not affecting all aspects of liver function.

G. L. Blackburn: (USA) One of my colleagues (Mainl) reported a series of patients before the Association for Academic Surgeons[2]. He found the problem mostly in septic individuals. He found striking impairment of BSP retention as the most sensitive parameter, often in patients who were not yet jaundiced. He got dramatic reversal in the BSP clearance and resolution of the liver failure profile by interrupting the feeding, and also orally feeding those patients. He did not withdraw the protein because the patients were in protein malnutrition.

D. E. F. Tweedle: (UK) We must not get too worried with the data that have been presented on patients on intravenous feeding as Dr Allardyce and Dr Sitges-

Creus have emphasized that it could be multi-factorial. Dr Blackburn's comment about the importance of sepsis may be crucial. It is vital that someone tries to present data demonstrating that there is an increased incidence of cholestatic jaundice in these patients who have intravenous feeding, in comparison with similar patients who do not have intravenous feeding. Until that is done, we have no indication whatever that the problem is due to intravenous feeding.

H. F. Woods: (UK) It has become obvious that so far as this adverse reaction to therapy is concerned, there must be more than one basis for its production. We have already heard people implying that amino acid solutions may be involved. Others have suggested that it only occurs in those patients who have received dextrose, and it is well recognized, from the work of Thompson and others[3], that the intravenous administration of fat can be associated with liver damage.

However, it has also been well-described that other carbohydrate sources, because of their pathways of metabolism, can cause liver damage. Schumer's group[4], Thomas's group[5] in Australia and others[6] have shown that both fructose and xylitol can acutely alter hepatic function. The cases which I find convincing, taking up Mr Tweedle's very good point, are those in which the attending physician or surgeon has withdrawn therapy and then reintroduced therapy, and again caused disturbances of liver function. In the cases from Dr Sitges-Creus and the cases from Hammersmith, which were associated with sorbitol infusion—withdrawal of therapy resulted in liver function tests returning to normal, and the reintroduction of therapy again caused liver damage.

References

1. Mauginello, F. P., Kok, E. and Javitt, N. B. (1977). *Ped. Res.*, **11,** 446
2. Mainl, B. (1976). *J. Surg. Res.*, **20,** 515
3. Thompson, S. W. (1974). *The Pathology of Parenteral Nutrition with Lipids.* (Springfield, Illinois) Ch. 5
4. Schumer, W. (1971). *Metabolism*, **20,** 345
5. Thomas, D. W., Edwards, J. B., Gilligan, J. E., Lawrence, J. R. and Edwards, R. J. (1972). *Med. J. Aust.*, **1,** 1238
6. Woods, H. F. and Alberti, K. G. M. M. (1972). *Lancet*, **ii,** 1354

31
The importance of parenteral nutrition as an adjunct to cancer treatment

E. M. COPELAND III AND S. J. DUDRICK

INTRODUCTION

Basal energy requirements are between 1300 and 1500 kcal/day and are increased by most illnesses which alter the metabolic demand for energy substrates. Cancer does not appear to significantly increase basal energy requirements; but chemotherapy, radiation therapy and surgery limit nutritional intake for varying periods of time, and repeated therapy can lead eventually to undernutrition. Chemotherapy and abdominal radiation almost always result in a loss of appetite, and often produce nausea and vomiting throughout weeks of treatment. No doubt a growing neoplasm extracts nutrients from the host and can result in host catabolism, particularly if the host does not ingest nutrients in quantities sufficient to supply the demands of the host and the neoplasm. Absorption of foodstuffs via a functional gastrointestinal tract is the best means of obtaining adequate nutrition; however, delivery of nutrients to the gut does not always result in rapid restoration of nutrition in the malnourished patient. In severe undernutrition, the gastrointestinal columnar mucosal cells become cuboidal, and the brush border is reduced in height. Decreased production of mucosal cells and decreased migration from the crypts occurs, gastrointestinal motility diminishes and overgrowth of facultative and anaerobic bacteria results[1]. Absorption of protein, fat and glucose may be greatly impaired. All of these morphological, microbiological and absorptive abnormalities are reversible following enteral protein-calorie replenishment. The process, however, is slow because adequate enteral nutrients are poorly absorbed at first, and the uncomfortable symptoms of nausea, diarrhea, bloating and abdominal pain limit the patient's desire to eat or obtain nutrients via nasogastric, gastrostomy or jejunostomy feeding tubes. Thus, malnutrition can result in a spectrum of malabsorptive defects and can produce a vicious cycle in that malnutrition begets malabsorption which limits the patient's capacity to digest and assimilate the necessary nutrients to correct nutritional deficits and overcome malabsorption.

The importance of the relationship between nutrition and disease has been recognized for many years, but not until the successful clinical application of intravenous hyperalimentation[2] and chemically defined (elemental)[3] diets did the physician have the ability to favourably alter this relationship in the seriously ill patient. Nutritional replenishment is now possible in almost all patients. The significant roles that amino acids, carbohydrates, vitamins, minerals and fats play in the management of chronic illnesses are being recognized and appreciated. Although cancer is not truly a chronic illness, the disease and the treatment do extract an identifiable and measurable nutritional toll from the patient. Using intravenous hyperalimentation, the importance of nutritional rehabilitation of the patient with cancer both before, during and after treatment is now being evaluated. Intravenous nutritional replenishment has interrupted the vicious cycle created by malnutrition because adequate nutrients can be provided as adjuvant support during therapy, and, if the cancer responds to treatment, appetite returns and weight gain is maintained.

Observations made by our group during the treatment of patients with head and neck malignancies would suggest that the gastrointestinal absorptive defects associated with malnutrition might be corrected by intravenous nutritional support. Three patients with severe malnutrition 4–6 weeks after major head and neck surgical procedures were unable to tolerate any oral food. The administration of various blenderized regular diets, formula diets or chemically defined diets caused profuse diarrhoea. These patients were fed intravenously and during 4–5 weeks, strength and general well-being improved. After nutritional rehabilitation, they were able to absorb, assimilate and digest regular foodstuffs since enteral feeding resulted in one or two formed bowel movements per day and in maintenance of weight.

The metabolic relationships between cancer and the host are not fully understood. Once cancer disseminates, there appears to be a direct correlation between the volume of cancer and the magnitude of weight loss. To explain this relationship, several investigators have postulated that the tumour acts as a 'nitrogen trap' because amino acids which gain access to the tumour cells ostensibly are never released again to participate in the hosts' amino acid pool[4]. Similarly, protein-calorie malnutrition occurs in some animal-tumour models even though the animals remain in positive nitrogen balance[5]. One theory proposed to explain this observation is that energy for protein metabolism is derived from host protein stores through gluconeogenesis, and the nitrogen liberated during this process is utilized by the tumour for protein synthesis and is not available for use by the host's body, thus leading to host protein-calorie depletion[6]. Cancer cells appear to be more dependent on glycolysis as a major source of their energy supply than do normal cells, possibly because of the cancer cells' enzymatic make-up and limited oxygen supply[7]. The partial pressure of oxygen in some human cancers has been shown to be reduced by as much as 50% when compared with normal tissue. The end product of anaerobic glycolysis is lactic acid, and production of this compound results in lowering of the pH within the tumour environment. The administration of dextrose to rats bearing transplanted tumours was demonstrated to reduce tumour pH, whereas the pH in normal tissues did not change[7]. Also, lactic acid concentrations have been demonstrated to be quite high in patients with extensive tumours[8]. Reichard and his co-workers[9] have demonstrated that almost all lactic acid generated from anaerobic glucose metabolism by tumour cells enters the blood to be resynthesized into glucose by the liver. Only 2 moles of adenosine triphosphate (ATP) are generated by glycolysis, and 6 moles of ATP are required by the liver to resynthesize glucose from lactic acid. Therefore, the metabolism of 1 mole of glucose by the cancer is accomplished at the expense of 8 moles of ATP from the host because the 2 moles of ATP generated by tumour metabolism are not available for host use, and 6 moles of ATP are required from the host for lactic acid metabolism. Inherent in this negative energy system is the fact that for each mole of glucose metabolized by the tumour, a mole of glucose is lost to the host for energy metabolism via the tricarboxylic acid cycle.

The metabolic rate of cancer cells is probably fixed within a narrow range of adaptability, and host anabolism can be achieved if nutrients are supplied in quantities necessary to meet the requirements of the host and the cancer. In an attempt to further define the effect of nutritional repletion on host and tumour metabolism, Ota and co-workers[10] investigated the effects of protein depletion and subsequent repletion on host liver enzymes and protein content, and compared these effects with those obtained from a Morris hepatoma growing as a transplant in the flank of a Buffalo rat. Protein-depleted, tumour-bearing rats were randomly put into three groups and either continued to ingest a protein-free diet, resumed a regular protein diet or were fed intravenously. Host and tumour metabolism were evaluated by measuring fructose-1,6-diphosphatase (FDPase), an enzyme in the gluconeogenic pathway between pyruvate and glucose, and by measuring glutamate-oxaloacetate transaminase (GOT) and glutamate-pyruvate transaminase (GPT). These latter two enzymes specifically degrade aspartate and alanine to oxaloacetate and pyruvate, respectively. In the protein-depleted host liver, FDPase activity was elevated significantly, whereas protein content, and GOT and GPT activities, were significantly reduced. Protein repletion by either intravenous feeding or a regular protein diet converted all of these activities toward normal. Depressed protein content in the host liver during protein depletion indicates that the host liver is giving up its protein for other uses. Increase in the FDPase activity indicates that one of these functions is to form new glucose. The low transaminase activity in the livers of the protein-depleted rats suggests that the amino acid enzyme-degrading pathways are reduced in order to conserve the diminished hepatic protein reserves. In the hepatoma, FDPase activity and protein content were unchanged by varying the protein in the diet, but GOT and GPT activities were increased significantly after a period of protein depletion. The tumour apparently had the ability to obtain the necessary protein moieties in order to maintain protein content even when host protein intake was negligible. Possibly, the increase in tumour GOT and GPT activities might represent a compensation by the tumour for the protein deficiency of the host. If so, the hepatoma might be in a better condition than the host liver to compete actively for amino acids to be utilized as energy substrates and nitrogen sources. Although protein repletion had no effect on tumour FDPase activity or protein content, GOT and GPT activities were lowered significantly. These data suggest that nutritional repletion of the malnourished host can result in more normal gluconeogenic enzyme activities and return of host protein stores to normal, while potentially decreasing tumour utilization of alanine and aspartic acid.

Cancer was once thought to unmask 'latent diabetes' and cause abnormal glucose tolerance secondary to depressed insulin output[11]. Malnutrition results in a similar pattern of abnormal glucose metabolism. Solomon *et al.*[12] investigated the possibility that the mild diabetes thought to be induced by cancer might actually reflect a state of malnutrition rather than cancer growth. These investigators studied eight malnourished patients with metastatic cancer. Oral glucose tolerance tests were done before intravenous nutritional repletion and after 7–10 days of intravenous nutritional therapy. Immunoreactive, serum growth hormone and insulin levels were determined. The results were compared with values from a group of fifteen normal subjects of similar ages. Of the eight cancer patients, five showed diabetic glucose tolerance tests before intravenous feeding, and each test returned toward normal afterwards. Six patients had a hypoinsulinaemic response to glucose load before, but insulin levels returned to normal after intravenous feeding. Fasting levels of growth hormone (GH) were elevated in five of the eight patients, and short-term intravenous feeding reduced these levels towards normal. Similarly, the paradoxical rise in GH following glucose load was reduced after nutritional repletion. These data confirm the altered glucose metabolism associated with cancer; however, all of these patients had an altered nutritional status secondary to their disease process, and nutritional repletion resulted in more normal glucose metabolism. In this small series of patients, it is likely that malnutrition contributed much more to the unmasking of 'latent diabetes' than did cancer growth.

The clinical situation encountered commonly is that of a malnourished patient who is immunosuppressed and has a growing malignant neoplasm. Intravenous feeding in this clinical setting may result in at least two problems:

(1) stimulation of tumour growth by the concentrated nutritional solutions; and (2) sepsis from the indwelling central venous feeding catheters. To study the effect of intravenous feeding on tumour growth and the effect of malnutrition on immune reactivity, we sensitized a group of Buffalo rats to PPD by inoculating them with complete Freund's adjuvant. After PPD reactivity was established, a cell suspension of Morris hepatoma was injected subcutaneously into the flank of each animal. When the tumour reached 1 cm in size, the animals were placed on a high carbohydrate, protein-free diet. They began almost immediately to lose weight, and after 2 weeks, 70% of the animals had negative reactions to PPD. This experimental model of weight loss, viable growing tumour and absence of a delayed cutaneous hypersensitivity response mimicked the clinical situation we were attempting to reproduce. Animals were then randomly put into three dietary groups: (1) continued high carbohydrate, protein-free diet, (2) normal rat chow diet, or (3) intravenous hyperalimentation. After 1 week on these diets, the rats again were injected with PPD and 48 h later they were killed. No animals fed the protein-free diet regained PPD reactivity, whereas almost all animals receiving the normal oral or intravenous diet became PPD reactive at the end of 1 week. All rats in the protein-free diet group continued to lose weight (average −23 g), and the average tumour weight at death was 9.9 g. Animals on normal diet also continued to lose weight (average −17 g), and tumour weight at death was 11.7 g. Rats fed intravenously gained weight (average +14 g), and average tumour weight at death was 12.9 g. Although tumours in the nutritionally repleted animals were larger, tumour weight to body weight ratios were not significantly different in all groups. Thus, tumour growth had not been stimulated out of proportion to the non-tumour host nutritional repletion by either a normal or intravenous diet. Moreover, the animals fed intravenously gained weight, whereas animals on normal diet continued their gradual decline in weight. Nevertheless, both nutritional repletion groups looked much healthier and were more vigorous than the protein-free diet animals and were immunocompetent[13].

From these animal studies, we extrapolated that the use of intravenous hyperalimentation in human beings was predictably safe and potentially efficacious. Dudrick and co-workers[14] have shown previously that proper aseptic management of the indwelling catheters and the intravenous delivery system, and aseptic mixing of the solutions by the pharmacist minimized septic complications to an acceptable level in a non-cancer patient population. Utilizing the same techniques, intravenous feeding was used to treat ninety-three patients with a wide variety of malignant diseases[15]. At the termination, each catheter tip was cultured for anaerobic and aerobic bacteria and fungi. The average period of central venous catheterization was 24.8 days, and one-half of the patients in this study received chemotherapy. Leucocyte counts below 2500 cells/mm^3 occurred in 50% of the patients and lasted for an average of 7.2 days. No organisms were grown from the catheters in place for less than 10 days, and eight positive cultures (7.3%) were obtained from catheters in place longer than 10 days. In only two patients could the catheter be incriminated as the source of infection (2.2%), and in both patients, *Candida albicans* was cultured from the catheter and the blood stream. This low rate of microbial complications showed that intravenous feeding could be used successfully in cancer patients if strict adherence to aseptic techniques was effected. Each of these ninety-three patients was considered a poor candidate for any form of oncologic therapy because of the increased risk of complications during treatment due to malnutrition. Nevertheless, these patients tolerated a therapeutic course of chemotherapy or radiation therapy or a major surgical procedure which might have been potentially fatal without nutritional rehabilitation.

No doubt, the low rate of microbial complications was secondary to proper technique, but return to normal function of an immune system depressed because of malnutrition might have been partially responsible. In an attempt to define what part malnutrition plays in immune suppression associated with cancer therapy, forty-seven cancer patients who were malnourished or whose treatment would result in malnutrition were skin tested during intravenous nutritional replenishment[16]. All patients received 0.1 ml each of dermatophytin, dermatophytin-O, Varidase, mumps and PPD skin test antigens intradermally into the forearm prior to the initiation of intravenous feeding and at 7-day intervals throughout treatment by chemotherapy, radiation therapy or surgery. Skin tests were read 48 h after injection, and a reaction of 10 $\times$ 10 mm of induration was considered a positive result. Previous negative results were considered to have converted to positive if at least 10 $\times$ 10 mm induration existed and if there was a 100% increase in the diameter of induration when compared with reactions before treatment. Of the twenty-three patients who received chemotherapy, seventeen initially had negative skin tests. Thirteen of these patients converted at least one skin test to positive in an average period of 11.4 $\pm$ 5.5 days of parenteral nutrition. The average weight gain was 6.5 $\pm$ 6.0 lb. The patients received parenteral nutrition for 2–7 days prior to starting chemotherapy, and eleven patients converted skin tests to positive during chemotherapy administration. Of the evaluable patients who converted skin tests to positive, 40% responded to chemotherapy, and 75% of evaluable patients who retained positive skin reactivity responded to chemotherapy. However, none of the patients whose skin tests remained negative during parenteral nutrition responded to chemotherapy.

Ten patients received intravenous feeding as support during major surgical procedures. The six patients who had positive skin tests both preoperatively and postoperatively had an uncomplicated postoperative recovery. Three patients had negative tests throughout treatment, and one patient's skin tests converted from positive to negative postoperatively. Two of these negative reactors died postoperatively, and the other two had prolonged postoperative recovery periods complicated by pneumonia, ileus and lassitude. Of seven patients who received radiation therapy, five continued to have negative tests throughout the course and two had tests that converted from positive to negative. Nutritional repletion during radiation therapy was considered satisfactory in each of these patients as indicated by an average weight gain of 5.8 ± 2.9 lb during an average of 22.4 ± 7.4 days of parenteral nutrition, and a rise in serum albumin concentration from an average of 3.0 ± 0.3 g% to 3.4 ± 0.2 g% ($P < 0.025$). There were no septic complications in any of the forty-seven patients whose skin test became positive or remained positive during treatment. From these data, four trends were apparent:

1. Absence of established delayed hypersensitivity in the cancer patient who is treated with chemotherapy may be secondary to malnutrition, and established cell-mediated immunity may be restored by proper nutritional replenishment.
2. Only those patients who developed or retained positive skin tests responded to chemotherapy.
3. Patients with positive skin tests preoperatively had an uncomplicated postoperative recovery, whereas 50% of the patients with negative tests died and the remainder had a prolonged period of recovery complicated by multiple septic episodes.
4. During radiation therapy, no patient maintained or developed positive skin tests, although weight gain and tumour response were obtained.

Parenteral nutrition was responsible for nutritional repletion which, in turn, was probably responsible for the return of positive skin test reactivity. If the body's immune mechanism is expected to eliminate those cancer cells remaining after oncologic therapy, it should be provided with the nutritional prerequisites to react properly.

The conclusion from the animal experiments and limited studies in human beings was that intravenous hyperalimentation results in host nutritional repletion without a disproportionate stimulation of tumour growth. Septic complications are uncommon if a proper aseptic technique is observed. Immunocompetence returns in many malnourished cancer patients whose treatment programmes include chemotherapy and surgery.

CLINICAL MATERIAL

In the past 4 years, more than 1000 adult patients have received intravenous nutrition as adjuvant therapy for malignant diseases at the M. D. Anderson Hospital and Tumor Institute. Nutritional depletion was defined as a recent loss of 10 lb or more of body weight, a serum albumin level of less than 3.4 g% and/or a negative reaction to a battery of recall skin test antigens. Patients who satisfied these criteria and who had a reasonable chance of responding to appropriate oncologic therapy were candidates for intravenous feeding. Similarly, patients who had been treated previously and were incapable of adequate enteral nutrition because of the malnutrition imposed by previous therapy were candidates for intravenous rehabilitation. Also, nutritionally healthy patients whose treatment plan necessitated multiple courses of chemotherapy, possibly combined with radiation therapy or surgery, were candidates in order to maintain their optimal nutritional status during treatment. The use of parenteral nutrition in this latter group of 'healthy' patients has allowed the safe delivery of intensive chemotherapy and radiation therapy without weight loss, and major complications have been reduced.

The response to chemotherapy or radiation therapy was defined as a 50% or greater reduction in measurable malignant tissue mass. With the exception of patients with cancer of the colon who received high doses of 5-fluorouracil (5-FU), no attempt was made to administer maximum tolerated doses of chemotherapy, but rather a dose which was considered therapeutic. Intravenous hyperalimentation was used as described previously, and insertion of the subclavian vein catheters and management of the regimen were the responsibility of the nutritional care team[17].

CHEMOTHERAPY

Intravenous hyperalimentation was utilized as an adjunct to chemotherapy in 175 patients[18] (Figures 31.1 and 31.2) and was used for an average period of 22.8 days resulting in an average weight gain of 5.6 lb. Often, the patients did not need to go home between courses of chemotherapy to recover nutritionally because nutrition was maintained intravenously, and the next course of chemotherapy could begin immediately following return of the leucocyte count to normal, usually in about 7–10 days. A tumour response was obtained in 27.8% of the patients (Table 31.1). Responding patients survived an average period of 8.2 months, whereas patients who did not respond survived

Table 31.1 Tumor response

Site of origin	*No. of patients*	*Percentage response*
Breast	18	25
Lung	34	29
Testicle	34	50
Gastrointestinal tract (no 5-FU)	9	11
Gastrointestinal tract (5-FU)	16	31
Head and neck	16	30
Lymphoma	12	25
Leukaemia	10	20
Sarcoma	13	23
Miscellaneous	13	20

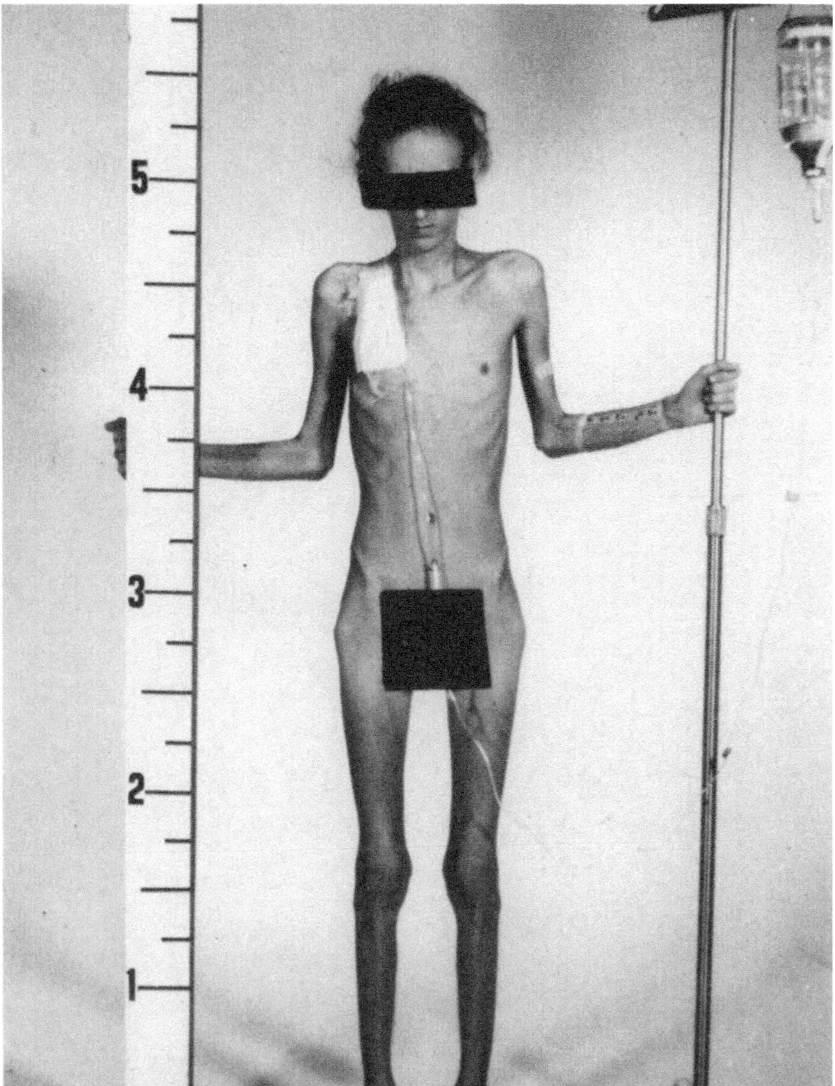

Figure 31.1 Seventeen-year-old male with acute lymphoblastic leukaemia was treated with multiple courses of vincristine and prednisone without remission. Subsequently, three courses of adriamycin and Ara-C were given and were followed by severe myelosuppression and multiple infections each time. Prior to the last course of chemotherapy, bone marrow cellularity responded with a fall in lymphoblasts from 92% to 24%, but the patient had lost weight from 122 lb to 88 lb

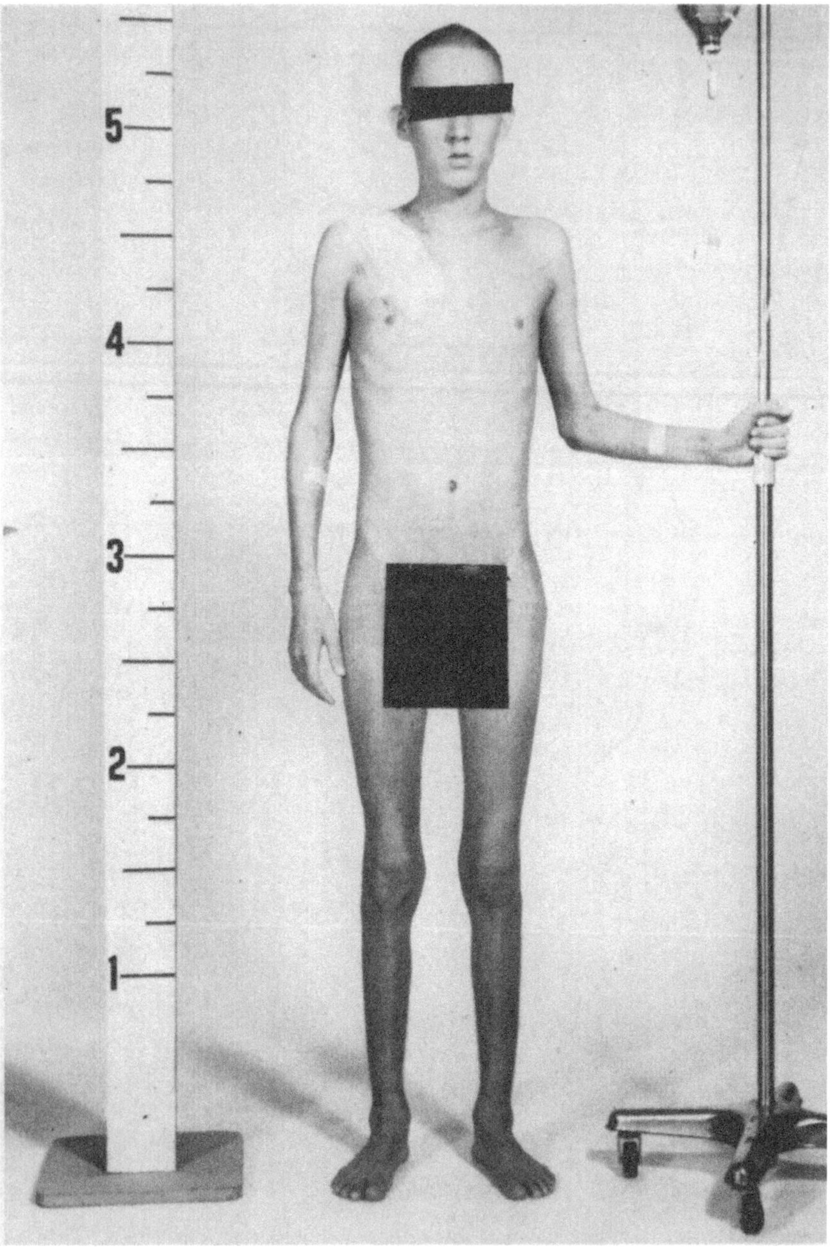

Figure 31.2 Intravenous hyperalimentation was begun, and during the next 40 days, the patient gained 21 lb while receiving the fourth course of adriamycin and Ara-C. He was discharged with 21% lymphoblasts in the bone marrow and was eating a normal diet

only 1.9 months. Only those patients whose malignant diseases were potentially responsive to chemotherapy were selected for intravenous hyperalimentation. Patients who had received all reasonable oncologic treatment and failed to respond were not considered. As a preventive measure against malnutrition, intravenous feeding and chemotherapy were begun almost simultaneously; however, if significant malnutrition existed before chemotherapy, then intravenous feeding was administered at least 7–10 days prior to beginning chemotherapy. Whether or not mucositis and the symptoms of nausea and general malaise were reduced during parenteral nutrition depended somewhat upon the chemotherapeutic regimens employed. For example, gastrointestinal symptoms secondary to 5-FU administration were reduced, whereas vinblastine and bleomycin continued to produce severe stomatitis. Leucocyte depression below 2500 cells/mm^3 occurred in 51.5% of patients for an average duration of 7.7 days. Neither the nadir nor duration of leucocyte depression appeared to be affected by nutritional support. Only four pathogenic organisms were cultured from 212 consecutive subclavian vein catheters. Only three patients had simultaneous positive blood and catheter cultures, and the incidence of catheter-related sepsis was 1.4%.

There was a positive correlation between nutritional status and response to chemotherapy in thirty-five patients with non-oat cell carcinoma of the lung who received the same treatment (bleomycin, cyclophosphamide, 5-FU, methotrexate and vincristine)[19]. Our hyperalimentation team was asked to evaluate and replenish fifteen of these patients nutritionally prior to and during chemotherapy. Each patient had lost more than 15% of his body weight prior to treatment. Seven patients responded to chemotherapy and experienced an average weight gain of 8% while receiving intravenous nutrition. Patients who did not respond increased their weight an average of only 2%. The remaining twenty patients in this series were not treated by the hyperalimentation team. Twelve of these patients had lost more than 6% of their usual body weight and did not respond to chemotherapy. The other eight patients had lost less than 6% of their usual body weight, and six of these patients did respond to chemotherapy. Thus, 75% of the patients with good nutritional status responded to chemotherapy, whereas no nutritionally depleted patients responded. When nutritionally depleted patients were restored, 47% responded. The better responses of the patients in good nutritional condition could not be explained on the basis of doses or courses of chemotherapy or by the distribution of histologic tumour types, symptom status, prior treatment or metastatic sites. The results imply that responses were achieved in patients who were adequately nourished at the outset of chemotherapy or who were nutritionally replenished during chemotherapy.

Since the advent of parenteral nutrition and the concept of 'bowel rest', it has been possible to reduce significantly the mechanical, physical and chemical trauma produced by the passage of food, digestive juices and faeces through the gastrointestinal tract. Application of intravenous nutrition as an adjunct to cancer chemotherapy with 5-FU should theoretically reduce both the incidence and the degree of severity of gastrointestinal toxicity. The concept of increased tolerance to 5-FU during bowel rest and nutritional maintenance was tested initially in Sprague-Dawley rats[20]. Two groups of rats received 5-FU in doses of 15 mg/kg/day intraperitoneally for 7 days. One group of rats was nourished entirely intravenously, and the other group was allowed to eat by mouth *ad libitum*. All orally fed rats were obviously ill by the third day of 5-FU injection, and 80% were dead by the tenth day of the experiment. Two surviving rats were killed on day 21, and microscopic evaluation of the small and large bowel showed necrosis of the villi, a marked inflammatory response and mucosal ulceration. In the group of rats receiving all their nutrients by vein, the first death was recorded on the sixth day; and by the tenth day of the experiment, 67% of the rats were still alive. All symptoms and signs of toxicity had abated by the seventh day. The average weight loss of the animals in this group was only 10%, and autopsies of the surviving animals killed on day 21 showed only nonspecific gastrointestinal lymphoid hyperplasia with no pathologic changes in the villi or mucosa.

Results of this experiment stimulated us to initiate a chemotherapeutic programme of 5-FU therapy in malnourished patients who had been nutritionally replenished intravenously. The limits of tolerance for 5-FU infused as the maximum recommended dose were studied in twenty-six cachectic, poor-risk patients with identifiable metastatic adenocarcinoma of the colon[18]. Sixteen of these patients were started on intravenous feeding 7 days prior to instituting 5-FU (15 mg/kg/day in 50 ml of 5% dextrose in water) infused daily over a 1 h interval. As in the rat experiments, drug toxicity was manifested initially by mild diarrhoea, often accompanied by stomatitis and nausea. These symptoms cleared within 24 h of discontinuing 5-FU therapy. The average total dose of 5-FU administered was 7.4 g during an average period of 8.6 days of treatment. Overall weight gain in these patients during 5-FU administration and parenteral nutrition was 8.5 lb, and five patients (31%) responded with a greater than 50% reduction in measurable tumour volume. The administration of 5-FU had no effect on weight gain and nitrogen balance once positive nitrogen balance was established. Perineal, pulmonary, sacral and intra-abdominal metastases were among the responding lesions. The ten patients not given intravenous nutrition lost an average of 4.2 lb during 5-FU administration and experienced vomiting, nausea, diarrhoea and stomatitis in an average of only 4.4 days of chemotherapy. The average total dose of 5-FU administered to these control patients was 3.8 g. Only one control patient responded to chemotherapy. All non-responding patients were dead within 3 months of treatment, whereas the average survival time for responding patients was 9.4 months. Conclusions from this study must be guarded because the patient groups were small; nonetheless, the application of 'bowel rest' and total parenteral nutrition did appear to increase the tolerance to 5-FU both in rats and man. Moreover, those malnourished patients who were replenished nutritionally prior to 5-FU experienced a greater response to chemotherapy (31%) than did those patients who were not replenished (10%). These results are similar to those obtained in the group of patients with non-oat cell carcinoma of the lung treated with a common chemotherapy protocol and concomitant intravenous feeding referred to earlier.

Parenteral nutrition has been used as a prophylaxis against weight loss induced by treatment with vinblastine and bleomycin[18]. Using this combination and parenteral nutrition, a 50% complete response rate has been obtained in a group of adult, nutritionally healthy males with metastatic embryonal cell carcinoma of the testicle. Throughout multiple back-to-back chemotherapy courses, weight loss was prevented and strength was maintained even though symptoms of stomatitis and general malaise were severe. When these data were compared with tumour response data in similar patients with the same disease treated according to the same drug protocol but who did not receive intravenous nutrition, it was noted that the response rates were the same, as were the survival times of the responding patients; however, the survival times of the non-responding intravenously fed patients were significantly greater than those of the non-responding patients who did not receive intravenous nutrition during chemotherapy. In the latter group, weight loss from 10 to 40 lb occurred during chemotherapy, and these patients were exposed to the side effects of nutritional depletion as well as advancing malignant disease. Undoubtedly, the patients who were nutritionally sound could deal better with the problems of increasing tumour mass than could their debilitated counterparts, and thus then enjoyed a longer survival. There was no difference in the response rates between the fed and starved patients, probably because both groups were intact nutritionally at the beginning of treatment. The importance of intravenous hyperalimentation in this study was the prevention of profound weight loss secondary to the toxic effects produced by high doses of the chemotherapeutic drugs used.

SURGERY

One hundred patients received intravenous feeding preoperatively and/or postoperatively as nutritional support for a general or thoracic surgical procedure[18]. Major organ resection or bowel anastomoses were performed in sixty-six of these patients, whereas thirty-four patients underwent palliative or diagnostic procedures involving major surgical intervention (Figures 31.3 and 31.4). Fifty-two percent of the patients had curative resections which included total gastrectomy, oesophagectomy and abdomino-perineal resections (Table 31.2). Without intravenous nutritional rehabilitation, recovery from these surgical procedures would have been questionable. The average age of the patients was 56.5 years, intravenous feeding was given for an average period of 24.2 days, and the average weight gain was 4.2 lb. In

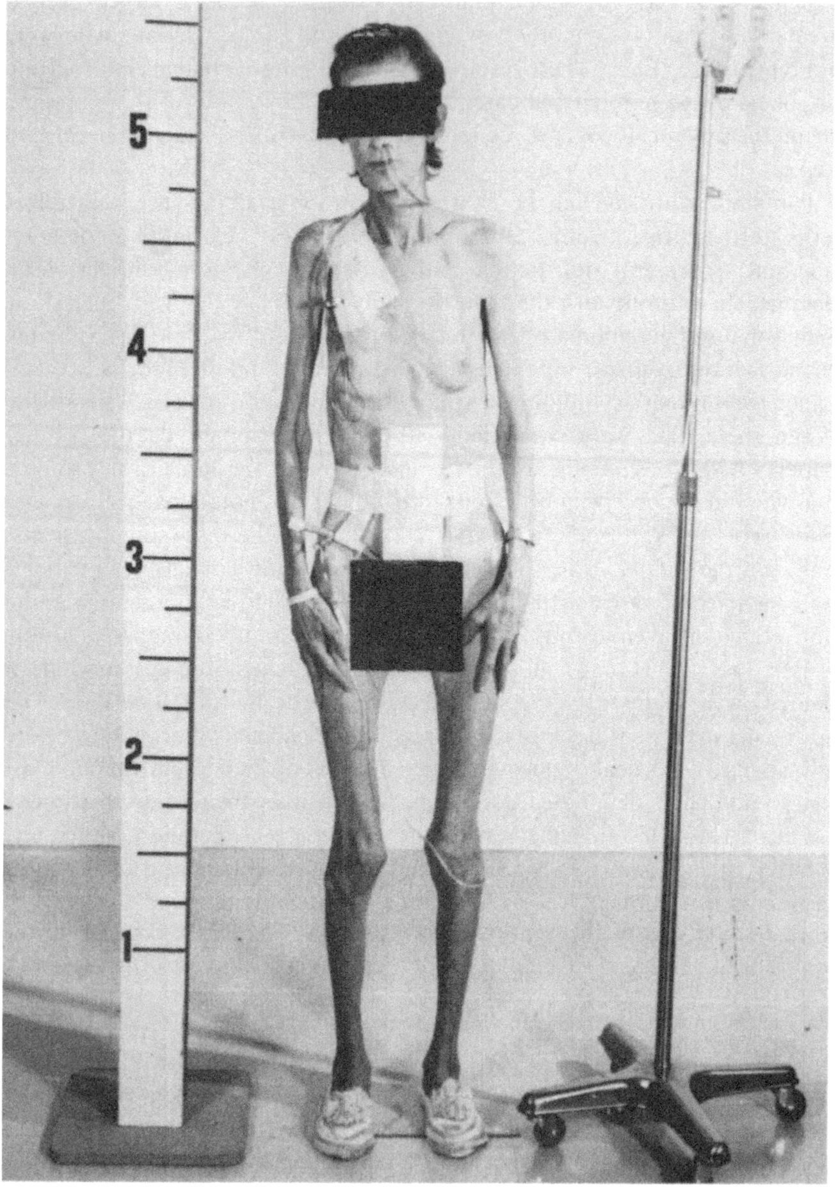

Figure 31.3 A 48-year-old woman had a partially obstructing squamous cell carcinoma of the upper one-third of the oesophagus treated with 6000 r in 6 weeks. Prior to radiotherapy, she had lost weight from 112 lb to 102 lb, and her serum albumin concentration was 3.6 g%. She was given chemically defined liquid diets during treatment, and by the end of radiotherapy, she weighed 96 lb and her serum albumin was 3.2 g%. Friability of the oesophagus prevented dilation, and 4 months later her weight had fallen to 76 lb and her serum albumin was 3.1 g%. A Stamm gastrostomy was performed, but 6 days postoperatively the wound dehisced and the gastrostomy feedings regurgitated around the tube. The patient weighed 76 lb and her serum albumin was 2.8 g%

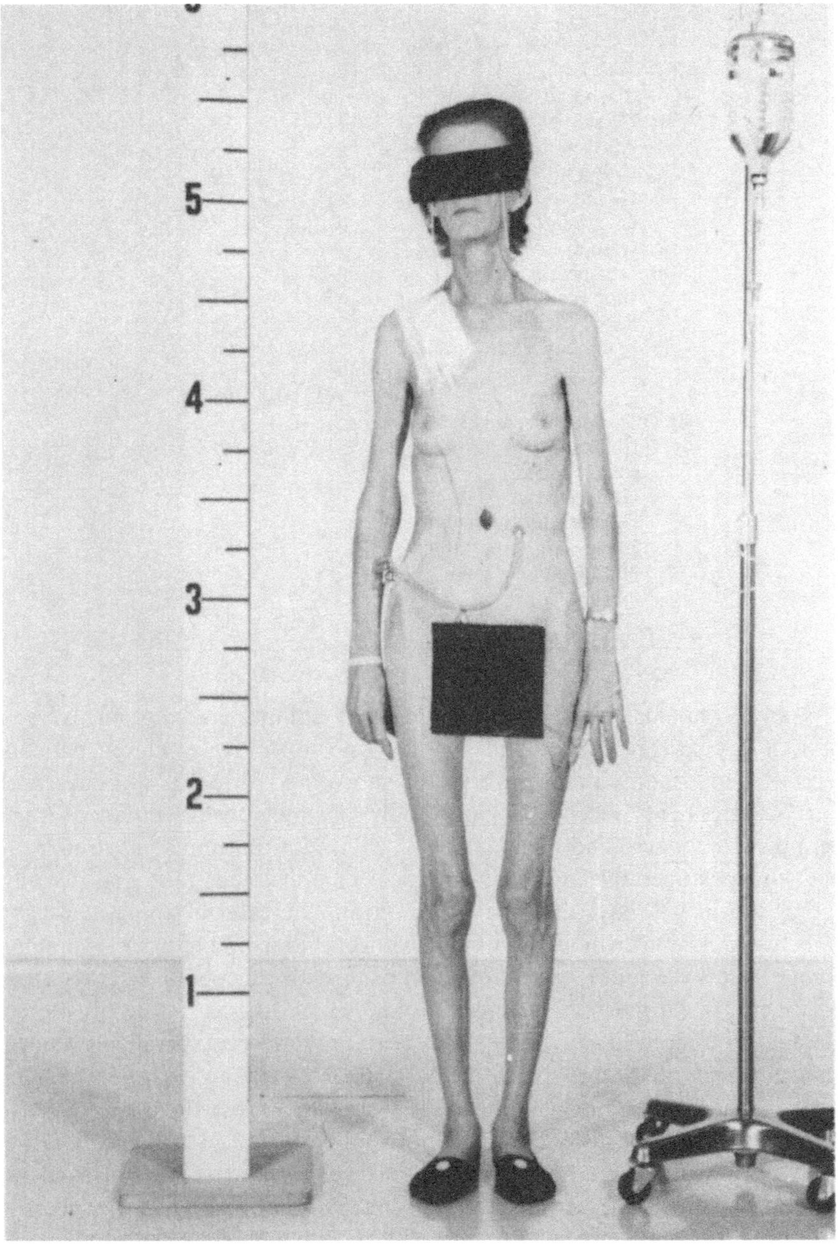

Figure 31.4 The nutritional care team was consulted, and parenteral nutrition commenced, over the next 18 days she gained 12 lb in weight and the serum albumin rose to 3.2 g%. The fistula tract around the gastrostomy tube healed, and tube feedings became practical by the eighth day of therapy. The wound dehiscence healed without operation. The patient was discharged on tube feedings, and 2 months later weighed 104 lb. Serum albumin concentration had risen to 4.1 g%

Table 31.2

Surgical procedure		*No. of patients*
A. Major organ resection or anastomosis		
Colectomy		14
Abdominoperineal resection		8
Colon interposition		10
Gastrectomy		10
Gastroenterostomy		9
Oesophagogastrectomy		5
Oesophagectomy		2
Whipple's operation		3
Pelvic exenteration		2
Small bowel resection		3
	Total	66
B. Diagnostic or palliative		
Colostomy		10
Biliary bypass		2
Gastrostomy		4
Celestin tube insertion		4
Exploratory laparotomy		13
Hip disarticulation		1
	Total	34

fifty-seven patients, intravenous feeding was administered for an average of 12.3 days preoperatively and 13.9 days postoperatively. Eleven patients received support only preoperatively for an average period of 18.1 days, and thirty-two patients received support only postoperatively for an average period of 18.9 days. Those patients who received intravenous nutrition both pre- and postoperatively had few surgical complications and were usually eating within 4–5 days after bowel resection. Increase in strength, weight gain, a significant rise in serum albumin concentration and return of immunocompetence were much easier to accomplish with preoperative rather than postoperative intravenous feeding (Table 31.3). Forty-six of the fifty-seven patients who received intravenous nutrition pre- and postoperatively gained an average of 8.0 lb during treatment; 11 patients lost an average of 3.8 lb. Average serum albumin concentration before treatment for those patients who gained weight was 3.23 ± 0.41 g% and rose to 3.77 ± 0.79 g% ($P <$ 0.05) prior to surgery. Postoperatively, at the termination of intravenous nutrition, the average serum albumin concentration was 3.45 ± 0.60 g%. The eleven patients who lost weight had an initial average serum albumin concentration of 2.84 ± 0.71 g% which rose to 3.24 ± 0.62 g% (not significant) immediately prior to operation. Serum albumin level was unchanged at the termination of intravenous feeding postoperatively. In patients who received parenteral nutrition both pre- and postoperatively, there were increases in weight and serum albumin during the preoperative period, but there was no further increase in serum albumin or weight postoperatively; in fact, when weight loss occurred, it was in the postoperative period. Thus, nutritional repletion and rehabilitation were much easier to accomplish preoperatively rather than postoperatively when one of the complications of malnutrition, such as an anastomotic breakdown or fistula, occurred. The patients' failure to gain weight postoperatively might be indicative of the magnitude of stress associated with surgery, and without intravenous nutrition weight loss and major complications would have been expected

Table 31.3 Weight and serum albumin changes

A. PRE- AND POSTOPERATIVE

	No. of Patients	△ *Weight (lb)*	*Serum albumin (g %)*† *Before IVH (Column 1)*	*Before surgery (Column 2)*	*After IVH (Column 3)*
Weight gain	46	+7.96	*3.23 ± 0.51	3.77 ± 0.79	3.45 ± 0.60
Weight loss	11	−3.82	**2.84 ± 0.71	3.24 ± 0.62	3.34 ± 0.69

*Weight gain: Column 1 vs. Column 2, $P < 0.005$; Column 2 vs. Column 3, $P > 0.05$; Column 1 vs. Column 3, $0.05 < P < 0.10$

**Weight loss: No significant differences between Column 1 and Column 2 or Column 2 and Column 3; Column 1 vs. Column 3, $0.05 < P < 0.10$

B. PRE- OR POSTOPERATIVE

	No. of patients	△ *Weight (lb)*	*Serum albumin (g %)*† *Before IVH*	*After IVH*
Preoperative only	11	+7.73	3.32 ± 0.37	3.50 ± 0.44 (NS)
Postoperative only				
Weight gain	16	+5.86	2.72 ± 0.59	3.44 ± 0.51 ($P < 0.01$)
Weight loss	16	−4.47	3.25 ± 0.52	3.11 ± 0.11 (NS)

IVH = Intravenous feeding
NS = Not significant
† An average of 15 g of exogenous serum albumin was given intravenously to surgical patients daily, but exogenous administration did not necessarily correlate with a rise in serum albumin concentration

because of the degree of malnutrition. Because these patients had so few surgical complications, we recommend that measures to correct malnutrition be instituted before operation instead of waiting until a catastrophic post-operative complication has occurred. Four patients in this series died. Two died of pneumonia: one patient had undergone a right colectomy and died 13 days later; the other patient had undergone an oesophagectomy and died 21 days postoperatively. Two patients died of myocardial infarctions, 4 and 14 days postoperatively, following exploratory laparotomy and bypass of a radiation-related enteric fistula. Thus, the mortality rate in these 100 consecutive surgical patients was only 4%, a low figure considering the magnitude of the surgical procedures and the debilitated condition of these patients. Only one patient had a simultaneous positive blood and catheter culture.

FISTULAE

Our experience with the management of fistulae in cancer patients has been rewarding. Fistulae present several unique problems because there may be cancer within the fistula tract, the fistula may involve an area of irradiated bowel or abdominal wall, and the patient's life expectancy may be so short that the physician does not think that the time needed to heal the fistula is justified unless the fistula is life-threatening. Overall, twenty-three patients with gastrointestinal fistulae have been treated with parenteral nutrition. Spontaneous closures have occurred in 44% of these patients, and after closure was achieved, each patient was discharged from the hospital and was able to lead a productive life for a time. In two patients, spontaneous closure occurred even though malignant disease was present in biopsies from the fistula tract. Six of the patients developed pharyngocutaneous fistulas after radical head and neck surgery. Two of these fistulas closed spontaneously after 17 and 20 days of intravenous feeding. The remaining four fistulae were closed surgically after 21–47 days of nutritional support, and the average weight gain during this period was 15 lb. In three patients, attempted surgical closure had failed prior to instituting intravenous feeding. Fistula management was easier during parenteral nutrition because salivary and mucosal secretions decreased when the nasogastric feeding tubes were removed[18].

NUTRITIONAL SUPPORTIVE CARE

Ten patients were admitted to the hospital for nutritional supportive care 1.5–24 months following major head and neck surgical procedures or radiation therapy. Intravenous hyperalimentation was used for an average period of 25.1 days, and the patients achieved an average weight gain of 8.7 lb. Four patients were discharged eventually from the hospital on nasogastric tube feeding regimens, two patients required gastrostomy feeding during long-term ambulatory nutritional maintenance, and four patients who responded favourably to head and neck muscular rehabilitation were discharged and were able to ingest food orally.

Rehabilitation after head and neck radiation therapy is important to prevent temporomandibular joint fibrosis and to strengthen the muscles of mastication. If the patient fails to perform his exercises, eating may become progressively more difficult and painful as jaw function becomes limited. Five patients received intravenous nutritional support during the convalescent period while rehabilitation of jaw function was accomplished. It was psychologically easier for these poorly motivated patients to be nutritionally rehabilitated if they were not burdened by nasogastric feeding tubes.

Three patients had pharyngeal incompetence following either a partial glossectomy, posterior pharyngeal wall resection or tongue excision. Pharyngeal incompetence was thought to be secondary to muscle weakness and reversible muscle injury. Deglutitory muscular rehabilitation was begun while nutrition was maintained intravenously. Weight gain of 8–26 lb was achieved and, concomitant with the return of general body muscle strength and tone, swallowing returned after 18–48 days of intravenous nutritional support[21].

Twenty-four patients were admitted to the hospital specifically for convalescent nutritional rehabilitation[18]. Seventeen of these patients had completed a course of chemotherapy or radiation therapy as outpatients and were unable to recover from the inanition that occurred during the therapy. Seven patients had not recovered sufficiently from a major abdominal surgical procedure before their release from the hospital and could not regain their lost weight as outpatients. Parenteral nutrition was used for a period of 13.4 days, the average weight gain was 13.9 lb, each of the twenty-four patients improved symptomatically and was discharged from the hospital capable of eating and assimilating a regular or soft diet. The vicious cycle of malnutrition–anorexia–further malnutrition was interrupted by intravenous nutrition. We do not know whether the gastrointestinal digestive and absorptive process was improved by parenteral nutrition or whether the patients were psychologically better motivated to eat because of the improvement in general well-being; in any case, hunger returned and anorexia disappeared.

RADIATION THERAPY

Trier and Browning[22] demonstrated in man that, by the end of the first week of radiation therapy, oedema began to collect in the submucosa of the bowel wall, and as radiation progressed, mucosal cells assumed a cuboidal shape, lymphocytes diminished in the lamina propria and polymorphonuclear cells accumulated in greatly increased numbers. When more than 3000 r were delivered, these lesions were still present as long as 4 months after therapy. Hugon and Bounous[23] demonstrated that the small bowel mucosa of radiated rats fed an elemental glucose–amino acid diet recovered more rapidly and had a higher mitotic index than did the small bowel mucosa of radiated rats allowed to eat regular rat chow. They postulated that radiation therapy impaired the small bowel's capacity for absorption of sugars and peptides, and a better nutritional mileu surrounded the damaged cells of the animals fed an elemental diet; also better cellular regeneration was stimulated. The delivery of calories, amino acids, vitamins and minerals intravenously should also provide appropriate nutrients for damaged mucosal cells and should aid the healing of radiation stomatitis and pharyngitis. Usually some degree of radiation enteritis or stomatitis must be accepted, in order for an adequate tumour dose of radiation therapy to be delivered to a malignancy that lies adjacent to or within the gastrointestinal tract. These patients often become anorectic, and the mucositis secondary to radiation therapy can produce pain on deglutition, crampy abdominal pain, nausea and diarrhea. The consequent oedema of the bowel wall may result in obstruction of an already partially compromised gastrointestinal lumen. The net result of acute radiation enteritis is that the patient ingests less food and is less able to digest and absorb those nutrients that do reach the small intestine.

Thirty-nine malnourished patients required treatment with intravenous hyperalimentation in order to complete a planned course of radiation therapy[24]. Intravenous feeding was used for an average period of 37.6 days, and the average weight gain was 7.8 lb. Anorexia, nausea and vomiting disappeared unless the patients attempted to eat, in which case all the symptoms recurred. The average dose of radiation delivered was 3827 r in an average of 3.5 weeks. Ninety-five percent of the patients completed their planned course of radiation therapy and improved symptomatically. Fifty-four percent of the patients responded with a greater than 50% reduction in tumour size. As with the chemotherapy patients, those patients responding to radiation therapy were able afterwards to maintain the weight gained during parenteral nutrition, but non-responding patients promptly lost weight. Responding patients gained an average of 13.0 ± 6.4 lb during intravenous nutrition (average 36.2 days) and radiation therapy (average 3832 r), whereas non-responding patients gained only 4.9 ± 8.8 lb ($P < 0.001$) (average 42.8 days) and radiation therapy (average 3819 r). Serum albumin rose from 3.12 ± 0.49 g% to 3.51 ± 0.68 g% ($P < 0.05$) during treatment of responding patients but did not rise significantly from 3.09 ± 0.48 g% in non-responding patients. The conclusions from the study of these 39 patients were: (1) parenteral nutrition allowed a planned course of radiation therapy to be delivered to a group of poor-risk, malnourished cancer patients; (2) a correlation between tumour response and nutritional status was identified; and (3) symptoms of radiation stomatitis and enteritis were reduced or eliminated as long as 'bowel rest' was maintained.

COMPLICATIONS

In a series of 406 patients, 428 consecutive catheters were cultured for anaerobic and aerobic bacteria and fungi. Pathogenic organisms grew on cultures from nineteen catheters (4.4%) (Table 31.4)[18]. However, simultaneous positive blood and catheter cultures were obtained for only ten patients (2.3%). A primary source of septicaemia other than the catheter was identified for three of these ten patients. For the remaining seven patients, temperature returned to normal within 48 h of catheter removal and antibiotics were not necessary. It was in these seven patients (1.6%) that the catheter was incriminated as the source of infection. In three of the nine remaining patients with pathogens on the catheter cultures, temperature returned to

Table 31.4

Pathogenic organism	*No. of positive cultures*
Candida tropicalis	5*†
Staphylococcus aureus	2*†
Kleb. pneumoniae	2
E. coli	2*†
Enterococcus	2†
Alpha streptococcus	1
Candida albicans	1
Proteus mirabilis	1†
Pseudomonas aeruginosa	1†
Enterobacter cloacae	1†
Corynebacterium xerosis	1
Total	19

* Simultaneous positive blood culture, same organism, temperature unchanged after catheter removal.
† Simultaneous positive blood culture, same organism, but temperature down immediately after catheter removal

normal immediately after catheter removal. The catheter could be incriminated as a cause of septicaemia in these patients even though a positive blood culture was not obtained. Therefore, at most, catheter-related sepsis occurred in only 2.3% of patients and was resolved promptly after catheter removal. In the six remaining patients whose catheter cultures grew pathogenic organisms, there were no associated febrile or septic episodes and the catheters were removed electively because of termination of intravenous feeding. Consequently, these positive catheter cultures were considered coincidental.

Four of the 406 patients developed fluid overload and transient pulmonary oedema caused by over-zealous use of peripherally administered parenteral fluids while the patients were simultaneously receiving intravenous nutrition. Since this experience, the hyperalimentation team of physicians have assumed the responsibility for all fluids prescribed for and delivered to patients on parenteral nutrition, and complications related to fluid administration have been minimized. Four patients developed subclavian vein thrombosis. The only treatment required was catheter removal, and heparinization was not necessary. Oedema of the arm resolved within 7 days of catheter removal, and no long-term sequelae were identified. Jugular vein thrombosis occurred in one patient because the tip of the catheter traversed the innominate vein to lie at the orifice of the left jugular vein. Since this complication occurred, we feel the only acceptable position for the tip of the feeding catheter is in the middle of the superior vena cava. Hyperchloraemic metabolic acidosis occurred in one patient. This complication resolved quickly after the concentration of administered chloride was reduced. One patient developed symptomatic hypophosphataemia while recovering from a head and neck surgical procedure. Metabolic complications such as these were few because of rigorous metabolic monitoring.

COMMENT

Nutritional support of patients receiving antineoplastic therapy has proved effective in allowing adequate treatment programmes to be carried out in a series of patients who otherwise might not have been candidates for any form of oncologic therapy. Tumour growth was not enhanced, and septic complications were minimal. There appeared to be a correlation between adequate nutrition and the potential for tumour response to chemotherapy. There was an increased tolerance for certain chemotherapeutic drugs, particularly 5-FU, and tumour response to these drugs might have been improved because more of the drug could be delivered per unit time. Established delayed hypersensitivity often could be restored by the proper use of intravenous hyperalimentation.

Cancer cachexia should no longer be a contraindication to adequate oncologic therapy. Adequate nutritional replenishment should be undertaken prior to the indicated antineoplastic therapy. Nutrients supplied in excess of the needs of the cancer should be available for use by the host to heal wounds, phagocytase cancer cells, repair immunologic mechanisms, replete protein stores and restore enzyme systems to normal. Malnutrition is harmful to cancer patients because a cachectic patient has a narrower safe therapeutic margin for most chemotherapy and radiation therapy. The therapeutic doses of these agents may be much closer to the lethal dose for normal tissues in the malnourished patient than in the well-nourished one. Attention to proper metabolic, physiological and nutritional repletion and maintenance can minimize the complications of oncologic therapy. Inadequate nutritional status must be recognized, and proper treatment must be individually selected for each patient. An enlightened approach to the therapy of the malnourished cancer patient is to rehabilitate him nutritionally with intravenous hyperalimentation before, during and/or after all forms of therapy whenever this goal cannot be accomplished by enteral means. With this treatment programme, optimal nutritional and antineoplastic results can be expected.

Acknowledgement

This work was supported in part by the National Institutes of Health Grants CA5831 and CA16672. Figures 31.1 and 31.2 are reproduced by courtesy of Modern Medicine Publications, Minneapolis.

References

1. Viteri, F. E. and Schneider, R. E. (1974). Gastrointestinal alterations in protein-calorie malnutrition. *Med. Clin. North Am.*, **58**, 1487

2. Dudrick, S. J., Wilmore, D. W., Vars, H. M. and Rhoads, J. E. (1969). Can intravenous feeding as the sole means of nutrition support growth in the child and restore weight loss in an adult? An affirmative answer. *Ann. Surg.*, **169**, 974
3. Greenstein, J. P., Otey, M. D., Birbaum, S. M. and Winitz, M. (1957). Quantitative nutritional studies with water soluble, chemically defined diets. *Arch. Biochem. Biophys.*, **72**, 396
4. Mider, G. B., Tesluk, H. and Morton, J. J. (1948). Effects of Walker carcinoma 256 on food intake, body weight and nitrogen metabolism of growing rat. *Acta de l'Union Inter Contre le Cancer*, **6**, 409
5. Sherman, C. D., Morton, J. J. and Mider, G. B. (1950). Potential sources of tumor nitrogen. *Cancer Res.*, **10**, 374
6. Gold, J. (1968). Proposed treatment of cancer by inhibition of gluconeogenesis. *Oncology*, **22**, 198
7. Shapot, V. S. (1972). Some biochemical aspects of the relationship between the tumor and the host. *Adv. Cancer Res.*, **15**, 253
8. Waterhouse, C. (1974). Lactate metabolism in patients with cancer. *Cancer*, **33**, 66
9. Reichard, G. A., Moury, M. J., Hochella, N. J., Patterson, A. L. and Weinhouse, S. (1963). Quantitative estimation of the Cori cycle in the human. *J. Biol. Chem.*, **238**, 495
10. Ota, D. M., Copeland, E. M., Strobel, H. W., Daly, J. M., Gum, E. T., Guinn, E. and Dudrick, S. J. (1977). The effect of protein nutrition on host and tumor metabolism. *J. Surg. Res.*, **22**, 181
11. Weisenfield, S., Hect, A., Goldner, M. G. (1962). Test of carbohydrate metabolism in carcinomatosis. *Cancer*, **15**, 18.
12. Solomon, N., Copeland, E. M., MacFadyen, B. V., Jr., Dudrick, S. J. and Samaan, N. A. (1974). Intravenous hyperalimentation and growth hormone in cancer patients. *Surg. For.*, **25**, 59
13. Daly, J. M., Copeland, E. M., Guinn, E. and Dudrick, S. J. (1976). Relationship of protein nutrition to tumor growth and host immunocompetence. *Surg. For.*, **26**, 113
14. Dudrick, S. J. and Copeland, E. M. (1973). Parenteral hyperalimentation. In Lloyd M. Nyhus (ed.). *Surgery Annual: Nineteen Seventy-Three*, pp. 69–95. (New York: Appleton-Century-Crofts)
15. Copeland, E. M., MacFadyen, B. V., Jr., McGown, C. and Dudrick, S. J. (1974). The use of hyperalimentation in patients with potential sepsis. *Surg. Gynecol. Obstet.*, **138**, 377
16. Copeland, E. M., MacFayden, B. V., Jr. and Dudrick, S. J. (1976). Effect of intravenous hyperalimentation on established delayed hypersensitivity in the cancer patient. *Ann. Surg.*, **184**, 60
17. Copeland, E. M., III, MacFadyen, B. V., Jr., Lanzotti, V. J. and Dudrick, S. J. (1976). Nutritional care of the cancer patient. In R. Lee Clark and C. D. Howe (eds.). *Cancer Patient Care at M. D. Anderson Hospital and Tumor Institute*, pp. 607–628. (Chicago: Year Book Medical Publishers, Inc.)
18. Copeland, E. M. and Dudrick, S. J. (1976). Nutritional aspects of cancer. In R. C. Hickey (ed.). *Current Problems in Cancer*, Vol. 1, No. 3, pp. 1–51. (Chicago: Year Book Medical Publishers, Inc.)
19. Copeland, E. M., III, MacFadyen, B. V., Jr., Lanzotti, V. J. and Dudrick, S. J. (1975). Intravenous hyperalimentation as an adjunct to cancer chemotherapy. *Am. J. Surg.*, **129**, 167
20. Souchon, E. A., Copeland, E. M., Watson, P. and Dudrick, S. J. (1975). Intravenous hyperalimentation as an adjunct to cancer chemotherapy with 5-fluorouracil. *J. Surg. Res.*, **18**, 451
21. Copeland, E. M., MacFadyen, B. V., Jr., MacComb, W. S., Guillamondegui, O., Jesse, R. H. and Dudrick, S. J. (1975). Intravenous hyperalimentation in patients with head and neck cancer. *Cancer*, **35**, 606
22. Trier, J. S. and Browning, T. H. (1966). A morphologic response of the mucosa of human small intestine to x-ray exposure. *J. Clin. Invest.*, **45**, 194
23. Hugon, J. S. and Bounous, G. (1972). Elemental diet in the management of the intestinal lesions produced by radiation in the mouse. *Can. J. Surg.*, **15**, 18
24. Copeland, E. M., Souchon, E. A., MacFadyen, B. V., Jr., Rapp, M. A. and Dudrick, S. J. (1977). Intravenous hyperalimentation as an adjunct to radiation therapy. *Cancer*, **39**, 609

Discussion

I. D. A. Johnston: (UK) One of the features of tumour regression when an endocrine background is altered is that pain disappears very rapidly, often before signs of regression can be detected. Is there any evidence that pain or other symptoms related to tumour bulk are altered by nutritional support, and is this an early pointer to success?

E. M. Copeland: (USA) No. Tumours do not regress rapidly but patients become candidates for therapy if they are nutritionally replenished.

In the radiation therapy group, patients with acute radiation enteritis have all the symptoms of enteritis when they ingest food; and if they do not ingest food, they are reasonably comfortable. These patients can be maintained parenterally, and the radiation therapy can be continued.

A. B. Jones: (Canada) The cancer patients that responded often gained weight, and those that did not respond lost weight. Is the weight gain or loss related to tumour regression? If they are losing weight, and more calories or nitrogen are given, could this immunological competence be changed, or if they are losing weight continuously is it that they will not respond?

Copeland: I am being asked whether nutritional improvement can be used as a parameter of potential response to chemotherapy. I am afraid we cannot say that.

D. W. Wilmore: (USA) The animal data suggested that as the animal is fed, the tumour is fed too. I would assume that the cell turnover of that tumour is being stimulated, and since drugs are taken up during the replicate cycle, one of the mechanisms by which this tumour would be made more sensitive to chemotherapy would be that an increased cell turnover is being stimulated.

Secondly, have any cell kinetic studies, half-life or turnover studies been done? Is the liver changed to metabolize the drug in another way, or is it that the patients can tolerate more of the drug?

Copeland: We are doing such studies at the moment. We speculated that if the tumour was being stimulated and getting larger, and the host was getting larger also, that the tumour:body weight ratio would stay the same. If during that period of 'stimulation' the animal was to be treated with chemotherapy, is that a point in time when the tumour growth would have been manipulated to one's own benefit?

We thought originally that we might be able to use cell cycle specific drugs better in a situation of hyperalimentation and potential tumour growth or tumour stimulation. It turns out that that is not true. The response rate between those that have been hyperalimented and those who have not been hyperalimented appears to be the same.

Johnston: I do not believe that there are data to suggest that intestinal cell kinetics as such are nutritionally related.

Wilmore: Steiger and his colleagues[1] about 18 months back, in an animal model showed that fed rats had turnover rates in the tumours that were increased, compared to starved rats.

The comment about chemotherapeutic agents is a much wider comment and applies to all sorts of drugs. The drug kinetics can be markedly changed when their turnover rates in people that undergo intravenous feedings are compared with patients who are starved.

H. K. Woods: (UK) There is quite a lot of evidence in animals concerning the effect of nutritional status on the degree to which drugs are metabolized.

If the nutritional status of the patient is improved, and if a drug is used that depends on an active metabolite for its action on the tumour, then one could postulate that the increased response in the fed group is a direct result of increasing the capacity of the patient to metabolize the drugs.

I know of only one recent study from the Middle East concerning the effect of malnutrition on drug metabolism. It used antipyrene half-life and showed that there was a prolongation of antipyrene half life in the really malnourished patient. There is, however, plenty of animal work, Basu and Dickerson[2], which shows that there is a very intimate relationship between the nutritional state of an animal and the speed with which it can produce metabolites. I have a feeling that a lot of the improved responses in patients who are undergoing drug therapy, especially for cancer, may well be directly related to the fact that their drug metabolism is altered to that which is comparable with the normal individual's.

A. B. Jones: (Canada) Dr. Copeland measured disaccharidases and a variety of other things in his rats. Does he attribute the decrease in disaccharidase activity etc. solely to the fact that the bowel was not in use, and that normal bowel hormones were not released, or to the nutritional state. What was the nutritional state of the rats? I gather that rats have to be given a lot of nitrogen because their nitrogen requirements are very great.

E. Copeland: (USA) The answer, I am afraid, is complex. The nutritional state of the animals was good and they gained weight. We used as our controls animals drinking the hyperalimentation solution and we measured nitrogen balance. They were in positive nitrogen balance, and they gained weight and were healthy. They did not, however, gain as much weight as animals eating regular rat chow. This was why we used hyperalimentation solutions orally as the control. They were then in positive nitrogen balance, potassium balance, etc.

Gut rest was what we wished to assess. The reason for the diminished disaccharidase enzymes as well as the diminished small bowel weight is probably twofold. We infused pentagastrin into another set of animals under the same experimental conditions and we did not get a fall in disaccharidase enzymes. There was also no fall in oxyntic gland area weight, nor any fall in pancreatic weight.

Dr. Lennard Johnston in our institution has felt for many years that the hormone gastrin is trophic for the small bowel, and he may be right. The addition of small doses of pentagastrin to the hyperalimentation solution prevented all of the changes shown with one exception. It did not prevent the increase in the peroxidase enzyme content. I find that particularly interesting; peroxidase is an enzyme of leucocytes which is diminished in the lamina propria. This means that leucocytes are diminished in the lamina propria in an animal that receives hyperalimentation. In an animal that feeds, it goes up. This may mean eating or assimilation and digestion stimulates an inflammatory response. Does this play any part in permitting the intestine of patients with Crohn's disease to rest and heal?

I. D. A. Johnston: (UK) Is there any evidence that the reduction in absorptive ability in the rested gut, apart from Crohn's disease—will be restored to normal when the intestine is stimulated again? There is evidence in some patients after massive small bowel resection that unless the intestine is constantly stimulated, the normal capacity for absorption does not return after a period of rest.

Copeland: In dog experiments following 6 weeks of hyperalimentation an immediate oral meal of regular dog food produced one formed stool a day and no diarrhoea. I Often feed patients intravenously who are debilitated after operation, particularly for various head and neck malignancies, and I have challenged these patients following 6–8 weeks of bowel rest with blended regular diets that they would not tolerate prior to hyperalimentation. They were able to take these diets after hypralimentation without developing diarrhoea. I thought that many of the enzymes, particularly the dipeptidases, might very well be protein moieties and nutritional replenishment might replenish those enzymes in the brush border, thus improving absorption. The rat enzyme systems respond to stimulation, and I suspect that may also be true of the human. If a human is fed a high concentration of maltose, maltase activity goes up rather dramatically and rapidly in the small bowel, so the enzymes can be induced. There appears to be no degree of malabsorption because of the diminished disaccharidase and probably dipeptidases, or the other findings such as diminished pancreatic weight, etc.

D. W. Wilmore: (USA) Would Dr. Copeland tell us about his studies of microflora and how the microflora changes. Some of his observations on inflammation may really be a reflection of alterations in microflora in the bowel.

Copeland: It may very well be. The microflora of the rat bowel diminishes, while the microflora of the human bowel has been found not to change significantly. However the quantitative bacterial counts diminish, but we have not found any qualitative changes. The bacteria are the same. There are not quite as many of them but they are there in sufficient quantity to be infectious.

W. P. T. James: (UK) Could I come back to the point about re-feeding rapidly patients who have not been on oral feeding for some time. I am rather intrigued that there have never been any complications. The story going back over 40 years is that with malnourished babies, there is no way in which a normal energy and protein requirement can be given instantly without producing the most profound diarrhoea. This may be a reflection of the diminished or limited colonic reserve for dealing with the overload coming down from the ileum. The stories of people emerging from concentration camps after the Second World War indicate that there was a very high death rate in those who were re-fed instantly. There are many stories from ex-concentration camp victims of the way in which they recognized the syndrome and refused to ingest normal amounts of food until 3, 4, 5 or perhaps 7 days after they were given free access.

Is there any evidence that there is no malabsorption in Dr. Copeland's patients, as distinct from overt diarrhoea?

Secondly, are there patients who for one reason or another have somewhat limited colonic reserve so that small intestinal events may be differentiated from large intestinal events?

Copeland: I have none of the data that have been asked for, but we are carrying out the necessary studies. However, I can give anecdotal and clinical observations. In the dog, we fed a bolus meal immediately and had no diarrhoea. In the clinical setting we have fed patients by nasogastric tube after head and neck cancer surgery, and they were able to tolerate the tube diet after hyperalimentation whereas they could not prior to it. However, we have done no malabsorptive studies on these patients, although we plan to do them.

When dealing with malabsorption obviously lactose intolerance and many other factors have to be ruled out, particularly in children. Where a patient has malabsorption secondary to malnutrition I do think that the malnutrition can be eliminated by intravenous nitrition.

G. L. Blackburn: (USA) Allan Walker, of the Boston Children's Hospital, who is a pediatric gastroenterologist, is concerned about antigen absorption during and after bowel-rest, even in well-nourished subjects. Perhaps one of the speakers might comment.

I also wanted to ask about the pharmacological effect of hypertonic glucose on intestinal fluxes, glucose conversion to lactate and lipogenesis. The metabolism of an intravenous nutrient is important beyond any provision of calories alone. We have been most impressed with the resuscitative effect of hyperalimentation in sepsis and shock.

Copeland: I am not sure that I am qualified to deal with this question. I can mention some of it in terms of manipulating a cancer cell.

The absorption of an antigen, particularly in an infant, in a hyperalimentation situation could potentially be a real problem. The parasite work suggests this. It is nice that the animals were able to expel the worms in their immunized state, but the worms were still accepted, and grew. We have yet to work with potentially sub-lethal infections. If 10^8 was sub-lethal and 10^9 was lethal, then had we given the animals 10^8, potentially they would have grown to 10^9 and killed the animal even though the animal was in an immunized state because it was hyperalimented. That is a study that we are about to do. It is a real fear, particularly in a very young infant who may be immunologically suppressed because of age.

S. J. Karran: (UK) What about the safety of the recall antigens, particularly on repeated challenge? Are they completely safe?

Copeland: We have had no problem. We have not had, for example, anyone strongly reactive to PPD ulcerate an arm in our patient population. We have had some large reactions, but almost all our patients are skin tested and in our group, we have not had ulceration from any of these skin tests. It may be that the doses that we use are 'proper' and that that is one of the reasons for our freedom from problems.

References

1. Steiger, E., Gram Smith, J., Miller, E., Kuo, L. and Vars, H. M. (1975). *J. Surg. Res.*, **18,** 455
2. Basu, T. K. and Dickerson, J. W. T. (1974). *Chem. Biol. Interactions*, **8,** 193

32
Artificial nutrition and the gastrointestinal tract: some clinical and experimental data

Y. A. CARPENTIER AND Ph. JANNE

Fistulae of the gastrointestinal tract—and particularly those involving the small bowel—undoubtedly represent surgical conditions whose prognosis has been improved dramatically during the last decade, with the use of total parenteral nutrition (TPN). Between 1960 and 1969, despite adherence to generally accepted principles of therapy, mortality rates of small bowel fistulae ranged between 50 and 75%[1-3]. Despite the suggestion of the usefulness of parenteral alimentation in 1948 by Thomas and Rose[4], the first results of TPN in a series of patients with small bowel and pancreatic fistulae were not reported until 1970 by Dudrick and co-workers[5]. Since then, these encouraging results have been confirmed by others and the position of TPN in the treatment of small bowel fistulae has been established. The mortality rate reported in recent series ranges from 21% to less than 10%[6-9]. The death rates were lower than those reported by teams using an enteral nutrition with a liquid elemental diet in similar conditions[10-12].

Because of the obvious improvement achieved using TPN on the prognosis of small bowel fistulae it is not possible from an ethical point of view to compare two randomized groups of patients receiving the same treatment—one with, and the other without, TPN.

CLINICAL STUDY

We have reviewed the course of twenty-six patients with one or more intestinal fistulae. These patients have been treated consecutively in our surgical department during a 12-month period. Nutritional support has been given to each patient and TPN was used in eighteen cases. Enteral nutrition, using a liquid elemental diet, was given alone to four patients. Both techniques were combined in four other cases. The twenty-six patients have been separated into two groups:

Group I (*'good prognosis'*)
This group is composed of eight patients with fistulae considered to have a satisfactory outcome. The cause of the fistulae, as well as the primary surgical procedures, are detailed in Table 32.1. While fistulae such as these do not usually require very special nutritional support, the patients in this study were considered to have a poorer prognosis, either because of poor nutrition or because of large losses from the fistula.

Group II (*'poor prognosis'*)
This group includes eighteen patients with one or more intestinal fistulae considered to be high-risk conditions. The daily output from the fistulae was always more than 500 ml. The thoracic oesophagus was involved in one patient, while the other seventeen patients had small bowel fistulae. The cause of the fistulae and the previous surgical procedures are detailed in Table 32.1.

Table 32.1 Intestinal fistulae

Level	*No.*	*Cause*	*Primary procedure*
Group I (good prognosis)			
Duodenum	2	Incomplete closure of stump	B. II gastrectomy
Caecum	2	Suture leak	Appendicectomy
Left colon	4	Anastomotic leak	Left colectomy
Patients	8		
Group II (poor prognosis)			
Oesophagus	1	Iatrogenic perforation	Oesophagoscopy
Oesophagus–jejunum	2	Anastromotic leak	Total gastrectomy
Duodenum	1	Anastomotic leak	B. II gastrectomy
	1	Anastomotic leak	Choledoco–duodenostomy
	1	Duodenal necrosis	Choledocotomy
Jejunum–ileum	11	Anastomotic leak	Small bowel resection
	1	Needle puncture	Laparoscopy
Patients	18		

In Group I, the nutritional support was commenced in six patients immediately the diagnosis of fistulae had been made. Two patients in this group were transferred from elsewhere and nutritional support was not started until at least 1 week after the diagnosis of fistula had been made.

In Group II, for similar reasons, nutritional support was started early in thirteen patients and late in five. As shown in Table 32.2, both techniques of alimentation (TPN and elemental diet) were used in Group I while TPN was given mainly in Group II. The elemental diet consisted of standard Vivonex (Eaton) and the mean duration of enteral feeding was 22 days.

Because of the high glucose content and high osmolarity of the mixture (500–600 mOsm for the usual dilution 25% w/v) the liquid diet was never taken orally but given through a thin paediatric nasogastric tube or a jejunostomy tube. This enteral feeding provided the patients with 1400–2400 cal. (mean: 1940 cal.) and 5–8 g of nitrogen (mean: 6.1 g/day). We also used high nitrogen Vivonex (Eaton) in which the amino acid content is doubled. The addition of medium chain triglycerides makes it possible to provide a daily intake of 4000 cal. and 20 g of nitrogen, in 3 litres.

Table 32.2 Intestinal fistulae—choice of nutritional therapy

Level	*No.*	*TPN*	*Elemental diet*	*Combined (TPN + ED)*
Group I				
Duodenum	2	2	—	—
Caecum	2	—	2	—
Colon	4	1	1	2
Group II				
Oesophagus	1	1	—	—
Oesophagus–jejunum	2	1	—	1
Duodenum	3	3	—	—
Jejunum–ileum	12	10	1	1
Total	26	18	4	4

Intravenous alimentation alone was infused for a mean of 19 days. TPN provided 2350–4000 cal. (mean: 2850 cal.) and 8.6–20 g of nitrogen (mean: 12.1 g/day). The energy intake was provided by glucose 20–50% solutions (Travenol) and Intralipid 20% (Vitrum), the fat emulsion accounting for 30–40% of the total calorie intake. Vamin 7% (Vitrum) was the regular amino acid solution infused. Electrolytes were added according to requirements. Trace elements, water and fat-soluble vitamins were administered as recommended by Wretlind[13]. The nutrients were given through a silicone rubber catheter inserted into the superior vena cava through the basilic vein[14]. Other points in management included the provision of adequate drainage, gastric fluid suction (in jejunal fistulae) and skin protection.

In twelve Group I 'early fed' patients, the fistulae closed spontaneously within 5 weeks (mean: 20 days); the thirteenth patient who had had radiation therapy died. A fistula had appeared at an oesophagojejunal anastomosis and never showed a tendency to heal. Of the five patients in whom nutritional support was delayed, only two survived; one closed spontaneously and the other after further surgery under ideal conditions; the three other patients died of sepsis, intestinal bleeding, and renal failure.

These results confirm the role of nutritional support in the treatment of patients with intestinal fistulae; moreover, they emphasize the necessity of starting it without delay. Wolfe and co-workers[15] examined the effect of elemental diet and intravenous alimentation on the output of experimental intestinal fistulae in dogs at different levels of the alimentary tract; from their results, it seems reasonable to use TPN for small bowel fistulae and an elemental diet for caecal or colonic fistulae.

The effect of TPN on the proximal gastrointestinal tract has been studied in rats by Johnson and co-workers[16,17] and Castro and co-workers[18], and in dogs by Thor and co-workers[19]. We have investigated the effect of a liquid elemental diet (Standard, Vivonex Eaton) on the weight, crypt cell number and proliferative parameters of the colon of rats[20]. Thirty-six male Wistar rats were randomized into two equal groups, the experimental group was given an elemental diet and the control group received *ad libitum* a rat chow diet (Protector, Brussels). The growth curve was normal in both groups. After 1, 2 and 4 weeks, six animals from each group were anaesthetized, weighed and killed; the colon and the small intestine were removed, opened rinsed in ice-cold saline, blotted and weighed; the liver, kidneys and testes were removed, rinsed in ice-cold saline, blotted and weighed. The results are shown in Table 32.3. The weight of the colon decreased from the first week of

Table 32.3 Mean weight after 1, 2 and 4 weeks of Vivonex (expressed as percentage of controls)

	1 *Week*	2 *Weeks*	4 *Weeks*
Colon	58.9*	56.9*	56.3*
Small intestine	83.6	96.0	110.3
Kidneys	95.1	85.9	96.4
Testes	107.5	95.5	106.1
Liver	85.8	98.8	113.0
Body weight	100.0	96.7	109.3

* $P < 0.01$

treatment. After 4 weeks of treatment, six rats from each group were killed; a 0.5 cm colonic segment was taken 15 cm from the ileocaecal junction, washed in ice-cold saline and fixed in Bouin's solution. Paraffin sections, 4 μm thick, were stained with haematoxylin and eosin. Thirty axially sectioned crypts and thirty cross-sectioned crypts were examined. The number of cellular spaces was measured in each glandular section. As shown in Table 32.4, the values of the crypt column length and the column count (both

Table 32.4 Effect of 4 weeks of Vivonex

	Normal diet (6 *rats*)	*Elemental diet* (6 *rats*)	*P*
Crypt column length	45.7 ± 3.9	23.3 ± 2.9	<0.01
Column count	24.6 ± 2.7	13.4 ± 1.1	<0.01
Total crypt cell population	1188.6 ± 23.6	287.8 ± 16.9	<0.01

expressed as mean number of cells) were decreased by approximately 50% in the experimental group; the total cell population per crypt (as estimated by the product of the column length and the count) was decreased by 76% in the experimental group.

After 1 and 2 weeks of treatment, six rats from each group were injected intraperitoneally with 1 μCi of [^{3}H]thymidine (Radiochemical Centre, Amersham, England) per g of body weight, and 1 h later, the animals were killed. A 1 cm colonic segment was taken 15 cm from the ileocaecal junction subdivided into small fragments, fixed in 2.5% glutaraldehyde and embedded in Epon 812. They were oriented in such a way that the mucosal glands could be cut longitudinally. Sections 1 μm thick were prepared and stained with periodic acid-Schiff. They were covered with nuclear emulsion (Ilford K5) developed 30 days later and counterstained with 1% toluidine blue in borax buffer (pH 9.2). The percentage of labelled cells and mitotic figures was determined in the progenitor area of twenty well-oriented crypts for each animal. As shown in Table 32.5, a considerable decrease in both labelling and mitotic index was observed after 1 week of elemental diet and more marked after a second week.

Table 32.5 Proliferation parameters of the colonic mucosa

	Normal diet	*Elemental diet*	*P*
1 *week*			
L.I.	11.961 ± 1.022	6.942 ± 0.291	< 0.01
M.I.	1.474 ± 0.212	0.814 ± 0.099	< 0.01
2 *weeks*			
L.I.	13.335 ± 0.994	5.483 ± 0.581	< 0.01
M.I.	1.548 ± 0.080	0.423 ± 0.094	< 0.01

These data show that oral administration of an elemental diet induces significant and selective colonic atrophy in rats. Considerable depletion and a decreased cellular proliferation have been demonstrated. The fall in the daily secretion of bile salts observed during the administration of an elemental diet[21] may be a possible factor in the atrophy of the colonic mucosa[22].

References

1. Edmunds, L. H., Jr., Williams, G. M. and Welch, C. E. (1960). External fistulas arising from the gastrointestinal tract. *Ann. Surg.*, **152**, 445
2. Chapman, R., Foran, R. and Dunphy, J. E. (1964). Management of intestinal fistulas. *Am. J. Surg.*, **108**, 157
3. Lorenzo, G. A. and Beal, J. M. (1969). Management of external small bowel fistulas. *Arch. Surg.*, **99**, 394
4. Thomas, P. O. and Ross, C. A. (1948). Effect of exclusive parenteral feeding on the closure of a pancreatic fistula. *Arch. Surg.*, **57**, 105
5. Dudrick, S. J., Wilmore, D. W., Steiger, E., Mackie, J. A. and Fitts, W. J., Jr. (1970).

Spontaneous closure of traumatic pancreatoduodenal fistulas with total intravenous nutrition. *J. Trauma*, **10**, 542

6. Aguirre, A., Fischer, J. E. and Welch, C. E. (1974). The role of surgery and hyperalimentation in therapy of gastro-intestinal–cutaneous fistulae. *Ann. Surg.*, **180**, 393
7. MacFayden, B. V., Jr., Dudrick, S. J. and Ruberg, R. L. (1973). Management of gastrointestinal fistulas with parenteral hyp ralimentation. *Surgery*, **74**, 100
8. Kaminsky, V. M. and Deitel, M. (1975). Nutritional support in the management of external fistulas of the alimentary tract. *Br. J. Surg.*, **62**, 100
9. Graham, J. A. (1977). Conservative treatment of gastrointestinal fistulas. *Surg. Gynecol. Obstet.*, **144**, 512
10. Bury, K. D., Stephens, R. V. and Randall, H. T. (1971). Use of a chemically defined liquid elemental diet for nutritional management of alimentary tract. *Am. J. Surg.*, **121**, 174
11. Voitk, A. J., Echave, V., Brown, R. A., McArdle, R. A. and Gurd, F. N. (1973). Elemental diet in the treatment of fistulas of the alimentary tract. *Surg. Gynecol. Obstet.*, **137**, 68
12. Rocchio, M. A., Mocha, C. J., Haas, K. F. and Randall, H. T. (1974). Use of chemically defined diets in the management of patients with high output gastro-intestinal cutaneous fistulas. *Am. J. Surg.*, **127**, 148
13. Wretlind, A. and Lee, H. A. (1975). Non-protein energy sources in parenteral nutrition. Presented at the *Xth International Congress of Nutrition*, August 3–9, Kyoto (Japan).
14. Mendes da Costa, P., Janne, Ph. and Carpentier, Y. A. (1976). Parenteral nutrition. Long-term catheterization. *Acta Chir. Belgica*, **75**, 530
15. Wolfe, B. M., Keltner, R. M. and Willman, V. L. (1972). Intestinal fistula output in regular elemental and intravenous alimentation. *Am. J. Surg.*, **124**, 803
16. Johnson, L. R., Copeland, E. M., Dudrick, S. J., Lichtenberger, L. M. and Castro, G. A. (1975). Structural and hormonal alterations in the gastrointestinal tract of parenterally fed rats. *Gastroenterology*, **68**, 1177
17. Johnson, L. R., Lichtenberger, L. M., Copeland, E. M., Dudrick, S. J. and Castro, G. A. (1977). Action of gastrin on gastrointestinal structure and function. *Gastroenterology*, **68**, 1184
18. Castro, G. A., Copeland, E. M., Dudrick, S. J. and Johnson, L. R. (1975). Intestinal disaccharidase and peroxidase activities in parenterally nourished rats. *J. Nutr.*, **105**, 776
19. Thor, P. J., Copeland, E. M., Dudrick, S. J. and Johnson, L. R. (1977). Effect of long-term parenteral feeding on gastric secretion in dogs. *Am. J. Physiol.*, **232**, E39
20. Janne, Ph., Carpentier, Y. and Willems, G. (1977). Colonic mucosal atrophy induced by a liquid elemental diet in rats. *Am. J. Dig. Dis.* (In press)
21. Hill, J. L., Mair, W. S. T., Edwards, J. P. and Goligher, J. C. (1976). Decreased trypsin and bile acids in ileal fistula drainage during administration of a chemically defined liquid elemental diet. *Br. J. Surg.*, **63**, 133
22. Raicht, R. F., Deschner, E. and Salen, G. (1975). Bile acids regulate intestinal cell turnover. *Gastroenterology*, **68**, 979

Discussion

I. D. A. Johnston: (Belgium) The elemental diet used had amino acids and no peptides. I wonder if the same results would be obtained if diets which contained peptides, as distinct from amino acids, were used. There is evidence that peptides are perhaps preferentially absorbed by the normal small bowel and are essential for more effective nitrogen absorption from the gut than amino acids alone. Information such as this is required in ill patients to enable the better formulation of elemental diets for the future.

Y. A. Carpentier: (Belgium) We know that it is not because this diet is a liquid diet, that we see atrophy. We know that a liquid hypercaloric diet produces this kind of atrophy, but we have no information about what happens with peptides.

J. T. Harries: (UK) Dr Carpentier showed that human beings do not like elemental diets. How was he able to ensure an isocaloric intake between the control group of rats and the rats that were fed an elemental diet?

Carpentier: We started with a preliminary study which defined if the rats liked or did not like an elemental diet. I know of other laboratories where there have been problems in feeding rats an elemental diet, but we had no problem and we had to limit the intake of the elemental diet to provide an isocaloric diet compared to the average intake of the rats fed with usual rat chow.

Harries: I am interested in your speculation that there may be a defect in bile salt synthesis or secretion into the intestinal lumen. What is the evidence that bile salts are not secreted, or are poorly secreted during periods of elemented diet?

Carpentier: We have not done the experiments in man. However, they have been done in animals—using an experimental fistula. The content of the bile salts in patients having an ileostomy has been studied by comparing a group of patients fed an elemental diet with a control group.

A. W. Goode: (UK) Hill in Leeds has quantitated the effect of elemental diets on bile acid production as measured by the bile salt excretion in established ileostomies. He found a reduction of approximately 35% after about 7 days.

We have had a fair experience at managing patients with intestinal fistulae with elemental diets. The big problem has been that although the elemental diet will help the fistula to close, and we would agree that the lower down the gastrointestinal tract it is, the quicker the closure. When patients go back to normal food, we found that in seven out of ten cases it tended to open again.

J. M. Kinney: (USA) Is that a suggestion that the quality of healing is different, and that they might have healed better if they had had TPN?

Goode: It may be so. The other possibility is that as they return to food, their gastrointestinal enzyme output is increased, and leakage occurs through a partially healed fistula.

Kinney: Which might have happened either way, whether they had TPN or a chemically formulated diet.

Carpentier: There have been some prospective studies in the healing of colostomy, comparing a group fed by a chemically defined diet with controls. It was impossible to show a significant difference between the groups.

R. K. Ausman: (USA) I was curious as to whether any changes of a similar kind were seen in the small bowel. I wondered whether they had been looked at, or was it assumed that they were no different because the weights were not different?

Carpentier: That is right. We were not interested in the small bowel because of the absence of difference in the weight, but we tried to study cell proliferation and we are still analysing that data. However, from preliminary data, we saw no significant difference in the proliferation rates. Studies of the proliferation of the small intestine are much more difficult than the same studies in the stomach and in the colon.

Section X
Parenteral Nutrition and Body Composition: Assessment of Therapy

33
The tissue composition of surgical weight loss

J. M. KINNEY

Weight loss is a commonplace accompaniment of major illness or injury, which has been one of the earliest physical signs to be recognized by friends and relatives even before it is evident to the patient himself. The extent of the weight loss is generally proportional to the severity of the illness or injury. Adult subjects vary in the rate of weight loss after injury, in relation to age, sex, body size and previous nutrition. The young adult male who is heavily muscled will have the most rapid and extensive weight loss after a given injury, in contrast to the female, the elderly, and the poorly nourished whose weight loss tends to be less for a given injury. It is of interest that weight loss is so commonly recognized and yet receives relatively little attention in clinical management. Some of the reasons are self-evident. The medical history of a hospital patient seldom includes a careful history of body weight; in fact, the patient may be too ill or too poorly informed to provide such information upon admission. The physical examination often fails to include a body weight (especially emergency admissions) or may have a single weight with no information as to whether this was before or after urination, what clothing was worn, etc. The accuracy of most hospital scales is questionable because of infrequent adjustment and calibration.

Every patient should have a reference or 'ideal' weight entered in his hospital chart along with his actual weight. The more critical the patient's problem, the more serial body weights should be a part of daily management. Accurate bed scales have made this requirement much easier to achieve. However, the body weight is seldom considered one of the 'vital signs' until the gain or loss is sufficiently extreme to have produced associated signs or symptoms (basal lung râles with water loading or marked weakness and fatigue with tissue loss). The gain or loss of body weight is the sum of changes in three body components: protein, fat and water. Because the body content and daily fluctuation for water is so much larger than for body fat or protein, there is a general feeling that body weights usually are not worth the effort, since they only show fluctuations in body water which are well tolerated in most cases. The purpose of this presentation is to review evidence which indicates that the use of body weight can be of greater importance in patient care than is usually thought and, with increasing experience, the use of body weight can provide 'red flags' to alert the physician to the need for associated measurements of daily balance or body composition to identify and treat undesirable trends in water retention or tissue loss.

WATER RETENTION

It is generally agreed that part of the metabolic response to injury includes a tendency towards water and salt retention immediately following the injury. This is thought to be a matter of a few days at most until a spontaneous diuresis will occur to rid the body of the extra salt and water when no longer needed. A reasonable clinical rule is that the patient should not have this tendency to water retention aggravated by intentionally producing water loading as part of treatment *unless* this is necessary to support the circulation. Consider four clinical examples: (1) the patient undergoing elective operation should not ordinarily gain weight, but will not show any significant weight loss for a period of 1–3 days because of the stimulus to fluid retention; (2) the patient in acute shock who has required fluid loading (including blood, colloid and crystalloid) will often have an increase of 5% or more of his regular body weight which will be excreted spontaneously in 2–5 days unless complications occur; (3) the patient with a major burn will often require fluid loading in excess of 10% of his pre-burn weight and will not have returned to his pre-burn weight until the second week or longer following the burn; and (4) patients who are fluid loaded for the treatment of shock, and develop complications such as peritonitis, will often fail to excrete this fluid load for as long as 3 weeks or more. The use of body weights can never be a guide to the amount of fluid to administer; that depends upon haemodynamic measurements and vital organ function. But the careful use of serial body weights can alert the physician to the failure of a patient to excrete a fluid load[1]. It is our clinical impression that the patient with unsuspected retention of a fluid load is at significant risk of pulmonary failure, should additional fluid loading be required in the treatment of a late complication. Only by serial body weights will the extent of the fluid retention be recognized, and the careful use of diuretic agents considered before interstitial pulmonary oedema has become a serious problem.

BODY COMPOSITION

The normal adult human body can be considered in terms of tissues and organs or of chemical phases. It is of interest that the vital organs and blood volume constitute roughly 15% of a normal adult male and it is this fraction which gets all the attention in the early treatment of the acute surgical patient. But as methods and techniques for resuscitation have become more successful, we are forced to turn our attention to the metabolic reserve represented by the muscle and adipose tissue which together represent approximately two-thirds of the adult body weight. It is these tissues which represent expendable amino acid and energy reserves, as long as some threshold of critical loss is not exceeded. A few features should be noted concerning the mythical 70 kg male with an average body composition[2]. The adult male body has an average composition of 40% organic material, 55% body water and 5% skeleton, with the organic material having an average content of 15% crude protein and 25% fat. Total protein is around 15% of body weight, or 10.5 kg, which includes three categories, tendon, dermis, bone matrix, etc. (approximately 45% or 4.7 kg) which has a relatively slow turnover rate, muscle protein which is estimated to be around 40% (or 4.2 kg) and is extensively degraded following injury, and the visceral protein (approximately 15% or 1.55 kg) with rapid turnover rates but which may be protected from the depletion more than the muscle protein after injury.

RATES OF WEIGHT LOSS

The monumental study of human starvation by Keys and co-workers[3] included review of some 3000 references in the world literature as well as the data from their own study of partial starvation. They made estimates of the approximate rate of weight loss to be expected when the caloric intake was reduced to some fraction of the intake needed to maintain a normal adult body weight. These estimates of weight loss with partial starvation are shown in Figure 33.1 when plotted as a percentage of body weight against days of partial starvation. The weight loss of total starvation in the famous Benedict study[4] is included to emphasize how much faster the weight loss occurs when compared with the intake of only 20% of the estimated daily need.

A group of four critically injured patients were resuscitated from shock and studied in our Surgical Metabolism Unit with daily resting calorie and nitrogen balance for periods up to 50 days. Each of these four patients began to take some oral nutrition by the fourth day and was considered to be making a satisfactory convalescence. However, when the data from the research dietician were reviewed, it became evident that daily intake always fell in the range of 40–60% of their estimated daily needs. The weight loss of these four patients with major injury is compared in Figure 33.2 with the

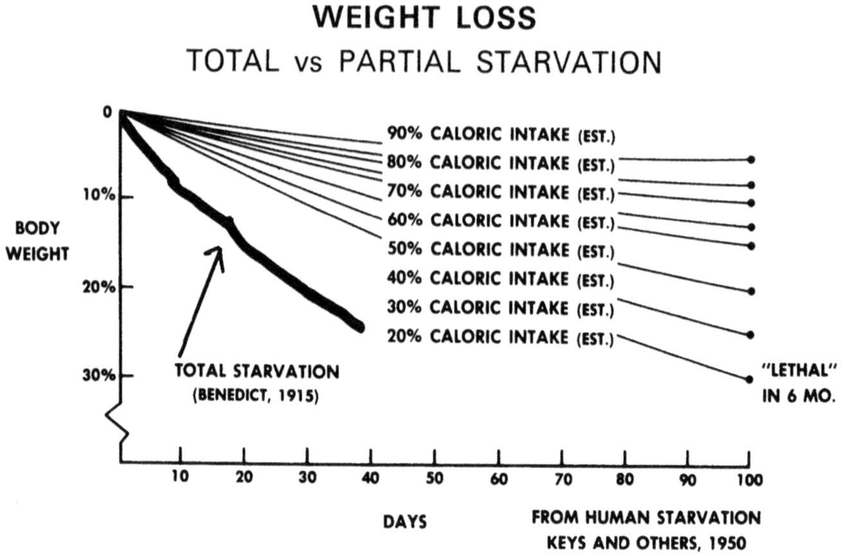

Figure 33.1 The loss of body weight which occurs with progressive levels of decrease in calorie intake is shown for 100 days, according to the estimates of Keys and co-workers[3]. The more rapid rate of weight loss with total starvation is shown from the study of Benedict[4]

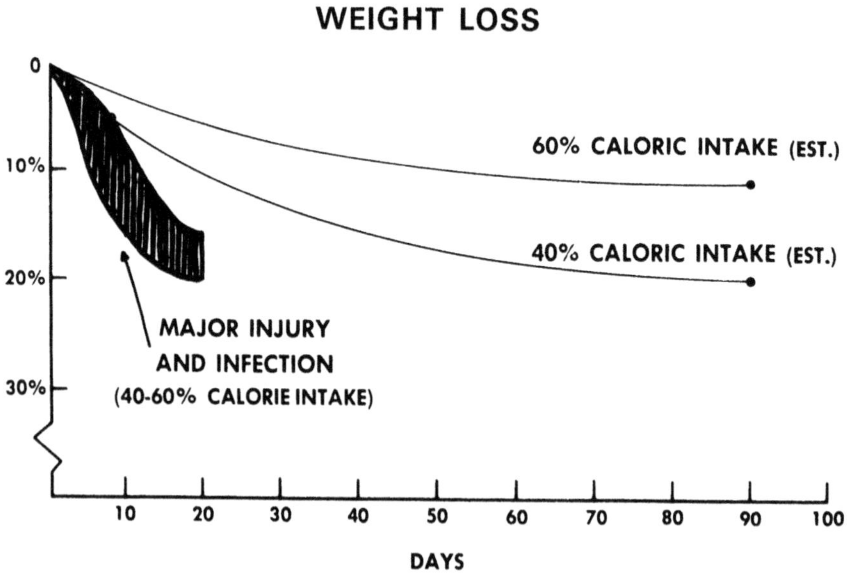

Figure 33.2 The estimated loss of weight with partial starvation is compared with that of cases of major injury which received an approximately similar range of oral nutrition

much slower weight loss estimated by Keys and co-workers for a similar limitation of intake but without injury. It is of particular interest that the rate of weight loss after major injury with 40–60% of estimated calorie and nitrogen needs is of the same rapidity as that of Benedict's subject with total starvation and no injury. While the rate of weight loss is similarly rapid, the most important aspect is whether the composition of the weight loss is similar. Will the injured patients have a much higher proportion of protein in their weight loss?

ANALYSIS OF WEIGHT LOSS

It is clinically obvious that when there is a major weight loss which is observed in a matter of hours to a few days, this change is mainly a change in body water. The sustained losses which continue for weeks to months, represent some balance between the losses of hydrated lean tissue and of anhydrous fat. Various methods have been introduced into the literature for analysing weight loss. The loss of protein is one of the easier measurements because of the Kjeldahl measurement of nitrogen. Fat loss is more difficult to measure. One can estimate changes in body fat by the serial use of skin calipers. One can do serial measurements of body water and calculate changes in body fat by difference. One can perform serial measurements of gas exchange with nitrogen excretion and arrive at the energy expenditure from indirect calorimetry. One can estimate the energy expenditure by the Newberg formula. This is based on measuring the insensible weight loss (and hence the insensible water loss) and converting this to calories of heat loss, which is assumed to be one-quarter of the total heat loss under carefully controlled thermoneutral conditions.

A knowledge of the energy intake together with the energy expenditure can be converted to a daily resting calorie balance. A negative calorie and nitrogen balance over days can be converted into grams of body fat and body protein, with the remainder of the weight loss over this period assumed to be loss of body water. This approach is extremely variable when applied to short-term measurements over only a few days. However, measurements made continuously over 10–14 days or more are surprisingly consistent.

COMPOSITION OF WEIGHT LOSS

Our first effort to study the composition of surgical weight loss was directed towards elective patients undergoing abdominal operation for peptic ulcer disease[5]. These patients received only 5% dextrose by vein until they were allowed to begin an oral diet on the third or fourth day after operation. The females lost 4–6% of their starting weight while the males lost 6–8% of their body weight by the time of hospital discharge at around 10 days. We were surprised to find that the protein breakdown contributed only 6–8% of the total weight loss. This work was delayed because of our clinical belief that the protein content of the weight loss must be larger.

Subsequent study of four critically injured patients who entered in shock revealed a loss of body weight between 14 and 18% in the first three weeks of convalescence. None of these patients received total parenteral nutrition since they began to take some oral intake by the fourth day and received between 40 and 60% of the calories and nitrogen which they were presumed to need. Surely these patients would demonstrate a much higher proportion of protein in their weight loss than the postoperative patients. The cumulative loss of protein and fat, as calculated from performing daily calorie and nitrogen balances, revealed approximately 12% protein and 14% fat when averaged over 3 weeks[6]. A careful analysis of the daily trend in the calculation of each component showed erratic shifts in the water balance for the first ten days. However, these shifts became less marked during the second and third weeks, and the contribution of protein and fat to the weight loss tended to fall into relatively narrow ranges of 10–14% for the protein and 14–24% for fat. While these findings need to be confirmed in a larger number of cases, the

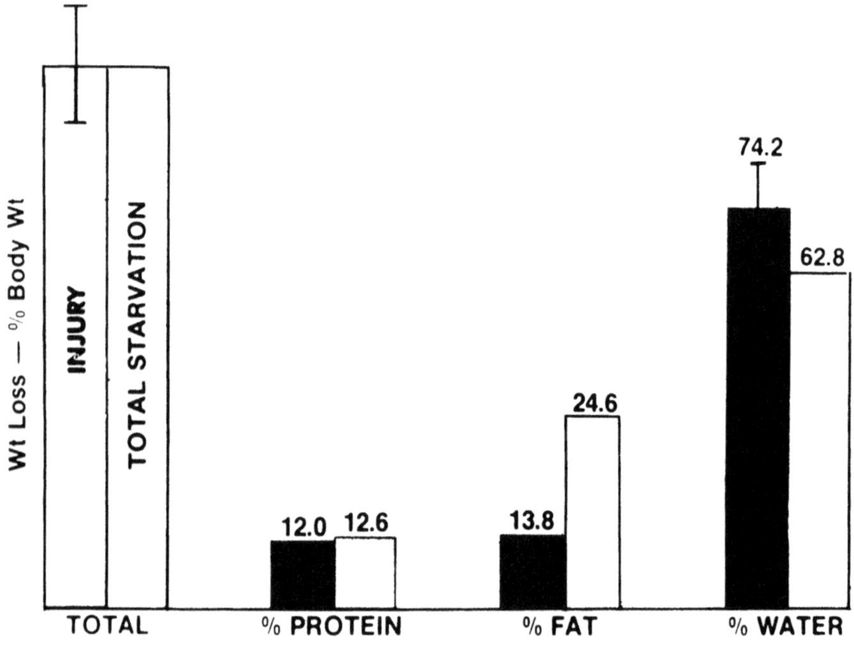

Figure 33.3 The tissue composition of the cumulative weight loss over 21 days for four cases of major injury (black bars) is compared with that of total starvation (white bars) in Benedict's study. Note that the protein content is essentially the same for similar degrees of weight loss, while the fat content is strongly influenced by the calorie intake. See text for details

consistency of the findings raises the question: Are these proportions different from what is found in total starvation or other conditions not associated with the increased nitrogen loss of injury or infection?

The weight loss sustained during total starvation by the adult male in Benedict's study was analysed for comparison with our injury patients, since the data are available for the gas exchange and nitrogen excretion throughout the month of fasting. The first 3 days is associated with a period of diuresis and rapid weight loss, followed by a surprisingly steady rate of weight loss of around 300 g/day. Examination of the protein and fat contribution to the weight loss revealed that the protein content of 6–8% during the first few days rose to an average of 12.6% for the first 21 days while the fat contributed approximately 26% for the first 3 weeks as shown in Figure 33.3.

Confirmation of the early weight loss having only about 10% protein is found in the data of Impietro and co-workers[7] who studied two groups of six men each of whom lived for 14 days in a chamber at 60 F. The first group received 600 cal/day with a mean weight loss of 5.66 kg while the other group were completely starved and lost 8.5 kg. The tissue composition of weight loss was nearly identical in both groups with protein providing 9.7% in the 600 cal group and 11.4% in the starved group. The contribution of body fat was 39% of the weight loss in each group.

The clinical data discussed in this presentation suggest that certain statements can be made about weight loss in general:

1. Total starvation is usually associated with a diuresis period during the first 3–5 days, followed by a relatively uniform but slower rate of weight loss.
2. Weight loss during the early days after injury or infection is unpredictable because of variable amounts of water retention.
3. The contribution of protein to sustained weight loss over periods of 3 weeks is remarkably similar (10–12%) regardless of whether the weight loss is occurring from total starvation, partial starvation, mild cold exposure, or multiple injury. The extent of protein loss is mainly a function of total weight loss, rather than the underlying reason for the weight loss.
4. The proportion of fat in the weight loss is obviously dependent upon the caloric intake, with the fat loss over 3 weeks of starvation being approximately 25% while it can be down to 14% with partial calorie intake.

References

1. Gump, F. E., Kinney, J. M., Long, C. L. and Gelber, R. (1968). Measurement of water balance—a guide to surgical care. *Surgery*, **64**, 154
2. Moore, F. D., Olesen, K. H., McMurrey, J. D., Parker, H. V., Ball, M. R. and Boyden, C. M. (1963). *The Body Cell Mass and its Supporting Environment*. (Philadelphia and London: W. B. Saunders Company)
3. Keys, A., Brozek, J., Henschel, A., Mickelsen, O. and Taylor, H. L. (1950). *The Biology of Human Starvation*. (Minneapolis: The University of Minnesota Press)

4. Benedict, F. G. (1915). A Study of Prolonged Fasting. Washington Publ. No. 203, p. 416
5. Kinney, J. M., Long, C. L., Gump, F. E. and Duke, J. H., Jr. (1968). Tissue composition of weight loss in surgical patients: I. Elective operation. *Ann. Surg.*, **168,** 459
6. Kinney, J. M. (1976). Surgical diagnosis, patterns of energy, weight and tissue change. In A. W. Wilkinson and D. P. Cuthbertson (eds.). *Metabolism and the Response to Injury*, p. 121. (Kent: Pitman Medical)
7. Iampietro, P. F., Goldman, R. F., Mager, M. and Bass, D. E. (1961). Composition and caloric density of weight loss during caloric restriction in cold. *J. Appl. Physiol.*, **16,** 624

Discussion

G. L. Blackburn: (USA) The correlation between major injury and starvation, in which both had some protein loss (12–16 %), has led to most of the commercially available solutions being designed to restore about 12–16 %.

The question is whether in hypercaloric feeding after major injury the composition makes any difference. I presume that there is no role for metabolic adaptation and after providing the nitrogen any other hypercaloric feeding will not make a difference to the body composition. Is there any impact on body composition of a hypercaloric feeding beyond the protein component?

J. M. Kinney: (USA) If Dr Blackburn is asking whether the difference between carbohydrate and fat makes any difference, or in other words is a calorie always a calorie, my own feeling is that a certain amount of glucose is needed, but once beyond that point, (100–150 g) any energy source can be utilized. I think that it is a great mistake not to give some carbohydrate and I would favour glucose.

Blackburn: Could Professor Kinney tell what he would expect the addition of 100 or 150 g glucose to the protein to do? Do we know the effect of adding carbohydrate to hypocaloric feeding on the utilization of the protein?

Kinney: In patients who will have a positive calorie balance from feeding, I made a reference that there should be some proportion as carbohydrate. My own feeling is that the difference between giving some carbohydrate, such as 100 g peripherally, plus peripheral amino acids, is uncertain from the data that I have seen. I do think that there may be some benefit in preserving liver glycogen, remembering that the liver can withstand all sorts of noxious influences when it had some liver glycogen. It seems to me that for that reason, it may be beneficial, but I do not think that we know the real answer.

34
Research in malnutrition and its application to parenteral feeding

W. P. T. JAMES

For the last 30 years nutritionists in developing countries have been working on the problems of identifying those malnourished children and adults in greatest need of nutritional support. A number of advances have been made, particularly when treating malnourished children, which are of direct relevance to physicians and surgeons in developed countries when they are dealing with very similar problems in patients in hospital. There is the same need to develop practicable, cheap and reliable tests for assessing the nutritional state and to evolve methods of treatment which are both cost-effective and safe.

ASSESSING NUTRITIONAL STATE

Measurements relating to body composition

Soon after World War II it became apparent that the traditional methods for assessing nutritional state by clinical examination were useful for identifying the severely affected cases but this method was a poor discriminator of the more moderate degrees of malnutrition. Observer error was also considerable. Recording a subject's weight was obviously important but seemed inexact because of the wide range in weights in a normal population. Relating weight to height has been accepted for decades in adult medicine but this has only recently been applied as a useful anthropometric relationship when assessing malnutrition in growth-retarded children[1]. Despite the narrow range of weights for heights in healthy children and adults there is still the problem, when confronted with a patient for the first time, of knowing if he is undernourished. There is a need to develop more specific tests.

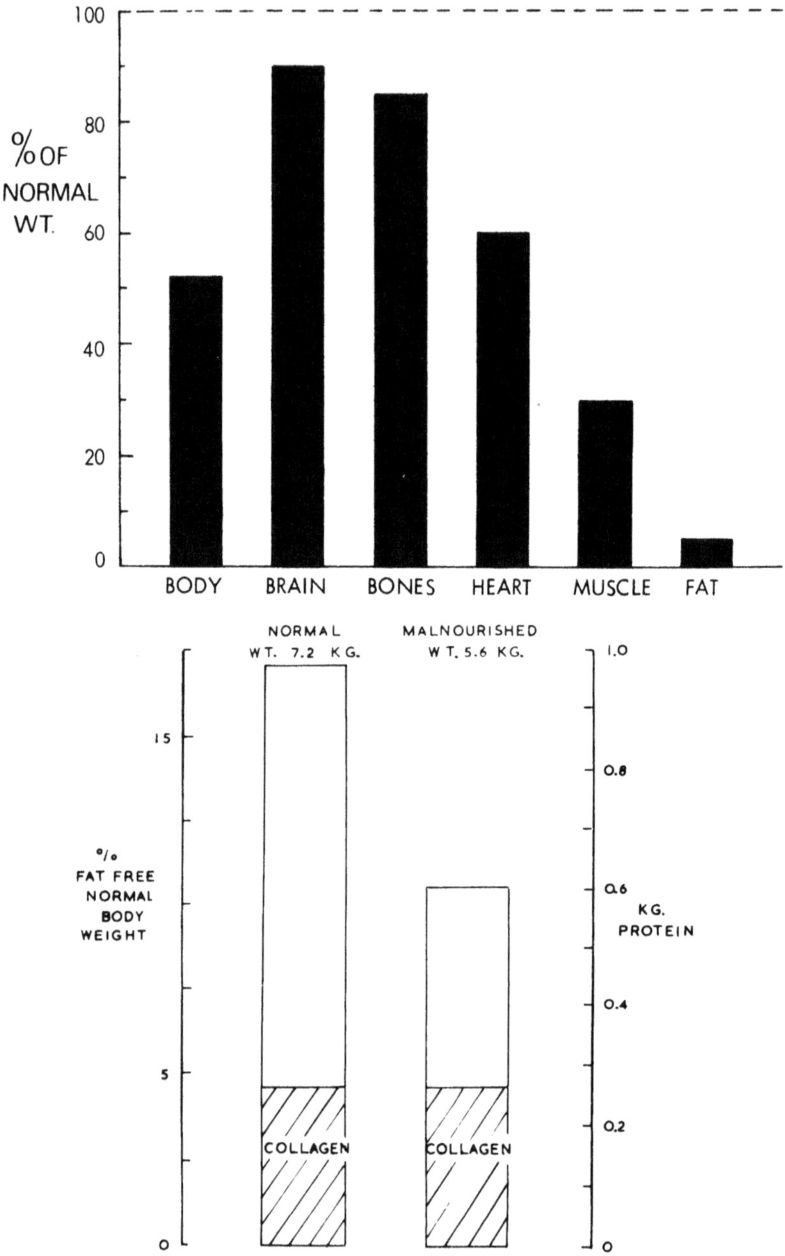

Figure 34.1 Body compositional changes in protein-energy malnutrition

(a) The body composition of a child dying of marasmus in whom the total weight of different organs was obtained by dissection and is expressed here as a percentage of that found in a child of normal nutritional state and of the same height.

(b) The amount of body protein, divided into collagen and non-collagen fractions in normal and malnourished children.

Data recalculated from Picou *et al.* (1966)[2]

Tests for nutritional state are based usually on a direct or indirect assessment of body composition. Figure 34.1 illustrates some of the body compositional change which occur in protein-energy malnutrition (PEM). The organ weights of a child dying of prolonged semi-starvation and marasmus show considerable differences between organs. With a body weight of only 50% of that of a normal child of equivalent height, Garrow and his co-workers[3] found the body fat amounted to only 5% of the normal and muscle weight was reduced to 30%. Further studies[3,4] showed that all tissues were remarkably depleted of protein; children died of malnutrition when they had lost 30% of their total protein mass[4]. There was, however, a disproportionate loss of the non-collagen proteins which fell to 50% of the normal level. The analyses suggested that muscle served as the major protein reserve of the body. This view was later confirmed by the elegant investigations of Cahill, Felig and their colleagues[5,6], who studied the interrelationships between the visceral tissues and skeletal muscle, and established the role of muscle in providing substrates for gluconeogenesis in starvation. From this evidence it became clear that tests aimed at monitoring the progressive changes in muscle mass could be useful indices of nutritional state. Only recently, however, has an appropriate test of muscle mass been introduced, i.e. the creatinine–height index, which relates the 24 h excretion rate of creatinine to the height of the child or adult[7]. This is less easy to use in children but should prove an excellent index in adults, despite some doubt over the long-term constancy of creatinine excretion in relation to muscle mass if subjects are put experimentally on a creatinine free diet.

Indices of body protein turnover

A more senstitive test might be found if an index were obtained which reflected the body's attempts to preserve its body protein. Two derivatives of the amino acids, proline and histidine, may prove useful. Picou *et al.*[8] showed that malnourished children had low rates of hydroxyproline excretion, compatible with a slowing down in the turnover of collagen and the preservation of collagen mass as malnutrition developed. The urinary output of hydroxyproline rose as the children recovered and this rate was associated with increasing creatinine excretion. Other workers[9,10] related the urinary concentration of hydroxyproline to that of creatinine in order to produce a simple index which provided information on the body's state of adaptation without the need to collect a full 24-h specimen of urine. The derivation of this index seemed helpful since it was low in children with kwashiorkor and rose to normal on treatment. Hydroxyproline–creatinine ratios and indices, however, obscure important nutritional changes since both metabolites are reduced in the urine in malnutrition, the one indicating the reduced turnover rate of a major component of body protein (collagen), and the other reflecting the degree of depletion of the largest reserve of non-collagen protein in the body. Logically, therefore, both should be measured as absolute excretion rates to give the most information. Daily urine collections are much more practicable in adult surgical patients than in children living in the community but there remains the problem of measuring hydroxyproline by techniques which are difficult to automate. There is also the possibility that an infected patient may have marked increases in hydroxyproline output since Whitehead[11] found anomalous results with marked fluctuations in hydroxyproline output in association with infections. Creatinine–height indices are, however, being used successfully and the early studies showed that they were low in all forms of malnutrition (Table 34.1).

Table 34.1 A comparison of anthropometric and biochemical indices in the assessment of the nutritional state of three groups of malnourished children

Clinical form of malnutrition	*Weight for age*	*Weight for height*	*Creatinine–height index*	*Hydroxy-proline 24 h excretion*	*3-methyl-histidine 24 h excretion*
			% Normal		
Kwashiorkor	65.8 ± 1.4*	77.0 ± 2.3*	52.8 ± 4.4(8)*	—	17.5(5)‡
Marasmus–kwashiorkor	49.9 ± 1.7*	71.1 ± 1.7*	48.5 ± 2.6(17)*	—	33.3(3)‡
Marasmus	45.5 ± 2.8*	61.7 ± 3.5*	61.2 ± 8.2(6)*	—	8.8(3)‡
Protein-energy malnutrition	—	73.6 ± 2.9†	64.3(10)†	26.5(10)†	19.3(11)‡

Results calculated from:
* Viteri and Alvarado, 1969[7]
† Picou, Alleyne and Seakins, 1965[8]
‡ Rao and Nagabhushan, 1973[13]

The number of subjects studied is shown in parenthesis. Of the ten Jamaican subjects studied by Picou *et al.*, eight were classified as marasmus–kwashiorkor. The data of Viteri allow separation into the categories of malnutrition defined by the Wellcome system; see *Lancet* (1970) **ii,** 302; the Indian classification may not have conformed with this system. Normal values are taken in the Jamaican values for creatinine and hydroxyproline from data obtained on children recovered from malnutrition.

Of considerable interest is the possibility of developing a test of myofibrillar protein turnover as a more sensitive monitor of changing nutritional state. Following Young's[12] suggestion that 3-methyl-histidine excretion be used, measurements were first applied to the study of malnutrition[13]. The excretion rate was very low or even absent in both marasmus and kwashiorkor. The results shown in Table 34.1 suggest that the excretion of both hydroxyproline and 3-methyl-histidine are likely to be much more sensitive indices of changing nutritional state than any anthropometric parameter or the creatinine–height index. These tests, which reflect the turnover of individual proteins, may therefore prove important in providing information about the response not only to the stress of trauma but to the efficacy of therapy in surgical patients.

Total body protein turnover

Whole body protein turnover can be assessed more directly by the use of labelled amino acids. Waterlow and his colleagues have undertaken a series of studies in malnutrition[14,15] and in patients undergoing surgery[16,17]. A low protein diet induces a fall in protein synthesis and a steady decline in protein breakdown rates[18]. Malnourished children, when first admitted to hospital, have low turnover rates which rise rapidly in response to feeding[15]. The increase is much more rapid than the rise in hydroxyproline and 3-methylhistidine output and these differences in the rate of response probably reflect the dominance of liver protein synthesis during the early recovery phase. Increased rates of albumin synthesis have been observed in treated malnourished children[19] and total body protein turnover rates are also elevated[15].

We found in surgical patients with tracer infusions of [1-^{14}C]L-leucine, that the total of protein synthesis in the body tended to fall after surgery if dextrose-saline was infused post-operatively: only one of the four patients showed an increase in the protein breakdown rate. More extensive studies with [^{15}N]glycine[17] confirmed these observations which are summarized with other data on turnover in Table 34.2. The form of therapy used post-operatively seems important since we found that the provision of amino

Table 34.2 Body protein turnover rates: changes in response to malnutrition, low protein intakes and surgery

Subjects	Total protein turnover: Synthesis	Total protein turnover: Breakdown
Studies with [^{15}N]*glycine*		
1. Children:	(g/kg/day)	
Malnourished	4.0 ± 0.5	3.8 ± 0.5
Recovering	6.9 ± 0.9	4.9 ± 0.8
Recovered	6.6 ± 0.5	4.4 ± 0.4
2. Surgical patients[17]	(g/kg/day)	
Pre-operatively	3.83 ± 0.73	3.88 ± 0.66
After surgery	2.94 ± 0.83	3.66 ± 0.65
3. Surgical patients[20]:		
Pre-operatively	276	299
After surgery	242	302
Studies with ^{14}C-L *amino acids*		
4. Obese adults[32]	(g/day)	
Diet (a) 70 g protein intake	400 ± 122	400
(b) zero protein intake	194 ± 86	228

* Golden, M., Waterlow, J. C. and Picou, D. (personal communication)

acids rather than glucose-saline was accompanied by maintenance of the normal rate of body protein synthesis and nitrogen balance[30].

Williamson and his colleagues[21] have confirmed recently that most patients subjected to severe trauma do not have an increase in muscle breakdown rates as has traditionally been assumed to occur in association with the

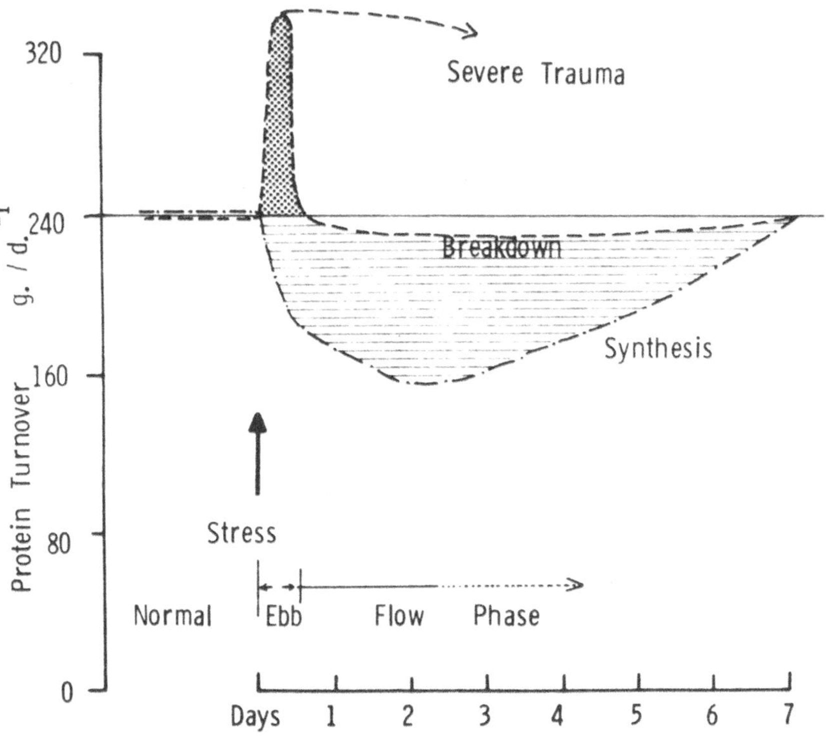

Figure 34.2 The responses in the rates of body protein synthesis and breakdown following surgery or trauma

The initial acute rise in breakdown rates is considered to result from the physical trauma to tissues during injury. The usual physiological response in breakdown rates is small so that the degree of protein loss depends on the extent to which synthesis falls. If there is severe injury then physical trauma with autolysis of tissue will increase the inflow of amino acids to the liver for catabolism; some non-ketotic subjects also show an increase in breakdown rates.

A low protein diet leads to an adaptive fall in body protein breakdown rates, thus minimizing the loss in body protein when synthesis is suppressed.

increased output of urinary nitrogen. A group of subjects with very severe trauma did, however, have a rise in 3-methyl-histidine output. This group had a higher excretion of urinary nitrogen and did not develop ketosis. Circulating ketones limit[22] amino acid efflux from muscle and Williamson's results suggest that ketones directly or indirectly affect the breakdown rates of myofibrillar protein in addition to any changes which they may induce in protein synthesis.

The so-called 'catabolic' response to surgery should perhaps be viewed differently, therefore. Figure 34.2 illustrates the main features of what may occur post operatively. We envisaged originally[20] that the increase in breakdown rates occurred only as a result of the physical trauma to tissues during surgery or in an accident. But Williamson's results on 3-methyl-histidine output do suggest that true increases in muscle turnover rate can occur. Figure 34.2 shows that the problem in achieving nitrogen balance is more difficult if total breakdown rates increase since the synthesis rate of body protein needs to be increased to supranormal levels, despite the insulin resistance which often develops post-operatively.

Serum proteins

It has been recognized for years that the two extreme forms of malnutrition, kwashiorkor and marasmus, are distinguishable not only by their clinical features but by differences in serum albumin concentrations. Children with kwashiorkor have low levels which play an important part in the pathophysiology of their oedema. Oedema is also seen in surgical patients, and monitoring the serum albumin concentration has become a useful measure of nutritional state. It should be remembered, however, that in starvation and marasmus albumin levels may be normal.

The availability of amino acids for hepatic synthesis is affected not only by the supply of dietary protein but by the balance between anabolic hormones, e.g. insulin, and catabolic hormones, e.g. cortisone and glucagon. Whitehead[23] has suggested that the difference in albumin concentration between kwashiorkor and marasmus may relate to the effect of insulin which tends to divert amino acids to muscle in children with kwashiorkor, thus depriving the liver of substrate for albumin synthesis. The concentration of plasma cortisol is elevated in marasmus and can thus exert its catabolic effect on muscle protein[24].

The normal response to the stress of surgery involves the mobilization of peripheral amino acids for gluconeogenesis and the synthesis of hepatic proteins. The use of glucose infusions post-operatively may then simulate those conditions found during the development of kwashiorkor when insulin levels tend to be high as albumin levels fall. It is not yet clear whether the differences in the metabolic responses of individuals after surgery or trauma are the consequence of differences in the type of stress, the result of different nutritional practices or a reflection of intrinsic differences between individuals in their response to a similar diet and stress. A similar problem is found when trying to unravel the differences in the aetiology of kwashiorkor and marasmus. In India it is claimed that children may develop either kwashiorkor or marasmus when consuming the same type of diet and the data shown in

Table 34.1 suggest that there may be very important differences in the response of the body to nutritional stress. Children who succumb to kwashiorkor rather than marasmus may adapt poorly but not in the way originally suggested. Thus children with kwashiorkor have a greater deficit in muscle mass yet continue to break down the myofibrillar proteins at a higher rate than the well-adapted marasmic child. The greater loss of body protein in children with kwashiorkor may then be of prime importance in the failure to maintain albumin synthesis since we have shown that a reduced intake of protein leads to a much greater fall in albumin synthesis once body protein reserves are depleted[19]. The capacity to reduce the rate at which body protein breaks down may therefore be a vital part of the adaptive process to nutrition stress. In surgical patients on intravenous therapy it would therefore be far more important to provide protein in addition to energy if muscle mass were small and the creatinine–height index low.

The choice of serum proteins for monitoring nutritional states

Many serum proteins have been measured in malnourished children in an attempt to find proteins which are reliable and sensitive discriminants of deteriorating nutrition, but none has emerged as superior to serum albumin, the concentration of which is known to have prognostic significance.

One possible disadvantage of using albumin as an index of changing nutritional status is that there is a considerable degree of adaptation in albumin metabolism as serum albumin concentrations fall[19]. Recently it has been suggested that measuring serum transferrin may be better since it shows a greater fall in children with kwashiorkor[25]. This greater sensitivity may relate to its faster turnover rate and different catabolic characteristics. However, transferrin synthesis is increased in response to stress and in iron deficiency so that its concentration may not alter in parallel with changes in

Table 34.3 A comparison of the relative sensitivity of four circulating proteins as indices of nutritional state in children with kwashiorkor or marasmus–kwashiorkor

		Duration of treatment	
	On admission	*1 week*	*3 weeks*
Albumin (g%)	1.74(53)	2.10(64)	3.22(98)
Transferrin (mg%)	131(39)	214(63)	445(131)
Thyroxin-binding pre-albumin (mg%)	6.38(29)	13.09(59)	22.31(100)
Retinol-binding protein (mg%)	1.62(32)	3.53(70)	5.41(107)

Numbers in parenthesis indicate the values as a percentage of those obtained in a control group of children

From Ingenbleek *et al.* (1975)[26]

body protein. An erratic response in serum transferrin was indeed seen in children recovering from kwashiorkor[26] and measuring transferrin levels seems of little value in children with marasmus.

Of greater interest is the recent suggestion by Belgian workers[27] that retinol binding protein or pre-albumin is more sensitive to dietary protein supply and that it may be a useful test for screening both forms of malnutrition, marasmus and kwashiorkor. Table 34.3 compares the relative sensitivities of albumin, transferrin, retinol binding protein and pre-albumin in malnutrition. The last two proteins have very fast turnover rates and a high tryptophan content[26]: these characteristics may explain their usefulness as nutritional tests. Whether these proteins prove to be too responsive to dietary manipulations, as became apparent when attempts were made to use simple ratios of plasma amino acid concentrations as appropriate tests, is uncertain, but this work deserves wider application in the assessment of surgical patients.

THE THERAPY OF MALNUTRITION

Considerable attention has been paid to the problem of assessing the requirements of patients recovering from malnutrition. Protein requirements are increased in children compared with adults because of the need to supply amino acids for the deposition of additional protein during growth. The same needs apply to malnourished surgical patients who have to restore their body protein mass. A normal adult's non-collagen protein contains about 50% of essential amino acids, but he needs only about 20% of his dietary protein as essential amino acids. Recycling and conservation of essential amino acids are greater than for the non-essential amino acids. Although a malnourished subject has an enhanced ability to reduce amino acid catabolism and achieve nitrogen balance on low intakes, to replenish non-collagen proteins with their high content of essential amino acids requires an appropriate supply of dietary or intravenous essential amino acids.

Balance studies in children[28] also suggest that the energy cost of new tissue formation may be considerable. If depletion of fat as well as protein has occurred then to replenish these requires as much as 48 kJ (10 kcal)/g tissue. A weight loss of 10 kg is common in post-operative patients who have developed complications and 480 MJ or 100 000 kcal are probably then needed in addition to basal requirements, to return the subject to his normal nutritional state. On this basis alone it is not surprising that 'convalescence' is protracted after severe illness.

The intake of energy has to be increased gradually since a very ill patient has adjusted to a reduced energy intake and the sudden influx of energy may precipitate acute changes in fluid balance. Malnutrition is often accompanied by increases in total body sodium and water with a variable impairment of sodium pump activity. Rapid transfer of intracellular sodium and water to the circulation may then overwhelm the kidney's capacity to excrete and precipitate extracellular overhydration and oedema[29].

ADDITIONAL NEEDS IN MALNOURISHED PATIENTS

The supply of energy and protein alone does not cover the needs of a malnourished patient. Potassium[30] and zinc deficiency are common and can have wide-ranging effects on hormonal secretion and nitrogen metabolism. Vitamin supplementation, particularly with folate, is also important if the characteristically impaired immune systems of a malnourished patient are not to be jeopardized further. The recognition of essential fatty acid deficiency as a component of the picture of infantile malnutrition parallels its need in patients being fed intravenously[31].

CONCLUSIONS

The emergence of parenteral feeding as an accepted measure of nutritional therapy in severely ill patients has focussed attention on the practical benefits which can accrue from a study of the principles of nutrition. These principles have been tested over many years in children from tropical environments. These studies suggest that urinary creatinine, hydroxyproline and 3-methylhistidine may prove useful indices of nutritional state, particularly if combined with monitoring serum albumin and pre-albumin or retinol-binding protein concentrations.

References

1. Waterlow, J. C. (1973). Note on the assessment of the classification of protein energy malnutrition in children. *Lancet*, **ii,** 87
2. Picou, D., Halliday, D. and Garrow, J. S. (1966). Total body protein, collagen and non-collagen protein in infantile protein malnutrition. *Clin. Sci.*, **30,** 345
3. Garrow, J. S., Fletcher, K. and Halliday, D. (1965). Body composition in severe infantile malnutrition. *J. Clin. Invest.*, **44,** 417
4. Alleyne, G. A. O., Halliday, D., Waterlow, J. C. and Nichols, B. C. (1969). Chemical composition of organs of children who died from malnutrition. *Br. J. Nutr.*, **23,** 783
5. Cahill, G. F. (1970). Starvation in man. *N. Engl. J. Med.*, **282,** 668
6. Felig, P. (1975). Amino acid metabolism in man. *Annu. Rev. Biochem.*, **44,** 933
7. Viteri, F. E. and Alvarado, J. (1970). The creatinine height index: its use in the estimation of the degree of protein depletion and repletion in protein calorie malnourished children. *Pediatrics*, **46,** 696
8. Picou, D., Alleyne, G. A. O. and Seakins, A. (1965). Hydroxyproline and creatinine excretion in infantile protein malnutrition. *Clin. Sci.*, **29,** 517
9. Whitehead, R. G. (1965). Hydroxyproline creatinine ratio as an index of nutritional status and rate of growth. *Lancet*, **ii,** 567
10. Allison, D. J., Walker, A. and Smith, Q. T. (1966). Urinary hydroxyproline:creatinine ratio of normal humans at various ages. *Clin. Chim. Acta*, **14,** 729
11. Whitehead, R. G. (1969). The assessment of nutritional status in protein-malnourished children. *Proc. Nutr. Soc.*, **28,** 1
12. Young, V. R. (1970). The role of skeletal and cardiac muscle in the regulation of

protein metabolism. In H. N. Munro (ed.). *Mammalian Protein Metabolism*. Vol. IV, p. 586. (New York and London: Academic Press)

13. Rao, B. S. N. and Nagabhushan, V. S. (1973). Urinary excretion of 3-methyl-histidine in children suffering from protein-calorie malnutrition. *Life Sci.*, **12,** 205
14. Waterlow, J. C. and Alleyne, G. A. O. (1971). Protein malnutrition in children: Advances in knowledge in the last ten years. *Adv. Protein Chem.*, **25,** 117
15. Picou, D. and Taylor-Roberts, T. (1969). The measurement of total protein synthesis and catabolism and nitrogen turnover in infants in different nutritional states and receiving different amounts of dietary protein. *Clin. Sci.*, **36,** 283
16. O'Keefe, S. J. D., Sender, P. M. and James, W. P. T. (1974). 'Catabolic' loss of body nitrogen in response to surgery. *Lancet*, **ii,** 1035
17. Crane, C. W., Picou, D., Smith, R. and Waterlow, J. C. (1977). Protein turnover in patients before and after elective orthopaedic operations. *Br. J. Surg.*, **64,** 129
18. Garlick, P. J., Millward, D. J., James, W. P. T. and Waterlow, J. C. (1975). The effect of protein deprivation and starvation on the rate of protein synthesis in tissues of the rat. *Biochim. Biophys. Acta*, **414,** 71
19. James, W. P. T. and Hay, A. M. (1968). Albumin metabolism: effect of the nutritional state and the dietary protein intakes. *J. Clin. Invest.*, **47,** 1958
20. O'Keefe, S. J. D., Sender, P. M., Clark, G. C. and James, W. P. T. (1974). The effect of varying the post-operative parenteral regime on the dynamics of protein metabolism following operative trauma. In C. Romieu, C. Solassol, H. Joyeux and B. Astruc (eds.). *International Congress on Parenteral Nutrition*, pp. 333–339 (University Montpellier)
21. Williamson, D. H., Farrell, R., Kerr, A. and Smith, R. (1977). Urine 3-methyl-histidine in man as a measure of muscle protein catabolism after injury. *Clin. Sci.*, **52,** 17P
22. Sherwin, R. S., Hendler, R. G. and Felig, P. (1975). Effect of ketone infusions on amino acid and nitrogen metabolism in man. *J. Clin. Invest.*, **55,** 1382
23. Whitehead, R. G. and Alleyne, G. A. O. (1972). Pathophysiological factors of importance in protein-calorie malnutrition. *Br. Med. Bull.*, **28,** 72
24. Alberti, K. G. M. M. and Johnston, D. G. (1977). Cortisol and catabolism: a new perspective. *Clin. Sci. Mol. Med.*, **52,** 333
25. McFarlane, H., Ogbeidi, M. I., Reddy, S., Adcock, K. J., Adeshima, H., Gurney, J. M., Cooke, A., Taylor, G. O. and Mordie, J. A. (1969). Biochemical assessment of protein-calorie malnutrition. *Lancet*, **i,** 392
26. Ingenbleek, Y., Van den Schrieck, H-G., De Nayer, P. and De Visscher, M. (1975). Albumin, transferrin and the thyroxine-binding pre-albumin/retinol-binding protein (TBPA-RBP) complex in assessment of malnutrition. *Clin. Chim. Acta*, **63,** 61
27. Ingenbleek, Y , De Visscher, M. and De Nayer, P. (1972). Biochemical assessment of protein-calorie malnutrition. *Lancet*, **ii,** 106
28. Ashworth, A., Bell, R., James, W. P. T. and Waterlow, J. C. (1968). Calorie requirements of children recovering from protein-calorie malnutrition. *Lancet*, **ii,** 600
29. Patrick, J. (1977). Death during recovery from severe malnutrition and its possible relationship to sodium pump activity in the leucocyte. *Br. Med. J.*, **1,** 1051
30. Mann, M. D., Bowie, M. D. and Hensen, J. D. (1972). Potassium in protein-calorie malnutrition. *S. African Med. J.*, **46,** 2062
31. James, W. P. T. (1977). Kwashiorkor and marasmus: old concepts and new developments. *J. Roy. Coll. Phys.*, **70,** 611
32. Sender, P. M., James, W. P. T., Garlick, P. J., Heard, C. R. C. and Waterlow, J. C. (1974). The effect of dietary energy and protein restriction on tyrosine and leucine metabolism in obesity. In A. Howard (ed.). *Rec. Adv. in Obesity Research.*, p. 83 (Newman Publishing, Ltd.)

Discussion

A. W. Goode: (UK) 3-methyl-histidine seems to be becoming more and more used as an index for protein turnover. Is it subject to the same errors as hydroxyproline, e.g. infection and other events distorting the results?

W. P. T. James: (UK) It is quite possible that it may prove to change in the same way as hydroxyproline. If Williamson's finding that it increases in certain patients is correct, then clearly we are in a situation where muscle protein breakdown can indeed increase. Whether or not this is associated with infection I do not know. Perhaps there are data already to suggest that. That would indicate that one has to be very careful in assessing repletion studies if the patient has any evidence of infection, because hydroxyproline and 3-methyl-histidine will then change. In normal people, or people in a stable state from the nutritional point of view, even though they are malnourished, we have found very reproducible excretion rates of 3-methyl-histidine, and they appear to progress in the expected manner.

G. L. Blackburn: (USA) Wannamaker and Beizel at the Infectious Disease Command of the US Army have shown increased 3-methyl-histidine losses with infection. Through a variety of nutritional pertubations in post operative patients 3-methyl-histidine seems to be the same steady state, one exception is burns, where there is true increased muscle protein breakdown, and tripling or quadrupling of the 3-methyl-histidine losses can occur.

I wanted to ask about the use of the very short half-life secretory proteins such as pre-albumin and retinol binding protein (RBP) whether with or without malnutrition post-surgically there is rather a dramatic drop in the short half-life protein. I wonder if we shall not get a lot of false positives using these early post operative values. This sensitivity is one reason why we prefer transferrin measurement to assess efficacy of nutritional therapy.

James: I may have overstated that. I meant to point out that this may have such a short half-life that it may end up in the same sort of place as the amino acid ratio work, where it is so responsive.

However, it seems to be a pretty good index of liver dysfunction. In that sense it may be well worth monitoring as an early sign of change in liver function.

H. F. Woods: (UK) One of our most recent patients in whom we are trying to assess these various indices was somebody with advanced thyrotoxicosis who was brought into us severely wasted, and who had to be fed intravenously.

Could Dr James suggest what index of muscle protein breakdown could be used in this case? Our Scandinavian colleagues have shown very nicely that thyrotoxicosis is a very good cause of increased hyroxyproline excretion, and our calculations for creatinine height index and other indices are totally spurious because of the effect of hormonal factors on muscle turnover.

James: I am not familiar with the concept of creatinine height index changing necessarily with turnover. Certainly it was well recognized some 30–40 years ago that the administration of thyroid hormone is associated with changes in body protein turnover. We would be in trouble looking at indices of protein turnover as an index in that unusual circumstance.

I am surprised that the creatinine height index did not work out, but that therefore suggests that we may be back to square one in those particular cases, looking for a more sensitive index.

P. Vinay: (Canada) If I remember, the *creatine* excretion rises very rapidly when muscle wastage occurs, and creatinine excretion stays quite stable, so there seems to be no reason why the creatinine height ratio should not work. Of course both urinary and plasma creatinine should be considered here.

James: There is also the question of the extent to which creatinine is an absolutely reliable index of muscle mass, particularly when one gets to a very protein-depleted state. There are studies suggesting that in anyone on a creatine-free diet for a long time progressive falls in creatinine excretion can take place which seem unrelated to muscle mass. Creatinine output can then be modulated by altering the protein, particularly the glycine intake.

For the moment the creatinine height index seems to be the best that we have as a static index of body compositional change.

35
The use of body composition measurements to assess the efficacy of parenteral nutrition

H. M. SHIZGAL

INTRODUCTION

The importance of parenteral alimentation has been recognized for many years. Robert Elman, in 1939, pointed out that 'Intravenous alimentation becomes important whenever the nutritional needs of the body cannot be met by oral feeding; it becomes essential when death threatens because of nutritional deficiencies which can be remedied in no other way'[1]. In the same paper he reported the first successful intravenous infusion of amino acids, obtained by the acid hydrolysis of casein to which was added 2% tryptophan and cystine. The importance of infusing carbohydrate with the amino acids was also recognized at that time, as the authors point out that 'dextrose was always added, not only because of its caloric value but also because there is considerable evidence that the utilization of amino acids is enhanced by the presence of carbohydrate'. Elman's work was rapidly taken up and repeated all over the world both with his Amigen solution, an enzymatic hydrolysate of casein and pancreas, and with a variety of other hydrolysed proteins which had become available. Despite the widespread availability of both amino acid and hypertonic glucose solutions, the importance of total parenteral nutrition (TPN) was not generally accepted, primarily because its efficacy had not been demonstrated. Francis D. Moore, in his classic book, *The Metabolic Care of the Surgical Patient*, published in 1959, emphasizes the importance of a central venous catheter for the administration of hypertonic glucose solutions. Yet he stated that 'We have never seen a patient gain solid tissue weight and pass into indubitably significant and lasting anabolism on the basis of parenteral nutrients alone'[2].

The efficacy of parenteral nutrition was not generally accepted until

Dudrick *et al.*[3] demonstrated normal growth and development of a group of beagle puppies, who received all of their nutrition by the parenteral route. Subsequently, a large number of reports appeared in the literature testifying to the clinical benefits of TPN[4–6]. An excellent example are papers reporting a significant reduction in mortality with the use of TPN in patients with small bowel fistula. Prior to the introduction of TPN, the mortality rate of patients with small bowel fistula ranged from 20%[7] to 54%[8]. With the addition of TPN, mortality rates in the range of 8%[9] to 14%[10] have been reported. Studies of this nature have demonstrated the benefits of TPN. However, the data obtained measured efficacy in a qualitative rather than quantitative manner. As a result, these data have a large variance, and are therefore almost impossible to utilize in testing and comparing the efficacy of TPN systems.

The measurement of nitrogen balance is widely employed to measure the efficacy of TPN, since it is a measure of the net effect of protein anabolism and catabolism. Under steady state conditions, positive nitrogen balance is indicative of anabolism, while negative balance occurs in the presence of catabolism. However, there is considerable error associated with nitrogen balance measurements as Vinnars has so nicely described[11]. Nitrogen intake is usually overestimated while output is underestimated. The experimental error of the difference, i.e. nitrogen balance, is therefore large, especially when this difference is small, which is usually the case. In addition this error is cumulative.

To avoid the considerable difficulties associated with nitrogen balance determinations, body composition measurements have been employed instead to quantify the efficacy of TPN. The body composition measurements employed in our laboratory in recent years are described and used to determine (a) the presence and severity of malnutrition, (b) the effect of amino acid solutions on protein sparing following major operations, (c) caloric requirements of the patient receiving TPN and (d) the efficacy of TPN with lipid as the major caloric source.

BODY COMPOSITION MEASUREMENTS

The body cell mass is the total mass of living, energy-exchanging, and oxygen-consuming cells of the body. It is therefore that component of body composition which TPN is intended to maintain, in the normal patient, and to restore in the patient with malnutrition. The efficacy of TPN can therefore best be measured by monitoring the body cell mass.

The size of the body cell mass is estimated by measuring total exchangeable potassium (K_e), since a linear relationship exists between K_e and the body cell mass[12]. Isotope dilution with a radioactive isotope of potassium would be the method of choice for measuring K_e. Unfortunately the commercially available radioactive isotope of potassium, ^{42}K, decays rapidly with a half-life of

12.5 h. Clinical studies involving an isotope with such a short half-life are expensive and logistically inconvenient. Total exchangeable potassium can also be measured with the whole body counter. However, it is an expensive installation and its calibration remains a difficult problem[13]. To overcome these problems an indirect technique for the measurement of K_e was developed in our laboratory. The description of this technique and its experimental validation have been given elsewhere[14]. A multiple isotope dilution technique was subsequently developed which measures the various components of body composition[15]. The isotopes employed and the parameters measured are listed in Table 35.1.

Table 35.1 Body composition measurements

Isotopes injected	*Parameters measured*
^{125}I labelled albumin	Plasma volume (PV)
^{51}Cr tagged red cells	Red cell volume (RBC)
^{22}Na	Extracellular water volume (ECW)
	Na_e
Tritiated water	TBW

Parameters calculated

Blood volume = PV + RBC
Lean body mass (LBM) = TBW/0.73
Body fat = Body weight − LBM
Intracellular water volume = TBW − ECW
K_e = TBW × R* − Na_e
Body cell mass (BCM) = K_e × 0.00833
Extracellular mass = LBM − BCM

* R = the sodium plus potassium content divided by the water content of a sample of whole blood.

Body weight can be partitioned, as illustrated in Figure 35.1, into body fat, and the lean body mass. The determination of the lean body mass is based on the assumption that 73% of its mass is water; thus the lean body is equal to total body water (TBW) divided by 0.73[15]. The lean body mass is composed of two major compartments: the extracellular mass and the body cell mass. The former is the extracellular, supporting, non-living component of body composition, in contrast to the body cell mass which is the living, functioning, oxygen-consuming, energy-exchanging component. The size of the extracellular mass is estimated by measuring total exchangeable sodium (Na_e) and/or the extracellular water volume; two parameters which are measured independently of each other. Similarly K_e and the intracellular water volume are measured independently of each other and thus provide two independent measures of the body cell mass.

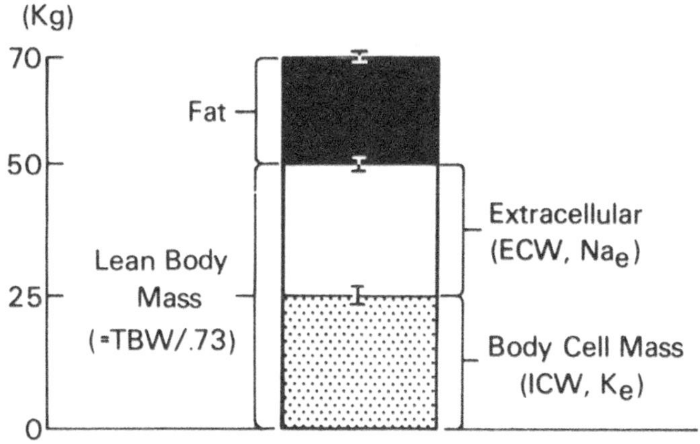

Figure 35.1 The mean body composition of twenty-five normal volunteers. Body weight is the sum of body fat and the lean body mass. The latter is divided almost equally into the extracellular mass and the body cell mass

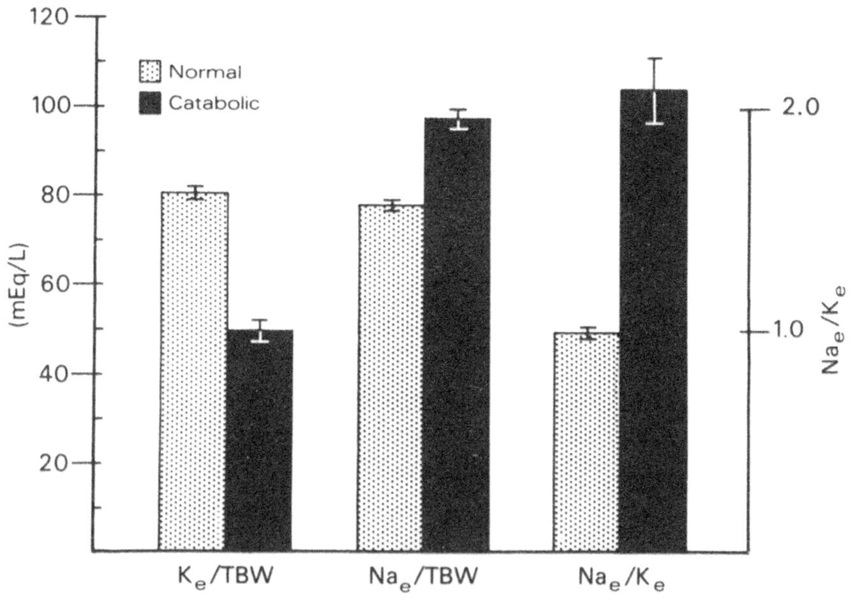

Figure 35.2 The mean ± standard error of the mean of Na_e/TBW, K_e/TBW and Na_e/K_e in twenty-five normal volunteers and in eighteen patients who were in a chronic catabolic state and starved. Na_e/TBW and K_e/TBW are a measure of the extracellular mass and the body cell mass respectively

MALNUTRITION

The effect of malnutrition on body composition is illustrated in Figure 35.2. Body composition measurements were obtained and compared to similar data obtained in twenty-five normal volunteers. The size of the extracellular mass and of the body cell mass was estimated by the measurement of Na_e and K_e respectively. To allow for variation in body size, these parameters were expressed as a function of TBW. Moore *et al.* have demonstrated that TBW is a more accurate independent parameter of body composition than body weight[12]. There was a significant decrease in the body cell mass, as expected, in the patients who are in a chronic catabolic state and starved (Figure 35.3). This was accompanied by an expansion of the extracellular mass. Thus the ratio Na_e/K_e rose significantly (Figure 35.2). This ratio has proved to be a sensitive index of nutritional status because of the reciprocal changes in the body cell mass and the extracellular mass which occur with malnutrition[15,16]. In the normal population the mean ratio is 0.98 with minimal variance (SD = 0.12, SEM = 0.02).

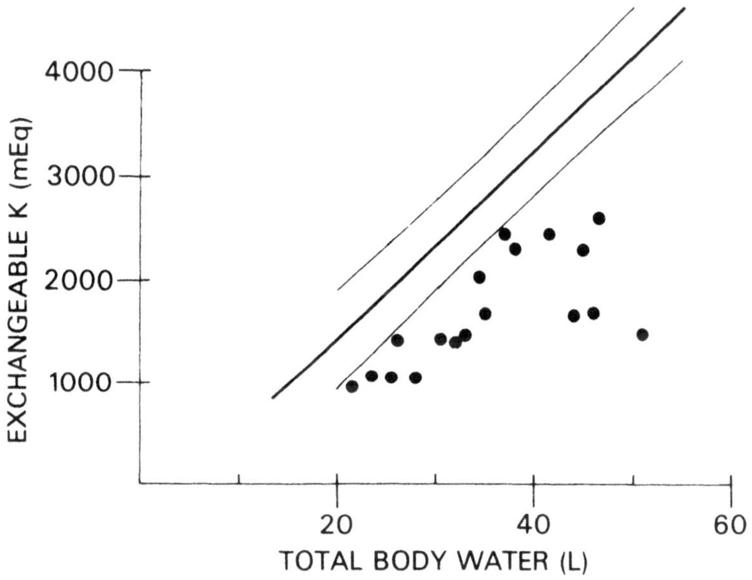

Figure 35.3 Exchangeable potassium, a measure of the body cell mass, was plotted as a function of TBW, to normalize for variation in body weight. The data were obtained in eighteen patients who were in a chronic catabolic state and starved. The normal range is indicated by the 95% confidence limits about the regression, which were calculated from data obtained in twenty-five normal volunteers

PROTEIN SPARING FOLLOWING MAJOR SURGERY

A catabolic state develops following any operation of moderate to major severity which, in the absence of postoperative complications, persists for

Table 35.2 Protein sparing following major surgery*

	Number	Glucose			Amigen		
		Pre-Op.	*Post-Op.*	*Change*	*Pre-Op.*	*Post-Op.*	*Change*
Body weight (kg)	19	66.2 ± 1.9	63.5 ± 1.8	−2.6†	68.1 ± 3.9	66.2 ± 3.7	−2.0†
Lean body mass (kg)	19	47.8 ± 1.8	47.1 ± 1.6	−0.8	48.0 ± 2.5	49.8 ± 2.4	+1.8†
Body fat (kg)	19	18.3 ± 1.5	16.5 ± 1.5	−1.9†	20.1 ± 2.1	16.4 ± 2.3	−3.7†
Na_e (mEq)	19	2685 ± 95	2822 ± 95	+137†	2737 ± 123	2828 ± 155	+91
Extracellular water (l.)	10	14.9 ± 0.9	15.4 ± 0.8	+0.5	14.8 ± 1.1	14.5 ± 1.0	−0.3
K_e (mEq)	19	2774 ± 178	2384 ± 167	−391†	2743 ± 184	2857 ± 151	+114
Intracellular water (l.)	10	18.6 ± 1.5	17.9 ± 1.1	−0.6	18.2 ± 2.0	19.4 ± 2.0	+1.2
Na_e/K_e	19	1.04 ± .08	1.29 ± 0.11	+0.25	1.03 ± 0.04	1.00 ± 0.03	−0.4

* Mean ± standard error of the mean
† Significantly ($P < 0.05$) different by Student's paired *t* test

several days. This postoperative catabolic state is characterized by a breakdown of body protein, and can therefore be measured as either negative nitrogen balance or a loss of the body cell mass. Blackburn and Flatt were the first to propose that this postoperative loss of body protein could be prevented by the infusion of amino acids during the postoperative period[17].

To test this hypothesis, body composition measurements were performed, in two groups of nineteen patients each, prior to, and on the fifth day following, a major operation. All the patients underwent either a gastrectomy or colon resection. One group of patients received all of their intravenous fluids and electrolytes as a 5% glucose solution. The second group received the same volume of water and electrolytes, as a 5% casein hydrolysate (Amigen, Baxter Laboratories, Malton, Ontario, Canada) solution. Thus, isocaloric solutions were administered to both groups.

The results obtained are listed in Table 35.2. The postoperative loss of body weight was statistically significant and of the same order of magnitude in both groups. The mean loss of body weight in the group receiving glucose,

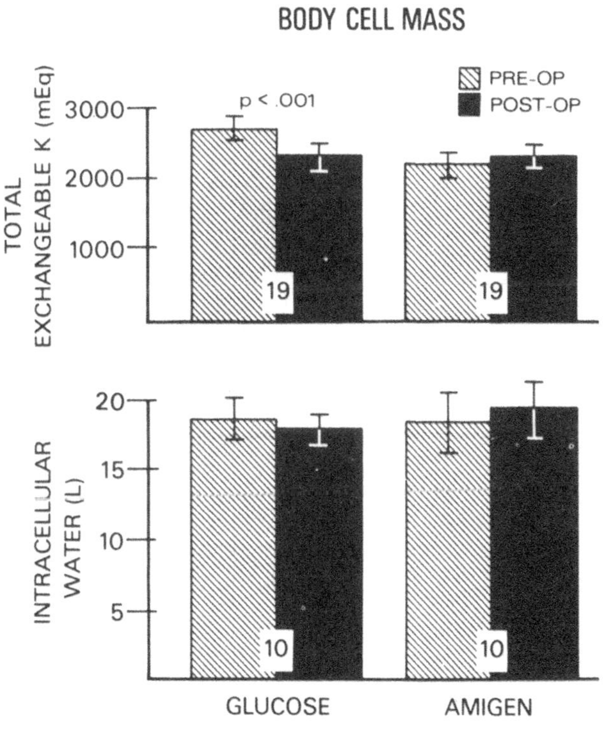

Figure 35.4 The mean ± standard error of the mean of K_e and intracellular volume, which are both a measure of the body cell mass. The measurements were performed preoperative and on the 5th post-operative day in both patient groups. The numbers within the bars indicate the number of patients in whom the measurements were performed

was 2.6 kg. This weight loss resulted from a 1.9 kg loss of body fat and a 0.8 kg loss of lean body mass. In contrast, the weight loss in the patients receiving Amigen resulted entirely from a loss of body fat.

Striking differences between the two groups were observed in the post-operative lean body mass. In the glucose group, there was a post-operative decrease in the two parameters which measure the body cell mass, i.e. K_e and the intracellular water volume (Figure 35.4). This was accompanied by an expansion of the extracellular mass as measured by Na_e and the extracellular water volume (Table 35.2). Thus, by the fifth post-operative day, in the patients receiving glucose, there was a contraction of the body cell mass accompanied by a relative expansion of the extracellular mass; changes characteristic of malnutrition and reflected by a significant elevation of the ratio Na_e/K_e (Table 35.2). These changes did not occur in the patients receiving 5% Amigen postoperatively (Figure 35.4, Table 35.2). In the latter patients, following operation there was a small but statistically insignificant increase in the body cell mass.

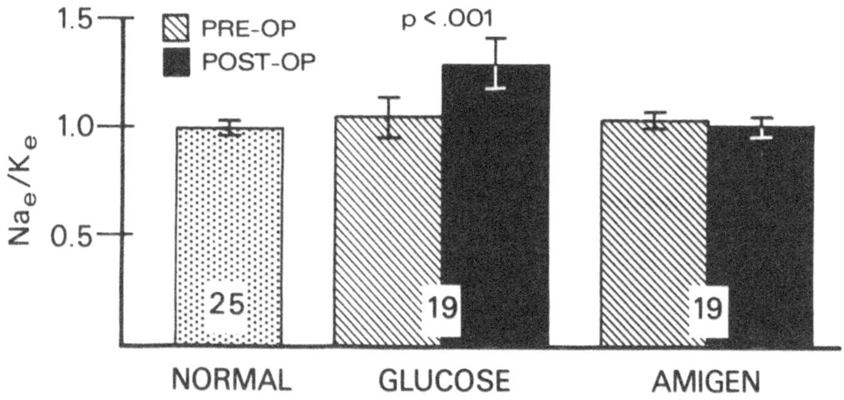

Figure 35.5 The mean ± standard error of the mean Na_e/K_e ratio in twenty-five normal volunteers and both preoperatively and on the 5th postoperative day in the two patient groups. The significance of the differences of the means was determined by an analysis of variance

The ratio Na_e/K_e, as pointed out previously, is a sensitive index of nutritional status. Preoperatively, in both groups, this ratio was normal (Figure 35.5). Postoperatively, it remained normal in the group receiving amino acids, but was significantly elevated in the patients receiving glucose. The data therefore demonstrate the postoperative protein-sparing effects of amino acid solutions.

CALORIC REQUIREMENTS OF PATIENTS RECEIVING TPN

In an earlier study[18], body composition measurements were performed in a group of severely ill patients to determine the efficacy of TPN. In these patients, who were in a chronic catabolic state, TPN prevented the decrease in the body cell mass and the concomitant expansion of the extracellular mass, which occurred in similar patients not receiving TPN. However, TPN did not result in a significant improvement in their body composition. Inadequate infusion of calories and/or protein was a possible explanation for this lack of improvement. The patients studied had received a mean of 50.4 ± 4.8 kcal/kg/day, which was considered adequate at the time. However, there is very little information available regarding the caloric requirements of the patients receiving TPN. As a result the following study was performed to determine the caloric requirements of patients receiving TPN.

Body composition measurements were obtained at both the beginning and end of a course of TPN, in thirty-five patients. Eighteen patients received a 25% dextrose solution containing 2.5% crystalline L-amino acids (Travasol*, Baxter Laboratories, Malton, Ontario, Canada) for 14.5 ± 1.2 days. Ten patients received a 25% dextrose solution containing 5% casein hydrolysate for 19.0 ± 3.0 days (McGaw Laboratories). In the third group of seven patients, equal volumes of a 10% Intralipid solution (Pharmacia Canada Ltd, Montreal, Canada) and a 7% crystalline L-amino solution with 10% fructose (Vamin, Pharmacia Canada Ltd.) was infused for a mean of 11.6 ± 1.8 days. The mean number of kcal/kg/day infused was plotted against the mean daily

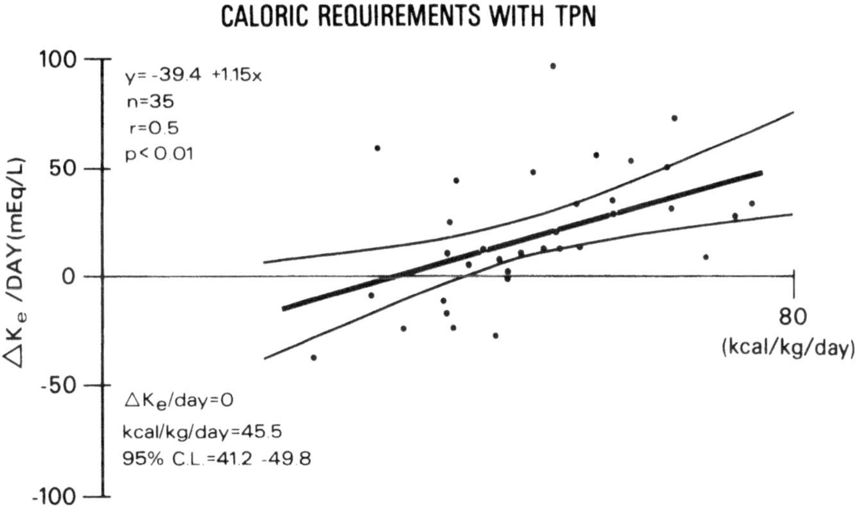

Figure 35.6 The mean daily change in K_e was correlated with the mean kcal/kg/day infused in thirty-five patients receiving TPN. The resultant regression line was statistically significant ($P < 0.01$) and intercepted the abscissa at 45.5 kcal/kg/day. The 95% confidence limits of this intercept are 41.2 and 49.8 kcal/kg/day

*Synthamin.

change in K_e (ΔK_e/day), a measure of the mean daily change in the body cell mass (Figure 35.6). The resulting regression line, which was statistically significant ($P < 0.01$), indicated that K_e, i.e. the body cell mass, remained constant when 45.5 (95% confidence limits = 41.2–49.8) kcal/kg/day was infused. In addition the data indicate that the infusion of calories in excess of this amount results in the rebuilding of a depleted body cell mass.

TOTAL PARENTERAL NUTRITION WITH LIPID

Total parenteral nutrition with lipid as the major caloric source, as opposed to hypertonic dextrose has several advantages. Lipid has a high caloric density, of 9 kcal/g, and is formulated as an isotonic solution. A central venous catheter is therefore not a necessity. In addition it can be administered simultaneously with an amino acid solution, by way of a Y connector, thus avoiding the necessity of mixing solutions prior to administration.

The efficacy of TPN with 10% Intralipid administered with equal volumes of a solution containing 7% L-amino acids and 10% fructose (Vamin) was determined. The latter was accomplished by performing body composition measurements prior to the onset, at 2-week intervals during, and at the completion of, a course of TPN. A total of 108 body composition measurements were performed, permitting the evaluation of 61 intervals of TPN, of 15.0 ± 0.4 days in duration. The mean ΔK_e/day was correlated against the kcal/kg/day infused. The resultant regression line was not statistically significant (Figure 35.7). The absence of a significant correlation between

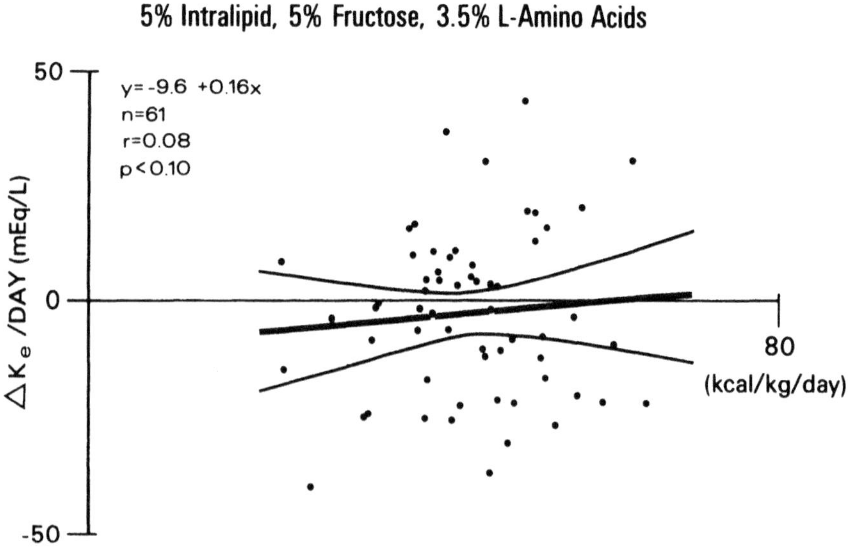

Figure 35.7 The mean Δk_e/day was correlated with the kcal/kg/day infused during sixty-one periods of TPN in a group of forty-seven patients. The resultant regression line was not statistically significant. Patients with and without malnutrition are included

the ΔK_e/day and the kcal/kg/day infused was attributed to the inclusion of numerous patients who did not have malnutrition at the onset of TPN. In the absence of malnutrition an increase in K_e, i.e. in the body cell mass, is unlikely, regardless of the amount of protein and calories infused. Consequently, the ΔK_e/day was correlated with kcal/kg/day infused only for those patients with malnutrition at the onset of TPN. Malnutrition was defined as a Na_e/K_e ratio which exceeded 1.22, which is the upper 95% confidence limit of our normal sample. The resultant regression line was statistically significant (Figure 35.8). The line interrupted the abscissa at 44.2 (95% confidence

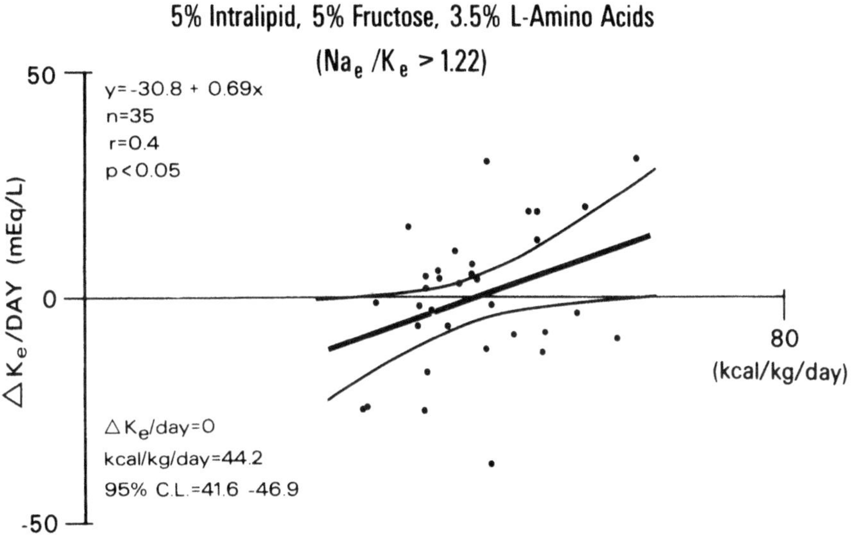

Figure 35.8 Similar to Figure 36.7 except that only patients with malnutrition are included. Malnutrition was defined by a Na_e/K_e ratio greater than 1.22. The regression line, which is statistically significant, intercepts the abscissa at 44.2 kcal/kg/day. The 95% confidence limits of this intercept are 41.6 and 46.9 kcal/kg/day

limits = 41.6–46.9) kcal/kg/day indicating that the body cell mass was maintained when calories were infused at this rate. However, the magnitude of the slope of the regression line was small (Figure 35.8), indicating that the infusion of calories in excess of this amount has very little effect on the body cell mass. This was demonstrated by dividing the patients into those with malnutrition ($Na_e/K_e > 1.22$) and those without malnutrition ($Na_e/K_e < 1.22$) at the onset of TPN. Each group was further subdivided according to whether they received more than, or less than, 44 kcal/kg/day; i.e. the amount of calories required to maintain the body cell mass (Tables 35.3, 35.4). The mean body composition of twenty-five normal volunteers, and of each of the four subgroups of patients receiving TPN is described in Figure 35.9.

In the patients without malnutrition at the onset of TPN, there was no change in their body composition following TPN, regardless of the number of calories infused (Figure 35.9, Table 35.3). Both the extracellular mass and the body cell mass remained normal. The patient without malnutrition was not expected to increase his body cell mass, regardless of the number of calories infused. Excessive administration of calories to a normal individual results in an increase in body fat without any change in the body cell mass. This has been documented in a group of morbidly obese patients in whom their excessive body weight resulted primarily from an increase in body fat while their body cell mass was normal[15].

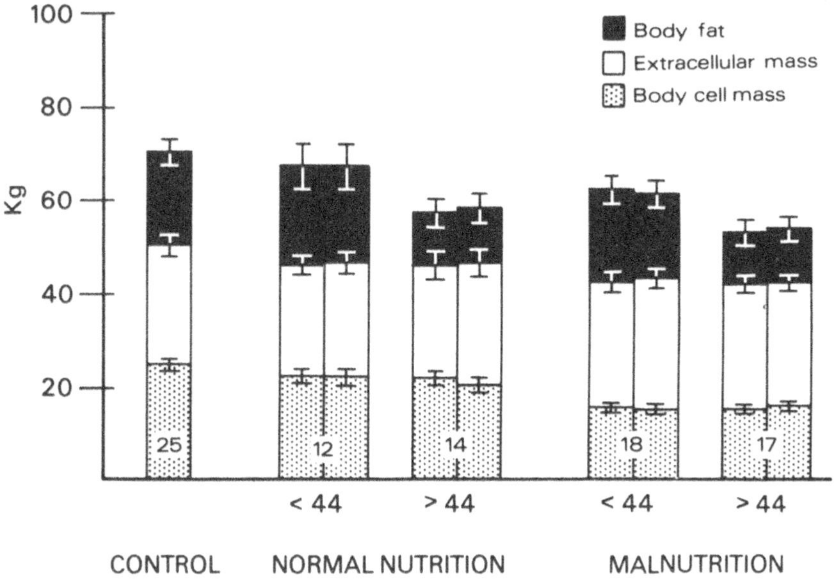

Figure 35.9 The mean body composition, before and following a course of TPN. The patients were divided into four groups according to the presence or absence of malnutrition and whether they received more than or less than 44 kcal/kg/day. The mean body composition of twenty-five normal volunteers is included

Parenteral nutrition with lipid did not significantly improve the body composition of the patients with malnutrition (Figure 35.9, Table 35.4). In the group III-A patients, who received a mean of 37.8 $\pm$ 0.9 kcal/kg/day for 14.6 $\pm$ 0.5 days, this was not surprising as they received less calories than was required to maintain their body cell mass. However, the group II-B patients similarly did not improve their body composition, in spite of receiving 50.9 $\pm$ 1.4 kcal/kg/day. The TPN administered to these patients effectively maintained the body cell mass but did not rebuild it. The slope of the regression curve, relating ΔK_e/day and the kcal/kg/day infused (Figure 35.8) had indicated this inability to increase significantly the size of a depleted body cell mass.

Table 35.3 TPN with lipid in patients without malnutrition*

	Normal volunteers	*Group II-A (<44 kcal/kg/day)*		*Group II-B (>44 kcal/kg/day)*	
		Pre-TPN	*Post TPN*	*Pre TPN*	*Post-TPN*
Number	25	18	18	17	17
Body weight (kg)	70.4 ± 2.5	62.4 ± 2.7	61.4 ± 2.8	53.0 ± 2.6	53.9 ± 2.3
Body fat (kg)	20.2 ± 1.4	20.0 ± 2.0	18.2 ± 2.5	11.1 ± 2.2	11.6 ± 2.1
Total body water (l.)	36.8 ± 1.4	30.9 ± 1.4	31.6 ± 1.5	30.6 ± 1.2	30.9 ± 1.0
Lean body mass (kg)	50.3 ± 1.9	42.4 ± 1.9	43.3 ± 2.1	41.9 ± 1.6	42.3 ± 1.4
Extracellular mass (kg)	25.6 ± 0.9	27.0 ± 1.4	28.3 ± 1.6	26.6 ± 1.0	26.5 ± 1.2
Body cell mass (kg)	24.7 ± 1.1	15.4 ± 0.8	15.0 ± 0.8	15.2 ± 0.7	15.8 ± 0.7
Na_e (mEq)	2869 ± 95	2855 ± 159	2892 ± 152	2849 ± 111	2816 ± 123
Na_e/TBW (mEq/l)	77.5 ± 0.9	92.1 ± 2.1†	91.7 ± 2.3†	93.4 ± 1.1†	91.0 ± 2.2†
K_e (mEq)	2955 ± 130	1844 ± 93	1795 ± 97	1826 ± 83	1894 ± 84
K_e/TBW (mEq/l)	80.0 ± 1.0	59.7 ± 1.8	57.3 ± 2.2†	59.7 ± 1.1†	61.9 ± 2.6†
Na_e/K_e	0.98 ± 0.02	1.57 ± 0.07†	1.64 ± 0.07†	1.58 ± 0.04†	1.54 ± 0.15†
Days on TPN		14.6 ± 0.5		15.6 ± 0.7	
Kcal/kg/day		37.8 ± 0.9		50.9 ± 1.4	
K_e/day		-4.0 ± 2.8		3.4 ± 4.3	

* Mean ± standard error of the mean
† Significantly different ($P < 0.05$) from normal by an analysis of variance and Scheffe's test
‡ Significantly different ($P < 0.05$) from pre-TPN measurement by paired Student's t test

Table 35.4 TPN with lipid in patients with malnutrition*

	Normal volunteers	*Group I-A (<44 kcal/kg/day)*		*Group I-B (>44 kcal/kg/day)*	
		Pre-TPN	*Post-TPN*	*Pre-TPN*	*Post-TPN*
Number	25	12	12	14	14
Body weight (kg)	70.4 ± 2.5	67.4 ± 4.5	67.3 ± 4.6	57.3 ± 2.9	58.3 ± 3.0
Body fat (kg)	20.2 ± 1.4	21.4 ± 4.1	20.8 ± 4.4	11.5 ± 1.9	11.9 ± 1.7
Total body water (l.)	36.8 ± 1.4	33.6 ± 1.4	33.9 ± 1.6	33.5 ± 2.0	33.9 ± 2.0
Lean body mass (kg)	50.3 ± 1.9	46.0 ± 1.9	46.5 ± 2.1	45.9 ± 2.8	46.4 ± 2.7
Extracellular mass (kg)	25.6 ± 0.9	23.8 ± 0.7	24.5 ± 1.0	24.2 ± 1.5	26.1 ± 1.5
Body cell mass (kg)	24.7 ± 1.1	22.2 ± 1.3	22.0 ± 1.6	21.7 ± 1.4	20.3 ± 1.5‡
Na_e (mEq)	2869 ± 95	2593 ± 106	2578 ± 137	2556 ± 153	2738 ± 163‡
Na_e/TBW (mEq/l)	77.5 ± 0.9	77.5 ± 1.8	76.2 ± 2.2	76.6 ± 1.2	81.2 ± 1.9‡
K_e (mEq)	2955 ± 130	2660 ± 161	2637 ± 189	2602 ± 167	2437 ± 182
K_e/TBW (mEq/l)	80.0 ± 1.0	78.7 ± 1.9	77.1 ± 2.6	77.5 ± 1.6	71.1 ± 2.6‡
Na_e/K_e	0.98 ± 0.02	0.99 ± 0.03	1.01 ± 0.06	1.00 ± 0.03	1.17 ± 0.07‡
Days on TPN		14.1 ± 0.4		15.6 ± 1.0	
Kcal/kg/day		34.6 ± 2.3		51.7 ± 1.5	
K_e/day		−1.3 ± 6.1		−9.7 ± 5.4	

* Mean ± standard error of the mean.
† Significantly different ($P < 0.05$) from normal by an analysis of variance and Scheffe's test.
‡ Significantly different ($P < 0.05$) from pre-TPN measurement by paired Student's *t* test.

The data do not however explain why the solutions infused were unable to increase the size of a depleted body cell mass. The use of lipid as the major caloric source is a possible explanation. Long *et al.*, on the basis of nitrogen balance measurements, have reported that only 20% or less of the energy requirements can be provided by lipid emulsions[19]. In contrast Jeejeebhoy *et al.* contend that lipid is an effective source of calories and reported positive nitrogen balance with a TPN system in which lipid provided 83% of the calories[20]. Another possible explanation is that insufficient calories were administered. The group II-B patients received a mean of 50.9 ± 1.4 kcal/kg/day (Table 35.4) which was only slightly in excess of the number of calories required to maintain the body cell mass, i.e. 44.2 kcal/kg/day. To infuse more calories would require that the patients receive more than 3 g/kg/day of lipid, which we had established as the upper limit. Intralipid is at present approved for a maximum administration rate of 2 g/kg/day. The poor results with the Intralipid and Vamin combination, as indicated by the body composition measurements, are nevertheless an important finding, regardless of the reason for the poor results.

The body composition data emphasize another difficulty with the use of nitrogen balance measurements to measure the efficacy of TPN. The ideal solution for TPN should maintain a normal body cell mass and rebuild one which is depleted. The infusion of such a solution would therefore result in nitrogen balance which is positive in patients with malnutrition, and zero in patients without pre-existing malnutrition. The interpretation of nitrogen balance measurements, without first determining the presence or absence of malnutrition, is therefore extremely difficult. The importance of a knowledge of nutritional status when evaluating the results of TPN was illustrated by the differences between the regression line in Figure 35.7, which included patients with and without malnutrition, and Figure 35.8, which included only patients with malnutrition.

SUMMARY

Advances in the field of TPN are possible only if the efficacy of this form of nutrition can be measured quantitatively. Nitrogen balance measurements have been widely utilized to determine the efficacy of TPN, as they are a measure of the net effect of protein anabolism and catabolism. However, large experimental errors are associated with the measurement of nitrogen balance. To avoid these difficulties body composition measurements were employed to determine the efficacy of TPN. A multiple isotope dilution technique was employed to estimate body fat, the lean body mass, and its two compartments: the extracellular mass and the body cell mass. The effect of malnutrition on body composition was determined in a group of patients who were in a chronic catabolic state and starved. Malnutrition was characterized by a loss of body cell mass, accompanied by an expansion of the extracellular mass, resulting in an increase in the Na_e/K_e ratio. This ratio has proved to be a sensitive index of nutritional status.

Body composition measurements were utilized to determine the efficacy of a 5% casein hydrolysate solutions (Amigen) to spare protein following a major elective operation. Body composition was measured before operation, and on the 5th postoperative day, in two groups of nineteen patients each. All of the postoperative fluids and electrolytes were administered as a 5% dextrose solution in the first group, and as a 5% casein hydrolysate in the second group. Postoperatively, in the glucose group, the body cell mass decreased while the extracellular mass increased. This did not occur in the patients receiving the amino acid solution, indicating significant protein sparing.

Body composition measurements were successfully employed to determine the caloric requirements of the severely ill patient receiving TPN. In thirty-five patients a statistically significant correlation was obtained between the kcal/kg/day infused and the ΔK_e/day, which is a measure of the mean daily change in the body cell mass. The data indicated that the body cell mass was maintained when 45.5 kcal/kg/day was infused and that the infusion of calories in excess of this amount resulted in the rebuilding of a depleted body cell mass.

Body composition measurements were employed to measure the efficacy of TPN with a 10% Intralipid solution administered simultaneously with an equal volume of a solution containing 7% amino acids and 10% fructose. This solution effectively maintains the body cell mass in patients without malnutrition. However, in the patient with malnutrition, this form of TPN did not rebuild a depleted body cell mass but was only capable of maintaining it.

References

1. Elman, R. and Weiner, D. O. (1939). Intravenous alimentation with special reference to protein (amino acid) metabolism. *J. Am. Med. Assoc.*, **112,** 796
2. Moore, F. D. (1959). *Metabolic Care of the Surgical Patient.* (Philadelphia and London: W. B. Saunders Co.)
3. Dudrick, S. J., Wilmore, D. W. and Vars, H. M. (1967). Long term total parenteral nutrition with growth in puppies and positive nitrogen balance in patients. *Surg. For.*, **18,** 356
4. Dudrick, S. J., Wilmore, D. W., Vars, H. M. and Rhoads, J. E. (1968). Long-term total parenteral nutrition with growth, development, and positive nitrogen balance. *Surgery*, **64,** 134
5. Freeman, J. B. and MacLean, L. D. (1971). Intravenous hyperalimentation: A review. *Can. J. Surg.*, **14,** 1
6. Vogel, C. M., Kingsbury, R. J. and Baue, A. E. (1972). Intravenous hyperalimentation. *Arch. Surg.*, **105,** 414
7. Roback, S. A. and Nicoloff, D. M. (1972). High output entero-cutaneous fistula of the small bowel. *Am. J. Surg.*, **123,** 317
8. Edmunds, Jr. L. D., Williams, E. M. and Welch, C. E. (1960). External fistula arising from the gastro-intestinal tract. *Ann. Surg.*, **152,** 445
9. Himal, H. S., Allard, J. R., Nadeau, J. E., Freeman, J. B. and MacLean, L. D. (1974).

The importance of adequate nutrition in closure of small intestinal fistulas. *Br. J. Surg.*, **61,** 724
10. Sheldon, E. F., Gardiner, B. M., Way, L. W. and Dunphy, J. E. (1971). Management of gastrointestinal fistulas. *Surg. Gynecol. Obstet.*, **133,** 385
11. Vinnars, E. (1971). Effect of intravenous amino acid administration on nitrogen retention. *Scan. J. Clin. Lab. Invest.*, **27** (Suppl.) **117,** 1
12. Moore, F. D., Olesen, K. H., McMurray, J. D., Parker, H. V., Ball, M. R. and Boyden, C. M. (1963). *The Body Cell Mass and Its Supporting Environment. Body Composition in Health and Disease.* (Philadelphia: Saunders)
13. Cohn, S. H. and Dombrowski, C. S. (1970). Absolute measurement of whole body potassium by gamma ray spectrometry. *J. Nucl. Med.*, **11,** 239
14. Shizgal, H. M., Spanier, A. H., Humes, J. and Wood, C. D. (1977). The indirect measurement of total exchangeable potassium. *Am. J. Physiol.* (In press.)
15. Spanier, A. H., Kurtz, R. S., Shibata, H. R., MacLean, L. D. and Shizgal, H. M. (1976). Alterations in body composition following intestinal bypass for morbid obesity. *Surgery*, **80,** 1971
16. Spanier, A. H. and Shizgal, H. M. (1977). Caloric requirements of the critically ill patient receiving intravenous hyperalimentation. *Am. J. Surg.*, **133,** 99
17. Blackburn, G. L., Flatt, J. P., Clowes, G. H. A., Jr., O'Donnell, T. F. and Hensle, T. E. (1973). Protein sparing therapy during periods of starvation with sepsis or trauma. *Ann. Surg.*, **177,** 588
18. Shizgal, H. M., Spanier, A. H. and Kurtz, R. S. (1976). Effect of parenteral nutrition on body composition in the critically ill patient. *Am. J. Surg.*, **131,** 156
19. Long, J. M., Wilmore, D. W., Mason, A. D., Jr. and Pruitt, B. A., Jr. (1974). Fat carbohydrate interaction: Nitrogen sparing effect of varying caloric sources for total intravenous feeding. *Surg. For.*, **25,** 61
20. Jeejeebhoy, K. M., Anderson, G. H., Nakhooda, A. F., Greenberg, G. R., Sanderson, I. and Marliss, E. B. (1976). Metabolic studies in total parenteral nutrition with lipid in man. *J. Clin. Invest.*, **57,** 125

Discussion

A. W. Goode: (UK) For maximal repletion, what is the calories per kg body weight which would produce the maximum anabolic effect?

H. M. Shizgal: (Canada) All we defined was the number of calories per kg per day required to maintain the body cell mass. This figure was 46 cal/kg/day.

Goode: I have no experience of multiple isotope techniques, but with exchangeable potassium as a single isotope it is reproducible to about plus or minus 3%. What is it when using two or three different isotopes simultaneously?

Shizgal: I suspect that it is increased as the number of isotopes used is increased. We have some indirect data to suggest that it is in the order of about 5%, with our methodology. It depends on how careful one is, how many duplicates are run, how much isotope is injected, how long one counts for. When we compare our indirect to direct measurement, we increase the variance of the measurement by only 2 or 3%.

P. Fürst: (Sweden) I have two diagrams that confirm Dr Shizgal's data. The results presented are obtained by direct measurements of muscle biopsy material in patients suffering from moderate or severe trauma respectively, compared with a control group. In the first illustration the water distribution is presented (Figure 1). The increase found in the extracellular water following moderate trauma was significant. Highly significant increases in total water and extracellular water content were observed in patients with severe trauma.

The electrolyte distribution in the different groups is presented in the second diagram (Figure 2). We found that the increase in the extracellular compartment was associated with an increased extracellular sodium and chloride content. Surprisingly, as we have heard, only in very severe trauma did we observe potassium depletion. When we plotted this group we found that some of the patients were depleted, and others were not. All these findings confirm the validity of the curves presented by Dr Shizgal. The low muscle potassium content in a patient with severe trauma was also associated with a moderate magnesium depletion.

The values presented were calculated with a membrane potential of —70 millivolts assuming a decreased potential in these patients. However, I would like to point out that for any assumed membrane potential the alterations which were observed are valid, confirming Dr Shizgal's data.

P. Vinay: Am I correct in thinking that these measurements, presented by Dr Fürst, were done by drying tissue and then measuring the electrolytes in a dry residue? What happens if for some reason a cell gets sick, and more sodium gets into the cell because the sodium pump is not working properly. This sick cell syndrome is well documented in several pathological conditions. When the sodium content inside the cell is higher than it should be, this will modify any conclusions that can be drawn from the various volumes inside and outside of the cell.

Fürst: The determinations of muscle sodium or potassium, are total determinations in the whole muscle tissue, and are independent of whether the potassium or the sodium is going in or out from the cells. The figures I showed were derived values, based on the Nernst equation. That is why I pointed out that by calculating with different membrane potentials the extracellular water presented for potassium and magnesium depletion and for an increased extracellular sodium are a reality. A decrease of the membrane potential to 55 mV will still give the changes mentioned above. The electrolyte measurements were performed using atomic absorption flamephotometry or activation analysis, which give extremely reproducible values.

Vinay: Is the cell potential actually measured, or is it calculated with an estimated value of around 70 for a normal cell potential? If it is not measured, then on what basis are the intra- and extracellular electrolytes separated?

Fürst: The normal cell potential is 87.2. We have not directly measured the cell membrane potential, but have used derived values.

Shizgal: We have taken care in doing these measurements not to rely on a single measurement of exchangeable sodium—and that is why! In a lot of studies we also measure extracellular water and intracellular water, and all these measurements are always made in parallel.

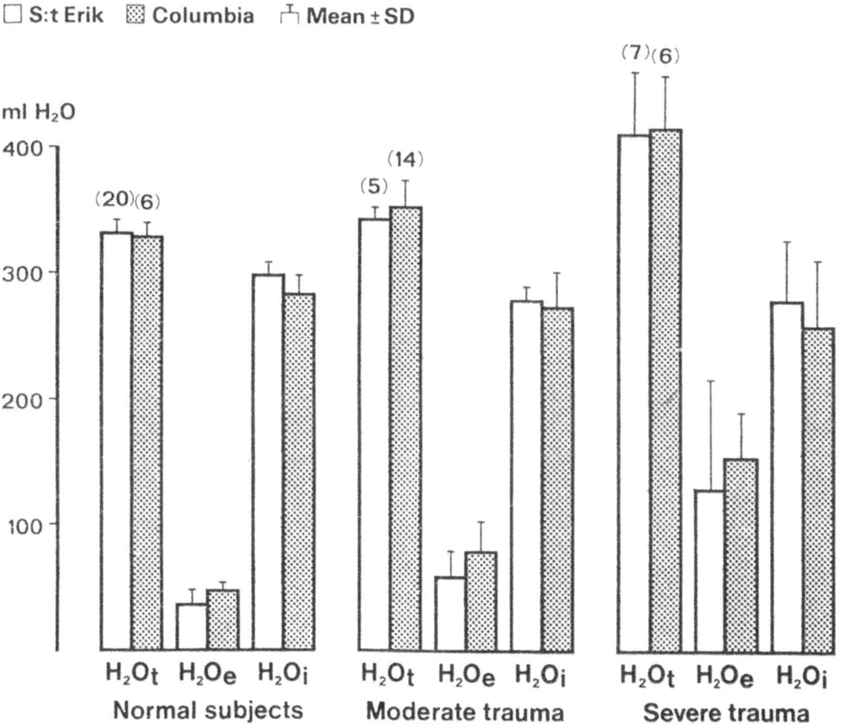

Figure 1 The water content and distribution in healthy subjects and in patients suffering from moderate or severe postoperative catabolism from Columbia University, New York and from St Eriks hospital, Stockholm (ml/100 g dry fat-free solids)

Vinay: The fact that several spaces that interact with each other are measured might confirm that when the increase in the total potassium exchangeable loss and the increase in total body water are seen together, one might be justified in saying that the body cell mass has actually increased. What concerns me is that the error made in estimating total body water or total body potassium, due to the time of exchange required to attain isotope equilibrium might be quite significant. That is why my question arises.

Most of the regression lines shown demonstrate that around a value of between 40–50 calories/kg is adequate. Most of them are based on a ratio of around 0.5 which means that only 25 per cent of the variation of the sample can be explained on the basis of the regression. This is unavoidable, and due to the technology. That is why I am concerned about the actual intracellular and extracellular volumes.

Shizgal: Dr Vinay asked a question about sodium measurement. There is a problem if sodium leaks into the cell. That problem does not exist for potassium because if a lot of potassium leaks out, one cannot survive. Extracellular potassium is a small fraction of total body potassium, and total body potassium is totally exchangeable. There is no potassium locked up in bone, so that is a fairly good measurement.

The point regarding the regression lines is the one that I tried to point out. Whenever one starts to look at the difference between two measurements, one will end up with a large experimental error, and

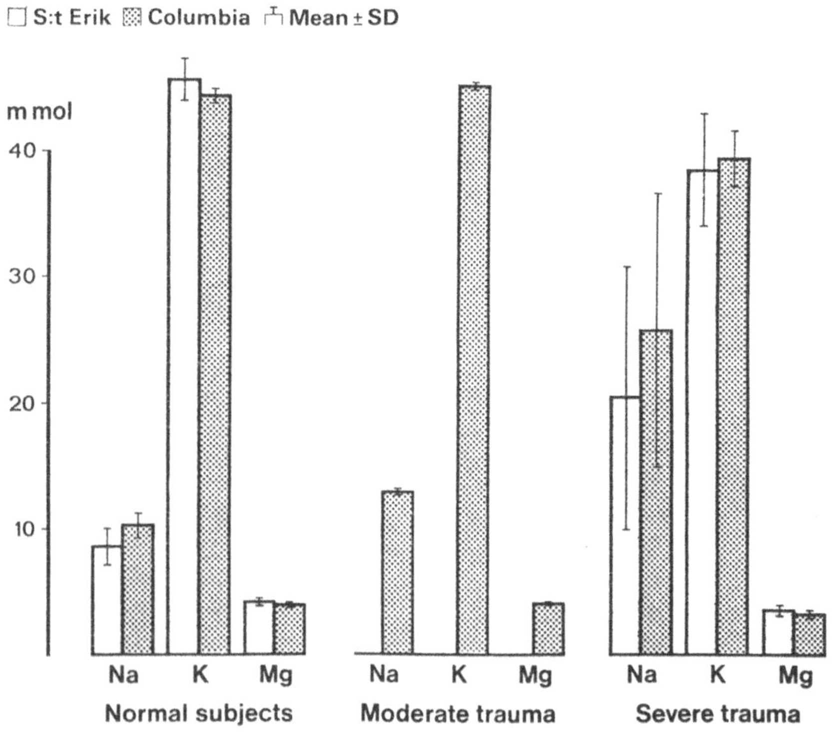

Figure 2 Electrolyte content in muscle tissue in healthy subjects and in patients with moderate or severe trauma as described in Figure 1 (mmol/100 g dry fat-free solids)

there is no such large error in our absolute-K measurements which are of the order of 5 %.

D. B. Allardyce: (Canada) In the group of patients supported with the calorie intake from Intralipid, and from fructose, Dr Shizgal failed to show any gain in the lean body mass over the five-day period. The patients described were similar to the patients that we treated, where we used Intralipid as a fairly major source of calories.

What percentage of the calorie intake was from Intralipid, and what percentage came from fructose?

Shizgal: In terms of non-protein calories, about 65–70% was from Intralipid.

Allardyce: I am a little concerned about what we are doing with Intralipid, because we use a lot of it. In our particular regimen we gave 10% Intralipid and 50% dextrose as a carbohydrate source, and the average patients would have received about 1500 calories from Intralipid and about 800 calories from dextrose, a total of 2300, which would be less than the recommended value for gain in lean body mass in those patients. In spite of getting only 2300 calories, they were getting 10% Travasol* and close to 18 g nitrogen per day, which I guess would be more than the patients on $3\frac{1}{2}$% amino acids were getting.

Our patients gained weight, and they showed obvious increase in depot fat, and they had a positive nitrogen balance. I grant that perhaps we overestimated this because we did not take gastrointestinal loss or skin loss into account.

Shizgal: We used the Vamin-Intralipid for the simple reason, that it allowed us to become independent of the pharmacists. I do not think that we can truthfully extrapolate our data to say that lipid is good or bad, or that fructose is good or bad. All that we can say is that by using our approach we can say what the efficacy of this combination is. I know that we used it for about two years, and during that time it was my own clinical impression that it was just as good as the other solutions that we were using.

R. K. Ausman: (USA) Dr Wilmore presented some information suggesting that in the early period following trauma, lipid was less useful than it is in the later period. As one went on in time treating those patients with the lipid, did the data change?

Shizgal: We have to look at patients spaced over an interval of time. Professor Kinney made the point earlier that nitrogen balance allows a day-to-day measurement, and it is very valid, but we cannot do it with these techniques. It would be almost impossible for us to dissect out early and late data.

The other problem was the quantitation of the degree of stress and trauma that these patients have. We all look at a patient and say that he is sick, he is not starving, or there is real stress here. But before we can make any meaningful statements we shall have to be able to quantitate that. We cannot do that at this point.

* Synthamin.

36
The use of ^{40}K counting and its relationship to other estimates of lean body mass

A. W. GOODE AND T. HAWKINS

There has been a recent increase in awareness of the importance of nutritional support in clinical practice and the methods available for the provision of such care. Parenteral nutrition is important in patients unable to be fed by the oral route, while elemental and supplemental diets are of great value when a patient can satisfactorily accept nutrition by mouth. Irrespective of the method used it is important that accurate assessment of the patient's nutritional status should precede therapy, and that a serial assessment of the response to feeding should be available. Frequently this is not the case, and as a result nutritional therapy is used in an uncontrolled manner with often erroneous clinical impressions of depletion or improvement.

Behnke[1] has shown that energy utilization is related closely to lean body mass but less so to body weight or surface area, suggesting that the vital metabolic functions are related directly to the lean body mass. Moore[2] refined this concept describing the work-performing, and energy-utilizing component as the body cell mass, the cellular component of which is hydrated and potassium- and nitrogen-rich in contrast to body fat.

In starvation the patient progressively loses weight as a result of the utilization of fat as the principal endogenous energy source, he loses lean body mass, clinically evident as muscle wasting, and there may be associated changes in hydration. Progressive loss of the lean body mass will result eventually in an inability to support vital body functions. Thus any assessment of nutritional depletion should ideally be a measure of the absolute loss of lean tissue and not simply loss of body weight. The usual assessment of depletion of lean body mass is nitrogen balance, but like all balance methods it is liable to compounding daily errors of collection from all sources of loss. It only gives an index of relative daily change and not absolute depletion or improvement with therapy.

Potassium is an element found in abundance in the body. Some 98 % of the total body potassium is within the lean tissue, the remainder being distributed at very low concentrations throughout the plasma, extracellular fluids and body fat. This simplified distribution, and the fact that potassium is weakly radioactive, has permitted the non-invasive assessment of total body potassium and its utilization as an index of the lean body mass (LBM). Of the potassium distributed throughout nature, including the human body, about one atom in ten thousand (0.012 %) is radioactive from the natural radioisotope ^{40}K. The remaining potassium is accounted for by the non-active isotopes ^{39}K (approximately 93 %) and ^{41}K (approximately 7 %).

The half life of ^{39}K is about thirteen hundred million years, and it decays into stable ^{40}K by the processes of beta particle emission (89 %) or electron capture (11 %). The latter route is accompanied by the emission of gamma ray photons of energy, 1.46 MeV. The small proportion of ^{40}K and still more its low gamma ray abundance means that just over 3 photons per second are emitted per gram of potassium. Other radioisotopes, both natural and artificial, contribute to the total gamma ray flux emitted by the body, though these are generally in much smaller quantities. Table 36.1 illustrates the typical levels of natural activity in the body in contrast to those used elsewhere in industry and medicine. It is thus apparent that a detector system of high sensitivity is required in order to measure the total body ^{40}K content with a reasonable accuracy.

Table 36.1 Levels of activity used in industry and medicine

Activity	*Used for*
100 000 Ci	Research; industrial radiation processes (e.g. sterilization of medical supplies)
1000 Ci	Teletherapy sources, ^{60}Co, ^{137}Cs (e.g. radiation therapy)
10 Ci	Industrial radiography (e.g. thickness and density gauging)
1–100 mCi	Radioisotope therapy (e.g. thyroid ablation using ^{131}I)
0.1–10 mCi	Radioisotope imaging techniques (e.g. localization of space occupying lesions)
1–100 μCi	Radioisotope tracer techniques (e.g. thyroid function using ^{131}I)
0.01–10 μCi	*In-vitro* diagnostic clinical tests (e.g. urine activity in electrolyte balance study)
10–100 nCi	Level of natural radioactive ^{40}K in the human body
$<$ 10 nCi	Low levels of other natural and artificial radioisotopes in the human body (e.g. ^{226}Rd; ^{137}Cs; ^{90}Sr)

Ci = 1 Curie = 3.7×10^{10} nuclear disintegrations per second.
mCi = millicurie = 10^{-3} Ci; μCi = microcurie = 10^{-6} Ci;
nCi = nanocurie = 10^{-9} Ci.

The development of such systems, whole body monitors, dates from about 1929 when Schlundt[3] reported the measurement of radioactive contamination *in vivo*. Monitors remained insensitive until Sievert[4] and Burch and Spiers[5] described their measurements of natural radioactivity in general and body potassium in particular. Miller[6] has outlined some of the desired features for monitors:

1. The counting sensitivity should be as high as possible in order to minimize the measurement time for patients.
2. The sensitivity should ideally be independent of the subject's body build or the distribution of radioactivity within the body.
3. The arrangement of the detectors should be independent of body build and the design should be such as to accommodate wide variations in habitus.
4. The monitor should have good energy resolution, energy stability and a low gamma ray background.

How far a monitor meets these demands will determine its capabilities, as the measurement of natural radioactivity within the body requires a higher sensitivity than studies in which radioisotopes are deliberately administered.

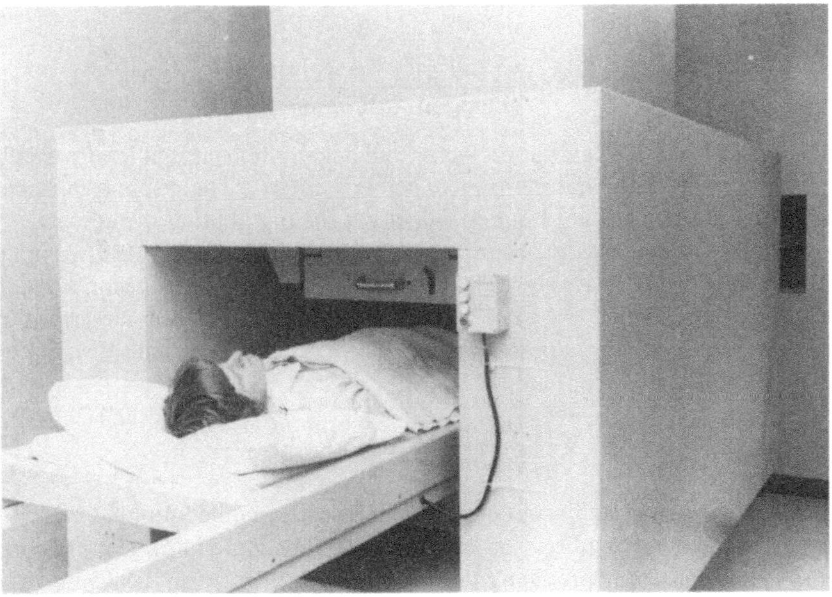

Figure 36.1 A shadow shield whole body monitor

A history of development of whole body monitors has been given elsewhere*. Presently a variety of designs exist, including those which use liquid

* Directory of Whole-Body Radioactivity Monitors, I.A.E.A., Vienna (1970.)

or plastic organic scintillation detectors or inorganic crystal scintillators, of which sodium iodide (NaI) is the most popular. Many substances have been adopted to act as a radiation shield including water, steel, lead, concrete, brick, chalk and soil. Monitors vary in weight from a few tons, for local or partial shielding, to the more elaborate steel rooms of a few hundred tons. The ancillary electronic systems vary in sophistication. Continued improvements in detection efficiency over the years have resulted in the evolution of a system for the non-invasive measurement of body potassium.

A view of the whole body monitor used in this present study is shown in Figure 36.1. It is of the shadow shield type described by Warner and Oliver[7] and has two opposing NaI (Tl) crystals, each 20.3 cm in diameter and 10.3 cm thick, their separation being 45.7 cm. The detectors and scanning bed are shielded by 14 tons of pre-1945 battleship steel, which is consequently relatively free from cobalt-60 and nuclear fall-out contaminants.

Monitor calibration

In principle the quantity of potassium in a subject can be obtained by measuring the gamma ray count rate and referring this to a standard mass of potassium in a phantom. The expression for total body potassium (TBK) may be written as:

$$\text{TBK (g)} = \frac{(\text{Subject } ^{40}\text{K cpm})}{(\text{Phantom } ^{40}\text{K cpm/g K})} \times \text{F} \qquad (1)$$

where F is a suitable calibration factor and its requirement is at least partially a consequence of the failure to meet Miller's criteria. The response of many monitors is not invariant but depends upon the distribution of radioactivity within the body. The problems of determining F for any individual is fortunately made relatively easy with the availability of a second radioisotope of potassium, ^{42}K. The calibration procedure has been described by others[5,8,9]. Following administration of ^{42}K to a patient and a phantom, then F is evaluated from

$$\text{F} = \frac{(\text{Phantom } ^{42}\text{K cpm}/\mu\text{Ci})}{(\text{Subject } ^{42}\text{K cpm}/\mu\text{Ci})} \qquad (2)$$

The method serves well when a single, or at least a limited number of, TBK determinations are required for an individual. Furthermore the same calibration factor will apply providing the subject does not alter physically between successive measurements. In many clinical situations it is the change in potassium which assumes importance—changes which occur in response to disease or therapy.

There then may be significant changes in body habitus and it is clearly laborious to redetermine F on each of several occasions. The calibration factor is expected to depend upon those physical characteristics of the patient which most influence the efficiency of measurement on the monitor. Many centres have considered weight and height to be particularly important and have used various combinations of them in arriving at regression equations allowing F to be predicted from these easily measured parameters. Our own calibration study was made using 115 healthy adults who were free from renal and cardiac disease. Each was given 45 μCi of ^{42}K and the necessary corrections were made before evaluating F. The relative importance of the anthropometric factors was determined using the standard 'analysis of variance' technique[10]. No significant improvement in regression was obtained by treating the sexes separately, neither was the inclusion of body density particularly helpful. The final equation considered best for practical routine use for predicting F was

$$F = (1131.4 + 5.29 \times (W\text{-}70) + 2.49 \times (H\text{-}170)) \times 10^{-3},$$

where W = body weight in kilograms
H = height in centimetres
Total body potassium is then obtained from equation (1).

Sources of error

The assessment of body potassium, like all objective measurements, is subject to experimental errors. For the monitor 'F' calibration procedure using ^{42}K these include Poisson statistical counting errors both in the subject and phantom; technical errors of dispensing; measurement of residual patient dose; urine assay and positioning errors on the monitor. The standard deviation from regression was 1.9% and when corrected for the known technical errors was 1.7%.

The final error is compounded from this and the errors of measurement of the ^{40}K in patients and phantom, 3.2% for a healthy adult male with 140 g K. Adding variances this yields a total final error of 3.6%. If, instead of using the predictive regression equation, F is obtained from individual ^{42}K measurements, then the compound errors were 3.3% (for 140 g K), a marginal improvement considering the extra technical work involved. The probable errors of a potassium estimate ultimately depend upon the detailed procedure followed, the design of the monitor, its characteristics and upon the numbers of subjects who comprised the calibration study. The figures given are fairly typical of the precision obtainable in total potassium measurements.

One interesting potential source of error arises from the measurement of monitor background radiation used to obtain the patient's net gamma ray flux. The background radiation is due to cosmic radiation; airborne ^{13}N, ^{41}Ar, radon and daughter products; intrinsic ^{40}K in the detector system and ^{60}Co, ^{226}Ra contaminants in the shielding which are all present to a greater or lesser degree in any monitor system. It has been observed that an inert mass placed in a whole body monitor will both attenuate and scatter environmental radiation[11,12]. We have investigated the effect on background counting rate of changing the mass of otherwise inert water-filled containers in the range 10–90 kg. The background counting rate was observed to fall progressively and significantly with increasing load[13].

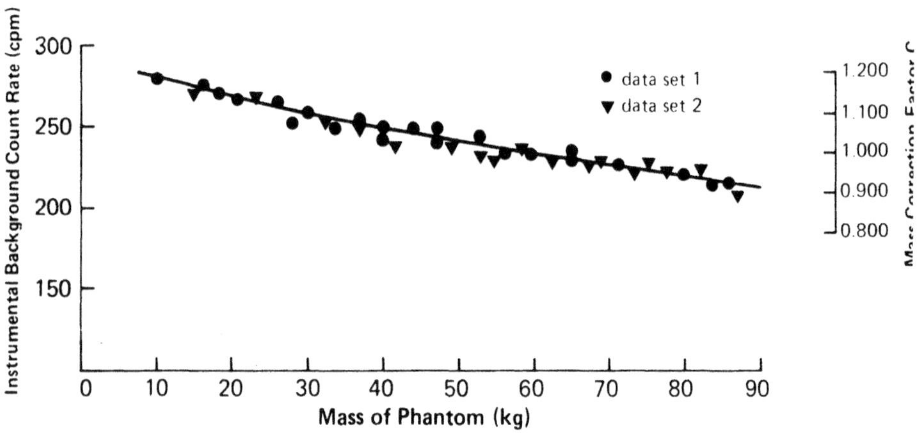

Figure 36.2 The effect of mass on monitor background count rate and the mass correction factor 'C'. $C = 1.000 - 3.285\,(M - 60) \times 10^{-3} + 1.139\,(M - 60)^2 \times 10^{-5}$

Extreme variations in the shape of the phantom were less important than its absolute mass. A simple correction factor 'C' was obtained by considering a 60 kg phantom to be the reference for background determinations and making the necessary allowance for subjects whose mass differed from 60 kg (Figure 36.2). Thus:

$$\text{True } ^{40}\text{K cpm} = \text{Observed } ^{40}\text{K cpm} - \frac{\text{Observed background cpm}}{\text{for 60 kg phantom}} \times \frac{\text{Subject's mass}}{\text{correction factor 'C'}}.$$

Others have reported similar disturbances in instrumental background[7,8,14,15], though very little detailed information appears in the literature either of its magnitude or correction technique. Perhaps the phenomenon is negligible elsewhere and our shadow shield system with its inevitable compromise in shielding is particularly vulnerable. However, it does seem a worthwhile cautionary note for those contemplating measurements of potassium to at least rule out possible influence from this potential source of error.

The prediction of normal total body potassium content

In clinical measurements of TBK, it may be important not only to know the changes which occur from one time to another, but also to know how 'normal' any particular value of TBK is. Several predictive equations for normal TBK have been cited in the literature[16–21].

Almost invariably they rely upon the simple parameters of patient sex, age, weight and height. Our own study has yielded such a regression equation which we now add to those already in use elsewhere.

Males

Total body potassium (TBK) =
$(30.84 \times W + 17.85 \times H - 8.14 \times A - 1402)$ mmol
Coefficient of variation was 6.9% of the mean.

Females

Total body potassium (TBK) =
$(23.81 \times W + 18.39 \times H - 1.72 \times A - 1887)$ mmol
Coefficient of variation was 8.9% of the mean,
with W = weight in kilograms
H = height in centimetres
A = age in years.

For individuals who are near average both in height and weight, agreement is generally very good amongst the predicted normal TBK values. With deviations from normal in either or both of these parameters, there is an increasing variation in the predicted total body potassiums. It is unfortunate that such anomalous conditions most frequently occur in patients with disease, the very group of subjects where a reliable potassium reference level is required. The predictive equations nevertheless give useful guidance to normal TBK.

Total exchangeable (Ke) and total body potassium

The exchangeable pool of potassium is still often utilized as an index of potassium status. Its measurement is made using the familiar 'dilution principle'[22] in which a known activity of the radioisotope ^{42}K or ^{43}K is allowed to equilibrate with the native potassium. A sample of body fluid, usually urine, or blood plasma is collected after an interval of about 24 h and is assayed both for its radioactivity content and its biochemical potassium concentration. These various factors combine to yield the exchangeable potassium value from the expression:

$$\text{Exchangeable electrolyte} = \text{Electrolyte space (l)} \times \text{Electrolyte concentration (mmol/l)}.$$

In our calibration study Ke was assessed at 22, 23 and 24 h. A comparison of Ke to TBK for each normal subject gave a mean value of 88.7% (range

75–114%). A similar mean of 87.9% (range 70.4–117.7%), was found in a clinical group of thirty grossly malnourished patients with normal renal function. The values agree reasonably well with other investigations[23–26]. In other disease groups, however, potassium equilibrium may be disordered; in patients with renal failure values for Ke/TBK of $60.7 \pm 3.3\%$ (24 h), $83.6 \pm 2.7\%$ (48 h), and $85.9 \pm 2.7\%$ (64 h) were found[27]. The difficulties of interpreting observed low exchangeable potassiums are clear: the problem is that of deciding whether the finding is genuine or an artefact arising from slow equilibration. Furthermore, in a total of 429 individual estimates of Ke, we found 30 (7%) which gave apparently aberrant results when viewed together with the other exchangeable and total body potassium data for each subject. This suggests that isolated measurements of Ke have a potential for error which may pass unrecognized. Potassium is thought to exchange slowly in bone, brain and red cells, which explains why Ke represents rather less than the total potassium content at the intervals of time normally considered.

The lean body mass

The use of weight to express the concentration of potassium in the body (mmol/kg body weight) remains useful in very many circumstances, but is open to criticism and may lead to anomalous results, particularly in disease[19,28,29]. The lean body mass (LBM) rather than body weight has been considered as a better reference for potassium status.

In the calibration series, LBM was obtained indirectly from total body water (TBW) in the relationship of Rathbun and Pace[30], LBM = TBW/0.732. Independent estimates of TBW were obtained from the regressions of Moore[2] and Hume and Weyers[31]. A further assessment of LBM was made from measurements of skinfold thickness at four sites and applying the regression formulae for body density of Durnin and Womersley[31,32]. Lean body mass follows from the body fat equation of Siri[33]. The mean value of potassium concentration in the lean tissue mass from our data is given in Table 36.2 together with those of other authors (Table 36.3). The agreement is reasonably good and it suggests that such values will serve as good reference standards for normality, and that LBM is a more reliable biological reference.

In the nutritional assessment of patients any 'bedside' method which gives a reasonable approximation of the lean body mass is of clinical use. From Table 36.2 the method using skinfold thickness (c) is in agreement with the general pattern of results. Durnin and Womersley[32] using Harpenden skinfold calipers[34] pointed out that in very lean subjects, particularly females, more data were required. However, despite this reservation we have found an excellent correlation ($P < 0.005$) in twenty patients between fat-free mass and lean body mass measured by total body potassium. This relationship does not hold in patients with clinical evidence of oedema or a low packed cell volume.

Table 36.2 Lean body mass (LBM) and potassium concentration derived from (a) Moore *et al.*[2], (b) Hume and Weyers[31], (c) skin-fold thickness

	(a)	*(b)*	*(c)*
Male LBM (kg)	54.7 ± 6.8	56.2 ± 6.1	57.4 ± 8.4
Female LBM (kg)	40.6 ± 3.6	42.8 ± 4.3	40.7 ± 4.8
Male mmol K/kg LBM	66.2 ± 4.5	64.4 ± 4.9	63.0 ± 3.7
Female mmol K/kg LBM	60.2 ± 5.8	57.2 ± 5.1	60.1 ± 4.9

Table 36.3 Potassium concentration in the lean body mass (mmol K/kg)

		Male	*Female*
Forbes *et al.*[35]		68.1	68.1
Boddy *et al.*[9]		64.5 ± 3.5	57.0 ± 4.1
Pierson *et al.*[36]		64.0 ±	54.0 ±
Von Dobeln[37]		69.9 ± 7.0	59.3 ± 6.0
Present series: mean of (a)(b)(c)		64.5 ± 4.4	59.2 ± 5.3
Burkinshaw *et al.*[38]	Series A	58.8 ± 3.3	58.2 ± 4.2
	Series B	64.3 ± 3.7	58.3 ± 3.1

The observation that the average potassium concentration (mmol/kg) in the lean body mass of males is consistently higher than in females has been made in numerous studies[23,37,39]. From a summary of the mean LBM (± 1 SD) and potassium concentrations (± 1 SD) estimated from our own series of 115 healthy adults statistical tests (Student's *t*; Wilcoxon's signed ranks), indicate a significant difference ($P < 0.001$) in potassium concentrations between the sexes. Such findings obviously have implications in the analysis of body composition.

For the organs and tissues as a whole there is, so far as we know, no evidence to suggest that similar tissues in the sexes differ in respect of their potassium concentrations. The skeleton forms a large part of the LBM. However its very low potassium content would require the skeleton to occupy a substantially larger proportion of the LBM in females to account for the observations. There is no evidence to support this suggestion. Moore *et al.*[2] found the ratio of dry skeleton to LBM to be on average 0.1039 for males and 0.1004 for females—a non-significant difference.

Studies of body composition show clearly that large variations occur in the proportion of fat in the body[40]. However the known difference between the average male and female in adipose content and the exceedingly low potassium content of this tissue correspond to differences of only approximately 120 mmol/kg or 2 kg LBM and may be justifiably ignored as a reasonable explanation for the observation.

The possibility that LBM is not of uniform composition within the sexes has often been noted, with the suggestion that there may exist a difference in the relative proportions of tissue. The LBM may be conveniently divided into the skeletal musculature and the remaining muscle free lean mass (MFLM)[2]. We may deduce with the aid of a realistic and simple example that differences in the muscle:MFLM ratio can account adequately for the observed facts.

In Table 36.4, columns (i) and (ii) show typical body weight and total potassium content of adult male and females, though the chosen values are not critical to the analysis. Column (iii) shows the distribution of the potassium in muscle and MFLM assuming that this may vary and that in healthy males and females the percentage of potassium located in muscle is 70% and 60% respectively. Considering the potassium content of muscle to be 82 mmol K/kg and in MFLM to be 41 mmol K/kg[17,41,42], then column (iv) indicates the total LBM to be expected. Finally column (v) shows the derived potassium concentration of the total LBM. Such values are broadly consistent with those observed. If the muscle:MFLM ratio is not allowed to vary then the LBM potassium concentration would be equal in male and female.

Table 36.4 Male and female, typical body weight (i) and potassium content (ii); relative proportion of potassium assumed to be in muscle and muscle free lean mass (iii); derived lean body mass (iv) and potassium concentration (v)

	(i) *Body weight* (kg)	(ii) *Total body potassium* (mmol)	(iii) *Muscle K*	*: MFLM K*	(iv) *LBM (kg)*	(v) *mmol K/kg LBM*
Male	70	3590 (140 g K)	2510 (70%)	1080 (30%)	56.9	63.1
Female	60	2560 (100 g K)	1540 (60%)	1020 (40%)	43.7	58.6

On this hypothesis the muscle mass represents some 54% of total LBM in males and 43% in females, values which follow closely the suggestion of Von Dobeln[37], that average muscle mass is 50% of LBM and that approximately 67% of the total potassium exists in the skeletal musculature. Furthermore allowing the proportion of potassium accounted for by muscle mass to increase to 80% would explain the high values of the LBM to body weight observed in studies of very fit athletes[43,44]. Additionally the low values of mmol K^+/kg LBM observed by us in a group of patients with Crohn's disease with severe wasting are accounted for by assuming a ratio of muscle to MFLM of 50:50 or less. We would endorse the statement that the skeletal musculature forms a highly significant variable in determining total body potassium[45].

The choice of values for mmol K^+/kg LBM are taken from separate sources and are not expected to be in substantial error despite the age of the reports. Independent and direct evidence of body composition (from X and gamma rays absorptiometry for example) would be needed to substantiate such hypotheses.

Where there is indeed a preferential change in the muscle content of total lean tissue in those diseases which drastically alter body composition, then the use of an average LBM concentration of potassium will consistently overestimate the actual gain or loss of lean tissue. It would thus be more correct to use a value of 82 mmol/kg. If the LBM was of constant composition then it would be both possible and advantageous to derive the LBM value from the total potassium content, thus avoiding the use of body water or body density which may be subject to some alteration in disease. However, in practice the variability in the relative proportions of lean tissue together with their substantial difference in potassium concentration would seem to limit the usefulness of such a relationship.

Total body potassium estimations in clinical practice

Factors which deplete potassium concentration in the lean body mass, such as hyperaldosteronism, diabetes and acid–base change, limit the interpretation of total body potassium estimations as an index of lean body mass. Recent work, however, suggests that diuretic therapy, either in the immediate post-operative period[46], or in long-term therapy[47] is not associated with depletion of total body potassium in the lean body mass. All our patient measurements have been made subject to the listed constraints, and the total body potassium has been used as a nutritional index, but the method is obviously not applicable in the immediate post-operative period.

The measurement of total body potassium by a whole body monitor allows a non-invasive reproducible index of loss of lean body mass prior to treatment by comparing the actual total body potassium with the predicted 'health' value. The response to treatment as measured by restoration of lean body mass from total body potassium measurements has been described by Bernard and Stahl[48] and Goode, Hawkins, Feggetter and Johnston[49]. Trials comparing the efficiency of different nutritional regimens in restoring lost lean body mass are now being performed, as the method allows controlled assessment of efficiency in comparable groups of patients.

The method may be used to identify patients at risk with preoperative malnutrition and to quantify the depletion. In a further trial ten adult patients were chosen as a random sample of patients about to undergo cardiac surgery for aortic or mitral valve replacement. Total body potassium was measured preoperatively and the deficit from predicted values used to identify loss of lean body mass and hence preoperative malnutrition. Four of the ten patients showed a significant degree of depletion with a mean loss of 18.2%, range 13–21%, loss of lean body mass, while the remaining six were not malnourished. Clinicians on clinical criteria alone were unable to identify the patients who were depleted. The depleted patients had a significantly longer convalescence and recovery time as measured by the time spent in hospital. The mean stay for the depleted patients was 29.5 days, range 18–59 days, compared with a mean stay of 16 days, range 14–19 days, for the well-nourished patients. There was no correlation between any other factor except preoperative nutrition which related to this postoperative morbidity.

The metabolic response to cardiac surgery has usually been measured by conventional nitrogen balance methods complicated by the many potential sources of loss. Manners[50] has suggested that the calculated response may be underestimated by this method and so the postoperative total body potassium was measured on the tenth postoperative day. The potassium loss reflecting loss of muscle tissue was calculated from the difference between the pre and postoperative measurements. The mean loss of lean tissue for the group was the equivalent of a negative nitrogen balance of 10.8 g/day. The metabolic response to cardiac surgery is about 30% greater when measured by the total body potassium method. This suggests that previous estimates have been too low as a result of the problems of complete collections of loss in such patients, and that the poor results obtained by Abel, Fisher, Buckley, Barnett and Austen[51] in the postoperative feeding of such patients may be due to consequent underestimation of requirements.

CONCLUSIONS

1. Clinical impressions of nutritional depletion or improvement are almost always unreliable.

2. Total body potassium estimated by a whole body monitor is a reliable method of individual nutritional assessment and a method of quantitating nutritional change. Potential sources of error in the method can be both identified and quantitated. For our system the error in measurement is 3.6% in a subject containing 140 g/K^+.

3. Direct exchangeable potassium estimations are typically 88% of total body values, and single exchangeable values interpreted in isolation may conceal gross error.

4. Skinfold caliper estimations of body fat to calculate fat free mass will provide a simple bedside method of estimating lean body tissue.

References

1. Behnke, A. R. (1953). The relation of lean body mass to metabolism and some consequent systematisations. *Ann. N.Y. Acad. Sci.*, **56**, 1095
2. Moore, F. D., Oleson, K. H., McMurray, J. D., Parker, H. V., Ball, M. R. and Boyden, C. M. (1963). *The Body Cell Mass and its Supporting Environment.* (Philadelphia: Saunders.)
3. Schlundt, H., Barker, H. H. and Flinn, F. B. (1929). First measurements of body radioactivity *in vivo. Metabolism*, **5**, 468

4. Sievert, R. M. (1951). Measurements of gamma radiation from the body. *Arch. Fysik*, **2,** 337
5. Burch, P. R. J. and Speirs, F. W. (1953). Measurement of gamma radiation from the human body. *Nature (Lond.)*, **172,** 519
6. Miller, C. E. (1962). An experimental evaluation of multiple crystal arrays and single crystal techniques. *Proceedings of the Symposium on Whole Body Counting*, pp. 81–120. (Vienna: I.A.E.A.)
7. Warner, G. T. and Oliver, R. (1966). A whole body counter for clinical measurements utilising the shadow shield technique. *Phys. Med. Biol.*, **11** (No. 1), 83
8. Burkinshaw, L. (1967). Measurement of body potassium calibration and inter comparison of two whole body radiation counters. *Phys. Med. Biol.*, **12,** 477
9. Boddy, K., King, P. C., Tothill, P. and Strong, J. A. (1971). Measurement of total body potassium with a shadow shield whole body counter: calibration and errors. *Phys. Med. Biol.*, **16,** 275
10. Fischer, R. A. (1925). *Statistical Methods for Research Workers*. 1st Ed. (Edinburgh: Oliver and Boyd)
11. Evans, R. D. (1937). Radium poisoning. The quantitative determination of the radium content and the radium elimination rate in living persons. *Am. J. Roent.*, **37,** 368
12. Speirs, F. W. (1962). *Whole Body Counting: An Introductory Review*, p. 3. (Vienna: International Atomic Energy Authority)
13. Hawkins, T. and Goode, A. W. (1976). The determination of total body potassium using a whole body monitor. *Phys. Med. Biol.*, **21,** (No. 3), 293
14. Kessler, W. V., Ziemer, P. L., Christian, F. E. and Shaw, S. M. (1968). A 4π liquid scintillation whole body counter—I. Design, operating characteristics and calibration. *Int. J. Appl. Radiation Isotopes*, **19,** 287
15. Johny, K. V., Worthley, B. W., Lawrence, J. R. and O'Halloran, M. W. (1970). A whole body counter for serial studies of total body potassium. *Clin. Sci.*, **39,** 319
16. Anderson, C. E. (1965). Determination of body potassium by 4π gamma counting. Second Symposium. *Radioactivity in Man*, p. 211. (Springfield, Ill.: Charles C. Thomas)
17. Oberhausen, F. and Onstead, C. O. (1965). Relationship of potassium content of man with age and sex. Radioactivity in man, pp. 179–185. (Springfield, Ill.: Charles C. Thomas)
18. Novak, P. L. (1972). Ageing, total body potassium, fat free mass and cell mass in males and females between ages 18 and 85 years. *J. Gerontol.*, **27** (No. 4), 438
19. Boddy, K., King, P. C., Hume, R. and Weyers, E. (1972). The relation of total body potassium to height, weight and age in normal adults. *J. Clin. Pathol.*, **25,** 512
20. Delwaide, P. A. (1973). Body potassium measurements by whole body counting: screening patient population. *J. Nucl. Med.*, **14,** 40
21. Ellis, K. J., Shukla, K. K., Cohn, S. H. and Pierson, R. N. (1974). A predictor for total body potassium in man based on height, weight, sex and age: applications in metabolic disorders. *J. Lab. Clin. Med.*, **83** (No. 5), 716
22. Corsa, L., Olney, J. M., Stenburg, R. W., Ball, M. R. and Moore, F. D. (1950). The measurement of exchangeable potassium in man by isotope dilution. *J. Clin. Invest.*, **29,** 1280
23. Remenchick, A. P. and Miller, C. E. (1962). The measurement of total body potassium in man and its relation to gross body composition. *Proceedings of Symposium on Whole Body Counting*, p. 331. (Vienna: I.A.E.A.)
24. Talso, P. J., Miller, C. E., Carballo, A. J. and Vasquez, I. (1960). Exchangeable potassium as a parameter of body composition. *Metabolism*, **9,** 456
25. Boddy, K., King, P. C. and Davies, L. D. (1973). The relationship between total body potassium and exchangeable body potassium measured at 24 hours and 44 hours after administration of ^{43}K. *Eur. J. Clin. Invest.*, **3,** 188
26. Surveyor, I. and Hughes, D. (1968). Discrepancies between whole body potassium content and exchangeable potassium. *J. Lab. Clin. Med.*, **71,** 464
27. Boddy, K., King, P. C., Lindsay, R. M., Winchester, J. and Kennedy, A. C. (1972). Exchangeable and total body potassium in patients with chronic renal failure. *Br. Med. J.*, **15** (No. 1), 140

28. Crooks, J., Bluhm, M. M. and Muldowney, F. P. (1959). The interrelationship between total exchangeable sodium, potassium, and chloride, and lean body mass in man. *Clin. Sci.*, **18,** 175
29. MacGillivray, I., Buchanan, T. J. and Billewicz, W. Z. (1960). Values of total exchangeable sodium and potassium in normal females based on weight, height and age. *Clin. Sci.*, **19,** 17
30. Rathbun, E. N. and Pace, N. (1945). Studies on body composition. I. The determination of total body fat by means of the body specific gravity. *J. Biol. Chem.*, **158,** 667
31. Hume, R. and Weyers, E. (1971). Relationship between total body water and surface area in normal and obese subjects. *J. Clin. Pathol.*, **24,** 234
32. Durnin, J. V. G. A. and Womersley, J. (1974). Body fat assessed from total body density and its estimation from skinfold thickness: measurements on 481 men and women aged from 16 to 72 years. *Br. J. Nutr.*, **32,** 77
33. Siri, W. E. (1956). University of California Radiation Laboratory Report 3349, p. 14. Donner Laboratory of Biophysics and Medical Physics.
34. Edward, D. A. W., Hammond, W. H., Healy, M. J. R., Tanner, J. M. and Whitehouse, R. H. (1955). Design and accuracy of calipers for measuring subcutaneous tissue thickness. *Br. J. Nutr.*, **9,** 133
35. Forbes, G. B., Gallup, J. and Hursh, J. B. (1961). Estimation of total body fat from ^{40}K content. *Science*, **133,** 101
36. Pierson, R. I., Lin, D. H. Y. and Phillips, R. A. (1974). Total body potassium in health: effects of age, sex, height and fat. *Am. J. Physiol.*, **226** (No. 1), 206
37. Von Dobeln, W. (1962). *Proceedings of Symposium on Whole Body Counting*, pp. 351–352. (Vienna: I.A.E.A.)
38. Burkinshaw, L. and Cotes, J. E. (1973). Body potassium and fat free mass: Correspondence section. *Clin. Sci.*, **44,** 621
39. Womersley, J., Boddy, K., King, P. C. and Durnin, J. V. G. A. (1972). A comparison of the fat free mass of young adults estimated by anthropometry, body density and total body potassium content. *Clin. Sci.*, **43,** 469
40. Widdowson, E. M., McCance, R. A. and Spray, C. M. (1951). The chemical composition of the human body. *Clin. Sci.*, **10,** 113
41. Brozek, J. (1965). Discussion 20. Second Symposium. *Radioactivity in Man*, pp. 272–277. (Springfield, Ill.: Charles C. Thomas)
42. Forbes, G. B. and Lewis, A. M. (1956). Total sodium, potassium and chloride in adult man. *J. Clin. Invest.*, **35,** 596
43. Novak, L. P., Hyatt, R. E. and Alexander, J. F. (1968). Body composition and physiologic function of athletes. *J. Am. Med. Assoc.*, **205,** 140
44. Boddy, K., Hume, R., King, P. C., Weyers, E. and Rowan, T. (1974). Total body plasma and erythrolcyte potassium and leucocyte ascorbic acid in 'ultra-fit' subjects. *Clin. Sci. Mol. Med.*, **46,** 499
45. Pierson, R. N., Lin, D. H. Y. and Phillips, R. A. (1974). Total body potassium in health: Effects of age, sex, height and fat. *Am. J. Physiol.*, **226** (No. 1), 206
46. Goode, A. W., Hawkins, T. and Feggetter, J. G. W. (1977). The effect of frusemide used for post-prostatectomy irrigation on total body potassium. *Br. J. Urol.*, **49,** 143
47. Davidson, C., Burkinshaw, L., McLachlan, M. S. F. and Morgan, D. B. (1976). Effect of long-term diuretic treatment on total body potassium in heart disease. *Lancet*, **ii,** 1044
48. Bernard, R. W. and Stahl, W. M. (1973). Total body potassium as a guide to IV alimentation. *Ann. Surg.*, **178,** 559
49. Goode, A. W., Hawkins, T., Feggetter, J. G. W. and Johnston, I. D. A. (1976). Use of an elemental diet for long term nutritional support in Crohn's disease. *Lancet*, **i,** 122
50. Manners, J. M. (1974). Nutrition after cardiac surgery. *Anaesthesia*, **29,** 675
51. Abel, R. M., Fisher, J. E., Buckley, M. J., Barnett, G. O. and Austen, W. G. (1976). Malnutrition in cardiac surgical patients. *Arch. Surg.*, **iii,** 45

Discussion

W. P. T. James: (UK) We have done an almost identical study and found similar relationships. We found that ($weight^2$/height)—in other words, an index of adiposity, is an important factor to be taken into account when calibrating the counter. Mr Goode implied that the dominant factor in his particular counter was height. Is this important, particularly in relation to his arguments relating to the 12% of potassium that is non-exchangeable. I had the impression from the way in which he derived his figures that the argument was circular in that he was not necessarily taking into account the self-absorption of ^{40}K that can come with subcutaneous fat. He started off by saying that he would calibrate this counter with ^{42}K. He then used the ^{42}K in the urine—an exchangeable value—and asked why there was a difference. Surely there is no difference, since that is the same measurement that is used to calibrate the counter.

They have shown in the West Indies that the dominant effect in terms of depletion of total body potassium relates to the loss of cell mass. Alleyne and Co.[1] found that it was only when the patient became very low in total body K/kg that there was objective evidence from muscle biopsies of a true depletion state within the body. However, there is the proviso that Mann[2], working with the whole body counter in Cape Town has published data whereby he derives values for the expected whole body potassium on the basis of skinfold thickness and has found with conditions such as pneumonia that an acute loss of potassium can occur in the early phase of illness which does not directly correlate with nitrogen loss, and that a child can be repleted —genuinely repleted—with potassium, acutely, over a matter of 2–3 days, suggesting the dual problem of genuine loss of cell mass, plus the potential for acute changes in potassium status within the cell.

A. W. Goode: (UK) I would agree with that. Certainly when measuring an individual parameter one has to be very careful of the factors which deplete such an index, and not read into potassium measurements things which may not exist.

The only comment I can make about the relationship of exchangeable to total body potassium is that this relationship of one being consistently less than the other has turned up in virtually every published paper on the subject.

S. J. Karran: (UK) Might I ask for more detail about the four patients who obviously did very badly. The range of hospital stay went up to over 50 days. Was that a fair spread, or was it just one patient who heavily weighted the series?

Goode: Of the four patients, one was in hospital for 18 days, one for 22 days, one for 37 days and the fourth for 56 days, so that one patient pulled the series out quite markedly. But even if he was taken out, the difference was still significant.

H. M. Shizgal: (Canada) Regarding the non-exchangeable component of total potassium, although most of the body counter-data tend to suggest this, no statistically significant difference has been found between the isotope method and the body counter method. The question is perhaps best answered by carcass analysis. When carcass analysis is compared to total exchangeable measurements using an isotope, a non-exchangeable pool has never been identified.

I should also like to comment on the use of regression lines from measurements of height, weight, and other such parameters. Dr Moore's data in his book, *The Body Cell Mass*, gives regression lines with which it is possible to predict all the parameters of body composition simply on the basis of weight, sex and age. When we compare our data to such regression lines, in many cases we get a very good correlation, and it works out extremely well in the normal. However, in the ill patient where one really wants to know the answer this regression analysis method is not helpful.

One more question, Mr Goode uses regression lines to calculate a lot of the constants, and there is no question that regression lines are highly significant statistically. But, one needs to know the error of each of the predictions as one goes through the calculations. Have the confidence limits for the population on which these regression lines are calculated themselves been calculated, and has the extent of error at the end of those calculations itself been determined?

Goode: The confidence limits are very strict. The reproducibility of the technique alone is plus or minus 1%. It is almost perfectly reproducible each time. I take the point—regression lines, regression equations, are as good as the interpretation placed upon them. But with that in view we have quite often carried out the whole calibration, again with an isotope, removing body weight, particularly in the depleted patients, and the agreement is still there.

James: On the exchangeable pool—David Halliday[3] in Jamaica had a whole body counter calibrated with ^{42}K. He put in children who died of malnutrition, measured their whole body K by this still indirect technique, then went on to analyse the whole child, and found practically identical values for the potassium content of those children.

References

1. Waterlow, J. C. and Alleyne, G. A. O. (1971). *Adv. Protein Chem.*, **25,** 117
2. Mann, M. D. and Hansen, J. D. L. (1972). *S. Afr. Med. J.*, **46,** 37
3. Halliday, D. (1967). *Uni. Sci.*, **33,** 365

Appendix

SI UNITS

The SI system of units (Systeme International d'Unites) was recommended for general use in 1960 by the international organisation responsible for units and measurements, the General Conference on Weights and Measures (CGPM).

The application of SI units to medicine has been studied by various international and national bodies, and during the last few years many

CONVERSION TABLE FOR SOME COMMONLY REPORTED NORMAL ADULT REFERENCE RANGES

	Traditional units		*SI units*		*Conversion factor*
Albumin (S)	3.4–5.0	g/100 ml	34–50	g/l	0.1
Bicarbonate (P)	22–29	mEq/l	22–29	mmol/l	no change
Calcium (S)	8.2–10.2	mg/100 ml	2.05–2.55	mmol/l	4.0
Carbon dioxide (pCO_2)	34–46	mmHg	4.5–6.1	kPa	7.52
Chloride (P)	96–106	mEq/l	96–106	mmol/l	no change
Copper (S)	70–160	μg/100 ml	11–25	μmol/l	6.37
Creatinine (P)	0.6–1.4	mg/100 ml	53–124	μmol/l	0.0113
Glucose (B)	60–90	mg/100 ml	3.3–5.0	mmol/l	18.0
Hydroxyproline (U)	10–35	mg/24 h	0.08–0.28	mmol/24 h	131.1
Iron (S)	Male 70–180	μg/100 ml	13–32	μmol/l	5.59
	Female 60–160	μg/100 ml	11–29	μmol/l	
Lactate (B)	6–18	mg/100 ml	0.65–2.0	mmol/l	9.0
Magnesium (S)	1.7–2.5	mg/100 ml	0.7–1.0	mmol/l	2.43
Oxygen (pO_2)	90–105	mmHg	12–14	kPa	7.52
Osmolality (P)	282–298	mOsm/Kg	282–298	mmol/kg	no change
Phosphate as inorganic P (S)	2.5–4.5	mg/100 ml	0.8–1.4	mmol/l	3.1
Protein total (S)	6.0–8.0	g/100 ml	60–80	g/l	0.1
Pyruvate (B)	0.3–0.9	mg/100 ml	35–105	μmol/l	0.0088
Sodium (P)	134–147	mEq/l	134–147	mmol/l	no change
Urea (P)	15–42	mg/100 ml	2.5–7.0	mmol/l	6.0

Key: (S) = Serum, (P) = Plasma, (B) = Blood, (U) = Urine
To convert traditional to SI units divide by conversion factor.
To convert SI to traditional units multiply by conversion factor.

With acknowledgements to Clinical Biochemistry Department, Royal Victoria Infirmary, Newcastle upon Tyne.

countries have begun the conversion from 'traditional' units. At the present time however, not all countries have converted totally to the SI system. As a consequence both traditional and SI units are used in this text.

To facilitate the inter-conversion of units, a conversion table is provided for some of the commonly reported normal adult reference ranges together with conversion scales for some general measurements used in medicine.

General Measurements

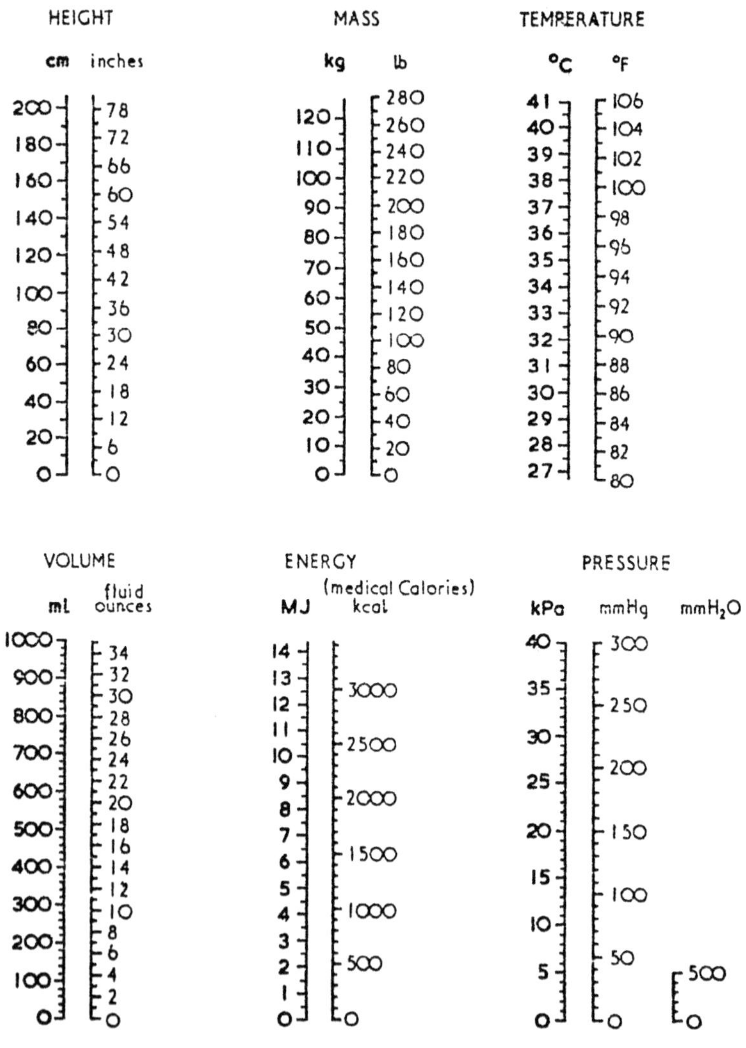

With acknowledgements to Professor D. N. Baron, and the *British Medical Journal.*

APPENDIX

For more detailed reviews of the subject consult:

1. Baron, D. N. (1974). *Br. Med. J.*, **4,** 509
2. B.S.I., The Use of SI Units. PD 5686, B.S.I., London, 1965
3. Royal College of Pathologists' Working Party (1970). *J. Clin. Pathol.*, **23,** 818
4. Young, D. S. (1974). *N. Engl. J. Med.*, **290,** 368

Index

GPSR Compliance

The European Union's (EU) General Product Safety Regulation (GPSR) is a set of rules that requires consumer products to be safe and our obligations to ensure this.

If you have any concerns about our products, you can contact us on ProductSafety@springernature.com

In case Publisher is established outside the EU, the EU authorized representative is:

Springer Nature Customer Service Center GmbH
Europaplatz 3
69115 Heidelberg, Germany

Batch number: 10823775

Printed by Printforce, the Netherlands